TEXTBOOK OF
OTOLARYNGOLOGY

TEXTBOOK OF
OTOLARYNGOLOGY

DAVID D. DeWEESE, M.D.

Professor Emeritus and Past Chairman of the
Department of Otolaryngology and Maxillofacial Surgery,
University of Oregon Medical School,
Portland, Oregon

WILLIAM H. SAUNDERS, M.D.

Professor and Chairman of the Department of Otolaryngology,
The Ohio State University College of Medicine,
Columbus, Ohio

SIXTH EDITION

with 646 *illustrations*

The C. V. Mosby Company

ST. LOUIS • TORONTO • LONDON   1982

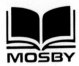

MOSBY

A TRADITION OF PUBLISHING EXCELLENCE

Editor: Eugenia A. Klein
Manuscript editor: Stephen C. Hetager
Design: Susan Trail
Production: Jeanne A. Gulledge

SIXTH EDITION

Copyright © 1982 by The C.V. Mosby Company

All rights reserved. No part of this book may be reproduced in any manner without written permission of the publisher.

Previous editions copyrighted 1960, 1964, 1968, 1973, 1977

Printed in the United States of America

The C.V. Mosby Company
11830 Westline Industrial Drive, St. Louis, Missouri 63141

Library of Congress Cataloging in Publication Data

DeWeese, David D. (David Downs), 1913-
   Textbook of otolaryngology.

   Bibliography: p.
   Includes index.
   1. Otolaryngology. I. Saunders, William H.
II. Title. [DNLM: 1. Otorhinolaryngologic
diseases—Diagnosis. 2. Otorhinolaryngologic
diseases—Therapy. WV 100 D516t]
RF46.D58 1982   617'.51   81-14162
ISBN 0-8016-1273-X   AACR2

GW/CB/B 9 8 7 6 5 4 3 2 1   01/C/010

The first three editions of this book
were dedicated to
Dr. Albert C. Furstenberg and Dr. James H. Maxwell
of the University of Michigan Medical School.
Both contributed much to medical education in all aspects
but particularly to postgraduate education in otolaryngology.
Both are now deceased.

The fourth and fifth editions were
dedicated to the medical student of the 1970s.

In the hope that it will continue to contribute to undergraduate medical education
as have the previous five editions
this sixth edition is dedicated to the medical student of the 1980s.

PREFACE

This book is designed primarily for the medical student and the general practitioner. Emphasis is on diagnosis and treatment. The discussions of anatomy and physiology contain adequate data for orientation but are not so detailed that the student is overburdened. The selected readings indicate sources of additional information.

Examination of the ears, nose, and throat requires special techniques and instruments. The first chapter emphasizes this fact. If students are not familiar with these instruments and techniques, and if they do not know normal appearances, they will not be able to diagnose or treat diseases of these parts.

In this edition, as in previous editions, attention is drawn to the new concepts of diagnosis, treatment, and rehabilitation that in the last three decades have broadened the scope of the specialty. Special emphasis is placed on diseases of the salivary glands, the facial nerve, tumors of the head and neck, and speech problems—areas and conditions of importance that are often overlooked. The continuing interest in otologic surgery and in the physiology of hearing has led to careful correlation of disease states and operative procedures with the anatomy and physiology of the ear. In some instances new drawings and photographs have been added or old ones have been replaced to clarify basic concepts.

In the past twenty years the trained otolaryngologist has become the physician who most often treats diseases of the head and neck, with the exception of the brain and the eyes. Therefore additional emphasis has been placed on the management of tumors of the head and neck, on trauma to the soft and bony tissues of the face and head, and on plastic surgery and reconstructive procedures.

The medical student is advised to read the entire book in continuity, since subsequent chapters enlarge on or complement prior chapters. The basic facts of otolaryngologic diagnosis are in this text. The discussions of treatment, which continues to change as a result of new research and new techniques, will require revision in future editions.

We wish to acknowledge the contributions of photographic material from our colleagues in otolaryngology and allied fields. Credit for these contributions is given in the legends. We wish to recognize the assistance of Jack A. Vernon, Professor of Otolaryngology and Director of the Kresge Hearing Research Laboratory of the Oregon Health Sciences University, for his suggestions in regard to the chapter on tinnitus and for his additions to that chapter. Robert E. Brummett, Professor of Otolaryngology, also of the Kresge Hearing Research Laboratory, was primarily responsible for the section on ototoxicity, and we acknowledge his contribution. We are indebted to Charles Von Wald of Portland, Oregon, for many of the photographs in this edition as well as in the previous editions. For original drawings we are indebted to Clarice Ashworth Francone and Fred Harwin of the University of Oregon Medical School and to Mary B. Meikle and Donna L. Himes of the Kresge Hearing Research Laboratory at the Oregon Health Sciences University. We are equally indebted to several illustrators from The Ohio State University.

David D. DeWeese
William H. Saunders

CONTENTS

TEXTBOOK OF
OTOLARYNGOLOGY

1 THE PHYSICAL EXAMINATION

Examination of the ears, nose, and throat is basically a study of epithelium. Using brilliant illumination, the physician is able to inspect directly or indirectly most parts of the upper respiratory passages. A few parts, such as the nasal accessory sinuses and the middle ear, cannot be visualized. Nevertheless, the examiner is usually able to infer their condition from the appearance of adjacent mucous membranes.

Lighting. A great many lighting systems are used. Some, such as the flashlight or otoscope, are entirely inadequate when used anywhere except in the ear. Others, such as electric headlights, are of variable worth, depending on their brightness.

The light par excellence is that reflected from the otolaryngologist's head mirror. A clear 150-watt light bulb provides the light source and is placed just behind and to the right of the patient.

More and more often, otologists are using the Zeiss operating microscope for diagnostic examination of the ear (Fig. 1-1) and sometimes for other parts of the otolaryngeal examination. This instrument provides brilliant illumination and also binocular vision and magnification. It may be used with the patient in either the sitting position or the supine position; and because of its delicate balance, it is as convenient to use as any other lighting system.

Adjustment of the head mirror. To adjust the head mirror, one should first place it well down over the left eye so that the back of the mirror actually touches the skin or glasses (Fig. 1-2).

The text for Chapter 1, with slight modifications, and Figs. 1-4, 1-8, 1-18, 1-25, and 1-30 taken from Saunders, W.H.: Ears, nose, and throat. In Prior, J.A., Silberstein, J.S., and Stang, J.: Physical diagnosis: the history and examination of the patient, ed. 6, St. Louis, 1981, The C.V. Mosby Co.

Then the right eye is closed and the light is focused on the patient's face to a small, brilliant spot. Too often the beginner fails to keep the light bright because he neglects to move his head toward or away from the patient. Obviously, since the focal length of the mirror is fixed, the only way the examiner can maintain a sharp focus is by adjusting his head position. Once the left eye is focused, the right eye may be opened for binocular vision. After a little experience, focusing becomes automatic and preliminary monocular focusing is not necessary.

If they wish, patients or students can observe part of their own examination (Fig. 1-7).

Use of the tongue depressor. The tongue depressor is held in the left hand (Fig. 1-3), so that the right hand is free to hold other instruments or to position the head. Tongue blades may be either the wooden type or the metal type. Most examiners prefer the wooden ones.

The blade should be placed on the middle third of the tongue. If placed too far anteriorly, it causes the posterior part of the tongue to mound up, obscuring rather than exposing the pharynx. On the other hand, most patients gag if the blade touches the posterior third of the tongue.

The correct maneuver depresses the tongue and scoops it forward at the same time. The blade is held in the corner of the mouth so that it will not be in the way of the instruments held in the right hand. The examiner should be careful not to press the patient's lower lip against the teeth.

The tongue is a strong, muscular organ. One need not (and occasionally cannot) depress the entire tongue at one time. Sometimes, in order to press more firmly, the examiner may use two tongue blades, one placed on top of the other.

1

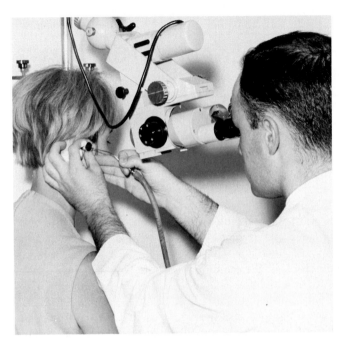

FIG. 1-1. Operating microscope used as a diagnostic instrument. Small aural suction tip aspirates serum or pus from the ear canal or middle ear.

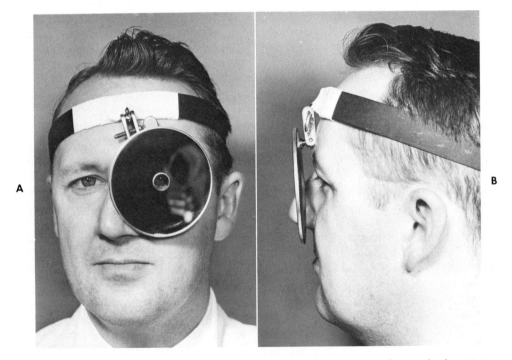

FIG. 1-2. A, Head mirror in position. Note that the mirror is worn *very close to the face.* It is directly in front of the pupil. **B,** Lateral view.

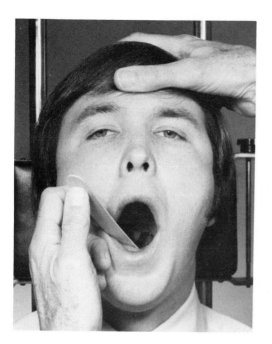

FIG. 1-3. Use of the tongue depressor. Note that the left hand is braced on the cheek; the right hand positions the head.

Warming the mirror. To prevent fogging, the examiner should use the flame of an alcohol lamp to warm the mirror to be used in examining the nasopharynx or larynx (Fig. 1-4). The glass surface is placed directly into the flame for a few seconds. The back of the mirror is then tested for warmth on the examiner's hand. Because children are sometimes frightened by the open flame, one may simply dip the mirror into a container of warm water before examining a child.

Patient's position. The patient's position is very important in otolaryngeal examinations. He should sit very erect, with knees together and head 10 to 12 inches from the back of the chair (Fig. 1-5). Many patients tend to slump and to slide their hips forward in the chair. The use of a headrest is discouraged because it fixes the head in one position and hinders the adjustments of the head position that are constantly required. The correct position is not restful, but the examination is not so long as to be tiring.

Cotton applicator. The cotton applicator is one of the most useful instruments in otolaryngeal examination. The examiner must learn to prepare his own, because commercial applicators

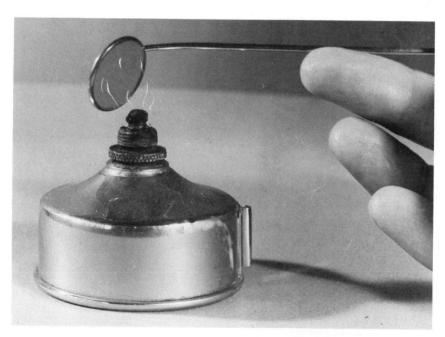

FIG. 1-4. Warming the mirror. The glass surface is placed directly over the flame.

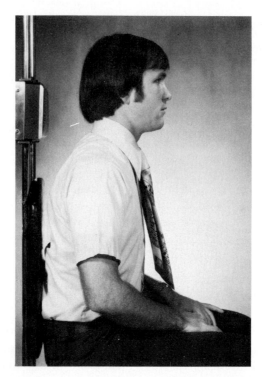

FIG. 1-5. Patient's position. The head and shoulders are drawn forward, with the hips against the back of the chair. Each patient must be positioned, often several times.

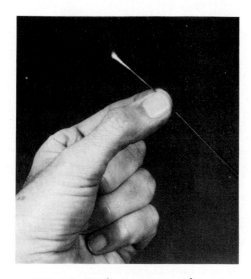

FIG. 1-6. Winding a cotton applicator.

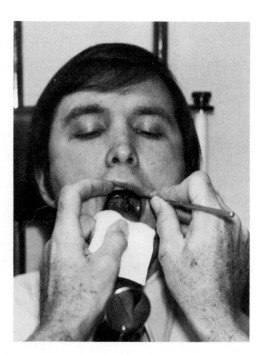

FIG. 1-7. By holding a large mirror, the patient can see his own larynx, nose, and nasopharynx.

are never satisfactory. A stiff wire is used, and a small piece of loose cotton is wound around it (Fig. 1-6). The tip of the wire is placed in the center of the cotton, and the cotton is twisted onto the wire, leaving a small tuft at the end. The tuft may be firmed or left loose as the situation demands. Beginners often make their cotton applicators too thick or fail to have a very small tuft at the tip.

EARS

Auricle. Conditions that affect the auricle are usually obvious and require little explanation. Some patients have congenitally deformed auricles that are too small (microtia) or too large (macrotia). Other ears stand out too prominently from the head (lop ears). Rarely, patients have no auricle at all, or a normal auricle may be associated with an atretic ear canal.

The examiner should inspect and palpate the auricle. Movements of the auricle and tragus are painful in external otitis but are not painful in otitis media. A postauricular scar indicates an old mastoidectomy.

A small dimple just in front of and slightly above the tragus is a remnant of the first branchial apparatus.

The need for inspection of the external ear is so obvious that it is frequently neglected, although it should require only a few seconds. Occasionally *tophi*, which are small white deposits of uric acid crystals that result from gout, are seen along the margins of the auricle. The gnarled, thickened *cauliflower ear* is the result of repeated trauma to the cartilage. Evidence of injury or congenital malformation is usually obvious.

Next, one inpsects the external auditory canal and the tympanic membrane. In physical diagnosis, the tympanic membrane, or eardrum, may be regarded as a translucent membrane through which the otologist views normal anatomy and also pathologic processes in the middle ear.

Cleaning the ear canal. The most important step in preparing to examine the eardrum is making sure that the ear canal and the surface of the drumhead are clean. Wax, particulate matter, and all pus and secretions must be meticulously removed. This caution seems ob-

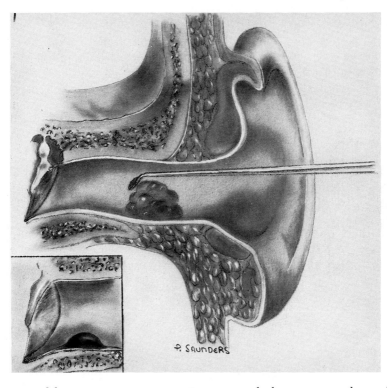

FIG. 1-8. Use of the cerumen spoon. *Inset,* Hematoma, which is easy to produce unless care is taken.

vious, but neglect of this preliminary is the rule. Actually, an experienced examiner may take several minutes to remove debris from the ear canal before he or she is ready to study the drumhead.

There are three methods of cleaning the ear canal. Often the simplest way is to remove particulate matter with a cerumen spoon (Fig. 1-8) or cotton applicator while working under direct vision through the ear speculum. The cerumen spoon should be inserted above the impacted wax; careful withdrawal of the spoon, which has been engaged in the wax, dislodges the wax. Because the epithelium covering the inner aspect of the ear canal is exquisitely sensitive, great care must be used in these manipulations to prevent pain and bleeding.

The second method of cleaning the ear canal is by irrigation (Fig. 1-9). Tap water is used—at body temperature, because water at any other temperature stimulates the inner ear and causes dizziness. If the cerumen to be removed is solidly impacted, and especially if it is dry and hard, irrigation may not be successful unless it is preceded by having the patient instill a few drops of mineral oil or so-called "sweet oil" in the ear for three or four nights. This oil softens the cerumen and makes it easy to remove by irrigation. Various proprietary preparations that will soften wax are also available. Most are harmless, although some have been known to cause a local inflammatory response.

The third method is by using a small, angulated suction tip to aspirate pus or other liquid material from the ear canal (Fig. 1-1). This method is especially useful when pus coming through a perforated drumhead fills the middle ear as well as the ear canal. Then, by carefully advancing the suction tip, the examiner may clean the ear canal and finally the middle ear space itself of pus so that the ear can be examined.

• • •

A good way to begin the examination is to pull the auricle upward and backward and the tragus forward (Fig. 1-10). This maneuver opens the meatus and may even provide a good view of the drumhead. It also lets the examiner select an aural speculum of proper size.

Examination with the aural speculum. Most otologists employ a metal ear speculum and a head mirror to examine the drumhead. Generally, other practitioners use an electric otoscope (Fig. 1-11). Whichever instrument is used, the principles of examination are the same. *The speculum selected should be the largest that will fit the canal.* The student usually makes the mistake of choosing a small speculum when a large one could be used.

The speculum is inserted to straighten and slightly dilate the cartilaginous ear canal (Fig. 1-12). About halfway to the eardrum the cartilage ends and the supporting wall becomes osseous. Here speculum pressure is painful. The epithelium lining the bony portion of the

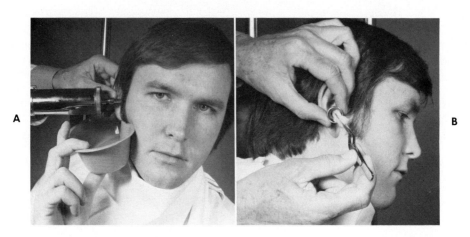

FIG. 1-9. A, Aural irrigation using tap water at body temperature. **B,** Drying the ear canal after irrigation.

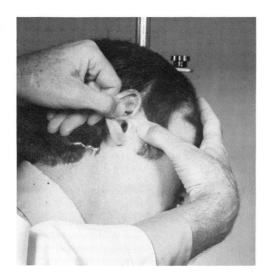

FIG. 1-10. Spreading the meatus—a preliminary step.

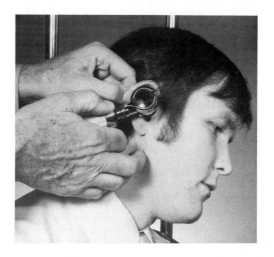

FIG. 1-11. Electric otoscope. Traction on the auricle straightens the canal.

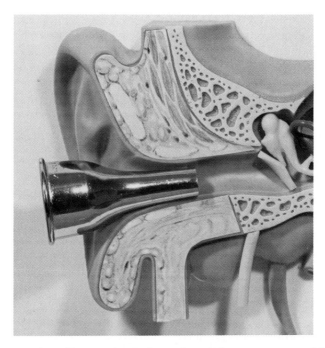

FIG. 1-12. The speculum dilates and straightens the cartilaginous portion of the ear/canal. If it is pressed against the inner, bony canal, it causes pain.

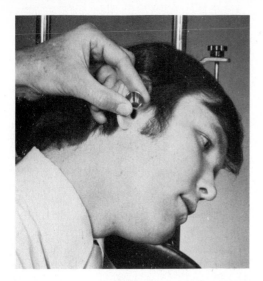

FIG. 1-13. Note that the head is tipped to one side. Also, note how one hand holds both the speculum and the auricle.

canal is very thin and exquisitely sensitive. One must be very gentle when cleaning the inner half of the ear canal—even more so than when cleaning the outer surface of the drumhead. In adults the ear canal may be straightened by pulling upward and backward on the auricle; in young children and infants it is straightened by pulling the auricle downward.

The position of the patient's head is important in aural examination (Fig. 1-13). One might think that with the patient's head perfectly upright the examiner could look directly into the ear canal and see the drumhead. This is a common error. Because of the oblique direction of the ear canal, the patient's head must be tipped sidewise (toward the opposite shoulder) for easy examination of the canal and drumhead. Students who neglect this step find that they are looking at the wall of the ear canal and not at the drumhead. It is usually necessary to change the head position several times in order to visualize all parts of the tympanic membrane.

Layers of the drumhead. There are three layers in the drumhead: an outer squamous epithelium, an inner cuboidal epithelium, and a middle fibrous layer. These layers constitute the structure of the pars tensa, which comprises almost all of the drumhead. In a very small part superiorly, known as the pars flaccida, the middle fibrous layer is absent.

When perforations heal in the drumhead, the area of perforation is often translucent or even transparent. The reason is that some perforations repair without formation of a fibrous layer. The healing also leaves that portion of the drumhead flaccid and therefore more easily moved by pneumatic pressure (through an otoscope) than the rest of the drumhead.

Color of the drumhead. The color of the drumhead is important because it is relatively constant in health. The normal drumhead is usually described as pearly gray. In disease the color may be amber (serum in the middle ear), blue (hemotympanum), dead white (pus in the middle ear), or red or pink (myringitis or infection of the middle ear). Ordinarily the tympanic membrane is quite shiny.

Dense white plaques representing deposits of calcium-like material are seen in some drumheads affected with tympanosclerosis. Other patients with tympanosclerosis have drumheads showing small white flecks scattered throughout the pars tensa. Ordinarily these minor changes merely indicate old, healed disease of the middle ear or tympanic membrane. They do not mean active disease.

Position of the drumhead. The position of the drumhead is oblique with respect to the ear canal. The upper posterior part of the drumhead is closer to the examiner's eye than is the lower anterior part. This obliqueness is more pronounced in infants than in adults. Sometimes all of the drumhead cannot be seen because the floor of the ear canal is at a higher level than the lowermost part of the drumhead. Also, the anterior part of the drumhead may be hidden by prominence of the bony wall of the ear canal.

The drumhead is also very slightly conical, with the concavity external. When pus forms in the middle ear because of otitis media, intratympanic pressures are raised and the drumhead actually bulges outward. Sometimes this bulging is in one part of the drumhead only; at other times the entire drumhead bulges so that none of the landmarks are seen.

A "retracted" drumhead occurs when intratympanic pressures are reduced. In such a situation, the entire drumhead is depressed by external atmospheric pressure, the malleus is left in sharp outline, and the malleolar folds are accentuated. This alteration of tympanic pressure is common. It occurs when the eustachian tube is obstructed (because of adenoiditis in the child, for example, or as a result of too rapid descent during air travel). Whatever the cause, the tube no longer ventilates the middle ear properly, and oxygen is absorbed from the middle ear and mastoid air cells into the bloodstream. A partial vacuum results. A transudate of blood serum may partially fill the middle ear to relieve the vacuum, and the drumhead appears amber. Also, an air-fluid level may be seen, or bubbles of air may appear in the amber fluid.

Landmarks. The landmarks visible in the normal drumhead (Figs. 1-14 and 1-15) vary with differences in its translucency. The *malleus* is the primary landmark. At its upper end the lateral or *short process* stands out as a tiny knob. The manubrium, or the handle of the malleus, extends downward from the short process to the *umbo.* Both the short process and the manubrium are embedded in the drumhead.

When bulging of the drumhead occurs, the manubrium and the short process become less and less well seen until they finally disappear. On the other hand, when the drumhead is retracted, the malleus stands out prominently and the white bone of the short process shines chalky white through the drumhead.

The *anterior* and *posterior malleolar folds* are seen superiorly and enclose between them the *pars flaccida* (Shrapnell's membrane). These folds or epithelium become more prominent when the drumhead is retracted.

The *annulus* is the peripheral fibrous ring of the tympanic membrane that fits in the tympanic sulcus. It looks whiter or denser than the rest of the drumhead. It is complete except superiorly, where it is deficient between the anterior and posterior malleolar folds. The importance of the annulus in aural diagnosis cannot be stressed too much. The examiner must follow the annulus completely around. It is at the periphery of the drumhead that important perforations often occur, and they will not be found unless the annulus is systematically examined.

The *light reflex*, or *cone of light*, reflects from the anterior inferior quadrant when the drumhead is in its normal position and its outer epithelium is normal. The light reflex extends inferiorly and anteriorly from the umbo. Some-times the reflex becomes broken or muddled, and sometimes it is missing altogether. Such changes usually indicate a disease state, but too much emphasis should not be placed on variations of the light reflex alone.

The *long process of the incus* is frequently visible posterior to the manubrium of the malleus. Whether or not it can be seen depends on the translucency of the tympanic membrane and the shape of the posterior wall of the bony ear canal. When the incus is seen, the examiner can be fairly certain of a normal middle ear.

Less frequently seen than the incus is the *chorda tympani nerve.* It crosses transversely behind the drumhead at about the level of the short process of the malleus.

Special examinations. Special examinations include demonstration of function of the eustachian tube, examination with the pneumatic otoscope, and examination of the temporomandibular joint.

DEMONSTRATION OF FUNCTION OF THE EUSTACHIAN TUBE. Function of the eustachian tube may be demonstrated by looking at the drumhead under magnification while the patient holds his nose and swallows. This maneuver reinforces the opening of the eustachian tube, which usually occurs during swallowing. At the moment of swallowing, the drumhead can be seen to flick outward and then inward again, a movement indicating patency of the eustachian tube. Also, the patient feels a sensation of pressure in one or both ears at the height of the swallow.

Demonstration of tubal patency is important in some patients who have certain symptoms (deafness, tinnitus, or dizziness) that may be due to occlusion of the tube.

EXAMINATION WITH THE PNEUMATIC OTOSCOPE. The pneumatic otoscope (Fig. 1-16) is a useful device that enables the examiner to compress air in the ear canal. This procedure exerts pressure against the drumhead, and it moves in and out as a bulb in the examiner's hand is alternately squeezed and released. Pinhole perforations that otherwise may not be apparent can be detected as middle ear secretions are drawn through them by suction. Certain drumheads will be found to be more flaccid than normal (usually because of healed perforations), and others will not move at all because they are perforated. Adhesions or fluid in the middle

Anatomy to consider

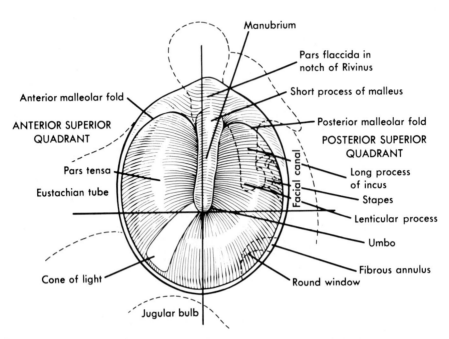

FIG. 1-14. Relationships of important middle ear structures. (From Saunders, W.H., and Paparella, M.M.: Atlas of ear surgery, ed. 2, St. Louis, 1971, The C.V. Mosby Co.)

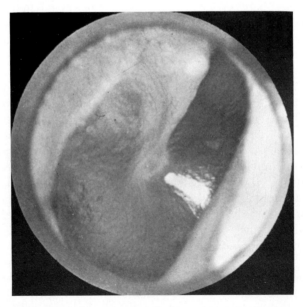

FIG. 1-15. Normal tympanic membrane. Note how the anterior wall of the ear canal obscures part of the drumhead. (From Buckingham, R.: What's New, No. 193, North Chicago, Ill., 1956, Abbott Laboratories.)

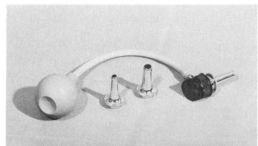

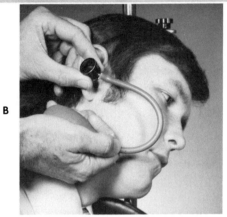

FIG. 1-16. **A,** Pneumatic otoscope. The speculum that fits this otoscope is attached. The magnifying lens may also be used with the usual type of speculum if magnification only is desired. **B,** Pneumatic otoscope in use. Note the lateral tipping of the head—the correct position for all otoscopic examinations.

ear may also prevent normal excursions of the drumhead. The pneumatic otoscope can be used to suck down secretions from the epitympanum or mastoid antrum in patients having chronic mastoiditis or to evacuate the middle ear of fluid after myringotomy.

EXAMINATION OF THE TEMPOROMANDIBULAR JOINT. It is common to see a patient with ear pain that is the result of referred pain from the temporomandibular joint. If the index fingers are pressed into the joint spaces as the patient opens his mouth widely, pain may be elicited (often only on one side) when he closes his mouth. This pain is commonly referred to the ear, and the patient complains not of a pain in his jaw joint but of otalgia. A common cause is malocclusion.

OROPHARYNX

The pharynx is divided into three parts—oropharynx, nasopharynx (epipharynx), and hypo-

pharynx. A patient complaining of sore throat might have a generalized pharyngitis involving all three parts; or only one part might be involved, as in carcinoma of the epiglottis, for example. It is necessary to use *different instruments* to see these three parts; and unless *all* parts of the pharynx are examined, the examiner cannot expect to establish a correct diagnosis for the patient complaining of sore throat.

Before any part of the pharynx is examined, the patient should remove his dentures. This is important, not only because the denture itself covers much of the mucosal surface to be examined but also because the lower plate tilts upward, causing gagging, and the upper plate often drops.

The tongue. The tongue is examined by both inspection and palpation. Palpation is necessary because some diseases of the tongue cause no surface manifestations and otherwise cannot be detected.

LINGUAL PAPILLAE. The filiform papillae are the most numerous. Keratinization of these papillae produces the well-known "coated tongue." Fungiform papillae are scattered throughout the filiform papillae and are especially abundant on the sides and apex of the tongue. These papillae look like small red dots because the underlying vascular connective tissue shines through the thin epithelium. The circumvallate papillae are arranged in an inverted V at the posterior part of the tongue. The apex of the V is at the foramen cecum. The circumvallate papillae are best examined with a laryngeal mirror.

VENTRAL SURFACE. The ventral surface of the tongue toward the floor of the mouth is smooth and shows large veins. In older persons these veins may become varicose.

FRENUM. The frenum is found in the midline under the tongue. Rather rarely, this structure is abnormally short and causes so-called tongue-tie. If the patient can protrude his tongue between his teeth, he should have no difficulty with speech.

GLOSSOPALATINE FOLD. The glossopalatine fold connects the tongue with the palate and is known as the anterior tonsillar pillar.

OTHER STRUCTURES. Other structures associated with the tongue are the lingual tonsils, the valleculae, and the glossoepiglottic folds. These structures are best seen with the laryngeal mirror and therefore will be described with the laryngeal examination.

Floor of the mouth. The floor of the mouth is another region where palpation is important. Tissues here are loose, and neoplasms sometimes are detectable only by palpation. The submaxillary salivary ducts may contain calculi that are best felt by palpation. Bimanual examination, using one gloved finger inside the mouth and the other hand outside, is best.

Submaxillary salivary gland. The submaxillary salivary gland empties into the floor of the mouth on either side of the frenum of the tongue. The orifices of the ducts are quite small, but they may be seen as small dark spots from which clear fluid can be expressed by pressure over the submaxillary gland. The orifices of the sublingual glands are not seen.

Teeth and gingivae. There are 32 teeth in the full adult dentition. The teeth are inspected for evidence of caries and malocclusion. Sometimes it is worthwhile to percuss a tooth to elicit tenderness in patients suspected of having a dental abscess.

The gums should be inspected and at times palpated. Bleeding from the gums is not unusual and at times is the sole cause of expectorated blood. In adults the gums gradually recede from the teeth and expose a larger and larger amount of tooth root.

Buccal mucosa. The parotid duct opens into the buccal mucosa opposite the upper second molar (Fig. 1-17). The orifice is larger than the submaxillary orifices and readily admits a probe. Pressure over the parotid gland produces a clear secretion.

In most adults yellowish glandlike structures may be seen shining through the buccal mucosa. They are sometimes mistaken for an abnormality, but they actually represent sebaceous glands lying directly under the squamous epithelium of the oral cavity.

Frequently there is a white line of parakeratin in the buccal mucosa adjacent to the occlusal surfaces of the molars. This results from invagination of the cheek between the teeth or from sucking on the cheek.

Palate. There is a distinct difference in color between the hard and soft palates. The soft palate is pink and shows fine vessels under the mucosa. The hard palate is whiter, more irregular, and has rugae running transversely. Scru-

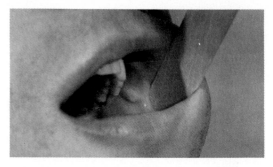

FIG. 1-17. Parotid (Stensen's) duct, opposite the second superior molar tooth.

tiny shows the orifices of ducts of mucous glands in the posterior part of the hard palate. In heavy smokers the duct orifices look like tiny red dots scattered throughout the hard palate. This is one form of nicotine stomatitis.

Uvula. The uvula is a muscular organ that varies greatly in length and thickness. It is sometimes bifid (Fig. 2-11). Frequently a small squamous papilloma is attached to the uvula, the free margin of the soft palate, or the anterior tonsillar pillar (Fig. 2-12).

Tonsils. Normally the palatine or faucial tonsils do not project much beyond the limits of the tonsillar pillars (Figs. 1-18 and 3-1). They are approximately the same color as the rest of the oral mucosa. There are crypts in the tonsils in which squamous epithelium exfoliates. Some patients have deep crypts; in such patients plugs of epithelial debris push toward the surface, where they appear as white spots on the tonsils. In other patients white spots on the tonsils may indicate follicular tonsillitis.

It is sometimes helpful to retract the anterior tonsillar pillar for better visualization of the tonsil. Palpation of the tonsil is important if a neoplasm is suspected.

Tonsillectomy is common. It is usually simple to tell when a patient has had a tonsillectomy because of the changes in the anterior or posterior pillars that occur with healing. Also, lymphoid nodules may remain in the tonsillar fossa and form so-called tonsillar tags.

Posterior pharyngeal wall. The posterior pharyngeal wall is the part of the pharynx that is visible when one uses only a tongue blade. Students are prone to speak of hyperemia or "injection" of the throat when they see any vessels on the posterior pharyngeal wall. Usually these small vessels are normal and do not represent

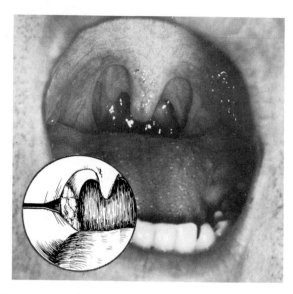

FIG. 1-18. Oropharynx. Note the anterior and posterior tonsillar pillars. *Inset,* Use of the pillar retractor in withdrawing the anterior pillar.

inflammatory changes. The same appearances may be seen on the tonsillar pillars and the soft palate.

Small, irregular spots of lymphoid tissue are common in the mucosa of the posterior pharyngeal wall. They are red or pink. The lateral pharyngeal bands are found behind the posterior pillar, running downward from the nasopharynx toward the base of the tongue. These pink bands are also composed of lymphoid tissue. The lymphoid elements in the pharynx—the adenoid, the lateral pharyngeal band, the faucial tonsil, and the lingual tonsil—are commonly known as *Waldeyer's ring.*

NASOPHARYNX

Technique of mirror examination. The best way to examine the nasopharynx is with the postnasal mirror. A No. 0 mirror is the correct size. Ordinarily, children above the age of 5 years and most adults can be examined without difficulty. Because of the small size of the mirror, all of the nasopharynx cannot be seen at one time. Instead, the mirror is rotated slightly to bring successive areas into view.

First, after the mirror is warmed, the tongue is depressed to create a large space in which to place the mirror (Fig. 1-19). The light must be focused sharply in the space next to the uvula, where the mirror will be placed. The mirror

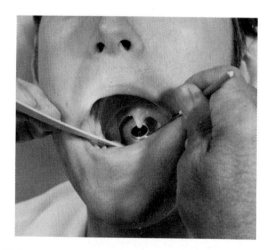

FIG. 1-19. Nasopharyngeal mirror in place. The key to this examination is *adequate tongue depression.*

is placed to one side of the uvula and *almost* touches the posterior pharyngeal wall. It is held in the right hand, and the fingers are braced against the patient's cheek to steady the hand. The left hand holds the tongue blade in the corner of the mouth so that it will not obstruct the examiner's view of the oral cavity.

The patient is instructed to breathe quietly through the nose so as to allow the soft palate to drop away from the posterior pharyngeal wall. Often the patient will protest, "I

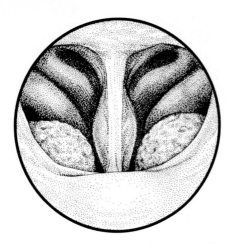

FIG. 1-20. Nasopharynx. The superior, middle, and inferior turbinates can be seen. Note hyperplastic mucosa on the septum and inferior turbinates (mulberry turbinates).

can't breathe through my nose with my mouth open!" but quiet reassurance and encouragement help to accomplish the desired palatal relaxation.

The beginner is likely to make two mistakes:

1. He fails to depress the tongue adequately, so that there is insufficient space in which to place the mirror.
2. He fails to focus his light sharply on the mirror.

Choana. The choanae are the posterior openings of the nose. Each choana is separated from the other by the posterior end of the vomer. The posterior ends of the turbinates can be seen in each side (Fig. 1-20). The turbinates (especially the inferior turbinate) vary greatly in appearance, even in normal noses. Sometimes they appear engorged with blood and look swollen and bluish. At other times the posterior tips are pale. Such changes may indicate an allergic or vasomotor disorder.

Posterior end of the vomer. Unlike the anterior part of the nasal septum, the posterior end of the vomer is always in the midline. However, it is not unusual to see a thickening of the vomer caused by hyperplastic mucosa.

Middle meatus. The middle meatus is an important space clinically because it is here that pus may be seen running from the maxillary sinus. Pus runs from the ostium (not visible) into the middle meatus and then drips over the posterior end of the inferior turbinate—a pathognomonic sign of maxillary sinusitis. The frontal and anterior ethmoid sinuses also drain into the middle meatus, but they drain higher and more anteriorly, and their drainage is best seen by means of the nasal speculum.

Inferior meatus. The inferior meatus is not well seen and has no clinical significance so far as its visualization with the postnasal mirror is concerned.

Superior meatus. The superior meatus (above the middle turbinate) blends with the region known clinically as the sphenoethmoid recess and is the site of drainage of the sphenoid sinus and posterior ethmoid cells.

Eustachian tubes. The eustachian tubes open laterally into the nasopharynx just under the torus tubarius. Over the torus is the fossa of Rosenmüller. The orifice of the tube usually looks a little pale or yellowish and is about as large as the eraser end of a lead pencil. Normally the tube is closed, but it opens whenever the patient swallows or yawns.

Adenoid. The adenoid (pharyngeal tonsil) is a collecion of lymphoid tissue present in every child and in some adults. It grows from the roof and posterior wall of the nasopharynx, extends into the fossa of Rosenmüller, and blends with that lymphoid tissue known as the lateral pharyngeal band. Sometimes the adenoid, particularly in adults, seems to be only a clump of lymphoid tissue that is centrally located.

In children the adenoid is prone to cause occlusion of the eustachian tube, which interferes with aeration of the middle ear. This causes deafness and predisposes a child to middle ear infection. Large masses of adenoid also produce nasal obstruction and mouth breathing in infants and young children.

Posterior aspect of the uvula and soft palate. The posterior aspect of the uvula and soft palate, and the lateral wall of the pharynx, are also visible in the postnasal mirror. Ordinarily no pathologic changes are found here except for nasopharyngitis, causing hyperemia and exudate formation. Many doctors fail to locate the site of the patient's sore throat because they fail to examine the nasopharynx. They use only a tongue blade to inspect the oropharynx, but the oropharynx may be normal even when the patient has a severe nasopharyngitis.

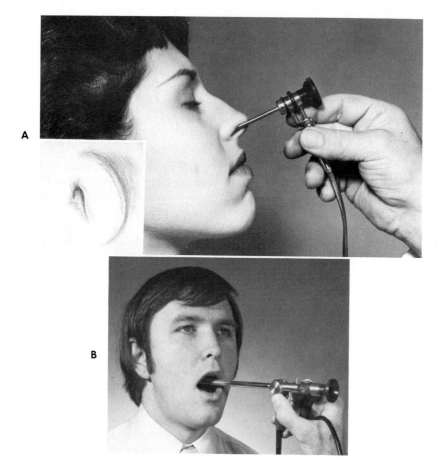

FIG. 1-21. **A,** Nasopharyngoscope. *Inset,* Eustachian tube as seen with the nasopharyngoscope. **B,** Pharyngoscope—shows either the nasopharynx or the larynx.

Other methods of examination. Other methods of examination include use of the nasal speculum, palpation, use of the nasopharyngoscope, use of the pharyngoscope, and use of the palate retractor.

USE OF THE NASAL SPECULUM. The nasal speculum may be used to see a small part of the nasopharynx by looking through the anterior nares. Such examination can be done in some patients without previous vasoconstriction, but in most patients a good look depends on careful shrinkage of the inferior turbinate. Anterior rhinoscopy is particularly useful in children who will not permit the use of a nasopharyngeal mirror. In adults it is a convenient route through which to remove tissue from the nasopharynx for biopsy.

PALPATION. Palpation of the nasopharynx is used in some instances. Usually better and less distressing methods are available. If one does use palpation, it is important to place several thicknesses of tongue blades between the patient's molars or to invaginate the patient's cheek between his teeth with the right index finger, to prevent the patient from biting the examiner's finger.

USE OF THE NASOPHARYNGOSCOPE. The nasopharyngoscope is a useful instrument that gives a view of one small area of the nasopharynx at a time (Fig. 1-21, *A*). The general physician, however, is usually unable to interpret what he sees through the nasopharyngoscope, and since the use of the postnasal mirror provides a better look anyway, the nasopharyngoscope is of limited importance to most physicians.

USE OF THE PHARYNGOSCOPE. A more useful instrument than the small nasopharyngoscope is the *pharyngoscope.* This larger instrument

(Fig. 1-21, *B*), which produces brilliant illumination, is held in the patient's mouth to give a
view of the nasopharynx (when the instrument
is turned upward) or of the hypopharynx and
larynx (when turned downward).

USE OF THE PALATE RETRACTOR. The self-
retaining *palate retractor* is a very useful instrument for the occasional patient in whom there is
insufficient space between the soft palate and
the posterior pharyngeal wall to afford an adequate view of the nasopharynx. It also is useful
when maximum working room is required—for
example, during the biopsy procedure.

HYPOPHARYNX AND LARYNX

The *approach to the patient* is exceedingly
important. The examiner must adopt a calm,
reassuring attitude and yet conduct the examination with firmness. Admittedly it is difficult
to cope with the "gaggy" patient, but annoyance
on the examiner's part only worsens the situation.

Topical anesthesia such as that provided by
4% cocaine, 1% tetracaine (Pontocaine), or 4%
lidocaine (Xylocaine) is permissible but is not
often needed by the experienced examiner.
One should avoid spraying with compressed-air
equipment because too much drug is likely to
be administered in this way. Using an atomizer
and bulb is safer.

Additional help in visualizing the larynx of
a patient who continues to gag even after careful reassurance and application of topical anesthetic can be obtained through the intravenous
administration of diazepam (Valium), 5 to 10
mg. over a 90-second period. One must be sure
to inject the drug into a large vein, since phlebi-
tis may result if a small vein is used. This medication greatly quiets the overactive psyche,
which seems responsible for the excessive gagging of certain patients. Its effect lasts about 20
minutes, after which time the patient is ready
to leave the office.

The *position* of the patient is of paramount
importance in this examination. The patient
must not be allowed to slouch or slump in the
chair. He must sit erect (in military posture).
The chin is drawn forward. Both feet are on the
floor, with the knees together. The head is not
placed in a headrest but is left free for adjustment during the examination.

The *tongue* is protruded as far as possible and
held firmly by the examiner in a piece of gauze.
First, the gauze is laid over the tongue and then
wrapped under it. This procedure keep the
gauze from wadding up on top of the tongue and
obscuring the examiner's vision. It also protects
the undersurface of the tongue from the sharp
lower incisor teeth. The tongue is then held by
the examiner between the left thumb and the
left middle finger while the index finger is
braced against the upper lip or the upper teeth.
If the patient cooperates and does not try to
retract the protruded tongue, it is not actually
necessary to pull on the tongue.

The *mirror* used for adults is a No. 5. The
glass surface is warmed over an alcohol lamp,
and the mirror back is tested on the examiner's
hand for heat. The mirror is held midway along
the shaft as a pen is held, not by the handle,
and the *fingers are braced* on the patient's
cheek.

The mirror is inserted into the mouth so that,
as the edge advances, the glass surface is flush
with the tongue. Thus the mirror is not introduced in its greatest diameter.

The mirror is placed with its back side against
the uvula (Fig. 1-22). The uvula and soft palate
are pressed upward in one smooth movement.
Once contact is made, the mirror is not shifted
about to any extent, although slight changes in
its position are necessary for seeing all of the
larynx. Touching the uvula and soft palate ordinarily does not cause gagging, but touching the
back of the tongue does. In the mirror, anterior
and posterior are reversed but right and left
remain the same.

The patient is asked to breathe quietly
through the mouth. He is told that as long as
he breathes regularly he will not gag. Sometimes, gaggy patients do best when they are
asked to "pant in and out like a dog." After the
examination has been completed during quiet
respiration, the patient is asked to sound a
high-pitched "e-e-e," "a-a-a," or, best of all,
"he-e-e." Almost all patients phonate too low
and must be told to make a sound high in pitch.
Most patients also phonate too briefly. A prolonged singing of "e-e-e" is desired—not a short
utterance, which does not give adequate time
for examination. The examiner makes the same
sound; in effect, the two sing a duet.

Some patients, when asked to phonate, will
remain aphonic and then shake their heads;

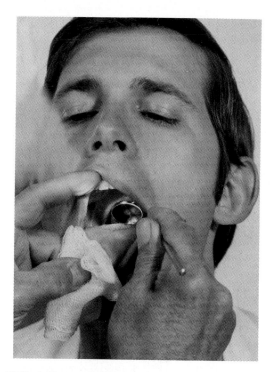

FIG. 1-22. Laryngeal mirror in place. *Inset* shows how mirror elevates the uvula. (1) Both hands are braced. (2) The instrument is held near the mirror end. (3) One finger retracts the upper lip.

others hold their breath. Careful explanation and quiet reassurance do much to obtain co-operation.

The following are the beginner's most common mistakes:

1. He does not explain what he intends to do before he does it.
2. He fails to position the patient properly.
3. He fails to focus his light brilliantly on the mirror.
4. He does not elevate the uvula and soft palate with the back of the mirror.
5. He does not insist on a prolonged, high-pitched "e-e-e."

Hypopharynx. The hypopharynx is above the level of the larynx but below the part of the pharynx that can be conveniently examined with a tongue blade. The following important structures are seen when one uses a laryngeal mirror.

CIRCUMVALLATE PAPILLAE. The circumvallate papillae are arranged in an inverted V, with the apex at the foramen cecum. The papillae vary considerably in size and prominence, and

patients sometimes mistake them for lingual tumors.

LINGUAL TONSILS. The lingual tonsils, visible in most adults, lie on either side of the dorsum of the tongue. They vary greatly in size and sometimes are extremely large. In the lingual tonsils one frequently sees small white spots that represent debris in crypts, or, if the patient has active lingual tonsillitis, follicular exudate. When the lingual tonsils are enlarged, there is often a deep cleft between them.

VALLECULAE. The valleculae are the cup-shaped spaces between the tongue and the epiglottis. They are separated from each other by the median glossoepiglottic fold. Large veins are frequently seen in the valleculae, and they are normal. Cysts may form here and are usually thin-walled and yellowish or white. To see the valleculae more distinctly, one asks the patient to phonate.

EPIGLOTTIS. The epiglottis is cartilaginous. Its shape, size, thickness, and color vary from patient to patient. The free edge of the epiglottis is usually thin and slightly curved. Sometimes (always in infants) the entire epiglottis is furled, in which case laryngologists speak of an "omega-shaped" epiglottis. The lateral glossoepiglottic folds and the median glossoepiglottic fold attach the epiglottis to the base of the tongue; the aryepiglottic folds attach it to the arytenoid cartilages.

The epiglottis (especially the tubercle) is usually in the way when the examiner wishes to see the anterior ends of the vocal cords. The patient is asked to phonate in a *high-pitched* "e-e-e" or "he-e-e" to draw the epiglottis out of the line of vision.

• • •

Although not a routine part of the examination, palpation of the hypopharynx with one finger is necessary in certain patients—not because visual examination is difficult but because tumors deep in the tongue or beneath the mucosa may not cause visible mucosal alterations.

The lateral and posterior walls of the hypopharynx are inspected along with the rest of the hypopharynx. Ordinarily nothing here confuses the examiner.

Larynx. In studying the larynx, the beginner too often fixes his attention on the true vocal cords alone, because these structures are so striking in their appearance and movement. But inspection of the true vocal cords is only part of the laryngeal examination.

FALSE CORDS. The false cords lie directly above and slightly lateral to the true cords. They are capable of contracting and closing the larynx, but generally they remain quiet during examination. Sometimes, however, the false cords are so active that they preclude a good view of the true cords. Ordinarily the false cords appear dull pink and look thicker than the true cords.

LARYNGEAL VENTRICLE. Directly under the false cords is a space called the laryngeal ventricle. It is not well seen by mirror laryngoscopy, but more of it can be seen by having the patient tilt his head sideward (ear toward shoulder).

TRUE VOCAL CORDS. The true vocal cords reflect light in such a way as to appear white and sharp edged in the laryngeal mirror. Of course, their color is not really white, and the edges are actually rounded.

Anteriorly the cords meet in the midline, where they are attached to the thyroid cartilage. Posteriorly they are attached to the vocal processes of the arytenoid cartilages. The anterior attachment is fixed, but the posterior attachment is mobile and allows the cords to open and close during respiration and phonation.

ARYTENOID CARTILAGES. The arytenoid cartilages form the posterior attachments for the true vocal cords. They are mobile and swing in and out with phonation and respiration. Their color is a dull red, and they appear as small mounds at the posterior end of the glottis (the space between the cords). The arytenoids also attach to the epiglottis via the *aryepiglottic folds*. In the aryepiglottic folds are smaller cartilages, the cuneiform and corniculate cartilages. The aryepiglottic folds, the false cords, and the true cords are the sphincters of the larynx. They protect the lower respiratory passages from foreign bodies and help to build up intrathoracic pressure for coughing and other functions.

From the standpoint of the surgeon—who needs to know as exactly as possible the site of origin of laryngeal tumors, because of different lymphatic distributions—the larynx is divided into (1) a supraglottic area (posterior or laryngeal surface of the epiglottis, ventricular bands or false vocal cords, ventricles, arytenoids, and

aryepiglottic folds), (2) a glottic area (true vocal cords), and (3) a subglottic area.

PYRIFORM RECESSES. The pyriform recesses are situated posterior and lateral to the arytenoids. They will dilate a little if the patient says "a-a-a" in a low voice. Secretions may gather here, but they should disappear when the patient swallows. If they do not disappear, the patient is said to have a "pooling" sign, which suggests obstruction or paralysis of the upper esophagus.

LARYNGEAL EXAMINATION. First, the cords are observed during quiet respiration (Fig. 1-23, *A*). They move only slightly, or not at all, and their color, configuration, and position are noted. The examiner also looks between the cords at the anterior wall of the trachea. In most patients a few tracheal rings can be seen, and sometimes the examiner can see all the way to the carina. He can do so best by kneeling on the floor in front of the patient and looking upward into the laryngeal mirror.

After the larynx has been inspected during quiet respiration, the patient phonates as previously described. Phonation (Fig. 1-23, *B*) causes adduction of the cords, which can be seen to vibrate as sound is produced. They become more tense and appear elongated. Normally there seems to be perfect approximation of the cords, but in the aged there is a small space that cannot be closed. This space produces the quavering voice of the old man. If one vocal cord is paralyzed, it will lie fixed while the opposite cord moves in and out.

Tumors of the true cords (Fig. 8-1) prevent accurate approximation during phonation and therefore cause hoarseness. Malignant tumors of the larynx have a very favorable prognosis if the patient sees a doctor as soon as he becomes hoarse and *if the doctor then examines the larynx*.

The greatest difficulty in examining the larynx lies in trying to see the anterior commissure, which is often hidden by the tubercle of the epiglottis. Rarely, it is necessary to apply topical anesthesia and to use a retractor to displace the epiglottis. Usually, proper phonation effects adequate retraction.

The attachment of the true vocal cords to the arytenoid process causes a slight, cup-shaped depression that is sometimes mistaken for an abnormality. Pellets of mucus resting on the

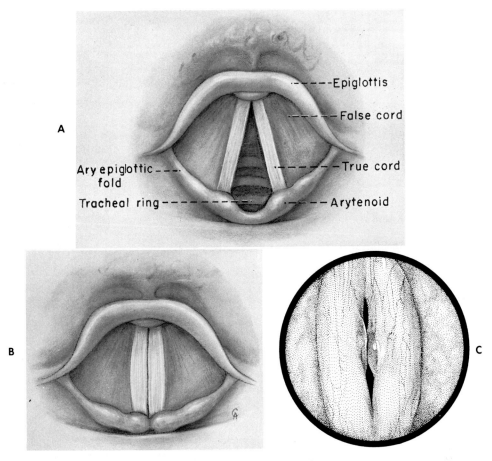

A

Ary epiglottic fold
Tracheal ring

-----Epiglottis
------False cord
------True cord
------Arytenoid

B

C

FIG. 1-23. A, Larynx in quiet respiration. **B,** Larynx during phonation. The mirror *reverses* anterior and posterior, but right and left remain the same. **C,** Bilateral vocal nodules. (See also Fig. 8-14.) A common condition to compare with the normal larynx as seen in **A** and **B.**

cords may look like small tumors. If the patient will cough, many of these "tumors" will disappear.

The area directly beneath the true vocal cords (conus elasticus) is not entirely visible by mirror (indirect) layngoscopy. Except for this area and the ventricle of the larynx, all parts of the larynx can be seen well with the laryngeal mirror.

Before the examination is completed, all parts of the larynx should be inspected during quiet respiration and phonation. Sometime during the examination the patient should be asked to turn the head and cough. A sharp cough indicates that the true vocal cords approximate. This functional test helps the examiner to differentiate between so-called hysterical aphonia and other causes of weak voice, or aphonia. Finally,

the beginner is again cautioned not to fix his attention on the true cords alone.

EXTERNAL LARYNGEAL EXAMINATION. Complete examination of the larynx calls for palpation of the neck. The shape of the thyroid cartilage is noted, and the space between the thyroid cartilage and the hyoid bone is palpated. This space is a common site for a thyroglossal duct cyst. The space between the thyroid and cricoid cartilages is also palpated. Sometimes a lymph node is felt in patients with carcinoma of the larynx. The cricothyroid space is the site where an emergency tracheotomy may be done with the least bleeding.

Because the cricothyroid muscle is the only laryngeal muscle innervated by the superior laryngeal nerve, the function of that nerve may be tested by having the patient say "e-e-e" in a high pitch. This action causes a contraction of the normal cricothyroid muscle, and the cricoid cartilage is drawn upward. These events fail to happen if the superior laryngeal nerve is not intact.

Laryngeal crepitation is elicited by grasping the larynx (thyroid cartilage) between the thumb and index finger and rocking it vigorously from side to side. This maneuver should cause crepitation that can be felt on either side. If crepitation does not result, a postcricoid neoplasm may be cushioning the movements of the larynx across the vertebral column.

NOSE AND PARANASAL SINUSES

Nose. The nasal chambers are examined by inspection. They are inspected anteriorly and posteriorly with the nasal speculum and the postnasal mirror, respectively. A metal applicator wound with cotton provides a useful instrument for light intranasal palpation.

Lighting is the same as already described. The light must be bright and focused to a small spot. Because the nasal chambers are several centimeters long, the position of the examiner's head that allows him to focus sharply in the nasal vestibule will not provide a bright spot of light in the posterior area of the nose. Therefore, to maintain adequate lighting, the examiner must constantly alter the relationship between the patient's head and his own.

Vasoconstriction (Fig. 1-24) is provided by topical application of 3% ephedrine in saline solution. Two percent cocaine has the added advantage of producing topical anesthesia. Shrinking the nasal mucosa (meaning the inferior turbinates in most instances) is necessary in many patients before complete intranasal inspection can be done.

Ephedrine may be sprayed from an atomizer, or it may be applied with wisps of cotton that have been wetted with the drug. The cotton wisps should be introduced along the inferior turbinate and left for several minutes. Sometimes it is important to obtain vasoconstriction in other areas, such as about the middle meatus and middle turbinate.

The *nasal speculum* is held in the left hand whether one is examining the left side or the right side of the nose (Fig. 1-25). The left index finger presses on the ala of the nose to anchor

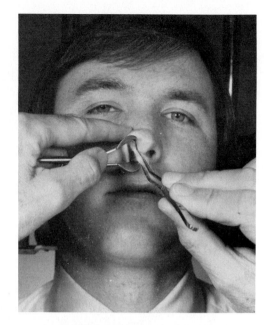

FIG. 1-24. Use of a vasoconstrictor. Most shrinkage comes by reducing the inferior turbinate. All intranasal manipulations are done under direct vision.

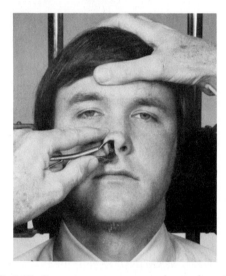

FIG. 1-25. Correct way to use a nasal speculum. Note the positions of the *thumb* and the *index finger*.

the upper blade of the speculum in place. The blades are inserted about 1 cm. into the vestibule. The speculum is opened vertically (not transversely) to avoid painful pressure against the nasal septum.

The *examiner's right hand* is the real key to intranasal inspection, because it positions the

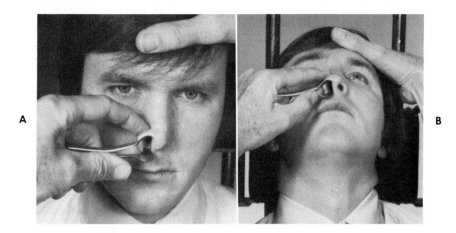

FIG. 1-26. A, Head position necessary to see the floor of the nose, the inferior turbinate, and the septum. Note how *widely* the blades are opened. **B,** Head position necessary to see the middle meatus, the middle turbinate, and the superior part of the septum. The *right hand* tips the head backward and thus is the real key to the examination.

head. Except when used for instrumentation, the right hand is placed firmly on the top of the patient's head and is used to change the head position from time to time (Fig. 1-26). Too much emphasis cannot be placed on this point. One must look at small areas successively. For example, with the patient's head erect the examiner can see the floor of the nose and the inferior turbinate, but he cannot see the septum well unless he turns the head sideways. Similarly, he cannot inspect the middle meatus until the head is tilted backward. Use of a headrest is discouraged because it fixes the patient's head and prevents proper use of the examiner's right hand.

Following are the mistakes every beginner makes:

1. He fails to adjust his head position to keep his light sharply focused.
2. He opens the nasal speculum too little. Actually, unless he opens the speculum as completely as the nose will permit (and often this means as fully as the speculum will open), it is better to use no speculum at all.
3. He fails to tilt and turn the patient's head with his right hand to see all parts of the nose.
4. He fails to use vasoconstrictors.

EXAMINATION. The examination should include the vestibule, the mucosa, the nasal sep-

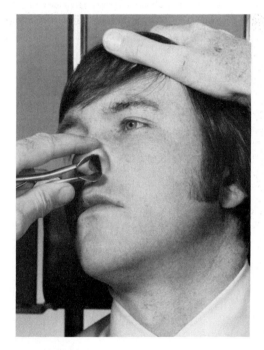

FIG. 1-27. Nasal vestibule. This part of the nose is lined with skin.

tum, the lateral wall of the nose, and the nasopharynx.

VESTIBULE. The vestibule of the nose is lined with skin and contains the nasal hairs, or vibrissae (Fig. 1-27). Except for folliculitis and fissures, no common diseases involve the nasal vestibule. The vestibule may be examined by tilting the tip of the nose upward with the finger. A nasal speculum is also useful.

MUCOSA. The nose is lined with respiratory mucosa except anteriorly, where there is skin, and far superiorly, where there is olfactory epithelium. The nasal mucosa is redder than the oral mucosa; therefore, students are prone to call normal nasal mucosa "hyperemic" or "injected."

NASAL SEPTUM. The nasal septum is composed of both cartilage and bone. In virtually every adult the septum is not straight. Instead it gradually deviates from the midline to a greater or lesser degree, or it has developed a sharp projection (a spur or ridge) or a more rounded projection (a hump). Sometimes the anterior end of the nasal septum is dislocated and projects prominently into one nostril. In any case, such irregularities of the nasal septum ordinarily cause no disturbance unless they are severe enough to obstruct the airway. Sometimes crusting occurs at the site of the nasal septal deviation or spur, and bleeding results.

There is an anterior plexus of blood vessels in the mucosa of the nasal septum, and one can often see small arteries and veins here. This is the most common site for epistaxis (nosebleed).

The posterior end of the septum is formed by the vomer and is best inspected by using a No. 0 nasopharyngeal mirror. Here the septum is normally thin, but sometimes inflammatory tissue gathered symmetrically on either side gives a plowshare appearance to the vomer.

LATERAL WALL OF THE NOSE. The important structures in the lateral wall of the nose (Fig. 1-28) are the inferior, middle, and superior turbinates and their respective meatuses.

The *inferior turbinate* is a separate bone; the middle and superior turbinates are parts of the ethmoid bone. The inferior, the largest turbinate, lies like a finger along the lower lateral wall of the nose. It is erectile and swells periodically. This swelling may cause alternating nasal obstruction, which is especially troublesome at night to some patients, who must turn from side to side to relieve the congestion caused by the dependent turbinate.

The two inferior turbinates are not the same size in most patients. When the septum is displaced to one side, the inferior turbinate on the opposite side is prone to swell and fill the concavity. Normally the turbinate is deep pink and similar to the color of the rest of the nasal mucosa, but in allergic states it becomes blue or pale and the tissue becomes boggy and swollen. Inflammation of the nasal mucosa causes redness.

The *inferior meatus* is not seen in its entirety because of the overhanging inferior tur-

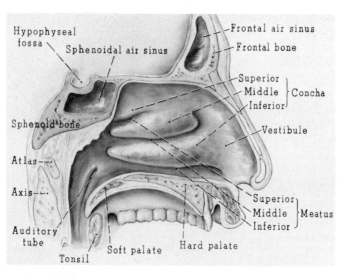

FIG. 1-28. Lateral wall of the nose. Each meatus lies under its respective turbinate. The eustachian (auditory) tube is posterior and at the level of the inferior meatus. (From Jacob, S.W., and Francone, C.A.: Structure and function in man, Philadelphia, 1970, W.B. Saunders Co.)

binate. The nasolacrimal duct, which opens into the anterior part of the inferior meatus, is not seen.

The *middle turbinate* is seen by looking into the nose anteriorly. Sometimes a deflection of the nasal septum partially hides the structure. Occasionally the middle turbinate contains an air cell that enlarges its anterior end. Ordinarily the middle turbinate does not contribute seriously to nasal obstruction.

The *middle meatus* is a very important area; it lies lateral to the middle turbinate. Appearing as a cleftlike space, it often is poorly seen because of encroachment by the adjacent middle turbinate. Vasoconstriction and careful positioning of the head will make the middle meatus visible. Secretions from the frontal, maxillary, and anterior ethmoid sinuses drain here. The ostia of the sinuses are not visible.

NASOPHARYNX. In most patients the examiner can look completely through the nose and inspect part of the nasopharynx. Sometimes this is possible on only one side, because of a deflection of the septum or an unusually prominent inferior turbinate. The use of vasoconstrictors greatly increases the number of patients in whom the nasopharynx can be examined in this manner.

Having the patient say "kick" or "k" causes the soft palate to fly upward. This movement orients the examiner as to how far posteriorly he is seeing. It also provides information about the mobility of the palate.

Paranasal sinuses. Examination of the paranasal sinuses is done more indirectly than other otolaryngeal procedures. One cannot see into any of the sinuses, and only rarely can one see a sinus ostium. Information about the condition of the sinuses is gained, first, by inspecting and palpating the overlying soft tissues (maxillary and frontal sinuses); second, by noting secretions that may drain from the sinuses; and, third, by transillumination (maxillary and frontal sinuses only).

PALPATION AND PERCUSSION. Palpation and percussion may be done over the maxillary and frontal sinuses (Fig. 1-29). Simultaneous finger pressure over both maxillae will demonstrate differences in tenderness (Fig. 1-29, A). Palpation under the upper lip may demonstrate fullness not appreciated by inspection.

The frontal sinuses are palpated by finger pressure directed upward toward the floor of the sinus, where the sinus wall is thin (Fig. 1-29, B). Tenderness may be discovered in this way. Swelling caused by tumors or retained secretions (mucocele) may cause a downward bulge in the floor of the frontal sinus. The ethmoid and sphenoid sinuses cannot be examined except by intranasal inspection.

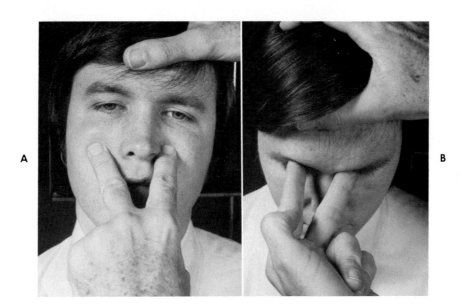

FIG. 1-29. A, Testing the maxillary sinuses for tenderness. **B,** Testing the frontal sinuses for tenderness.

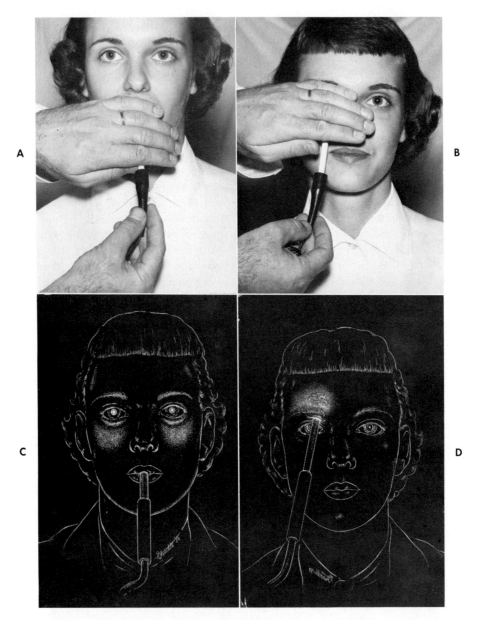

FIG. 1-30. A and **C,** Technique of transillumination. Both maxillary sinuses are transilluminated at once. Pupillary reflexes are pink, there are crescents of light under each eye, and cheeks glow diffusely pink. **B** and **D,** Technique of transillumination. Hand should shield entire transilluminator. Many normal frontal sinuses transilluminate poorly. Drawing shows a large, clear frontal sinus. (From Saunders, W.H.: Ears, nose, and throat. In Prior, J.A., and Silberstein, J.S., editors: Physical diagnosis: the history and examination of the patient, ed. 3, St. Louis, 1973, The C.V. Mosby Co.)

WHERE THE SINUSES DRAIN. It is possible to determine which sinus is infected by discovering where a purulent discharge appears in the nose. It is important to use vasoconstrictors and a sharply focused light if one is to see a small stream of pus in the nose.

FRONTAL AND ANTERIOR ETHMOID CELLS. The discharge is found well forward in the middle meatus and seems to come from high up.

MAXILLARY SINUS. The ostium is somewhat farther back in the middle meatus, and drainage occurs over the posterior end of the inferior turbinate. Therefore pus from the maxillary sinus often is seen best by using the postnasal mirror.

SPHENOID AND POSTERIOR ETHMOID CELLS. The drainage is far posterior. The examiner sees secretions from the posterior sinuses by using the nasal speculum or the postnasal mirror. The pus runs down between the middle turbinate and the septum.

TRANSILLUMINATION. By shining a bright light in the patient's mouth with the lips closed about a special bulb, the examiner transilluminates the maxillary sinuses (Fig. 1-30, A and C). The amount of light that passes through the bony walls and soft tissues covering the sinuses varies greatly from patient to patient. Therefore, differences in the degree of transillumination, without other findings, are not diagnostic. It is more important if one maxillary sinus transilluminates clearly and the other fails to do so than if both fail to transilluminate. The frontal sinus is transilluminated by shining a shielded beam of light through the floor of the sinus (Fig. 1-30, B and D). The ethmoid and sphenoid sinuses cannot be examined by transillumination.

WHAT TO LOOK FOR IN SINUS TRANSILLUMI-NATION

FRONTAL SINUSES. As transillumination is done, the face of each sinus becomes light. Because the frontal sinuses are rarely the same size, the examiner may see a considerable difference in light reflex. Often neither side transilluminates well even in normal patients.

MAXILLARY SINUSES. There are red pupillary reflexes and crescents of light under the eyes, and the faces of the sinuses glow pink.

• • •

Although most pathologic changes affecting the ears, nose, and throat are recognized readily after a careful history and a thorough physical examination, some conditions remain obscure and require functional and laboratory tests to establish a diagnosis. The physical examination, therefore, is often supplemented by audiometric examination, vestibular examination, and roentgenography. Cultures and biopsies are also common. Endoscopic examination of the trachea and bronchi and of the esophagus is carried out when necessary.

All these procedures are discussed in detail in the chapters that follow.

SELECTED READINGS

Becker, W., and others: Atlas of otorhinolaryngology and bronchoesophagology, Philadelphia, 1969, W. B. Saunders Co.

Mawson, S.: Diseases of the ear, ed. 2, Baltimore, 1967, The Williams & Wilkins Co.

FILMS

Saunders, W. H.: Physical diagnosis of the ear, nose, and throat (a 30-minute color-sound motion picture), Ohio State University, Departments of Photography and Otolaryngology, 1959.

Saunders, W. H. (consultant): The ears (an 18-minute color-sound motion picture), National Medical Audiovisual Center Production, Atlanta, Ga., 1970.

Saunders, W. H. (consultant): The nose (a 14-minute color-sound motion picture), National Medical Audiovisual Center Production, Atlanta, Ga., 1970.

2 LESIONS OF THE ORAL CAVITY

LESIONS OF THE TONGUE

Papillae. There are several different papillae on the tongue. The *circumvallate* papillae are arranged as an inverted V at the base of the tongue. Clinically they cause no trouble, except that some patients mistake them for tumors.

The *filiform* papillae give the tongue its coating; when heavily keratinized, they make the tongue look white. When they are stained by tobacco or by chromogenic organisms, the tongue may look brown or black; and if the papillae become elongated, we speak of a black, hairy tongue. If the filiform papillae desquamate, the tongue looks slick and red (vessels in the corium shine through). Such a condition is seen in geographic tongue and as a congenital disorder in median rhomboid glossitis.

Median rhomboid glossitis. Median rhomboid glossitis (Fig. 2-1), well named anatomically, is poorly named pathologically. In the embryo the tuberculum impar, occupying the middle third of the tongue, becomes depressed below the surface as the two lateral halves of the tongue join one another. Occasionally, when there is a minor developmental abnormality, the tuberculum impar persists as a surface structure. The absence of papillae permits the underlying blood vessels to shine through the mucosa, and the tongue looks red and slick.

Geographic tongue. Although not related embryologically to median rhomboid glossitis, geographic tongue (Fig. 2-2) bears some resemblance to that condition because certain areas of the tongue are denuded of papillae and the epithelium is very thin. These areas look reddish. The remainder of the tongue, with normal papillae and normal epithelium, has the usual appearance. The reddest areas are around the borders of the denuded regions, but centrally there is a regeneration of papillae. Alter-

nating regeneration and desquamation change the surface configuration from time to time—hence the synonym "migratory glossitis." In some patients the lingual pattern changes weekly; in others changes are slower, or the condition may remain healed for a year and then recur.

There is some justification for calling this condition glossitis, because microscopic sections do show infiltration of epithelium by leukocytes. Some patients complain of a slight burning of the tongue, but usually they have no complaint and often are even unaware of the unusual appearance of their tongues. Treatment is unnecessary.

Hairy tongue. So-called hairy tongue (Fig. 2-3) is another condition that is well named according to gross appearance but improperly named according to microscopic appearance. Patients with this condition look very much as if long hairs are growing on their tongues. The "hairs" are greatly elongated filiform papillae that are brown or black in color. Sometimes they are so long that the patient can actually comb his tongue.

Usually the cause is not apparent. Some patients develop the condition as a result of using penicillin lozenges or because of irritation from smoking or poor mouth hygiene. Many chronically ill patients have hairy tongue. Microscopically, colonies of yeast organisms are seen growing among greatly keratinized filiform papillae. A superficial glossitis may be present. Treatment is not always successful. Local measures, such as cleaning the back of the tongue with a toothbrush, applying oxidizing solutions (half-strength hydrogen peroxide), shaving the filiform papillae, and cautery with trichloroacetic acid, have all been used with some success. Measures designed to improve general health

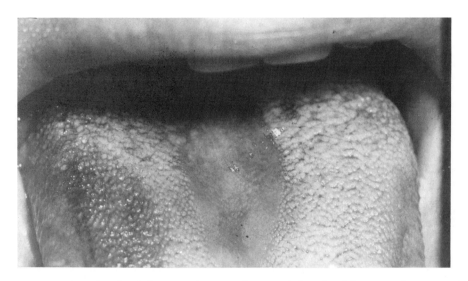

FIG. 2-1. Median rhomboid glossitis. The central area is slick and red because it has no papillae.

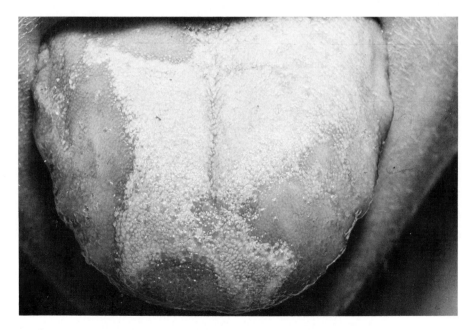

FIG. 2-2. Geographic tongue (migratory glossitis). Compare the denuded areas with those in Fig. 2-1.

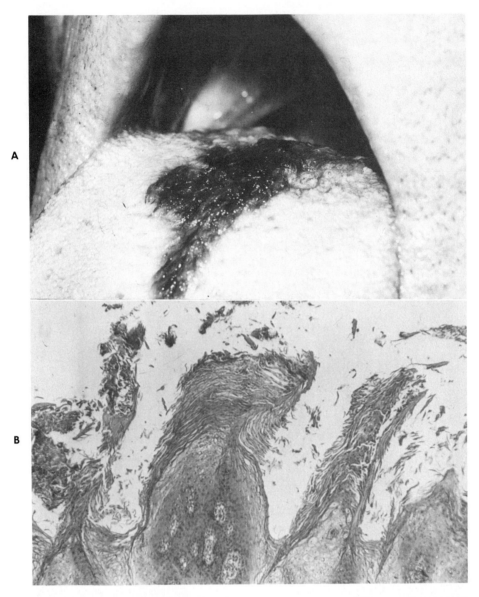

FIG. 2-3. A, Black hairy tongue, cause unknown. **B,** Hairy tongue. Note great keratinization.

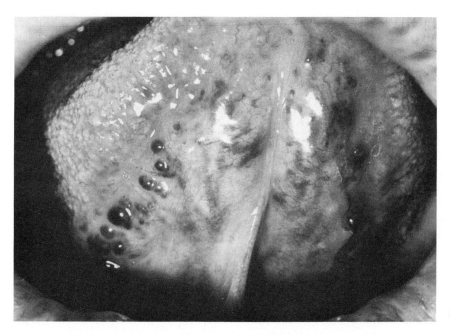

FIG. 2-4. Lingual varicosities.

are always suggested, and, of course, vitamins are recommended. However, the condition persists in many patients despite all treatment.

Varicose veins. Varicosities under the tongue (Fig. 2-4) are common in older people. They never bleed and are of no clinical significance, although certain medical textbooks relate the condition to cardiac decompensation. Varicosities are also found in the valleculae. They, too, never seem to cause bleeding. On the dorsum of the tongue there is occasionally a single varicosity containing venous blood.

Hereditary hemorrhagic telangiectasia. The small bright red lesions of hereditary hemorrhagic telangiectasia (Rendu-Osler-Weber disease) occur on the tongue as well as on other oral mucous membranes. They look as though they contain arterial blood. Similar lesions in the nasal mucosa cause serious bleeding, but in the oral cavity the telangiectasia is generally asymptomatic.

Fissured tongue. Fissured tongue (Fig. 2-5) is a familial, but not always a congenital, condition. It is also called scrotal tongue. The fissures are of variable depth and usually extend laterally from a median groove. There are no symptoms unless food and debris lodging in the depths of the fissures cause a mild glossitis. No treatment is necessary.

Tongue-tie. True tongue-tie (ankyloglossia), in a degree that produces symptoms, is not common. If the tongue protrudes to the teeth, there is no interference with speech. In the occasional patient requiring treatment, cutting the frenum may improve the condition.

Macroglossia. Macroglossia may be due to tumor, lymphangioma (Fig. 2-6), amyloid deposit, edema from lymphatic obstruction, or other causes. As an acute phenomenon, macroglossia may be caused by an allergic reaction such as is seen in angioneurotic edema, or it may result from hematoma or abscess. Some individuals simply seem to have more tongue tissue than others. It is difficult to examine their throats because of their large tongues.

Hypoglossal paralysis. As a result of certain infections (poliomyelitis, for example), injury, or cancer, the hypoglossal nerve may be paralyzed (Fig. 2-7). Then one half of the tongue begins to fibrillate and the muscle tissue atrophies. As the patient protrudes his tongue, the strong muscles of the normal side push the tongue toward the side of the paralysis. Usually neither speech nor swallowing is disturbed in unilateral paralysis if the other related cranial nerves are intact.

Amyotrophic lateral sclerosis. Amyotrophic lateral sclerosis is an uncommon disorder that

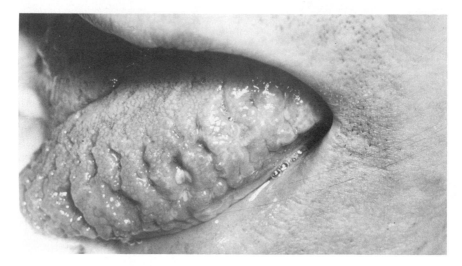

FIG. 2-5. Fissured tongue, asymptomatic.

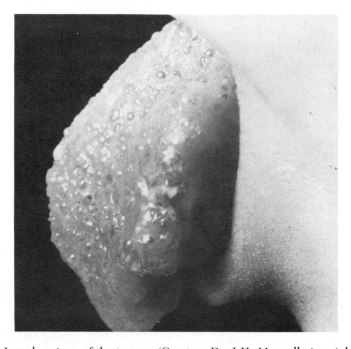

FIG. 2-6. Lymphangioma of the tongue. (Courtesy Dr. J.H. Maxwell, Ann Arbor, Mich.)

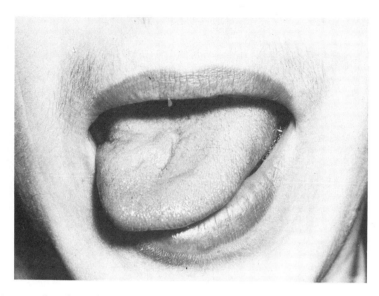

FIG. 2-7. Hypoglossal paralysis. Note atrophy of the tongue and deviation toward the weak side.

may produce a paralysis of the tongue as well as other muscles about the oral cavity and pharynx. At first the diagnosis is not suspected, and the patient complains only of occasional trouble with articulation or similar symptoms. As the disease progresses, the entire tongue fasciculates and becomes immobile, and there is drooling, weight loss, and complete loss of speech.

In the course of the disease weakness and fasciculation of various large muscles of the body develop, and the diagnosis becomes readily apparent. No effective treatment is possible, and the patient's condition gradually deteriorates toward death.

LESIONS OF THE PALATE

Torus palatinus. The bony exostosis of torus palatinus (Fig. 2-8), covered by thin epithelium, is a common finding in the midline of the hard palate. The torus palatinus is usually single and approximately in the midline. This tumor, the result of embryologic malfusion, is not a neoplasm, although it is frequently mistaken for one. It is entirely painless and asymptomatic until the patient discovers it and begins to wonder what it is. Then he may worry about cancer. Traumatic ulcers of the torus are seen occasionally. Rarely, it is necessary to remove the exostosis in order to fit a denture.

Torus mandibularis. The torus mandibularis (Fig. 2-9) is similar to the torus palatinus except that it usually occurs bilaterally. It is found on the lingual aspect of the mandible near the midline. Ordinarily these growths are much smaller than the torus palatinus. They are quite common but are usually overlooked. They are also asymptomatic but may confuse the examiner who does not understand their nature.

Elongated uvula. The normal uvula varies greatly in length and thickness. It is a muscular organ and contracts when the soft palate does. Some physicians believe that an abnormally long uvula (Fig. 2-10) may cause a chronic cough or gag a patient. On that basis, the excess length is sometimes amputated. Actually, the uvula probably causes no symptoms whatever, regardless of its length, and any apparent relationship between a long uvula and throat symptoms is likely to be coincidental.

Bifid uvula. Fairly common, the bifid uvula (Fig. 2-11) has some clinical significance because it means that the patient may have a submucous cleft palate. In other words, even though there is no apparent cleft palate (because epithelium is intact), the muscle tissue of the palate is deficient.

If an adenoidectomy is done in a child with a bifid uvula, he may have difficulty in closing off the nasopharynx. The reason is that his pal-

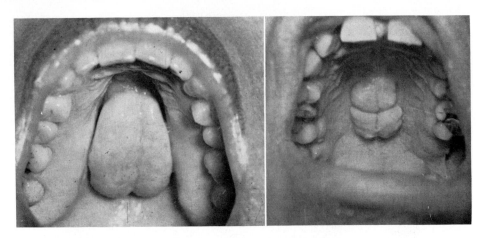

FIG. 2-8. Large tori palatini.

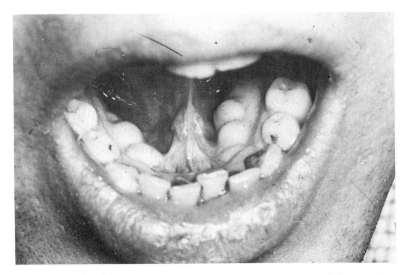

FIG. 2-9. Multiple mandibular tori. Large growths like these are unusual, but smaller ones are common.

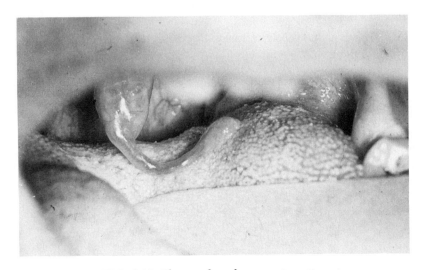

FIG. 2-10. Elongated uvula, asymptomatic.

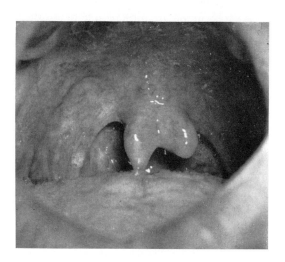

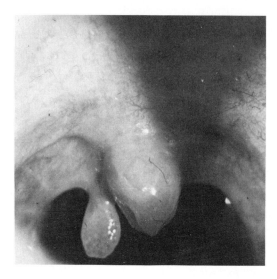

FIG. 2-11. Bifid uvula.   FIG. 2-12. Typical squamous cell papilloma.

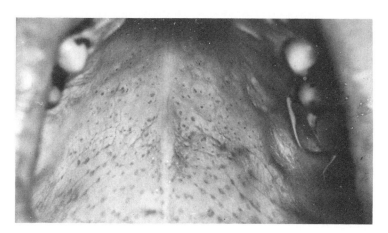

FIG. 2-13. Nicotine stomatitis.

ate, deficient in musculature, cannot approximate the posterior pharyngeal wall. This inability to approximate the palate and pharynx is common in many children after removal of large amounts of adenoid tissue, but the condition is temporary and nasal speech soon corrects itself. However, in patients with a bifid uvula and submucous cleft of the palate, nasal speech can be permanent.

Papilloma. Squamous cell papillomas (Fig. 2-12), presumably of viral origin, are common in the oral cavity. They are almost always attached by a pedicle to the uvula, the tonsillar pillars, or the free margin of the soft palate. The condition requires no treatment unless the patient requests that the lesion be excised. Their ap-

pearance is so characteristic that they are not likely to be confused with other lesions.

Nicotine stomatitis. Lesions of the palate due to smoking are common. In fact, anyone who smokes a pack of cigarettes a day may develop definite changes in the mucosa of the hard palate. The orifices of mucous glands in the hard palate are normally seen as small white dots scattered through the mucosa. In smokers these orifices become red and sometimes are actually umbilicated (because the surrounding tissue has swollen) (Fig. 2-13). One is often able to tell whether a patient is a heavy smoker by examining the palate.

Patients with advanced stages of nicotine stomatitis demonstrate a similar but more pronounced pattern. The surrounding palatal mucosa has a blanched or cooked appearance because of hyperkeratosis. Red, umbilicated nodules may stand out plainly against this pale background.

Smokers occasionally develop an ulcer in the hard palate that heals only when the patient stops smoking.

LESIONS OF THE GINGIVA

Pyorrhea. Pyorrhea, a form of periodontitis, is a slowly progressive disorder that causes the gums to regress from the teeth so that more and more tooth root is exposed (Fig. 2-14). Eventually the teeth become loosened and may even fall out. This disease begins as a gingivitis and later involves the periodontal membrane. Finally it destroys the alveolar bone.

Bacteria and other organisms commonly infect this lesion. In persons with pyorrhea there is a deposit of calculus (in the periodontal pocket), which irritates and ulcerates the epithelium and permits bacteria to enter the tissue. The gingivitis that precedes pyorrhea is usually reversible. Any patient with bleeding or swollen gums or with calculus formation should be advised to see his dentist immediately.

Gingival hyperplasia. Gingival hyperplasia may be the result of long-standing irritation. It may occur in a local area, or it may involve most of the gums of the upper and lower jaws. Phenytoin (Dilantin), used in the control of epilepsy, sometimes causes great connective tissue proliferation and progressive gingival enlargement (in tooth-bearing areas only).

Patients with leukemia may develop gingival hyperplasia. An infiltration of leukemic cells causes the swelling. In addition, small bleeding spots appear on the gums between the teeth. Infection frequently supervenes and causes a gingivitis that is difficult to control. When a patient is known to have leukemia, the diagnosis is evident and biopsy is not necessary. Therapy may be quite difficult; it depends largely on controlling the leukemic process. Gentle local treatment, which may include the use of antibiotics, is beneficial.

An ill-fitting denture may cause swollen gingival mucosa (Fig. 2-15). Red, soft, movable masses of tissue form on the gingiva. If the dentures are left out, the mucosal swelling improves greatly, although it may not disappear entirely. Mucosal reactions in the hard palate, caused by irritation of dentures, are often mistaken for allergic reactions. Actually, a contact allergic reaction of this sort is rare. A dermal patch test with scrapings from the dentures will settle the question.

Epulis. There are two types of epulides: the giant cell epulis (Fig. 2-16) and an epulis related to pregnancy. In the giant cell epulis there is usually a focus of osteomyelitis near a tooth root. Therapy is excision of the epulis and treatment of any bone infection. In the epulis associated

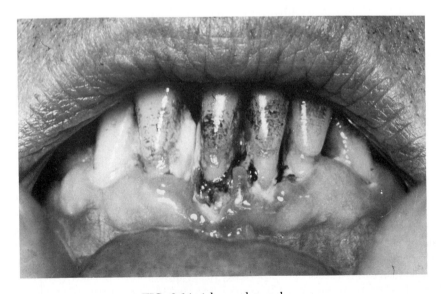

FIG. 2-14. Advanced pyorrhea.

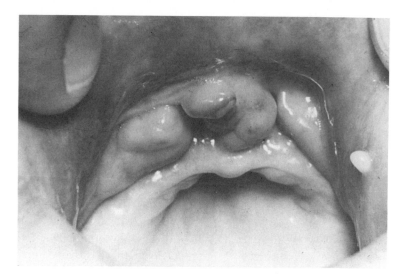

FIG. 2-15. Gingival hyperplasia caused by an ill-fitting denture.

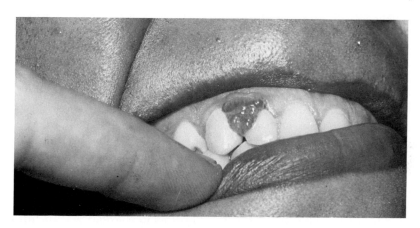

FIG. 2-16. Giant cell epulis.

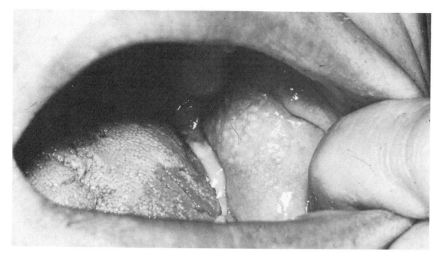

FIG. 2-17. Fordyce spots—normal sebaceous glands just under the buccal mucosa. They are seen in every adult.

with pregnancy, treatment is deferred until after delivery because the growths usually recur if they are removed sooner.

Amalgam tattoo. Amalgam tattoo results when a fragment of silver amalgam in a tooth breaks off during dental extraction and is incorporated into the gingiva. Later it shines through the mucosa as a black spot. The condition is quite common in edentulous patients.

Fordyce spots. Fordyce spots (Fig. 2-17) are seen under the buccal mucosa of every adult. These yellowish spots are sebaceous glands. They shine through the mucosa and are often mistaken for mucous glands or for an abnormal condition.

INFECTIONS

Herpetic stomatitis. Infection with the herpes simplex virus produces a vesicular eruption in the oral cavity and on the lips. In the acute stage the vesicles are often associated with fever, cervical lymphadenitis, pharyngitis, and malaise. Because they rupture so readily, they are usually not seen, and white ulcerated lesions take their place. These lesions are very painful, and the patient may refuse to eat.

After the initial infecton, the herpes virus remains in the tissue as a latent infection. It may become an acute infection again if the tissue is injured by trauma or if the host develops an upper respiratory infection. Because the host develops antibodies, the recurrent type of herpes is limited and is usually not associated with constitutional symptoms. Often when there are only one or two discrete lesions, they heal in about a week. When recurrent stomatitis produces a severe local reaction, the condition may be mistaken for a primary infection, but in the recurrent form there is no constitutional reaction.

Rarely, patients are seen who have constantly recurring stomatitis caused by the herpes virus. Apparently these patients cannot form antibodies effectively.

In the acute initial episode (usually in children) the infection may be severe. A topical anesthetic such as lidocaine (Xylocaine Viscous) or dyclonine (Dyclone) affords some relief of the oral pain. Aspirin or other analgesics help. Antibiotics are of no value.

Vincent's infection. Vincent's infection (trench mouth) is an ulceromembranous or necrotizing gingivitis. The cause is local irritation and invasion of the gingiva by organisms that make up the normal flora of the mouth. Vincent's organisms, part of the normal flora, predominate. In advanced forms of Vincent's infection, the gingivae are ulcerated and bleed readily when probed. A pseudomembrane can be stripped off. The breath has an unpleasant odor. Milder forms of the disease are more frequent. In a common localized type, a third molar erupts only partially and a pocket forms between the tooth and the flap of overlying gingiva.

Treatment consists of local applications of an oxidizing solution such as hydrogen peroxide (half strength). Also very important are scaling of the teeth and complete removal of any local irritant. Usually a dentist is best equipped to treat this oral infection.

Actinomycosis. The cervicofacial type of actinomycosis is much more common than either the abdominal form or the thoracic form. The causative organism, *Actinomyces bovis*, gains entrance through a break in the oral mucous membrane. An indurated swelling of the lower jaw and neck develops, and eventually multiple sinus tracts drain through the skin. Pathognomonic "sulfur granules" are found in the pus. Treatment of actinomycosis of the cervicofacial type is administration of penicillin or clindamycin (Cleocin), a derivative of lincomycin. The disease runs a protracted course but usually is not fatal. In differential diagnosis the important diseases to consider are tuberculosis, pyogenic osteomyelitis, and cancer.

Histoplasmosis. The first signs of histoplasmosis, a systemic fungal disease, may be lesions of the larynx and pharynx. The diagnosis is usually confused with other, more common diseases, such as tuberculosis or carcinoma. The primary infection may be subclinical or appear as a nonspecific respiratory illness, with cough, pleuritic pain, shortness of breath, and hoarseness. Irregular pyrexia, chills, and myalgia accompany the respiratory symptoms. Chest films usually show localized infiltrations or occasionally a diffuse miliary infiltration.

The lesions can occur anywhere in the larynx, oral cavity, pharynx, or nose, but the larynx and tongue are sites of predilection. There is no typical appearance of the lesions, but the most common finding is one or more nodular ulcers. Patients with histoplasmosis of the larynx and pharynx should be treated with the fungicidal drugs despite their inherent toxicity. Amphotericin B is currently the drug of choice.

Osteomyelitis. Chronic osteomyelitis may be produced by the tubercle bacillus or by fungi, but most often it is caused by a pyogenic bacterial infection.

The mandible is most commonly involved, but the maxilla and the small bones of the face can become infected. The massive suppurative process in the lower jaw that causes acute osteomyelitis most often comes from an infected tooth. Other oral infections, as well as external trauma, are occasionally responsible.

In the *acute stage* sepsis and high fever are the rule. As pus strips periosteum from cortex, the mandibular blood supply is cut off. Infection spreads throughout the marrow space. Finally, pus drains through the skin, and sequestrae may be extruded. Successful treatment depends on good drainage, removal of all dead bone, and adequate antibiotic therapy. In severe cases most of the mandible may be lost.

Chronic osteomyelitis causes a prolonged drainage of pus and induration of the jaw and neck. The condition may be confused with other infections of the neck or with malignant disease.

WHITE LESIONS

Lichen planus. Lichen planus is a dermatologic disease with oral manifestations, although often the lesions are present in the oral cavity but not on the skin. When skin lesions exist, generally on the flexor surface of the arms and legs, they appear as shiny purple papules that itch slightly. Oral lesions occur chiefly in the buccal mucosa (Fig. 2-18) and appear as fine white lines arranged in a lacelike or spiderweb pattern. They may also occur on the lower lip or tongue, where they tend to be round and not lacy. The lesions appear white because there is increased keratin on the mucosa. In the dermis there is an infiltration of lymphocytes, sharply limited to the upper corium, and liquefaction degeneration of the basal cell layer of epithelium, which causes small cystlike spaces.

The cause of the condition is unknown except that it is usually related to a psychosomatic disorder. The oral lesions frequently regress under almost any type of threapy, provided that strong reassurance accompanies the treatment. The condition may later recur without apparent cause.

Lichen planus of the oral cavity is asymptomatic, and the patient is usually unaware of its existence. Like many disorders, it causes anxiety only after it has been called to the patient's attention.

Leukoplakia. Leukoplakia is another of the white lesions of the mouth (Fig. 2-19). It is generally considered premalignant, but some authors say that they have only rarely seen carcinoma develop in a leukoplakia lesion. It is important to emphasize that not all authors agree on what leukoplakia (white plate) signifies. Perhaps the most reasonable position is as follows: "A white keratotic lesion which is not identifiable as some other entity (such as lichen planus, lupus erythematosus, solar cheilosis, white sponge nevus or carcinoma) is designated as focal keratosis if there is no significant histologic change in the epithelium, or leukoplakia if the epithelial changes suggest that carcinoma might develop in the area concerned."*

In contrast to lichen planus, the lesions of leukoplakia appear thick and plaquelike and do not show a fine, lacy pattern. The lesions may be on the tongue, the buccal mucosa, the gingiva, or the lip. An irritating denture or a jagged tooth often seems to be the cause of leukoplakia. Heat from a pipe stem, which may burn the lip, is a classic cause. Leukoplakia shows more hyperkeratosis than lichen planus, and epithelial changes suggesting premalignancy are to be expected.

Hyperkeratosis. Hyperkeratosis (Fig. 2-20) is the third of the white lesions commonly seen in the oral cavity. The condition may occur in almost any part of the oral cavity, but it is particularly common in the buccal mucosa and on the tongue. It is often caused by local irritation and is asymptomatic except for its appearance. There are no epithelial changes suggesting that the lesion might become malignant.

Linea alba. Linea alba is a common condition seen when the buccal mucosa becomes invaginated between the molars. The mucosa becomes slightly traumatized and forms a white line that runs horizontally from the posterior part of the buccal mucosa forward to the first

---

*From Color atlas of oral pathology, United States Naval Dental School, Philadelphia, 1956, J.B. Lippincott Co.

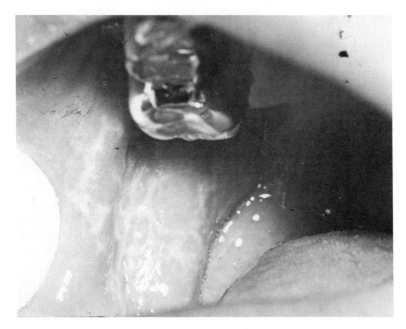

FIG. 2-18. Lichen planus in the buccal mucosa. Note the lacelike pattern. No skin lesions were present. The patient recovered without treatment, except reassurance, and then relapsed. He had no symptoms.

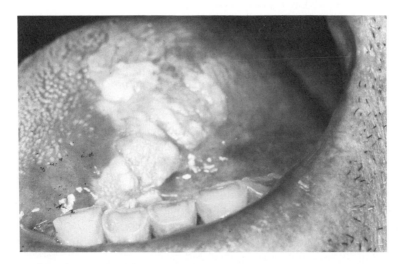

FIG. 2-19. Leukoplakia, side of the tongue. Tissue diagnosis was necessary to differentiate the condition from cancer.

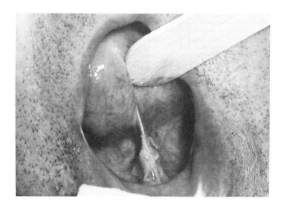

FIG. 2-20. Hyperkeratosis. This condition must be distinguished from leukoplakia and cancer.

molar. The lesion is white because the epithelium shows heavy parakeratin (the cornified layer retains its nuclei). Linea alba is so common that it can be considered a variation of normal.

Cheek nibbling. Some patients habitually nibble or chew their cheeks, much as a child sucks his thumb. The buccal mucosa looks white (as a result of hyperkeratosis) and rough; sometimes it becomes secondarily infected. Actual ulceration may occur.

Summary. The various white lesions of the mouth are not always clearly distinguishable from each other by either clinical or pathologic examination. Frequently, however, the nature of a lesion is very obvious, and there is no difficulty in differentiation. A wide difference of opinion exists as to what the term leukoplakia should signify and whether the word shoud be used to describe only lesions showing microscopic evidence of premalignancy. In case of doubt it is best to obtain tissue for examination by a pathologist.

TUMORS

In general, most tumors of the oral cavity are readily detectable by inspection, but some are not. For that reason palpation is an important diagnostic measure, since it may give a better estimate of the size of a tumor than inspection; in fact, palpation may be the only method by which some tumors can be detected.

Also of importance is the toluidine blue test for staining malignant tumors. An ulcerated lesion is dried and painted with toluidine blue. Areas that take up the dye are particularly suspicious. Satellite lesions adjacent to the major tumor may be found that otherwise would have gone undetected. See p. 61 for detailed instructions.

Fibroma. Fibromas of the oral cavity occur in the buccal mucosa or on the tongue. They usually result from injury to the cheek or tongue. Rarely, they may represent a primary neoplasm. Usually they are white and quite firm. Pain is not a symptom, and the patient does not complain unless he bites the lesion or feels it with his tongue. Since the clinician cannot differentiate accurately between the benign fibromas and other lesions (for example, sarcoma), it is best to remove fibromas for examination.

Mixed tumors. Mixed tumors of the salivary glands occur most frequently in the parotid gland, but sometimes they are found in the palate, on the lip, in the tongue, or wherever there is salivary tissue. They enlarge slowly. There is controversy concerning whether malignant degeneration occurs. A stong tendency exists toward recurrence—because of seeding at the time of excision, incomplete removal, or multicentric foci of origin. Treatment is surgical excision.

Squamous cell carcinoma of the lower lip. In the oral cavity squamous cell carcinoma varies greatly in its malignant potential. In general, of carcinomas about the oral cavity, lesions on the lower lip (Fig. 2-21) carry the most favorable prognosis and are also the most common. These lesions are usually successfully treated—by either irradiation therapy or excision. Metastases are to the submental or submandibular lymph nodes. Cancer of the lower lip is most often seen in men who work out-of-doors and thus excessively expose the lower lip to the sun.

Squamous cell carcinoma of the tongue. The tongue is the second most common site of oral carcinoma (Fig. 2-22). The prognosis is much less favorable than in lip carcinoma. The side or undersurface of the tongue is most frequently involved. Carcinoma of the base of the tongue (or of the posterior one third) has a poorer prognosis than has carcinoma of the anterior two thirds. Sometimes carcinoma develops in an area of previous leukoplakia (the same is true of the lip). The disease is very painful to most patients. Metastasis occurs early, and about one

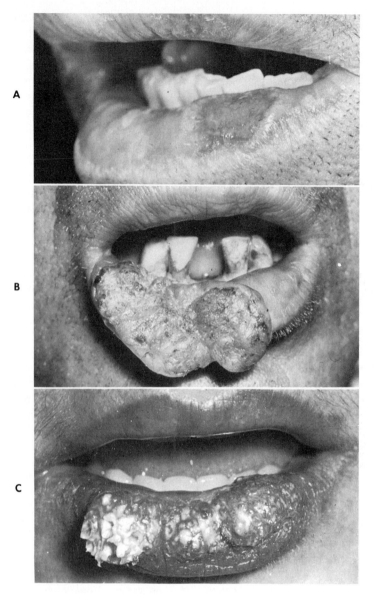

FIG. 2-21. A, Early squamous cell carcinoma. **B,** Far advanced squamous cell carcinoma. Bilateral cervical metastases were present. **C,** Superficial squamous cell carcinoma.

third of the patients have bilateral metastases. Carcinoma of the tongue is treated by either irradiation therapy or surgical excision. Often a radical neck dissection is done in continuity with a hemiglossectomy. Most patients manage both speech and swallowing very well after hemiglossectomy. Total glossectomy is sometimes required when tumor invades the entire base of the tongue. This operation is not as debilitating as one might expect; some patients who have total glossectomies are able to speak,

although indistinctly, and most of them can eat normally. An occasional patient may require total laryngectomy because of persistent aspiration.

Squamous cell carcinoma of other areas of the oral cavity. Other areas of the oral cavity, such as the floor of the mouth (Fig. 2-23), the palate, the buccal mucosa, and the tonsils and their pillars, are also sites of squamous cell cancer. The prognosis varies greatly, depending on the microscopic appearance of the tumor,

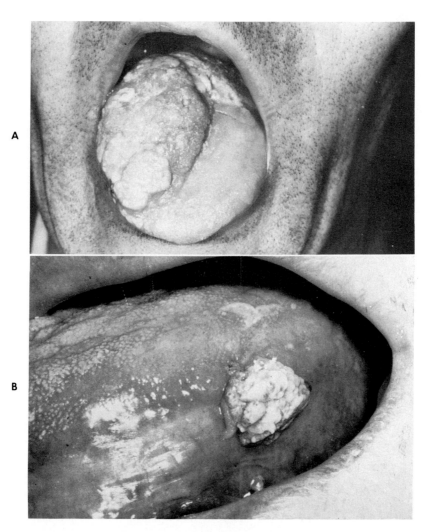

FIG. 2-22. A, Squamous cell carcinoma of the tongue. Treatment consisted of partial glossectomy and radical neck dissection. **B,** Exophytic squamous cell carcinoma—treated by wedge excision. (**B** from Saunders, W.H.: Ears, nose, and throat. In Prior, J.A., and Silberstein, J.S., editors: Physical diagnosis; the history and examination of the patient, ed. 3, St. Louis, 1973, The C.V. Mosby Co.)

host resistance, lymphatic drainage, and other factors.

Squamous cell carcinoma of the oral cavity is slow growing and may become quite large before it is recognized unless there is ulceration present. There is also a great tendency toward *multicentric origins* of oral squamous cell cancer. Multiple lesions may be adjacent but separate, and then later they may coalesce. At other times separate lesions may be at some distance from one another and even metastasize separately. Careful follow-up examinations utilizing *palpation* as well as inspection are imperative.

Basal cell carcinoma. Basal cell carcinomas are tumors of the skin but may spread to involve the oral cavity, especially the upper lips. Unlike squamous cell carcinoma, basal cell cancers do not metastasize. If they can be *widely* excised, almost all are curable. These lesions, which arise from the basal cell layer of squamous epithelium, are most common in the middle third of the face. Basal cell carcinoma is also known

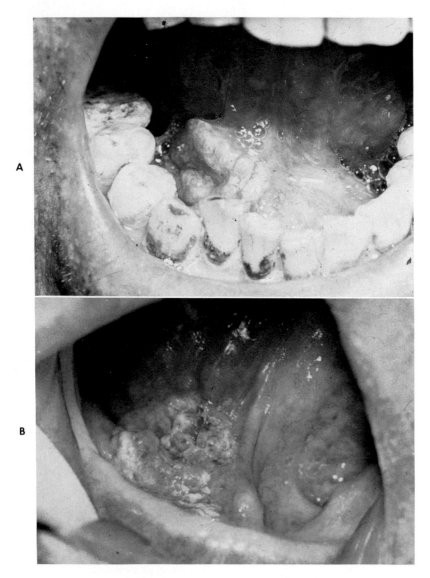

FIG. 2-23. A, Carcinoma of the floor of the mouth. Usually oral carcinomas ulcerate, but this one did not. Palpation of soft tissue may be necessary to discover some lesions. Treatment consisted of partial mandibulectomy and radical neck dissection. **B,** Ulcerated squamous cell carcinoma of the floor of the mouth.

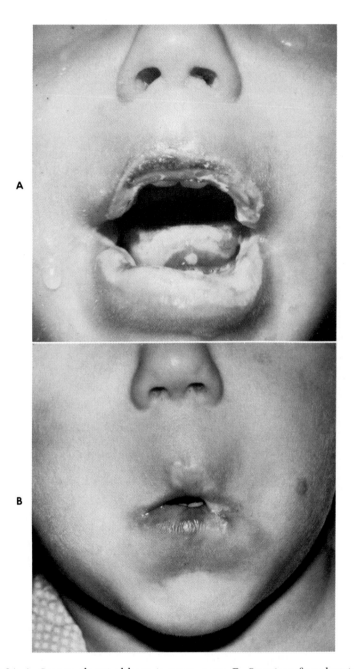

FIG. 2-24. A, Severe electrical burn in acute stage. **B,** Scarring after electrical burn.

as a "rodent ulcer." If not treated, the lesion undermines skin, ulcerates, and slowly spreads to destroy even bone. Then, of course, the prognosis is poor.

At an early stage the lesion often looks like a pimple with a scab, except that it fails to heal. Later there is a small ulcer with a raised border.

Other malignant tumors. Besides squamous cell carcinomas and basal cell carcinomas, there are many other malignant tumors that occur in and about the oral cavity. Adenocarcinomas, cylindromas, sarcomas, leukemic infiltrations, and lymphoepitheliomas are only the more common ones. Some of these lesions are responsive to irradiation or surgical removal. The location of the tumor, as well as its type, is of great importance in determining the prognosis. For more information on malignant tumors, see Chapters 31 and 32.

TRAUMA

Lacerations of the lip are usually easily repaired, but great care must be taken to match the vermilion border exactly. Otherwise, the cosmetic result will be very unsatisfactory. When cinders or dirt has been ground into abrasions or lacerations on the lip or face, one must use particular care in cleaning the wound. Otherwise, after healing, the face will be marked with a blue or black tattoo.

Laceration or perforation of the palate is fairly common. Usually it occurs in a child who falls while running with a stick or sucker in his mouth. Occasionally the hard palate may be perforated. If the laceration is deep, it should be sutured. The same is true of the tongue.

ELECTRICAL BURNS

Children are sometimes burned on the lips and tongue as a result of chewing on electrical wires. Adults may also have electrical burns of the mouth.

Electrical burns are classified as either arc or contact. Arc burns result in a charring of the soft tissues, while contact burns occur at the entry and exit sites. Most electrical burns involving the head and neck are of the arc type; they occur most frequently in children under 2 years of age. Most such burns are perioral, since they generally occur as a result of a child biting a live electrical cord. Moisture from the mouth lowers tissue resistance, resulting in an arc burn

that is usually full thickness. Damage results from extensive coagulation necrosis, which extends beyond the limits of the apparent injury. Electrical burns differ from thermal and chemical burns in that there is more deep-tissue involvement.

When small, easily treated areas of the lip are affected, treatment is early excision of the involved tissue to prevent sepsis and wound contracture. Burns that involve the commissures of the mouth are treated by waiting for spontaneous separation of the eschar, with healing, before definitive repair is done. Oral splinting is required to prevent microstomia. When a commissure is involved, treatment requires careful attention to *gentle cleansing* and prevention of secondary infection. Use of systemic antibiotics may be necessary. No other specific treatment is indicated. The burns are allowed to heal and often cause scarring and distortion of the lips; sometimes, severe partial stenosis results. After *complete* healing has taken place, plastic procedures may be necessary to provide an optimum cosmetic and functional result (Fig. 2-24).

SELECTED READINGS

Applebaum, E.L., and Sisson, G.A.: Squamous cell carcinoma of soft palate, Laryngoscope **87**:1151-1156, July, 1977.

Becker, W., and others: Atlas of otorhinolaryngology and bronchoesophagology, Philadelphia, 1969, W.B. Saunders Co.

Bull, T.R.: Color atlas of E.N.T. diagnosis, Chicago, 1974, Year Book Medical Publishers, Inc.

Butler, E.D., and others: Electrical injuries, Am. J. Surg. **134**:95-101, July, 1977.

Chanda, J.J., and Callen, J.P.: Erythema multiforme and the Stevens-Johnson syndrome, South. Med. J. **5**:566-570, 1978.

Converse, John M., and others: Facial burns, Reconstr. Plast. Surg. **3**:1595-1642, 1977.

Folsom, T.C., and others: Oral exfoliative study: reviews of the literature and report of a three-year study, J. Oral Surg. **33**:61, 1972.

Krull, E.A., Fellman, A.C., and Fabian, L.A.: White lesions of the mouth, Clin. Symp. **25**(2):1-32, 1973.

Noone, R.B., and others: Lymph node metastases in oral carcinoma, Plast. Reconstr. Surg. **53**:158, 1974.

Rothman, K., and Keller, A.: The effect of joint exposure to alcohol and tobacco on risk of cancer of mouth and pharynx, J. Chronic Dis. **25**:711, 1972.

Shedd, D.P.: Clinical characteristics of early oral cancer, J.A.M.A. **215**:955, 1971.

Strong, M.S., DiTroia, J.F., and Vaughan, C.W.: Carcinoma of the palatine arch, Trans. Am. Acad. Ophthalmol. Otolaryngol. **75**:957, 1971.

Trodahl, J.N., and Sprague, W.G.: Benign and malignant melanocytic lesions of oral mucosa; analysis of 135 cases, Cancer **25:**812, 1970.

Van de Heyning, J.: Levamisole in the treatment of recurrent aphthous stomatitis, Laryngoscope **88:**522-527, March 1978.

Vaughn, C.W.: Carcinogenesis in the oral cavity, Otolaryngol. Clin. North Am. **5**(2):291, 1972.

Wilkie, T.F., and Brody, G.S.: Surgical treatment of drooling: a 10-year review, Plast. Reconstr. Surg. **59:**791-798, June 1977.

Yap, B.S., and others: Oropharyngeal candidiasis treated with a troche form of clotrimazole, Arch. Intern Med. **139**(6):656-657, June 1979.

3 DISEASES OF THE PHARYNX

The pharynx is the space behind the oral cavity that extends upward from the larynx to the base of the skull. It is subdivided into the nasopharynx (epipharynx), that portion above the margin of the soft palate; the oropharynx, which is visible to the examiner when the tongue is depressed with a tongue blade; and the hypopharynx (laryngopharynx), which is inferior to the base of the tongue. The nasopharynx is discussed in Chapter 5.

The oropharynx is bounded posteriorly by the mucosa that covers the superior constrictor muscle and the cervical vertebrae. It communicates with the nasopharynx above and the hypopharynx below. Laterally it is bounded by the anterior and posterior tonsillar pillars, the palatine (faucial) tonsil, and the lateral pharyngeal bands (Fig. 3-1). Anterior to the oropharynx is the oral cavity, with the tongue below and the soft palate above.

The hypopharynx is bounded posteriorly by the superior constrictor muscle and the vertebrae. Below are the larynx and the pyriform fossae. Anteriorly it is bounded by the hyoid bone, the constrictor muscles, the base of the tongue, and the aryepiglottic folds. The upper free margin of the epiglottis projects into the hypopharynx.

The oropharynx and hypopharynx are essentially spaces surrounded by a muscular cone that supports the surrounding tissue and provides an open passageway for air, food, and fluids to be taken into the body. The specialized musculature of the constrictors of the pharynx and the suprahyoid and infrahyoid muscles make possible the act of swallowing. These muscles and their respective nerves act as protective organs for the air and food passages. When unwanted material threatens the airway or the throat, a reflex action of the nerves and muscles causes gagging and coughing. Both actions help in expelling any undesirable material that enters the throat. The important muscles and their attachments are shown in Figs. 3-2 to 3-5.

The lower air and food passages are further protected by a ring of lymphoid tissue that surrounds the opening of the oropharynx. Known as Waldeyer's ring, it is discussed with the tonsils and adenoids in Chapter 4.

ACUTE INFLAMMATIONS

Diseases of the upper respiratory system account for approximately 25% of the complaints of all patients who seek medical help. The throat, as well as the nose, is the first barrier to infection that may attack the respiratory system. Since diseases of this area are common and often serious, recognition of them is important.

Acute pharyngitis. The most common throat inflammation is acute pharyngitis, which may be viral or bacterial in origin. The inflammation may precede the common cold, and the usual symptoms are a mild sore throat, slight difficulty in swallowing, and mild fever. Unless the inflammation is complicated by other pathogenic bacteria, symptoms remain mild and the throat returns to normal in 4 to 6 days. Treatment consists of rest, warm saline-solution throat irrigations or gargles, and aspirin.

Acute follicular pharyngitis. Streptococcal (group A β-hemolytic) infection is by far the most common bacterial infection, especially in children. Staphylococci also may cause pharyngitis, but chiefly in debilitated patients. The onset of inflammation is usually abrupt and may be accompanied by chills and an elevation in temperature to 103° F. or higher. Headache, and muscle and joint pain may also be present at the onset. Examination of the throat reveals

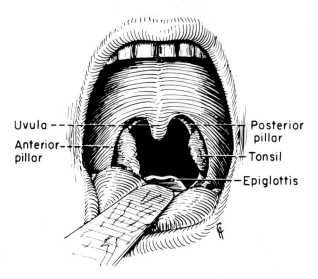

FIG. 3-1. Normal structures of the throat.

Uvula
Anterior pillar
Posterior pillar
Tonsil
Epiglottis

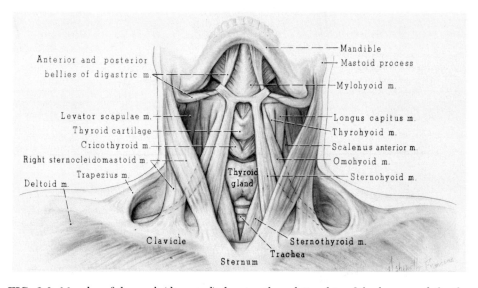

Anterior and posterior bellies of digastric m.
Levator scapulae m.
Thyroid cartilage
Cricothyroid m.
Right sternocleidomastoid m.
Trapezius m.
Deltoid m.
Clavicle
Sternum
Thyroid gland
Trachea
Sternothyroid m.
Mandible
Mastoid process
Mylohyoid m.
Longus capitus m.
Thyrohyoid m.
Scalenus anterior m.
Omohyoid m.
Sternohyoid m.

FIG. 3-2. Muscles of the neck (dissected) showing the relationship of the larynx and the thyroid gland. Note also the relation of the digastric muscles and the mylohyoid muscle to the floor of the mouth. (From Jacob, S.W., and Francone, C.A.: Structure and function in man, Philadelphia, 1970, W.B. Saunders Co.)

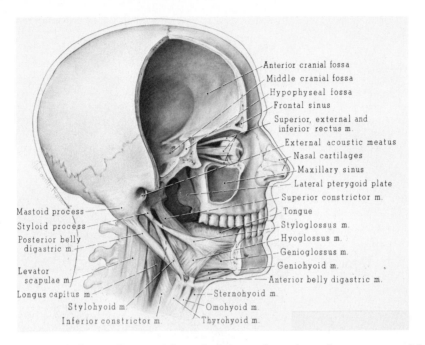

FIG. 3-3. Lateral (dissected) view of the styloid group of muscles and cut-out view of the relationship of the maxillary sinus, the orbit, and the anterior and middle cranial fossae. (From Jacob, S.W., and Francone, C.A.: Structure and function in man, Philadelphia, 1970, W.B. Saunders Co.)

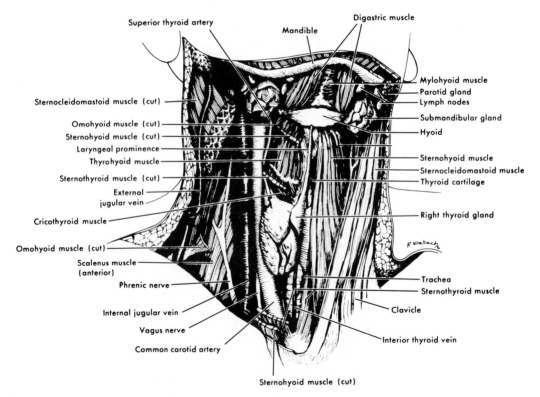

FIG. 3-4. Structures of the neck.

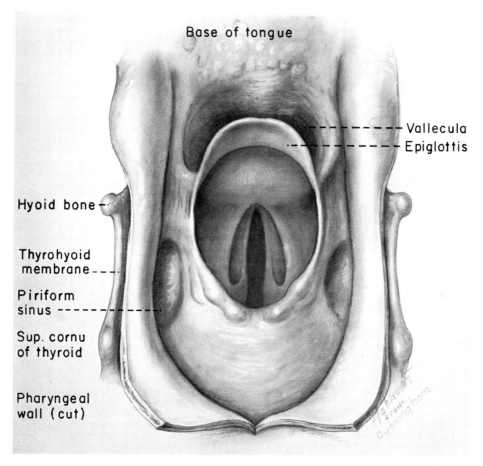

Base of tongue

Vallecula
Epiglottis

Hyoid bone

Thyrohyoid
membrane

Piriform
sinus

Sup. cornu
of thyroid

Pharyngeal
wall (cut)

FIG. 3-5. Hypopharynx as seen from the posterior view. Note the relationship of the hyoid bone, the thyroid cornu, and the pyriform fossa (sinus).

an acutely inflamed mucous membrane studded with white or yellow follicles. If the tonsils are present, most of the follicles will be found on the tonsils (acute follicular tonsillitis, Fig. 3-6, *A* and *B*). If the tonsils have been removed, the follicles appear on the individual lymph islands of the posterior wall of the pharynx. They may also be present on the lingual tonsils and in the nasopharynx. The follicular exudate is confined to the lymphoid areas of the throat and does not involve the tonsillar pillars or the soft palate.

Treatment requires bed rest, antibiotics, throat irrigations, and analgesics. Occasionally the throat will become so painful and swollen that adequate fluids cannot be taken. Hospitalization and maintenance of proper fluids by the intravenous route may be necessary for 24 to 72

hours, until the inflammation subsides. Because streptococci are the responsible organisms in most cases, the drug of choice is *penicillin*. Other antibiotics—for example, tetracyclines—are also effective, but about 20% of group A β-hemolytic streptococci are resistant to these drugs; and most *Staphylococcus aureus* organisms are resistant to tetracycline. Recurrence is common if antibiotics are stopped too soon. Antibiotics should be continued for 24 to 48 hours after the visible signs of infection in the throat have disappeared.

Acute epiglottiditis. Acute epiglottiditis is caused characteristically, but certainly not exclusively, by the *Haemophilus influenzae* organism. The disorder is especially common in young children, ages 1 to 5 years, but it is also seen in adults. In children it is especially dan-

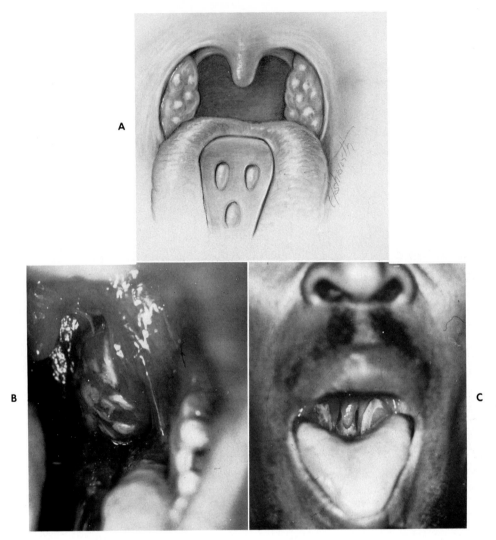

FIG. 3-6. **A** and **B,** Acute follicular tonsillitis. Note that the follicular exudate is confined to the tonsils. **C,** Membranous tonsillitis. Note that the membrane is confined to the tonsil. In diphtheria, the membrane may also cover the pillars.

gerous because the rapid swelling of the epiglottis can shut off the supraglottic airway surprisingly quickly, resulting in asphyxia.

Characteristically, respiratory difficulty begins 4 to 10 hours after the onset of illness (sore throat, dysphagia, fever), and shortly there is inspiratory stridor, cyanosis, accumulation of pharyngeal secretions, great anxiety, weakness, and disorientation. The child is desperately ill.

Treatment consists of establishing a diagnosis by indirect or direct laryngoscopy and inserting an intratracheal tube of the Portex type to ensure patency of the airway. At this point tracheotomy is recommended. Great care must be taken to ensure that the endotracheal or tracheotomy tube remains in place; the services of an experienced nurse are invaluable. A croup tent with oxygen, humidification, and tyloxapol (Alevaire) is used, and appropriate antibiotics are started. For *H. influenzae* the drug of choice is ampicillin or chloramphenicol. Usually ampicillin is given empirically until the results of a pharyngeal culture have been reported. In most instances extubation can be done in about 48 hours, when the swelling has diminished and the airway can be trusted.

Acute nasopharyngitis. The general symptoms of acute nasopharyngitis are the same as those for acute follicular pharyngitis except that there is little sore throat. Headache is often severe, and the patient complains of a full feeling behind the nose. On examination the throat appears to be normal. A nasopharyngeal mirror must be used to see the discrete follicles that characterize the disease. Treatment is the same as for acute follicular pharyngitis.

Lingual tonsillitis. Occasionally an acute infection of the pharynx involves only the lingual tonsils. The patient has all the generalized symptoms of acute throat infection. The pain in the throat is low, and often there is some difficulty in swallowing and a feeling as if there were a lump low in the throat. Diagnosis is often difficult when neither the faucial tonsils nor the oropharyx has follicles. Examination with a laryngeal mirror (Fig. 1-22) is necessary in order to make a correct diagnosis. Treatment is the same as for acute follicular pharyngitis.

Diphtheria. The incidence of diphtheria has rapidly decreased in the past four decades as a result of required immunization. However, the disease is still seen. Since 1965 there has been an increase in reported cases, probably because of developing complacency and less universal immunization. In diphtheria, a gray or white membrane forms in the throat. The membrane advances rapidly and may cover the entire oropharynx, nasopharynx, and laryngopharynx. It may extend into the trachea. It is never confined to the lymphoid areas of the throat alone. It is adherent to the underlying submucosal tissue, which it has ulcerated. Attempts to remove the membrane reveal a bleeding base. The patient's temperature is rarely higher than 101° F., but signs of toxicity are common. The pulse rate is usually high, and the pulse is thready. The patient appears more ill than one would expect from the appearance of the throat, particularly if the membrane has not advanced extensively. There is little or no acute inflammation of the tissues around the membrane.

The diagnosis must be suspected from the examination and proved by culture of throat secretions on special media. To be sure that an adequate sample of the secretions is obtained, the membrane should be lifted and a swab made from the bleeding base. Treatment requires intravenous and intramuscular specific anti-

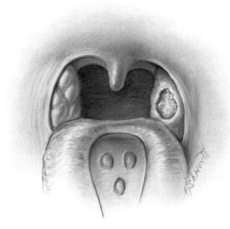

FIG. 3-7. Vincent's ulcer of the tonsil.

toxin and large doses of penicillin. If the airway is threatened by the advancing membrane, tracheotomy may be necessary to prevent death from asphyxiation.

Vincent's angina. The spirochetes and fusiform bacilli that cause Vincent's infection of the gum margins (trench mouth) may also infect the throat. The patient complains of a mild unilateral sore throat that increases in severity over several days. Often there is associated intermittent pain referred to the ear on the same side. There is no general toxicity. The patient may complain, in addition, of a bad taste in the mouth, and a slight fetid odor may be recognized. Examination most often demonstrates a deep, circumscribed ulcer of one tonsil (Fig. 3-7). The base of the ulcer is dirty gray and bleeds when scraped. There is no firm membrane over the ulcer. The ulcer crater does not involve the pillars on the tonsil. Vincent's angina rarely occurs in the throat if the tonsils have been removed. Vincent's infection of the gums often accompanies the ulcer in the tonsil.

A suspected diagnosis of Vincent's infection of the tonsil or gums can be established in the office. Less than 5 minutes is required. The only materials needed are a small metal ear spoon (or a small swab to collect a moist specimen), a glass slide, a flame, gentian violet stain, and a microscope.

The margin of the ulcer is scraped gently to remove the pseudomembrane. From the depths of the areas to be tested, a small amount of debris is removed and smeared on a glass slide. The slide is gently flamed. flooded with gentian violet stain for 30 to 45 seconds, washed off with tap water, and examined under oil immersion.

When Vincent's infection is present, one can easily see numerous spirochetes and fusiform bacilli. Often a single microscopic field will contain 20 to 30 spirochetes. A thick smear is desirable, and the specimen *must* be taken from the involved area since the organisms are anaerobic. Surface smears will ordinarily show only desquamated cells and nonspecific bacteria.

Treatment depends primarily on application of medication to the involved area. Since the spirochete of Vincent's angina is anaerobic, it is important to remove the membrane covering the ulcer crater and to treat the tissue at the base of the ulcer. This is best accomplished by local cautery of the base with phenol. Phenol is a strong caustic and must be used with caution. Two cotton applicators are prepared. One is moistened in full-strength phenol, and the other is moistened in 95% alcohol. The base of the ulcer is cleaned with a small curette. The phenol-moistened applicator is then applied to the bleeding base of the ulcer for a moment or two, and the caustic action of the phenol is immediately neutralized with the alcohol-moistened swab. This procedure prevents spreading of the tissue destruction from the phenol beyond the margins of the ulcer. Gargles and mouthwashes of sodium perborate or peroxide are prescribed for several days. One level teaspoonful of sodium perborate in half a glass of warm water is the most desirable mouthwash and gargle.

Vincent's infection is spread by direct contact through kissing or the common use of infected dishes and silverware. Therefore, a patient should be instructed to boil his dishes after eating, to use his own washcloth and towel, to avoid kissing, and to purchase a new toothbrush after the infection has cleared.

Infectious mononucleosis (glandular fever). Infectious mononucleosis often lowers a person's resistance to such an extent that an acute streptococcal pharyngitis superimposes itself on the mononucleosis. The presenting complaint in such a case is a severe sore throat. A low-grade, persistent sore throat is a common complaint of a person with infectious mononucleosis, even when secondary infection is not superimposed. The most common clinical findings in infectious mononucleosis are cervical lymphadenopathy, pharyngitis, splenomegaly, and fever. Ordinarily the disease is suspected when the anterior or posterior cervical lymph glands are enlarged out of proportion to the degree of pharyngitis. When this sign is accompanied by enlarged lymph glands in the axilla and groin, the diagnosis is almost assured. Not infrequently the throat may appear normal to routine examination, even when a sore throat is the complaint and the cervical glands are enlarged. In these instances examination of the hypopharynx with a laryngeal mirror will often show that the lingual tonsils are enlarged, particularly when the faucial tonsils have been removed.

Diagnosis is established by a differential white blood cell count, and a positive heterophil antibody test or Monospot test. The Monospot test is now more commonly employed than the heterophil antibody test, since it takes only a minute or two. Fresh stabilized horse erythrocytes are used to detect the specific heterophil antibodies associated with the disease. A differential white blood cell count showing a preponderance (50%) of lymphocytes and 10% to 15% atypical forms, plus a positive heterophil antibody test with a titer of 1:112 or higher, is considered diagnostic. Treatment is symptomatic and supportive. Bed rest may be required when toxicity is severe or liver damage is suspected. The superimposed acute pharyngitis should be treated with adequate antibiotics. Recent reports indicate that prednisone given in doses of 20 mg. daily for 2 or 3 days and then reduced to 5 mg. daily for 2 or 3 days often is followed by a prompt beneficial response.

Agranulocytosis and blood dyscrasia. When the white blood cell count is seriously reduced, as a result of either agranulocytosis or leukemia, acute sore throat often occurs. There is nothing characteristic about the appearance of the throat inflammation. The oral and pharyngeal tissues that are not inflamed may appear pale because of the coincident anemia. The patient's symptoms of toxicity, fatigue, and fever are usually more severe than would seem warranted by the appearance of the throat. Poor response to treatment or progression of the toxicity and local signs in spite of treatment should raise the sus-

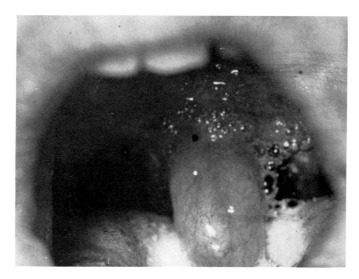

FIG. 3-8. Acute edema of the uvula as a result of aspirin sensitivity. More serious allergic edema may encroach on the airway and cause respiratory distress.

picion that a systemic disease is present. A complete blood cell count should be done for every patient.

Thrush. When the throat is infected with *Candida albicans,* discrete white patches form over the pharynx, the tonsils, the tonsillar pillars, and the base of the tongue. Formerly thrush was seen exclusively in children or in malnourished adults. Since the advent of antibiotics, it has occurred in people of all age groups regardless of their nutritional state. The prolonged use of antibiotics may destroy the normal bacterial flora of the oral cavity and allow the overgrowth of monilia, which are almost always present in the mouth. Thrush is persistent and annoying, but rarely serious. The characteristic chalk-white patches change daily and may become confluent. Sore throat is gradual in onset but may become severe.

Treatment requires local cleansing of the throat with saline irrigations and the use of nystatin (Mycostatin) for its fungicidal effect. Gentian violet (1% aqueous solution), painted on the throat lesions two or three times daily, appears to be beneficial.

Acute edema of the uvula (Quincke's disease). Occasionally a patient will complain of the sudden onset of fullness of the throat and a muffled voice without pain or fever. Examination reveals the uvula and soft palate to be swollen and pale. The uvula may be so large that it rests on the tongue and moves in and out of the oropharynx with respiration. The cause is often unknown but may be related to allergic phenomena. Treatment with epinephrine by injection may be necessary, and corticosteroids or antihistaminics also help. The edema usually subsides in 2 or 3 days, even without treatment (Fig. 3-8).

CHRONIC INFLAMMATIONS

Recurrent or chronic sore throat causes symptoms of mild degree. The discomfort is annoying, tends to disappear and recur, and is not accompanied by systemic symptoms. The physical signs are often minimal. Careful observation of slight changes in color and texture of the tissues of the throat is essential if the cause is to be found. Often a complaint of chronic sore throat, without local signs of inflammation of the throat, is evidence of systemic disease.

Chronic tonsillitis. Chronic infection of the tonsils is not so common as was once suspected. The term chronic tonsillitis has often been misused to indicate any kind of sore throat that occurs when the tonsils are still present. The diagnosis should not be made unless confirmatory signs are found.

The usual symptom of chronic tonsil infection is recurrent sore throat. Episodes of acute tonsillitis may be superimposed when resistance is lowered by fatigue or chilling. Between such episodes the throat remains uncomfortable. A feeling of malaise may also occur. The anterior cervical area may be tender. Exacerbations of acute infection are seen more commonly in children than in adults. Slight hypochromic anemia may accompany chronic tonsillitis.

Examination of the throat often shows enlargement of the tonsils, but an increase in size alone does not indicate infection. The mucosa of the anterior pillar may be inflamed. Under normal conditions the pink color of the buccal mucosa is continued onto the anterior pillar. If the tonsils are infected, a sharp line between the color of the buccal mucosa and the color of the pillar may be seen. The mucosa of the pillar is dusky red. The crypts of the tonsils may be enlarged and filled with exudate. Enlargement and tenderness of the anterior cervical lymph nodes are common. When both the tonsils and the adenoids are infected, enlargement of the glands of the posterior triangle of the neck is also expected. Unusual enlargement of the cer-

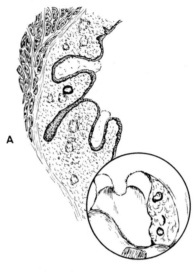

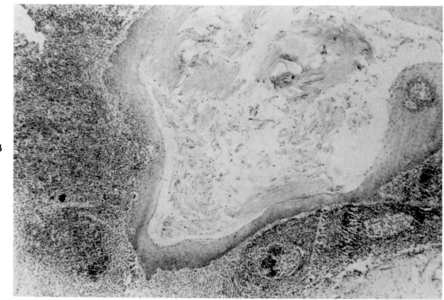

FIG. 3-9. **A,** Tonsillar crypts containing debris, chiefly desquamated squamous epithelium. **B,** Photomicrograph of a tonsillar crypt.

vical lymph glands should initiate investigation of the possibility that infectious mononucleosis, allergy, or blood dyscrasia may be present. Then tests to rule out these possibilities should be done.

When the history is compatible with a diagnosis of chronic tonsillitis, the most reliable sign is the presence of purulent matter in the tonsillar crypts. To prove the presence of pus, pressure must be exerted on the tonsil. A tonsillar pillar retractor or a wooden tongue blade can be used. Firm pressure is exerted on the anterior pillar while the tonsil is observed. Purulent material, which is usually deep in the crypts, will be expressed to the surface of the tonsil. When only material of a cheesy consistency can be expressed from the crypts, the diagnosis of chronic infection is not established. This material is often present in the crypts and represents epithelial debris and food particles (Fig. 3-9). When chronic infection of the tonsils has been proved, surgical removal is the only effective treatment.

Chronic lingual tonsillitis. Occasionally the lingual tonsils will be chronically infected. This is more common after the faucial tonsils have been removed. The primary symptom is a mild sore throat. A frequent symptom that accompanies lingual tonsillitis is a feeling of a lump in the throat. This may cause the patient to swallow frequently. In most instances the infection clears gradually. If it persists, removal of the lingual tonsils is necessary.

Chronic granular (hypertrophic) pharyngitis. The complaint of chronic sore throat may be accompanied by enlargement and mild inflammation of the individual lymphoid islands of the oropharynx. The cause is not always known. When persistent purulent postnasal discharge is the cause, treatment must be directed toward the nose or the sinuses. Allergy is sometimes responsible for granular pharyngitis, and the allergen must be found if management is to be effective. Granular pharyngitis (Fig. 3-10) is rarely seen when the tonsils are still present. It may therefore represent hypertrophy of the normal pharyngeal lymphoid islands in response to the need for lymphoid tissue after the faucial tonsils have been removed.

If an allergic cause has been ruled out, treatment consists of hot saline throat irrigations and the local use of 10% silver nitrate applied by the physician. This is an exception to the rule that local medication to the throat for infection is of little or no value.

Hypertrophy of the lymphoid islands of the pharynx is sometimes seen on examination when there are no symptoms, in which case no treatment is indicated. Occasionally a patient will be alarmed with he sees the granular islands in a mirror. Then reassurance regarding possible malignancy may be necessary.

Herpes simplex. Herpetic inflammation is caused by a virus. Although it is most commonly seen on the lips, the buccal mucosa or the pharynx may be involved. The lesions are discrete round vesicles that break to form shallow ulcers surrounded by a narrow zone of inflammation. Each lesion causes intense, localized tenderness. As one vesicle disappears, others form. When several are present over the palate and tonsillar pillars, pain during swallowing may be severe.

Allergy to certain foods, particularly chocolate, can produce lesions of the throat and palate that are identical to the lesions of herpes simplex. Except when allergy is known to be the cause and antihistaminics are indicated, treatment consists of cautery of the ulcer base with silver nitrate. Prompt relief of pain is accomplished, and the ulcer tends to heal more rapidly following cautery.

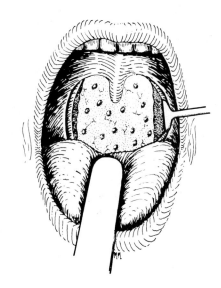

FIG. 3-10. Granular pharyngitis. The pillar retractor at the left exposes a prominent lateral pharyngeal band.

Pharyngitis sicca. Atrophy of the mucous and serous glands of the pharynx often accompanies atrophic rhinitis (see Chapter 15). Rarely, a similar atrophy is seen when no cause is apparent. The pharynx appears dry, smooth, and shiny. Crusts may form on the surface of the mucosa. Ulceration does not occur. There is no redness or inflammation. The only symptoms produced are a feeling of dryness in the throat and a desire to swallow or clear the throat more often than is normal.

Treatment is unsatisfactory in most patients. Some relief can be obtained by the oral administration of 50% potassium iodide (10 drops in water or milk twice daily) or ammonium chloride (5 gr. twice daily). Iodine and potassium iodide in glycerin (Mandl's solution) can be used locally for subjective relief.

Drug irritation. Chronic sore throat can be caused by medication. It is a reaction similar to dermatitis medicamentosa. The constant use of over-the-counter gargles can cause throat irritation in some patients. The use of medicated lozenges to ward off bad breath or to "prevent" colds may give rise to throat irritation. The use of hypertonic salt solution as a gargle for prolonged periods may prevent a self-limited inflammation from resolving. Antibiotic lozenges, particularly those containing penicillin, have been known to cause chronic throat irritation. In some instances the local sensitivity that develops during the use of antibiotic lozenges is so severe that ulceration is produced. Ammoniated tooth powders have been proved to cause throat irritation.

Treatment in each instance depends on an awareness of drug irritation, withdrawal of the drug being used, and sometimes the use of antihistaminics.

Fungus infection. The mouth and throat are occasionally infected by blastomycosis, sporotrichosis, or actimycosis. The occurrence of thrush (moniliasis), which is more common, has been discussed. Blastomycosis and sporotrichosis cause ulceration of the oral or pharyngeal mucosa, often with associated multiple small abscesses. Recognition by examination alone is difficult. The diagnosis is usually made when there are signs of associated systemic disease, when a biopsy of a persistent ulcer is done, or after a culture has been grown on special media. Actinomycosis produces an indolent, indurated sub- cutaneous swelling with slight inflammation. Tissue necrosis occurs slowly. Multiple sinus tracts may form in the buccal area. When the cervical glands are involved, these tracts are associated with the typical appearance of "lumpy jaw."

Treatment of blastomycosis and sporotrichosis depends on the response to treatment of the systemic disease. Amphotericin B, which has both a fungistatic and a fungicidal action, is the drug of choice for most systemic mycoses. Actinomycosis can be cured by operative removal of the lesions and systemic administration of penicillin or clindamycin (Cleomycin).

Syphilis. Syphilis may produce lesions in the throat during any stage of the disease. The primary lesion (a chancre) usually affects the tonsil and appears as a firm, indurated area with superficial ulceration. Frequently a single node in the neck accompanies a chancre. Since the primary lesion is self-limited, symptoms disappear in 5 to 10 days. Often the chancre is never seen. The secondary stage of syphilis causes, in addition to a transient skin rash and lymphadenopathy, the formation of "mucous patches" in the mouth or throat. The patches are slightly elevated, dull red lesions with a well-defined border. The lesions are shallow and transient. Tertiary syphilis of the mouth and throat causes the formation of gummas or sharply punched-out ulcers.

A biopsy and a positive serology test are necessary to establish the diagnosis. Treatment consists of the use of penicillin and is directed toward the systemic disease only.

Tuberculosis. Tuberculous infection of the pharynx or larynx is seen only in patients who have pulmonary tuberculosis. The ulcers produced are pale and shallow and are usually multiple. A white base, which may appear constructive, occurs at times. Diagnosis is established by proving the presence of pulmonary or tracheobronchial tuberculosis. When ulceration of the larynx involves the perichondrium, pain is severe. It is often referred to the ear through the tenth cranial nerve. Treatment is directed toward the systemic disease and consists of the use of modern antitubercular drugs. Formerly, the use of cautery for localized lesions of the pharynx was practiced, and procaine hydrochloride (Novocain) or alcohol injection of the superior laryngeal nerve was some-

times needed to control pain. Modern antitubercular medication, however, has made
these local treatments largely unnecessary.

THROAT IRRIGATIONS

Treatment of inflammation of the throat,
acute or chronic, is often aided by the cleansing
of the throat with warm normal saline solution.
Warm or hot saline solution is as effective as
any of the many drugs advocated for local use
in the throat. One level teaspoonful of salt in
1 pint of water, or $\frac{1}{3}$ teaspoonful of salt in an
ordinary drinking glass of water, will provide a
solution near isotonicity. The use of a warm
isotonic solution cleanses the throat and increases surface blood supply by causing vasodilation. Both cleansing and vasodilation are
beneficial in hastening the resolution of infection and, in addition, providing some relief from
discomfort.

The common practice of patients is to use salt
water as a gargle. Throat irrigations are more
effective. When a person gargles, the solution
used may not reach beyond the soft palate and

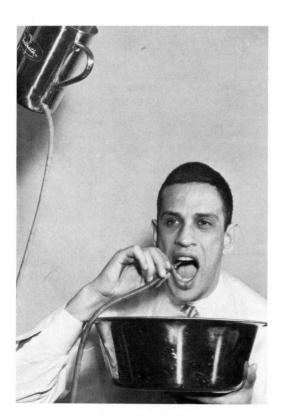

FIG. 3-11. Throat irrigation.

tonsillar pillars. Irrigation of the throat is easily
done by using a 1-quart douche can or a hot-
water bottle with a rubber tube attached. The
container is hung 2 or 3 feet above the patient's
head. The plastic or glass tip, attached to the
rubber tubing, is directed into the throat. The
patient leans over a washstand or holds a basin
(Fig. 3-11). Throat irrigation can be done at
home or in the hospital. In subacute conditions
irrigation two or three times daily is beneficial.
In acute conditions irrigation every 1 or 2 hours
while the patient is awake will hasten recovery.

SLEEP APNEA

Sleep apnea is a syndrome, not a disease.
It affects persons of all ages and both sexes but
occurs most commonly in men over 40. Sleep
apnea is the cessation of air flow in the upper
respiratory tract for more than 10 seconds while
a person is asleep. These episodes become
pathologic when they number more than 35 per
night. The disorder may be due to a central
failure of ventilatory effort or an anatomical
diurnal factor causing upper airway obstruction,
or a combination of these factors. The most frequent symptoms are somnolence, sleep attacks,
and drowsiness. Enuresis also occurs occasionally. A patient's spouse often says the patient
struggles or chokes during sleep. A common
habitus associated with the syndrome is the
pickwickian—short, thick neck and obesity.

A thorough otolaryngologic examination is essential to rule out correctable causes of sleep
apnea. In most cases, the results of an ear, nose,
and throat examination are relatively normal.
Anatomic causes such as micrognathia, macro-
gnathia, vocal cord paresis or paralysis, hypopharyngeal masses, congenital glottis, or hypertrophy of Waldeyer's ring may be corrected.
Videohypopharyngoscopy done while the patient is sleeping has shown a collapse or incoordination of hypopharyngeal musculature,
causing upper airway obstruction.

Diagnosis, which requires study in special
sleep laboratories, is based on polysomno-
graphic monitoring of air exchange, ventilatory
effort, heart activity, arterial oxygen saturation,
extraocular muscle movement, brain activity,
body temperature, and nocturnal penile tumes-
cence. Patients with severe cases may require
tracheotomy. For milder cases pharmacologic
treatment with protriptyline has been used.

MYASTHENIA GRAVIS

Myasthenia gravis is a neuromuscular disorder that affects transmission across the neuromuscular junction. The clinical manifestations are weakness and fatigability of voluntary muscles, similar to the situation found in curare poisoning. Myasthenia gravis most commonly presents to the otolaryngologist as dysfunction of the facial, ocular, laryngeal, pharyngeal, and respiratory muscles, producing symptoms such as dysphonia, dysphagia, aspiration, and weak voice. Symptoms appear to worsen with activity and to abate with rest.

The basic defect is a reduction in the number of available acetylcholine receptors at the neuromuscular junction; this defect is believed to result from an autoimmune phenomenon. Pyridostigmine bromide and neostigmine are useful for acute attacks as well as for maintenance therapy. Edrophonium (Tensilon) is used for diagnosis, as well as for treatment in severe cases; however, it is short acting. Corticosteroids are also used. Tracheotomy may be necessary to prevent aspiration, for pulmonary care, or if a patient requires mechanical ventilation. Thymectomies are occasionally performed in patients who do not respond to medical management or in those who have thymomas.

FASCIAL SPACE INFECTIONS

Peritonsillar abscess (quinsy). Acute tonsillitis, usually due to streptococci, may cause infection in the tissue between the tonsil and the fascia covering the superior constrictor muscle. A peritonsillar abscess forms. The patient has had a sore throat (tonsillitis) for several days and may seem to be improving, but then one side of the throat becomes increasingly painful. Soon he has trouble swallowing and sits with his mouth partially open so that he can drool. The voice is muffled ("hot potato voice"). Referred pain to the ear is common. The usual general symptoms associated with any infection are present.

Trismus may be present, but not always. The patient has a very sore throat; and rather than swallow, he drools. He must hawk up thick, ropy secretions. The tonsil is pushed toward the midline but also forward and downward. There is a tense swelling of the soft palate and anterior pillar above the tonsil. Usually one cannot tell by palpation whether there is fluctuation.

The uvula often rests against the tonsil or the swollen palate. If spontaneous rupture of the abscess occurs, there is drainage of pus—usually through the anterior pillar.

It is often difficult to know at first whether a peritonsillar infection represents an abscess or a cellulitis. Incision into the swollen tissue adjacent to the tonsil (at the intersection of a vertical line from the upper second molar and a horizontal line from the base of the uvula) will often yield pus. Spreading a pointed hemostat in the wound will then enlarge the incision and provide good drainage. It helps somewhat to spray the throat two or three times with a little topical anesthetic. Local anesthetic injected into the mucous membrane also helps, but some physicians object to using local anesthesia in infected tissue. Antibiotic therapy can be started before pus begins to form. After drainage the medication is continued. Hot saline irrigations are also useful and give symptomatic relief. Not all peritonsillar infections, either treated or untreated, go on to abscess formation. The patient can drink more easily if someone stands behind him and pulls upward on the sides of his head as he swallows. Finally, when all infection has subsided (usually at least a month is required), a tonsillectomy is done because peritonsillar infections tend to recur. Primary tonsillectomy with adequate chemotherapy has been successfully performed without complication.

Retropharyngeal abscess. Retropharyngeal abscess (Fig. 3-12) is not common but is important in understanding the fascial spaces of the head and neck. In infants and young children there are lymph nodes in the retropharyngeal space that atrophy or regress by young adulthood. Therefore, retropharyngeal abscess is seen almost exclusively in infants and young children. A special type, the "cold" abscess of tuberculosis (Pott's disease), may be seen at any age.

A child with a large retropharyngeal abscess has great difficulty breathing. There is stridor and nasal obstruction. The cry is muffled, and the patient lies with the head extended. There is a soft, red bulging of the posterior pharyngeal wall. The retropharyngeal abscess, unlike the peritonsillar abscess, is usually fluctuant. X-ray films show that the larynx is pushed forward and that there is a mass in the posterior portion of the pharynx (lateral view).

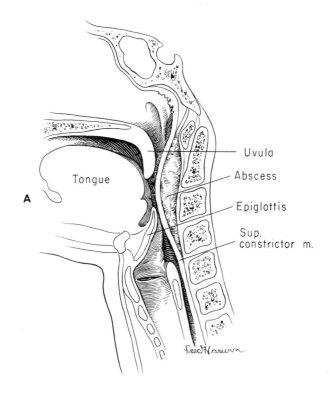

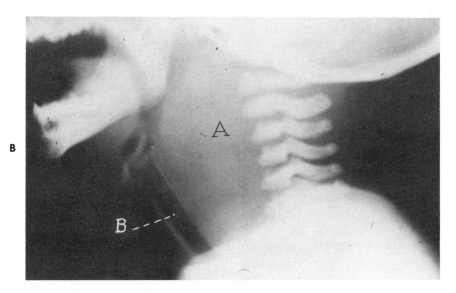

FIG. 3-12. A, Retropharyngeal abscess. **B,** Roentgenogram of a retropharyngeal abscess, showing the abscess *(A)* and the displaced tracheal air column *(B).*

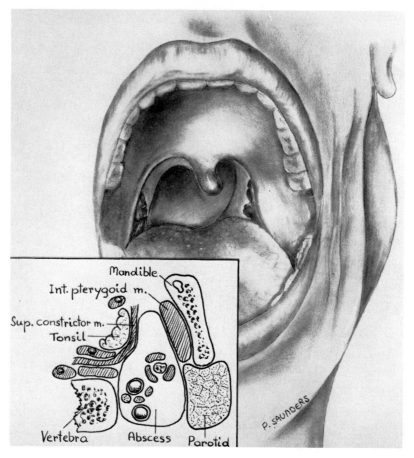

FIG. 3-13. Pharyngomaxillary (parapharyngeal) space infection. Note the external swelling as well as swelling in the pharynx. This condition often produces severe trismus, so that the patient cannot open his mouth. (Mouth is open here for illustrative purposes.)

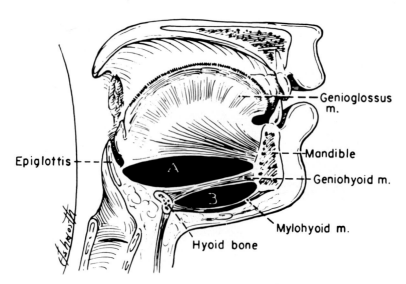

FIG. 3-14. Ludwig's angina. The black areas (*A* and *B*) indicate potential spaces in which infection may start. This condition is a phlegmon rather than an abscess.

Incision and drainage are important. If left alone, the abscess may rupture and asphyxiate the patient or infection may spread to another fascial space (chiefly the pharyngomaxillary space). The child is held with head extended over a table, and, usually without anesthesia, the fluctuant mass is incised. Suction apparatus is kept constantly in the mouth to aspirate pus as it wells out of the abscess.

Pharyngomaxillary space infection. The pharyngomaxillary (lateral or parapharyngeal) space is infected less often than the peritonsillar space but more often than the retropharyngeal space. Like all fascial spaces, the pharyngomaxillary space is a space only when it is filled with pus (or a tumor). In the normal patient fascial planes are always in contact; there are no empty spaces in the body.

Infection of the pharyngomaxillary space may develop directly by contamination with a needle (as in anesthesia for tonsillectomy) or by extension of an adjacent infection, such as a peritonsillar, retropharyngeal, dental, or parotid abscess.

The pharyngomaxillary space is deep and lies against the fascia of the parotid gland and internal pterygoid muscle laterally and against the fascia of the superior constrictor muscle medially. In it are the internal carotid artery; the jugular vein; the ninth, tenth, and twelfth cranial nerves; and the styloid process with its three muscles. The space connects with the retropharyngeal space and below continues downward along the great neck vessels into the superior mediastinum.

In advanced cases there is fullness or actual bulging of the normally concave angle behind the jaw and sometimes bulging inward of the entire lateral wall of the pharynx (Fig. 3-13). The swelling must be differentiated from a peritonsillar infection (in which there is usually tonsillitis and more superficial inflammation). Trismus is present because of irritation of the internal pterygoid muscle.

Incision and drainage are done through an incision under the jaw. The surgeon inserts a finger into the wound and pushes upward to the styloid process. If the infection has spread downward, the surgeon may follow along the carotid sheath with his finger to drain pus. Antibiotics are necessary. Blood transfusions are given if needed, and other systemic measures are taken to support the patient.

Masticator space infection. The masticator space is subperiosteal; it lies between the bone of the mandible and its periosteal covering. Infections of the masticator space usually arise from dental infections. A dental abscess may let pus into the subperiosteal space, so that swelling appears under and about the jaw. Because the masseter and internal pterygoid muscles attach to the mandible, there is usually trismus. The swelling in indurated and tender but not always fluctuant. Treatment is drainage through a wide, usually external incision. The infected tooth may be extracted then or at a later date.

Ludwig's angina. Ludwig's angina is a virulent infection in the tissue spaces of the floor of the mouth. It is usually a phlegmon, not an abscess. The tongue is pushed upward, and the submaxillary area is swollen, feels woody, and is very tender. The infection usually begins about a tooth root; and because the tips of the roots may extend below the mylohyoid line, the infection may start either above or below the geniohyoid muscle (Fig. 3-14). Later it involves all the tissues under the mandible and usually one or both submaxillary spaces. The boardlike swelling may extend downward to the clavicle. The condition is treated with systemic antibiotics and usually with drainage through a wide external incision. Tracheotomy should not be delayed if the patient's airway seems in danger.

TUMORS OF THE PHARYNX

Diagnosis of tumors of the pharynx usually is not difficult; when the patient is first seen, the lesion often is ulcerated and rather obvious. Also, cervical adenopathy caused by a metastatic lesion is common. Sometimes, however, there is no ulceration, and the tumor is much better appreciated by palpation than by inspection. Therefore it is *extremely important to palpate* the tongue and pharynx when a lesion is suspected.

Another aid in the diagnosis of lesions of the oral cavity, pharynx, and larynx is the toluidine blue test. Staining living tissue with toluidine blue is a simple, painless test that is helpful in distinguishing between oral malignancy and other conditions that may look malignant—for example, benign tumors, traumatic ulcerations, lichen planus, and leukoplakia. Carcinoma in situ and invasive carcinoma stain bluish, whereas other conditions generally do not. The test helps identify sites for biopsy and also indicates preoperatively the line of excision. False positives do occur.

The procedure is as follows:

1. The mouth is washed with water (the patient should take several sips).
2. One percent acetic acid (a mucolytic agent) is applied with a cotton-tipped applicator.
3. Fibrin and necrotic debris are removed.
4. One percent toluidine blue is placed on suspicious areas or over the entire mucosa.
5. The mouth is rinsed with water.
6. Areas showing blue staining, characteristic of carcinoma in situ or invasive carcinoma, are sites for biopsy.

This technique has also been used in the larynx to demonstrate areas of malignancy that otherwise might be unsuspected.

Malignant tumors. The clinical courses of malignant conditions of the pharynx vary greatly according to the histologic type and the site of the primary tumor. Often by the time the patient first sees a doctor, the lesion is so advanced that it is difficult to tell exactly where it started. On the other hand, some primary lesions metastasize early but themselves remain small. Sometimes a primary lesion cannot be found until months or years after a radical neck dissection.

POSTERIOR PHARYNGEAL WALL. When malignancy occurs on the posterior pharyngeal wall, which is rare, treatment consists of irradiation therapy. The prognosis is poor.

SOFT PALATE, UVULA, AND TONSILLAR PIL-LARS. Most malignancies of the palate, uvula, or tonsillar pillars begin on the anterior tonsillar pillar or in the supratonsillar region. The lesions are almost exclusively squamous cell carcinomas (Fig. 3-15). They spread to adjacent tissues, such as the pterygoid fossa, and onto the mandible, hard palate, and buccal mucosa. Symptoms are local pain, sometimes trismus, and often weight loss because of pain on swallowing. Metastases are to the upper cervical nodes. Treatment consists of surgical excision or irradiation. To be effective, surgical excision must be wide. Often it includes removal of part of the mandible and palate. A radical neck dissection is commonly done. Carcinoma of the anterior pillar has a particularly poor prognosis.

TONSILS. Malignancy of the tonsil is the second most common upper respiratory malignancy. Malignancy of the larynx is first. There are three types of tonsillar malignancies, and each differs clinically as well as microscopically. *Carcinomas* are usually poorly differentiated lesions and are most common in men. They spread anteriorly to the tonsillar pillar or upward into the soft palate. Early metastases are the rule. When first seen, most patients have a metastatic node in the upper neck. Local ulceration and otalgia are frequent symptoms. *Lymphoepitheliomas* often remain small, even in late stages, but neck metastases occur early and grow large. These tumors seldom ulcerate but remain submucosal. Digital palpation of the tonsil is helpful in locating the primary lesions. *Lymphosarcoma* of the tonsil produces a very large tonsil, but it usually does not ulcerate or cause pain. Neck metastases are found early;

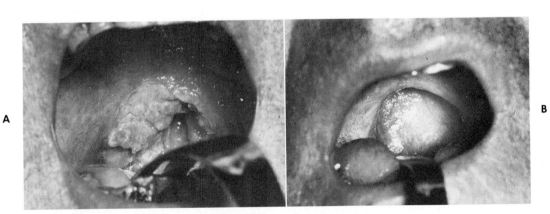

FIG. 3-15. A, Squamous cell carcinoma. **B,** After irradiation therapy and excision. The patient died of metastatic disease 1 year later.

soon other parts of the lymphatic system are involved.

Usually the treatment of all forms of tonsillar malignancy is irradiation therapy. The initial response is rapid; the tumors seem to melt away, but before long many recur locally or as distant metastases. Five-year survival rates vary between 15% and 40%, with the best figure given for lymphosarcoma.

BASE OF THE TONGUE. Malignancies of the base of the tongue are also carcinomas, lympho-epitheliomas, or lymphosarcomas. The same generalizations apply as in tonsillar lesions. The symptoms differ because involvement of the tongue musculature causes interference with speech. Patients often develop the so-called hot potato voice. Treatment is always difficult but not impossible. A typical patient with extensive involvement of the base of the tongue might require radical neck dissection and total glossectomy. Irradiation therapy, although palliative, is not likely to cure patients with carcinoma of the base of the tongue. Lymphosarcoma and lymphoepithelioma are best treated by irradiation.

Cryotherapy for head and neck cancer. Cryotherapy, although not a new method of treatment (it was used in England as early as 1851), is gaining in popularity for the treatment of rare advanced malignant lesions that cannot

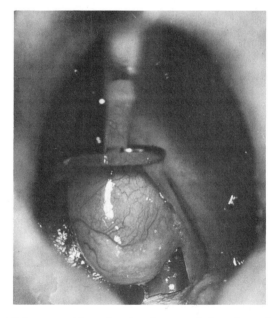

FIG. 3-16. Choanal polyp hanging below the soft palate.

be treated effectively by surgical excision or irradiation therapy. It has the advantages of little or no morbidity and minimal bleeding; treatment is possible even after extensive surgery and radiotherapy. Cryosurgery produces virtually total cell destruction that can be limited almost precisely to the diseased tissue. Because of the simultaneous destruction of sensory nerve endings, the method is relatively painless and the subsequent area of necrosis also is free of pain.

Benign tumors. *Simple inclusion cysts* (Chapter 32) are common in the vallecula, on the tonsillar pillars, or in the tonsils. They are usually asymptomatic. A mixed salivary gland tumor is occasionally found in the tongue or the palate. Benign squamous papillomas are common. Such a lesion is most often seen attached to the uvula, the tonsillar pillar, or the free margin of the soft palate (Fig. 2-12). Sometimes a choanal polyp, originating in the maxillary sinus or the posterior nasal cavity, is visible below the level of the soft palate (Fig. 3-16).

The majority of benign lesions are adequately treated by careful local excision. If they are small, they need not be removed.

SELECTED READINGS

Ash, J.E., and Raum, M.: An atlas of otolaryngic pathology, Rochester, Minn., 1956, American Academy of Ophthalmology and Otolaryngology.

Bachman, A.L.: Benign non-neoplastic conditions of the larynx and pharynx, Radiol. Clin. North Am. **16**(2):273-290, 1978.

Barrs, D.M., and others: Squamous cell carcinoma of the tonsil and tongue-base region, Arch. Otolaryngol. **105**(8):479-485, 1979.

Baysen, M.E., and others: Internal cysts and fistulae of branchial origin, J. Laryngol. Otol. **93**(5):533-539, 1979.

Becker, W., and others: Atlas of otorhinolaryngology and bronchoesophagology, Philadelphia, 1969, W.B. Saunders Co.

Bisno, A.L.: The diagnosis of streptococcal pharyngitis, Ann. Intern. Med. **90**(3):426-428, 1979.

Borowiecki, B., and others: Fiberoptic study of pharyngeal airway during sleep in patients with hypersomnia obstructive sleep-apnea syndrome, Laryngoscope **88**:1310-1313, August, 1978.

Bradenburg, J.H.: Neurogenic tumors of the parapharyngeal space, Laryngoscope **82**:1292, 1972.

Carpenter, R.J., and others: Cancer of the hypopharynx: analysis of treatment and results in 162 patients, Arch. Otolaryngol. **102**:716-721, December, 1976.

Chandler, J.R.: Anatomical variations of stylohyoid complex and their clinical significance, Laryngoscope **87**:1692-1701, October, 1977.

Clark, R.W.: Obstructive sleep apnea, Cleve. Clin. Q. **47**(1):3-7, 1980.

Davidson, F.W.: The antibody deficiency syndrome, Arch. Otolaryngol. **86:**685, 1967.

Drachman, D.B.: Medical progress: myasthenia gravis, N. Engl. J. Med. **298:**136-186, 1978.

Glass, R., and others: Inaccuracy of house staff in reading throat cultures, J.A.M.A. **240**(24):2651-2652, 1978.

Levitt, G.W.: Cervical fascia and deep neck infections, Laryngoscope **80:**409, 1970.

McCook, T.A., and others: Retropharyngeal masses in infants and young children, Am. J. Dis. Child. **133**(1):41-43, 1979.

Motta, J., and others: Tracheostomy and hemodynamic changes in sleep-induced apnea, Ann. Intern. Med. **89:**454-458, October, 1978.

Neely, J.G., and others: The otolaryngologic aspects of cystic fibrosis, Trans. Am. Acad. Ophthalmol. Otolaryngol. **76:**313, 1972.

Ogura, J.H., Biller, H.F., and Wette, R.: Elective neck dissection for pharyngeal and laryngeal cancers, Ann. Otol. Rhinol. Laryngol. **80:**646, 1971.

Rankow, R.M., and Abraham, D.M.: Actinomycosis: masquerader in the head and neck, Ann. Otol. Rhinol. Laryngol. **87:**230-237, March-April, 1978.

Saunders, W.H., and Gardier, R.W.: Pharmacotherapy in otolaryngology, St. Louis, 1976, The C.V. Mosby Co.

Schultz, A.R., and others: Dysphagia associated with cricopharyngeal dysfunction, Arch. Phys. Med. Rehabil. **60**(8):381-386, 1979.

Sprinkle, P.M., Veltri, R.W., and Kantor, L.M.: Abscesses of the head and neck, Laryngoscope **84:**1142, 1974.

Stefani, S., and Eells, R.W.: Carcinoma of the hypopharynx—a study of distant metastases, treatment failures, and multiple primary cancers in 215 male patients, Laryngoscope **81:**1491, 1971.

Tobin, H.A.: Radiation-induced pharyngeal stenosis: a report of two cases after planned postoperative radiation therapy, Arch. Otolaryngol. **105**(6):362-363, 1979.

Traff, B., and Tos, M.: Nasotracheal intubation in acute epiglottitis, Acta Otolaryngol. **68:**363, 1969.

4 THE TONSILS AND ADENOIDS

When it was recognized in the middle 1920s that local infection could affect distant organs of the body, attention began to be directed to the importance of infection of the lymphoid areas of the throat and nasopharynx. Soon undue emphasis was being placed on sequelae from infected tonsils and adenoids. During the early 1930s, removal of the tonsils and adenoids was the most common surgical procedure, comprising approximately 35% of all the operations being done. Tonsils and adenoids were often removed in children before they were 4 years old.

In spite of the increase in population and the improvement in surgical tools and techniques, fewer tonsillectomies and adenoidectomies are done today than were done during the 1930s. This is a healthy trend. It indicates that the medical profession has learned (1) that lymphoid structures of the throat play an important role in immunity, (2) that removal of the tonsils and adenoids does not significantly lower the incidence of upper respiratory disease, and (3) that indiscriminate removal of the tonsils and adenoids in the hope of some future benefit may actually be harmful to the patient.

The physician should recognize that the ring of lymphoid tissue surrounding the opening of the lower airway (Waldeyer's ring) is a protective barrier between the mouth and throat and the larynx, trachea, and lungs. Experimental work has shown that, in all probability, the lymphoid tissue of the throat plays an important role in the development of immune bodies. Development of immune bodies must, of course, be stimulated by bacterial infection. It is probable that each infection in the pharyngeal lymphoid tissue stimulates the further production of immune factors that will provide future protection. This reasoning is borne out by the

known fact that acute infections of the throat, and particularly of the tonsils, occur with decreasing frequency from infancy to adult life.

Absence or hypoplasia of tonsil and adenoid tissue in an infant or young child who suffers from frequent attacks of pharyngitis, bronchitis, sinusitis, and/or pneumonitis should be viewed with alarm and should raise a suspicion of possible hypogammaglobulinemia. However, in some antibody-deficiency syndromes (hypogammaglobulinemia, nodular lymphoid hyperplasia, and dysgammaglobulinemia) the tonsils may be enlarged. When medical examination indicates unusual frequency of infection, hypogammaglobulinemia, or dysgammaglobulinemia, it may be a mistake to remove the tonsils and adenoids. The same is true if relatives of the patient have evidence of immunoglobulin deficiency or if there has been a high incidence of collagen disease in the family.

Tonsils and rheumatic fever. A large amount of statistical and experimental work has been done in the past 30 years in an attempt to determine whether infection of the tonsils and adenoids alters the course of rheumatic fever. At one time it was thought that there is a direct relationship. It was believed that the streptococcus that causes rheumatic fever entered the body by way of the tonsils and that removal of the tonsils and adenoids would prevent the occurrence of rheumatic fever. This has been disproved.

It is reasonable to say that the incidence of the first attack of rheumatic fever is only slightly higher in children whose tonsils have not been removed than in those who have had a tonsillectomy and an adenoidectomy. Once a patient has had rheumatic fever, any intercurrent infection of the throat may lead to a second attack, an exacerbation, or carditis. If such a person is subject to recurrent tonsil infection, removal of the tonsils and adenoids will decrease the likelihood of future carditis. However, removal of the tonsils and adenoids does not prevent future rheumatic fever. The condition of each patient must be carefully evaluated before a decision is made to remove the tonsils and adenoids. No overall rules can be laid down.

Tonsils and poliomyelitis. During the early 1940s there was considerable concern regarding the possible relationship between poliomyelitis and tonsillectomy. After many statistical studies, no causal relationship was established. Since poliomyelitis has been practically eliminated by the use of vaccines, it is no longer a factor in the decision regarding tonsillectomy.

Waldeyer's ring. The lymphoid barrier surrounding the throat is called Waldeyer's ring. It is composed of four concentrations of lymphoid tissue that completely surround the entrance to the lower air and food passages.

The *adenoid* (pharyngeal tonsil) is a mass of lymphoid tissue in the nasopharynx. It extends from the roof of the nasopharynx almost to the free edge of the soft palate. Laterally it blends with lymphoid tissue in the fossa of Rosenmuller and with the lateral pharyngeal bands. The adenoid is present in all infants and children, starts to regress just before puberty, and is usually absent in the adult.

The *lateral pharyngeal bands* extend down the lateral wall of the pharynx from the adenoid, are located behind the posterior pillar of the caucial tonsil, and gradually thin out and disappear below the level of the faucial tonsil.

The *palatine (faucial) tonsil* is located laterally at the junction of the oropharynx and the oral cavity. It is partially hidden by the anterior pillar (palatoglossus muscle). The posterior pillar (palatopharyngeus muscle) lies between the faucial tonsil and the pharynx. The tonsil is composed of large lymphoid follicles and contains numerous crypts lined with squamous epithelium. It is surrounded by a distinct capsule and lies on the fascia of the superior constrictor muscle of the pharynx. Inferiorly a small triangle of tissue containing separate lymphoid follicles connects the tonsil to the base of the anterior pillar. This is known as the plica triangularis. The tonsillar and palatine arteries that supply the tonsil come from the external carotid system.

The *lingual tonsils* are two masses of lymphoid tissue. They are located on the dorsum of the tongue and extend from the circumvallate papillae of the tongue to the epiglottis. They usually are not seen during routine examination of the throat unless the tongue is protruded or a laryngeal mirror is used.

The *lymphatics* from Waldeyer's ring drain to the lymph nodes of the neck. The lymphatic drainage from the nasopharynx (adenoid) is to the posterior cervical lymph glands, whereas the drainage from the palatine tonsils and lingual tonsils is to the anterior cervical lymph glands. Malignant disease of the nasopharynx will often be discovered only after a metastatic lymph node is found in the *posterior triangle of the neck.*

Acute tonsillitis. Acute inflammation of the tonsils in children and in adults begins as a severe sore throat. It is accompanied by fever and often also by chills, headache, and muscular pain. The discomfort and malaise increase for 24 to 72 hours and then may slowly subside. The anterior cervical lymph glands usually become swollen and tender. Group A β-hemolytic streptococci are responsible for almost all tonsillitis and pharyngitis, particularly in children. Penicillin, therefore, is the treatment of choice. It may be given orally, in repeated intramuscular injections, or in one injection of benzathine penicillin G (Bicillin). Other antibiotics, such as erythromycin and tetracycline, also are effective.

At times tonsillitis is diffuse. Examination shows enlarged and brightly inflamed tonsils with diffuse inflammation of the pharynx. When streptococcal infection is the cause, the tonsils are usually studded with discrete yellow follicles, 10 to 20 on each tonsil (Fig. 3-6).

In the absence of complications, acute tonsillitis will in most instances subside in 7 to 10 days if the patient can go to bed, take adequate fluids, and irrigate the throat with hot saline solution several times a day. High fever and persistent unusual systemic malaise for more than 48 to 72 hours may be reason enough for administration of antibiotics in amounts appropriate for the age and weight of the patient.

When antibiotics are used, they should be continued 24 to 48 hours beyond the time of subsidence of symptoms. Too often an immediate beneficial response to the antibiotic causes the physician to discontinue its use after a day or two, a practice that leads to recurrence of the infection in a significant number of patients. Several recurrences may lead to chronicity of infection or to development of bacteria that are resistant to the antibiotic.

Recurrent acute tonsillitis may cause permanent changes in the tonsils but may leave no residual changes. Repeated attacks of tonsillitis do not indicate the need for removal of the tonsils unless signs of persistent infection remain.

Chronic tonsillitis is discussed on p. 53.

Adenoid infection. Acute infection of the adenoids rarely occurs alone. It almost always accompanies acute tonsillitis in children, and it would do so in adults if adenoid tissue were present.

In many children, repeated attacks of acute inflammation of the adenoids eventually lead to adenoid hypertrophy. When the adenoids remain, characteristic symptoms may develop. Nasal obstruction in varying degree is always present, leading to mouth breathing, poor rest at night, and a slight nasality of the voice. Chronic mouth breathing during the age when the facial bones are changing toward the adult configuration often produces a high arch in the hard palate, pinching in of the nose, shortening of the upper lip, and a staring expression in the eyes. The face becomes slightly elongated, and the upper teeth may be prominent. These changes constitute the *adenoid facies* (Fig. 4-1).

Prolonged hypertrophy of the adenoids may also produce changes in the eustachian tubes and in the ears. The most common change is partial blocking of the eustachian tube, with retraction of the eardrum and fluctuating hearing loss. In addition, fluid may form in the ears as a result of negative pressure. If chronic infection of the adenoids and hypertrophy are present, recurrent suppurative otitis media is often present, too. The combination of hypertrophy and chronic infection is the usual reason for recommending removal of the tonsils and adenoids. When adenoid hypertrophy is present *without signs of chronic infection of the tonsils*, removal of the adenoid tissue alone is indicated.

Tonsillectomy and adenoidectomy. Because of the importance of the adenoids, they are also considered in Chapter 5 (pp. 77 to 78).

INDICATIONS. The decision to remove the tonsils or adenoids, or both, should not be made

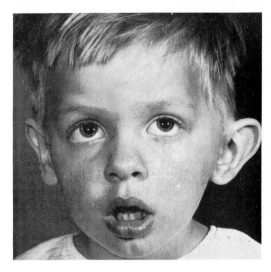

FIG. 4-1. Typical adenoid facies. Note the broad nose, staring eyes, and open mouth. This child also has a postauricular mastoid abscess on the left. Note how the ear protrudes.

without having first taken a careful history. It is necessary to question the patient or the parents regarding throat infections, ear infections, and hearing loss. It is also necessary to know whether the patient or members of his family have a tendency to bleed. When there is doubt regarding the nature of throat infections, it is wise to observe the patient during one or two episodes to be sure he has tonsillitis rather than diffuse pharyngitis.

Tonsillectomy and/or adenoidectomy is indicated if the history or personal past experiences with the patient disclose the following: (1) repeated attacks of tonsillitis; (2) peritonsillar abscess (quinsy); (3) hypertrophy of the tonsils and adenoids to the point of obstruction; (4) proof that the patient is a diphtheria carrier; (5) recurrent attacks of purulent otitis media; (6) fluctuating hearing loss due to serous otitis media associated with enlarged tonsils and adenoids (adenoidectomy alone may be indicated if the tonsils are not involved); (7) persistent enlargement of the cervical lymph glands (infections of the mouth and teeth, as well as lymphadenopathy from systemic causes, should be ruled out first); or (8) a definite relationship between attacks of tonsillitis and exacerbation of arthritis, iritis, rheumatic fever, or asthma.

CONTRAINDICATIONS. Since tonsillectomy and adenoidectomy are elective procedures,

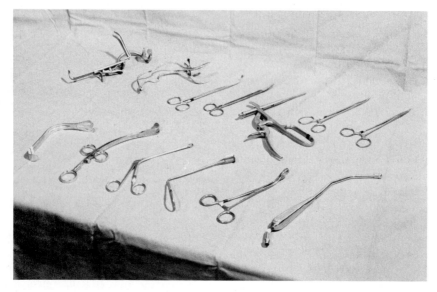

FIG. 4-2. Instruments for tonsillectomy and adenoidectomy. Note the self-retaining mouth gag and tongue depressor at the upper left and the standard mouth gag beside it.

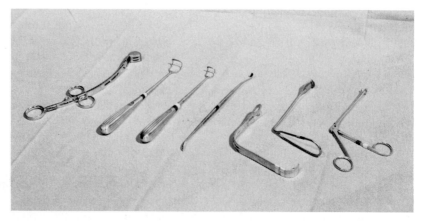

FIG. 4-3. Instruments for adenoidectomy. *Left to right*, Adenotome, two adenoid curettes, pillar retractor, tongue depressor, palate retractor, and adenoid punch forceps. An adequate suction tip is also necessary.

they should not be done when any acute infection is present. Neither tonsillectomy nor adenoidectomy should ever be done if the patient has leukemia, purpura, aplastic anemia, or hemophilia.

PREOPERATIVE PRECAUTIONS. The patient should be given an explanation of the reason for the operation, the hospital routine, and the expected postoperative course. If the patient is a child, he should always be told what is going to happen. This information is best given to the child by his parents. However, the physician must instruct the parents.

If there is no history of a bleeding tendency in the patient or his family, the results of routine tests for bleeding and clotting times are not reliable indications of possible postoperative bleeding. More reliable information is obtained from a careful history regarding bleeding tendencies.

The patient should not be taken to the hospital if an upper respiratory infection is present. If the patient has been hospitalized (usually a patient is hospitalized the evening before the operation) and there is any suggestion of a beginning upper respiratory tract infection, the operation should be postponed.

PREOPERATIVE MEDICATION. Tonsillectomy in an adult is most often done under local anesthetic. Therefore preoperative medication should consist of a barbiturate (Seconal or Nembutal, 3 gr.), a narcotic (morphine sulfate, ¼ or ⅙ gr., or meperidine [Demerol], 75 mg.), and atropine, ¹/₁₅₀ gr. When general anesthesia is used for tonsillectomy or adenoidectomy in an adult, the preoperative medication is the same as when any general anesthetic is given.

For children, anesthesia is preceded by atropine. The dose depends on the age and weight of the child. Children under 2 years of age should receive no medication preoperatively. It is desirable to have a child react quickly after the operation so that the cough and gag reflexes will prevent aspiration of secretions from the throat. Preoperative use of barbiturates delays recovery from anesthesia. Consequently, barbiturates are not recommended prior to tonsillectomy or adenoidectomy in children.

ANESTHESIA. Any accepted and safe general anesthetic may be used for tonsillectomy or adenoidectomy. Anesthesia administered by way of an oral intratracheal tube is almost universally recommended. Occasionally an intratracheal tube causes trauma to the vocal cords, particularly in children.

The depth of the anesthesia should be just enough to prevent activity of the muscles of the throat. If the level of anesthesia is too deep, aeration of the lungs is hindered and recovery following anesthesia will be delayed.

When local anesthesia is used, the anterior and posterior pillars and the peritonsillar tissues are injected with procaine hydrochloride (Novocain), 1%, or lidocaine (Xylocaine) hydrochloride, 1%; epinephrine 1:100,000 is usually given along with either drug.

OPERATIVE TECHNIQUE—TONSILLECTOMY. The most common method for removal of the tonsils is dissection and snare. This method can be used for all sizes of tonsils, whether they are in shallow or deep fossae. The steps of the procedure are as follows:

1. The tongue is depressed, and the tonsil is grasped with tonsil forceps.
2. A shallow incision is made through the mucous membrane around the tonsil and between the tonsil and the anterior and posterior pillars (Fig. 4-4, *A*).
3. The capsule of the tonsil, which is exposed by the incision of the mucous membrane, is grasped.
4. By means of blunt dissection with curved scissors, the capsule of the tonsil is separated from the fascia covering the superior constrictor muscle. The tonsil is freed from the anterior and posterior pillars by blunt dissection (Fig. 4-4, *B*).
5. A wire snare is passed over the tonsil forceps and over the tonsil and is then carefully tightened around the pedicle, which is still attached to the base of the fossa (Fig. 4-4, *C*). The snare is closed, and the tonsil is removed.
6. A gauze sponge is placed in the tonsil fossa and held with slight pressure for several minutes.
7. Bleeding points are located and are individually tied. The method of tying varies in different hands (Fig. 4-5). It is rarely necessary to use a "stick tie" with a needle.
8. When nonexplosive anesthesia is used, some surgeons control small bleeding vessels with electrocoagulation.

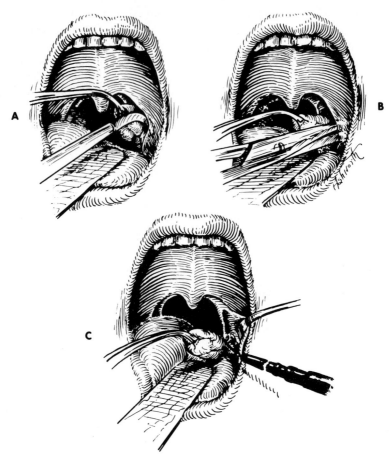

FIG. 4-4. Technique of tonsillectomy. **A,** Incision around the tonsil (shallow). **B,** Blunt dissection with curved scissors. **C,** Final removal with a wire snare. The same procedure is used whether local or general anesthesia is employed.

Some surgeons prefer to use the guillotine method of tonsillectomy (Fig. 4-6). The fenestrated end of the guillotine tonsillotome is placed over the tonsil. The tonsil is forced through the fenestra with the finger of the opposite hand, and the blade is slowly closed. Pressure around the base of the tonsil is maintained for several minutes before the blade is completely closed.

The guillotine method of tonsillectomy has disadvantages. It is not suitable for tonsils that are deeply recessed in the fossa or when there is heavy scar tissue in the peritonsillar space. Injury to the tonsillar pillars is more common with this method. The guillotine may not reach the base of the tonsil and thus will leave a tonsil tag, which must then be removed by dissection.

OPERATIVE TECHNIQUE—ADENOIDECTOMY.
Prior to removal of the adenoids, the nasophar-
ynx is examined by lifting the soft palate with a retractor. The nasopharynx can also be palpated with the finger. The steps in removal of the adenoids are as follows:

1. The main mass of adenoid tissue is usually removed with an adenotome. After the adenotome has been placed in the nasopharynx, the blade is opened, pressed backward, and then closed (Figs. 4-7 and 4-8, *A*).

   An adenoid curette can also be used to remove the main mass of adenoid tissue. The curette is place in the nasopharynx. While pressure is exerted on the posterior nasopharyngeal wall with the curette, a careful sweep is made from the vault downward (Fig. 4-8, *B*).

2. Residual adenoid tissue laterally can be removed with the adenoid curette.

3. The soft palate is elevated. All remaining

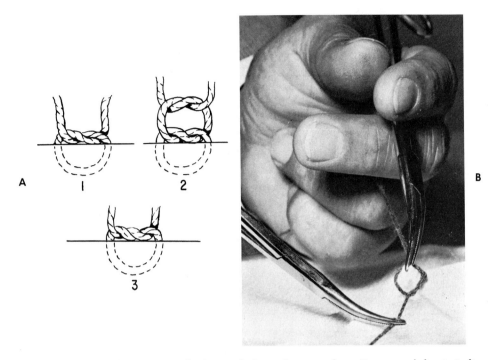

FIG. 4-5. A, Knots for tying vessels: *1,* Simple knot; *2,* square knot; *3,* surgeon's knot. A slip knot may also be used. **B,** Technique of tying with two sets of forceps deep in the throat. The lower forceps hold the suture while the knot is pulled tight with the fourth and fifth fingers. The upper forceps are on the bleeding point.

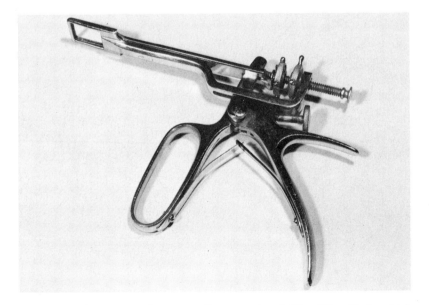

FIG. 4-6. Tonsil guillotine. Note the square, fenestrated end. The sliding blade, which severs the tonsil at the base, is closed by means of the worm-screw mechanism just above the handgrip.

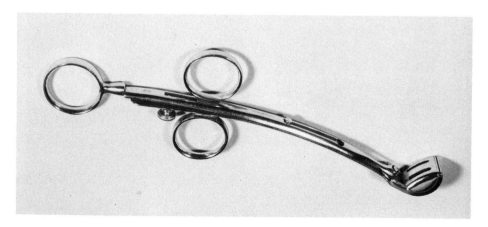

FIG. 4-7. LaForce adenotome. The curved basket end is pressed over the adenoid, and the sliding blade is closed by exerting pressure on the single ring.

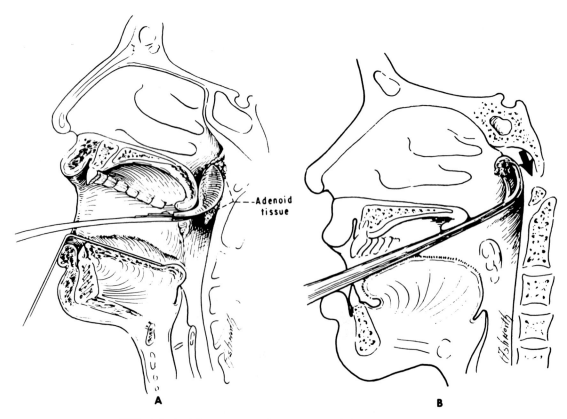

A   B

FIG. 4-8. A, Adenotome in place. **B,** Use of the adenoid curette.

adenoid remnants are inspected and carefully removed *under direct vision* with biting punch forceps. The punch forceps, with either a round or a flat cutting edge, is the only instrument that will allow adequate removal of the lymphoid tissue behind the eustachian tube and in the lateral gutter (Figs. 4-9 and 4-10).

This is the most important step in performing an *adequate* adenoidectomy. The older method of blind removal of rem-

nants with a curette rarely accomplishes complete adenoidectomy. Often it leaves tissue behind, contributing to rapid regrowth of adenoid tissue.

4. When the nasopharynx has been grossly cleaned of *visible* lymphoid tissue, a gauze sponge is placed in the nasopharynx and pressure is applied until bleeding stops. Sutures are unnecessary in the nasopharynx.

COMMENT. The tonsils can be removed first, and the adenoids are removed after the throat has dried. The order of removal can be reversed if desired. If the adenoids are removed first, a sponge is left in the nasopharynx while the tonsils are being removed.

Although removal of tonsils and adenoids is often called "minor surgery," the potential hazards are many. The operation should not be performed by an inexperienced person. *Bright light is essential during the procedure.* Considerable experience with the use of a head mirror or an electrically operated head light is necessary if adequate removal of tissue is to be accomplished. A common error is to attempt the operation with an overhead spotlight. This inevitably casts shadows from the lips and teeth and does not allow adequate vision. The use of an overhead light also increases the likelihood of leaving tonsil tags or pieces of adenoid tissue. Furthermore, with an overhead light there is a greater possibility that a shadow from the an-

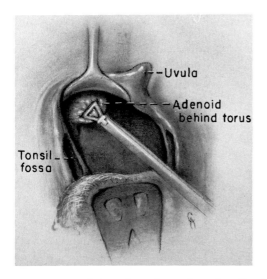

FIG. 4-9. Use of the adenoid punch under direct vision. Note the retractor holding the palate up.

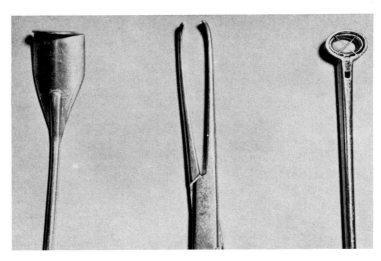

FIG. 4-10. Close-up of instruments. *Left to right*, Palate retractor, tonsil tag grasp, and adenoid punch.

terior pillar will obscure bleeding points behind it.

Another hazard is obstruction of the airway as a result of collection of secretions during the operation, including blood. Therefore, tonsillectomy and adenoidectomy should not be assigned to a student anesthetist until late in his or her training. The surgeon, as well as the anesthetist, must constantly be aware of the depth and character of respiration and of the color of the blood during operation. Carelessness on the part of either the surgeon or the anesthetist can lead to hypoxia, which may cause cardiac arrest, prolonged recovery, and excessive bleeding.

The operation can be performed with the patient supine or with his head extended over the operating table (Rose's position). In the former position the surgeon stands to the right or the left of the patient. In the latter position the surgeon is seated higher than the patient's head, and the anatomy he views is upside down. Advocates of the Rose position find it desirable because it allows the blood to collect in the nasopharynx rather than in the throat and because the mouth gag (Davis type) is fitted with a tongue depressor, thus freeing one of the assistant's hands.

POSTOPERATIVE CARE. Immediately following the operation done under general anesthesia, the patient is returned to bed and turned so that he lies with his face partially down and with a pillow under one shoulder. This position permits removal of any excess secretions from the mouth without aspiration. As soon as the patient is awake, he is permitted to take liquids, ice chips, or ice cream. Aspirin or narcotics can be used as needed. An ice collar may provide some relief from discomfort.

One of the changes in postoperative therapy in recent years is recognition of the fact that a young child who has had nothing to drink for 8 to 12 hours and who may have lost a considerable amount of blood during operation needs fluids. Inasmuch as an intravenous infusion has already been started by the anesthetist, it makes sense to continue giving fluids by this route until fluid loss has been replaced and the previous dehydration corrected. If the patient tolerates this reasonably well, even longer treatment by this route is advisable, since most children refuse to drink any substantial quantity of liquid on the day of surgery.

The throat remains sore for 5 or 6 days. During this time the diet is changed from soft to solid foods. In anticipation of the questions that are always asked by the patient or a relative, it is important to give patients a printed set of instructions for postoperative care. The following instructions are suggested.

INSTRUCTIONS FOR HOME CARE AFTER TONSILLECTOMY
First day (at home)

1. Eat liquid and very soft foods such as custards, gelatin, milk, broth, ice cream, or pureed vegetables (strained).
2. Drink enough water. (Lukewarm water is less irritating than cold water.)
3. Stay in bed part or all of the day, depending on how you feel.
4. Gargle the throat with warm salt water (1 level teaspoon of salt to 1 pint of water) every 2 hours during the day.
5. Chew Aspergum before meals for 15 minutes and between meals if needed for soreness. Some people prefer powdered aspirin. Two powdered tablets placed on the tongue and allowed to dissolve slowly will give relief.
6. Do not overexert yourself physically.
7. *Children need not gargle.*

Second day

Continue gargles, and aspirin or Aspergum. Add soft-boiled eggs to your diet (very soft cooked). You may also add soft milk toast if the crusts are removed from the toast and the toast is allowed to soak in warm milk until soft. Stay in bed or lie down part of the day.

Third day

Continue the use of aspirin as needed. Gargle if the throat feels stiff. You may add mashed potatoes, soft vegetables, and bread without the crusts to your diet. Get out of bed as desired.

Fourth, fifth, and sixth days

Continue the use of aspirin before meals. Gargle only as needed. Gradually add foods to your diet, including meat cooked well. Well-ground hamburger is well tolerated.

Seventh day

Come to the office for a checkup examination.

ADDITIONAL INFORMATION—
PLEASE READ CAREFULLY

1. The danger of serious bleeding is not over after you leave the hospital. In about 2% of people there is some bleeding after 5 or 6 days. If this happens, do not become excited, for this bleeding is usually slight. Be quiet, lie down, and spit the blood out gently. Gargle the throat gently with ice water and remain quiet. *If the bleeding does not stop promptly, call me.* If I am not available and bleeding continues, call another doctor promptly.

2. Avoid drinking orange juice, grapefruit juice, and tomato juice for several days after the operation, since they will make the throat burn. They are not harmful to you but will make you uncomfortable.

3. Two white patches will form where the tonsils were removed; do not be alarmed if you see them in the mirror. They are perfectly normal and are like a scab on the outside of the body. Most people have some pain in the ears for several days after the operation. This is usually controlled by the use of aspirin. It does not mean that there is an ear infection.

The throat is examined 1 week after the operation. Complete healing occurs in 14 to 21 days.

POSTOPERATIVE BLEEDING. Prevention of postoperative bleeding begins in the preoperative period. If the operation is not performed when the patient has an active upper respiratory infection, the possibility of postoperative bleeding will be decreased.

The most serious bleeding usually occurs a few hours after the operation. In most instances it is due to one of three errors:

1. The cleavage plane between the tonsil and the superior constrictor muscle has not been located, and dissection has been carried into or beyond the muscle.

2. Part of the tonsils or adenoids has not been removed. When tags of lymphoid tissue remain, the small blood vessels will not retract into the muscle bed and seal off, as they ordinarily do.

3. Inspection of the nasopharynx and the tonsil bed has been done carelessly, or the ties around vessels have been inadequately or improperly placed.

IMMEDIATE POSTOPERATIVE BLEEDING. When bleeding occurs in the immediate postoperative period, emergency measures may be necessary. As soon as excessive bleeding is recognized, the throat must be examined. If simple measures, such as pressure or local application of vasoconstrictors, do not stop the bleeding, it is necessary to anesthetize the patient again, inspect the pharynx carefully, and resuture the vessels as required. Medications for injection, such as carbazochrome (Adrenosem), oxalic and malonic acid mixture (Koagamin), or conjugated estrogenic substances (Premarin), are of no value. The bleeding that occurs at this stage is usually from a sizable vessel.

When the operation has been done under optimum conditions, when no remnants of tissue have been left, and when adequate hemostasis has been done, the incidence of bleeding in the immediate postoperative period should be less than 0.5%.

DELAYED BLEEDING. Bleeding can also occur after the immediate postoperative period. The usual time for occurrence of delayed bleeding is from the fifth to the tenth postoperative day. Bleeding at this time is caused by premature separation of the white "scab" that forms over the raw surfaces of the area from which the tonsils and adenoids have been removed. It may be precipitated by intercurrent infection, or it may occur when rough food is eaten too soon after the operation.

Delayed bleeding is rarely dangerous unless neglected, and then it may be fatal. Generally it comes only from capillaries, but sometimes a large vessel is involved—especially in cases in which a deep suture ligature was used to control bleeding during the tonsillectomy. Often a small clot will form slowly in a tonsil fossa at this stage. *Removal of the clot is essential* and may be all that is necessary to stop the bleeding. If bleeding continues, epinephrine, mild caustics, or pressure can be used locally. At this stage the medications for injection, which have already been mentioned, are of value, because their action affects the small capillaries and the clotting mechanism.

SELECTED READINGS

Bloor, M.J., and others: Geographical variation in the incidence of operations on the tonsils and adenoids, pt. I, J. Laryngol. Otol. **92**(9):791-801, 1978.

Bloor, M.J., and others: Geographical variation in the incidence of operations on the tonsils and adenoids, pt. II, J. Laryngol. Otol. **92**(10):883-895, 1978.

Carden, T.S., Jr.: Tonsillectomy—trials and tribulations: report on the NIT consensus conference on indications for T & A, J.A.M.A. **240**(18):1961-1962, 1978.

Cunning, D.S.: Poliomyelitis-tonsillectomy survey, 1948, Laryngoscope **59**:453, 1949.

Harlowe, H.D.: Complications following tonsillectomy, Laryngoscope **58**:863, 1948.

Hoppe, R.T., and others: Non-Hodgkin's lymphoma: involvement of Waldeyer's ring, Cancer **42**(3):1096, 1978.

Lawson, L.I., and others: Effects of adenoidectomy on the speech of children with potential velopharyngeal dysfunction, J. Speech Hear. Disord. **37**:390, 1972.

Mason, R.M.: Preventing speech disorders following adenoidectomy by preoperative examination, Clin. Pediatr. **12**:405, 1973.

Massumi, R.A., and others: Tonsillar hypertrophy, airway obstruction, alveolar hypoventilation and cor pulmonale in twin brothers, Dis. Chest **55**:110, 1969.

Pattern, B.M.: Human embryology, Philadelphia, 1946, The Blakiston Co.

Rynnel-Dagoo, B., Ahlbom, A., and Schiratzki, H.: Effects of adenoidectomy: a controlled 2-year follow-up, Ann. Otol. Rhinol. Laryngol. **87**:272-278, March-April, 1978.

5 DISEASES OF THE NASOPHARYNX

Acute nasopharyngitis. In the child naso-pharyngitis usually implies adenoiditis. In the adult, who may have no lymphoid tissue in the nasopharynx, the condition represents a mucous membrane infection. The cause may be either bacterial or viral. The common cold often begins as nasopharyngitis. The patient complains of a burning in the throat above the soft palate. Later, nasal symptoms appear. Nasopharyngitis may be an isolated infection limited to the epipharynx, or it may be part of a generalized pharyngitis due, for example, to streptococci. Another cause of nasopharyngitis, particularly in young adults, is infectious mononucleosis. As seen in the postnasal mirror, the mucosa is red, sometimes there are petechial hemorrhages, and often there is white exudate. The exudate and swelling may be so great as to obscure the usual landmarks.

In most patients with mild disease the condition clears up without treatment. In those who have fever and more severe local and general symptoms, systemic antibiotics are necessary for relief. Nasal irrigations are not advisable, because of the possibility of spreading the infection into the paranasal sinuses or middle ear.

Chronic nasopharyngitis. Much less common than acute nasopharyngitis, chronic nasopharyngitis is often associated with chronic rhinitis.

ATROPHIC RHINITIS. Atrophic rhinitis often extends posteriorly and involves the nasopharynx, so that there are green crusts and a dry mucous membrane that may bleed slightly when the crusts are removed. Treatment is discussed on p. 220. Sometimes the atrophic process extends downward and even reaches the larynx, but this is unusual.

PHARYNGITIS SICCA. Pharyngitis sicca is an ill-defined condition in which the nasophar-ynx, and usually the pharynx also, becomes very dry. The patient hawks out ropy secretions that are often brown. The mucosa may look glazed. The condition is not well treated, because it is not well understood. Symptomatic measures include use of nasal saline irrigations, instillation of oily nose drops (mineral oil), use of Mandl's paint, and other measures. In some patients thyroid extract or other hormonal therapy may help.

Adenoids. Although discussed in Chapter 4, the problem of the adenoids (pharyngeal tonsil) is so important to otolaryngology and pediatrics that additional comments are added here. The chief symptoms caused by the adenoids in young children are nasal obstruction and obstruction of the eustachian tube. A conductive type of hearing loss or purulent otitis media often occurs. The hearing loss is usually not the result of pus in the middle ear but of serum—serous otitis media. This condition causes an intermittent hearing loss of mild degree that often frustrates the parents and the teacher or school nurse. When the hearing loss is present, the child does not have an appointment with the doctor, and by the time he sees the doctor the adenoids have regressed and the serous otitis has resolved itself. *But the story of recurrent hearing loss in a young child with large adenoids is so characteristic that the doctor should suspect the cause.* Adenoidectomy may be necessary; it should be done if the condition has been persistent or recurrent in spite of proper medical management.

After adenoidectomy there can be recurrence of lymphoid tissue. This is especially true in children who come from families with allergic conditions. Probably the adenoids are *never* removed completely; unlike the palatine tonsil, the adenoids are not surrounded by the distinct capsule and thus cannot be dissected as completely. Remaining bits of adenoid tissue then hypertrophy or proliferate in some patients. It must also be recognized that removal of the adenoids is not done with equal care by every surgeon. What sometimes is described as a recurrence may be adenoid tissue that was never removed.

The parents should be instructed preoperatively that after adenoidectomy a change in voice may result. With the large adenoids gone, the palate cannot quite approximate the posterior pharyngeal wall, and therefore the patient "talks through his nose" for several weeks. The more the patient had needed adenoidectomy, the more nasal the voice may be.

Mouth breathing may persist after adenoidectomy even though the enlarged adenoids were the original cause. Apparently the child finds it difficult to close the mouth and breathe through the nose. It is well to advise parents preoperatively about this also.

Nasopharyngeal bursa. Rarely, a bursa is present in the posterior wall of the nasopharynx. This condition is also called Thornwaldt's disease. Some authors say that the bursa is common in children but that it later disappears. Others relate the bursa to remnants of Rathke's pouch. Whatever the origin, the symptoms are periodic crusting of the nasopharynx and a bad taste in the mouth. The cyst lining secretes a gummy material that collects in the bursa and then extrudes and forms a crust. When the crust is removed, a small probe can be passed into the opening. Treatment is excision of the cyst or its destruction by electrocoagulation.

Diseases of the turbinates. Normally the posterior tips of the inferior, middle, and superior turbinates are visible in the nasopharyngeal mirror (Fig. 5-1). The turbinates, especially the inferior turbinates, are erectile structures. They swell and diminish periodically, and the posterior ends of the inferior turbinates, particularly, look different from time to time. This normal variation in size is accentuated in certain abnormal conditions. Patients with allergic rhinitis, vasomotor rhinitis, certain forms of chronic rhinitis, or, of course, acute infections often complain of nasal obstruction, because the turbinates become so swollen. Obstructive swelling is usually limited to the inferior turbinates. In al-

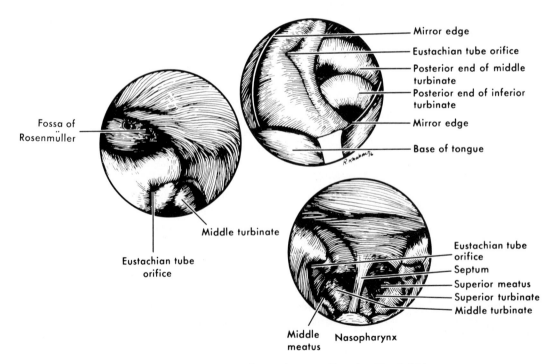

FIG. 5-1. Mirror view of nasopharynx. (See also Fig. 1-20.)

lergic rhinitis and in acute infections, usually the entire length of the inferior turbinate is swollen, but in other conditions (chronic rhinitis) only the posterior end may be enlarged.

The posterior ends of the inferior turbinates sometimes look bluish and irregular or pitted and have been likened to mulberries. At other times the inferior turbinates are pale and swollen. The term "hyperplastic rhinitis" is used in both instances.

In the treatment of nasal obstruction, when it is due to chronic enlargement of the turbinal structures, one must first discover and then treat the underlying condition—such as allergic rhinitis. Of course, not all inferior turbinates, just because they are enlarged or because their color is altered, require treatment. Some physicians pass a wire snare around the enlarged posterior tips of the swollen inferior turbinates and cut them off. Others use two-pronged (bipolar) electric needle to produce a submucosal fibrous reaction that will reduce the turbinate.

Another excellent treatment consists of submucous resection of the inferior turbinates. An incision is made along the length of the turbinate, and then a portion of the turbinate bone is removed. This procedure permits the turbinate to drop laterally against the sidewall of the nose, and the resultant scarring further retracts the turbinate tissue. If this operation is done, packing must be left in place 2 or 3 days; otherwise there is apt to be postoperative hemorrhage.

Finally, one may simply crush the inferior turbinate laterally against the sidewall of the nose.

Choanal polyp. A choanal polyp is a large nasal polyp that comes from the maxillary sinus. It often obstructs one or even both choanae completely (Fig. 5-2). Rarely, these polyps hang down to the level of the soft palate (Fig. 3-16). They look gray and shiny (like most nasal polyps), although some, because of infection and local irritation, may be red and meaty. Treatment is avulsion of the polyp, usually by means of an intranasal approach.

Choanal atresia. Choanal atresia is discussed on p. 221.

Juvenile nasopharyngeal fibroma. Juvenile nasopharyngeal fibroma, an uncommon neoplasm, arises from the periosteum of the occipital, sphenoid, or ethmoid bones (Fig. 5-3). It occurs almost exclusively in boys 8 to 15 years old and shows a tendency toward spontaneous regression after adolescence. The cause is unknown.

A nasopharyngeal fibroma, also known as an angiofibroma, consists of many thin-walled blood vessels coursing through masses of fibrous tissue (Fig. 5-4). The bleeding tendency of the tumor can be readily appreciated when a specimen is examined microscopically.

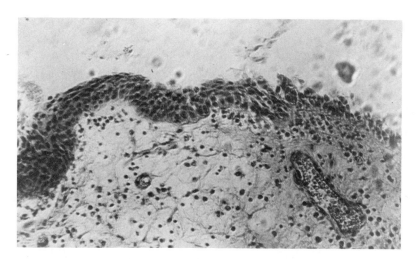

FIG. 5-2. Metaplasia of respiratory epithelium to squamous type, sometimes seen in polyps exposed to trauma.

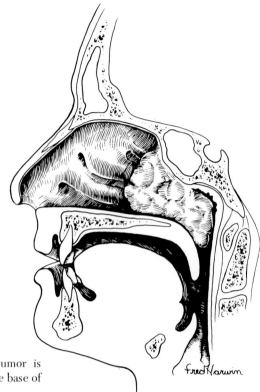

FIG. 5-3. Nasopharyngeal fibroma. The tumor is attached to the periosteum of the bones at the base of the skull.

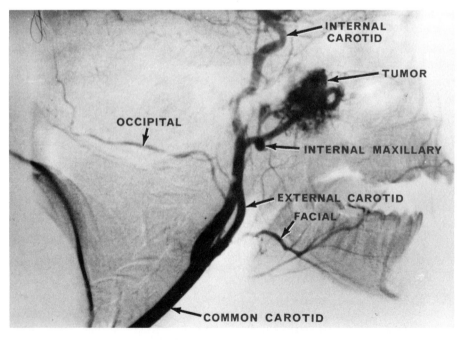

FIG. 5-4. Carotid angiogram (subtraction technique) of a patient with nasopharyngeal angiofibroma. Note the marked tumor staining, indicating extreme vascularity of the lesion.

The two principal symptoms are bleeding and nasal obstruction. Obstruction of the eustachian tube, causing serous otitis media, may produce hearing loss. Epistaxis is often profuse. Attempts to control it by packing the nose often make the bleeding worse. Patients do not die of epistaxis, but the repeated hemorrhages may cause serious anemia. Nasal obstruction may be unilateral or bilateral. The tumor usually extends anteriorly into one nasal cavity like a projecting finger, but most of the growth rests in the nasopharynx.

Severe nosebleeds in a boy with nasal obstruction should make one strongly suspect nasopharyngeal fibroma. The diagnosis is best made using a nasopharyngeal mirror. The tumor appears as a large mass completely obstructing one or both choanae. Usually at least one tubal orifice is not seen. The tumor mass may also be visible if one uses a nasal speculum. The tumor feels hard. If the diagnosis is suspected, it is best not to probe the growth very much, lest severe bleeding occur.

A carotid angiogram is an important step in the diagnosis. This examination shows well the exact size of the tumor, whether it is confined to the nasopharynx, whether it extends around the posterior aspect of the maxilla into the pterygomaxillary fossa, and whether there is intracranial extension. The CAT scan is also excellent for diagnosis and localization. Depending largely on the angiogram, the surgeon decides on the type of surgical exposure necessary and whether an operation is even feasible (Fig. 5-4).

Tissue for a biopsy may be taken either directly through the nose or through the mouth by reaching above the palate. Many authorities regard the tumor as so characteristic and so unlike any other condition that a biopsy is not done, thus avoiding bleeding, which can be severe.

Many surgical approaches have been described for removal of a nasopharyngeal fibroma. Perhaps the best, because it gives good visualization and is simple, is a transpalatal approach. The mucous membrane covering the hard palate is reflected posteriorly as far as possible. Then rongeurs are used to remove part of the bone of the hard palate so as to create a window through which the tumor can be inspected directly. Even when such a tumor is large and extends into the paranasal sinuses, often only the base is attached. Therefore, for the most part, when the base of the tumor is detached, removal of additional tumor that may have invaded adjacent cavities does not cause more bleeding.

At times it is necessary to approach large tumors by using a lateral rhinotomy incision or a combination of the Caldwell-Luc (see Fig. 16-11) and transpalatal incisions, to allow more adequate visualization. The incision is similar to that used for external ethmoidectomy, but it is not carried into the eyebrow or under the ala nasi, as in the Weber-Ferguson incision (Figs. 16-13 and 17-14).

Some authorities recommend preliminary treatment with a combination of sex hormones, which is said to reduce the vascularity of the tumor.

Hemorrhage is invariably excessive during avulsion of the tumor. Thus it is extremely important that the patient have an intratracheal tube in place and that two blood transfusions be started prior to the operation. A 10-year-old child may lose 4 to 8 pints of blood during the 10 or 15 minutes required to remove the growth. Use of the cryoprobe to freeze the tumor and reduce blood loss has been reported, but generally this method is not used. Once the tumor has been completely removed and the nasopharynx has been packed, hemorrhage usually is readily controlled. For that reason the tumor should be removed in toto whenever possible, and not piecemeal.

Embolization of the chief artery or arteries feeding the vascular mass, usually the internal maxillary artery, is a new technique designed to reduce bleeding during surgery. The procedure is done by a radiologist, who feeds tiny pieces of Gelfoam into the artery to produce thrombosis.

Irradiation therapy also produces resolution of the tumor. It may be that this method of treatment will become more prominent in the future. A tumor dosage of about 3,000 rads seems sufficient to cause symptomatic relief and to arrest the growth of the tumor after a few months to 2 years.

Nasopharyngeal malignancy. Malignancies in the nasopharynx are usually undifferentiated carcinomas or lymphoepitheliomas. They are uncommon tumors. *Local symptoms* occur

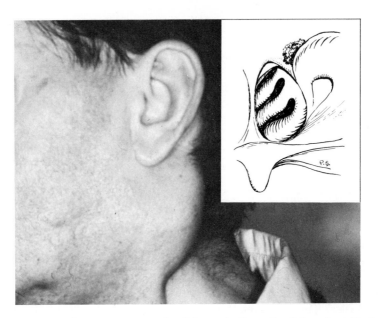

FIG. 5-5. Metastasis to the posterior triangle of the neck. *Inset,* Small lymphoepithelioma (the primary lesion). Both the primary and the metastatic lesions disappeared rapidly with irradiation therapy but recurred after 1 year.

when the tumor grows large enough to obstruct the choana; then the patient complains of nasal obstruction. If the tumor should compress or obstruct the eustachian tube, aural symptoms develop. The patient feels as if he has a "blocked" ear; there is loss of hearing and sometimes tinnitus. Fluid may form in the middle ear; any adult patient with persistent serous otitis media that is otherwise unexplained should be reexamined frequently to exclude the possibility of nasopharyngeal malignancy. The tumor may also bleed. Ordinarily pain is not a prominent symptom until the tumor ulcerates or invades bone at the base of the skull.

Remote symptoms include metastatic lesions in the neck and in the lung or other distant organs, and cranial nerve paralysis. Often the first symptom of nasopharyngeal malignancy is a lump in the neck. The lump, a metastasis from the primary nasopharyngeal tumor, appears most often in the posterior cervical triangle. Sometimes the metastatic lesion grows to be as large as a plum, whereas the nasopharyngeal lesion remains very small. In fact, the primary tumor may be invisible. Metastatic lesions in the lung or other distant organs are not unusual.

Intracranial extension of tumors of the nasopharynx occurs when a neoplasm grows upward through the foramen lacerum. There may be cranial nerve palsies; the abducent nerve, the longest of the cranial nerves, is the one that is most often paralyzed. Also, the oculomotor and the ophthalmic nerves are commonly involved. The patient's first complaint may be double vision or pain about the eye.

Often the first sign is a nontender, movable mass deep in the posterior triangle of the neck (Fig. 5-5). Usually the patient says it has grown rapidly. Mirror examination of the nasopharynx may show a large fungating tumor or only a very small lesion; sometimes no lesion is seen, and then months later the primary tumor grows larger and is discovered. Often part of the nasopharynx can be seen through the nose, especially after vasoconstrictors have been used. The nasopharyngoscope (Fig. 1-21, A) may be used to advantage in some instances, particularly to obtain a right-angle view of the eustachian tube. The diagnosis is made by biopsy. One should continue to take tissue for biopsy until a positive report is obtained or the suspicious lesion is gone. Sometimes, when a patient has a metastatic node in the neck, "blind" biopsies of the pharynx are made even though no obvious tumor can be seen or palpated.

Irradiation therapy is the only effective

treatment for malignancy of the nasopharynx. This treatment cures an occasional patient and palliates the disease in patients. Because the malignancies are usually lymphoepitheliomas and undifferentiated carcinomas, the initial response to irradiation is often good or even dramatic, but the recurrence rate is high. Metastases in the neck are also treated initially by irradiation, although surgery eventually may be required if there is not complete resolution of the neck mass.

Pituitary tumors. Pituitary tumors are mentioned here because occasionally a pituitary tumor grows large enough to appear in the nose or nasopharynx via the sphenoid sinus. The chromophobe adenoma grows particularly large. It invades the floor of the sella turcica and eventually fills the sphenoid sinus. Symptoms are described at length in ophthalmology and medical textbooks and will not be stressed here except to note that chromophobe tumors cause symptoms by replacing normal pituitary cells and by encroaching up on adjacent structures, whereas acidophilic and basophilic tumors produce symptoms by elaboration of their own particular hormones. Treatment is by surgical removal or irradiation. The least traumatic operation is done by the otolaryngologist through a transseptal approach. A submucous resection of the nasal septum is done. Then, working between the mucoperichondrial flaps, the otolaryngologist removes the rostrum of the sphenoid and enters the sphenoid sinus.

In another procedure, a Caldwell-Luc incision is made, and bone is removed from the anterior wall of the maxillary sinus. Then the floor of the sella turcica is removed and the tumor is removed. An equally good approach is through the maxillary sinus. This approach gives access to the sphenoid and the sella turcica and has the added advantage that the operating microscope can be used to provide brilliant illumination and magnification. The neurosurgeon may also approach pituitary tumors by means of a craniotomy.

Sphenoid sinus mucoceles (an uncommon entity) are often misdiagnosed as pituitary tumors. If the mucocele causes loss of vision, intracranial surgery may be performed rather than a more suitable intranasal or transsinal approach to the sphenoid.

Chordoma. Other tumors of the nasopharynx, all of them rare, include the chordoma, histologically a benign tumor but locally destructive. This tumor arises from remnants of the notochord and is found in the sacral area as well as at the base of the skull. The clinical signs of chordoma are similar to those in other slowly developing new growths in the area, such as meningioma and fibroma. Pronounced neurologic signs may be present, and an egg-sized mass may be present in the nasopharynx or posterolateral wall of the pharynx. Treatment is excision, since the tumor is not very responsive to irradiation therapy.

SELECTED READINGS

Batsakis, J.G.: Tumors of the head and neck: clinical and pathological considerations, Baltimore, 1974, The Williams & Wilkins Co.

Becker, W., and others: Atlas of otorhinolaryngology and bronchoesophagology, Philadelphia, 1969, W.B. Saunders Co.

Biller, H.F.: Juvenile nasopharyngeal angiofibroma, Ann. Otol. Rhinol. Laryngol. **87**(5, pt. 1):630-632, 1978.

Briant, T.D.R., Fitzpatrick, P.J., and Berman, J.: Nasopharyngeal angiofibroma: a 20-year study, Laryngoscope **88**:1247-1251, August, 1978.

Erich, J.B.: Juvenile fibromas of nasopharynx, Arch. Otolaryngol. **62**:277, 1955.

Fitzpatrick, P.H.: Nasopharyngeal angiofibroma, Can. J. Surg. **13**:288, 1970.

Fu, Y.S., and others: Nonepithelial tumors of the nasal cavity, paranasal sinuses and nasopharynx, Cancer **42**(5): 2399-2406, 1978.

Fu, Y.S., and others: Nonepithelial tumors of the nasal cavity, paranasal sinuses and nasopharynx, Cancer 43(2): 611-621, 1979.

Hall, B.D.: Choanal atresia and associated multiple anomalies, J. Pediatr. **95**(3):395-398, 1979.

McGrath, P.: Cysts of sellar and pharyngeal hypophyses, Pathology **3**:123, 1972.

Nugent, G.R., Sprinkle, P., and Bloor, B.M.: Sphenoid sinus mucoceles, J. Neurosurg. **32**:708, 1970.

Schnohr, P.: Survival rates of nasopharyngeal cancer in California: a review of 516 cases from 1942 through 1965, Cancer **25**:1099, 1970.

Some progress with nasopharyngeal carcinoma, editorial, Lancet **1**(8123):959-960, May 5, 1979.

Struton, S.D., and others: Carcinoma of the nasopharynx, Int. Abstr. Surg. **53**:1, 1970.

Tonkin, S.L., and others: The pharyngeal effect of partial nasal obstruction, Pediatrics **63**(2):261-271, 1979.

6 THE LARYNX—ANATOMY, PHYSIOLOGY, PARALYSIS

ANATOMY

The larynx is an arrangement of several cartilages held together by ligaments and muscles; it is connected above, through a wide opening, with the hypopharynx and below with the trachea. Outside the cartilaginous framework are the strap muscles of the neck. Behind the larynx are the fourth, fifth, and sixth cervical vertebrae. Anteriorly the thyroid cartilage protrudes as the Adam's apple. With the head extended, the cricoid cartilage, just below the thyroid cartilage, is readily seen in lean necks and can be palpated in any normal neck. Above the thyroid cartilage is the hyoid bone (not visible externally but readily palpable), which suspends the larynx and affords attachment to the tongue and other muscles.

Framework (Fig. 6-1). The *hyoid bone* (hyoid—U-shaped), although not a part of the larynx, is connected to it by the thyrohyoid membrane. Excision of the hyoid bone, even though it provides attachment to 20 muscles and ligaments, produces no great deformity or physiologic deficit. The superior laryngeal nerve and vessels perforate the thyrohyoid membrane.

"Thyroid" means shieldlike. The *thyroid cartilage* shields the intrinsic part of the larynx anteriorly and laterally. The vertebrae protect it from behind. The cartilage is incomplete posteriorly. At its top, in front, is the thyroid notch; and on either side, below the notch and flaring outward, are the two thyroid alae. Extending upward from each ala, posteriorly, is the superior cornu; and extending downward to meet the cricoid cartilage is the less prominent inferior cornu.

Behind the shielding framework of the thyroid cartilage are the internal parts of the larynx; the true vocal cords, the ventricles; the false vocal cords, their muscles and ligaments; and the arytenoid, cuneiform, and corniculate cartilages. The inferior constrictor muscle attaches to the external surface of the thyroid ala and sweeps backward to close the posterolateral part of the larynx.

The thyroid cartilage articulates only with the cricoid cartilage. For this purpose there are two articular facets, one on each inferior cornu. These facets meet with corresponding articular facets on the cricoid. The joint (enclosed in a synovial membrane) permits the cricoid to tilt slightly in relation to the thyroid.

The *cricoid cartilage* (cricoid—ring shaped), is the only complete ring of cartilage in the larynx. It has been likened to a signet ring, with the signet located posteriorly. It articulates with both the thyroid and *arytenoid* (jug-shaped) cartilages. The cricoarytenoid articulation is another synovial joint. The arytenoids swing in and out (medially and laterally) as though rotating about a fixed central point. This action opens and closes the glottis (space between the vocal cords), because the posterior end of the vocal cord is attached to the vocal process of the arytenoid and must move with it. The cricoid cartilage is attached to the thyroid cartilage by the cricothyroid membrane.

Besides the three major cartilages of the larynx (thyroid, cricoid, and arytenoids), there are two *corniculate cartilages*, one on top of each arytenoid cartilage, and two *cuneiform cartilages*, one in each aryepiglottic fold. Finally, the *epiglottis* is a cartilaginous structure

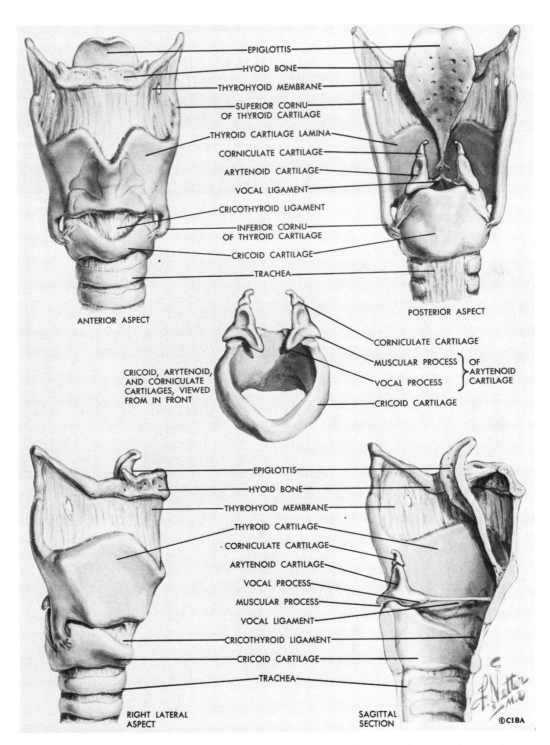

FIG. 6-1. Cartilages of the larynx. Note that only the cricoid is a complete ring. (Copyright 1964 CIBA Pharmaceutical Company, Division of CIBA-GEIGY Corporation. Reproduced, with permission, from the CLINICAL SYMPOSIA illustrated by Frank H. Netter, M.D. All rights reserved.)

attached to the thyroid and arytenoid cartilages and to the base of the tongue by ligaments and folds of mucous membrane.

• • •

In the operation called total laryngectomy, the hyoid bone is removed along with the larynx in order to remove the preepiglottic fat pad and its lymphatics. The superior laryngeal vessels may be isolated easily and ligated just external to the thyrohyoid membrane.

Anesthesia of the larynx is readily produced by holding a curved applicator in the throat so that it rests in the pyriform recess. Here, only mucosa separates the applicator with its local anesthetic from the superior laryngeal nerve.

Thyroglossal cysts may form just external to the thyrohyoid membrane, where they produce swelling in the anterior midline of the neck. The body of the hyoid is removed during the operation for excision of a thyroglossal duct cyst.

Although the larynx looks relatively unprotected, it rarely suffers severe injury. Sometimes, however, the thyroid or cricoid cartilage, or both, is fractured. Then mucosa and other soft tissues inside the larynx may be torn, or a hematoma may form. The airway is endangered, and a tracheotomy may be necessary.

Sometimes, because of infection or arthritis, the cricoarytenoid joint becomes immobilized and the patient is said to have *cricoarytenoid ankylosis.* The vocal cords cannot swing outward, because their posterior attachments are no longer free to rotate.

Because the airway is almost immediately subcutaneous at the cricothyroid membrane, and because this point is well under the level of the vocal cords, the cricothyroid membrane is a good place to make the incision for an emergency tracheotomy. On the other hand, a tracheotomy tube should not be left in the cricothyroid space too long, because it may irritate the undersurface of the cords and cause laryngeal stenosis.

Soft tissues. The *mucous membrane* lining the larynx is continuous with the mucosa and the pharynx above and with the trachea below. The epithelium is columnar in the ventricle, changes to stratified squamous along the vocal

cord, and becomes columnar again in the trachea.

The *laryngeal ligaments* (Fig. 6-1) *and mucosal folds* are important as supporting structures. For the clinician they provide ready anatomic landmarks. The epiglottis attaches to the tongue by the *median glossoepiglottic fold* and to the lateral walls of the pharynx by the two *pharyngoepiglottic folds.* Both of these folds are easily visible by mirror laryngoscopy. The two *aryepiglottic folds* join the epiglottis and the arytenoid cartilages. In these folds are a few muscle fibers and the cuneiform cartilages. The aryepiglottic folds, readily visible in the laryngeal mirror, are important as landmarks in physical examination.

Beneath the epiglottis the mucosa folds over the ventricular band (false cords), invaginates into the laryngeal ventricle, and comes out again to cover the true vocal cords before descending into the trachea.

The *true vocal cords* (Fig. 6-2) join anteriorly, where they attach to a fixed point, the inner surface of the thyroid cartilage; but posteriorly they attach to movable structures, the arytenoid cartilages. Thus the cords are held immobile anteriorly (the anterior commissure), but they can abduct and adduct posteriorly. By mirror laryngoscopy one gains a false impression of both the color and contour of the true cords. In the mirror the cords look very white and sharp edged, but when examined by other means (direct laryngoscopy or during laryngofissure), they are pink and their edges are rounded. Also, as seen in the mirror, the cords seem to have an outer (lateral) edge. Actually, they do not. The outer edge is merely a line made by the overlying false cord—the mucosa of the true cord joins that of the false cords after invaginating into the ventricle.

The *false cords* (ventricular bands) lie just above the true cords. They are attached anteriorly to the thyroid cartilage and posteriorly to the arytenoid (but not to the vocal process). They are folds of mucous membrane, covering fibrous tissue, glands, and a few muscle fibers.

The *laryngeal ventricle,* an invagination of mucosa between the true and false cords, extends upward a variable distance under cover of the thyroid cartilage. It is not visible by mirror laryngoscopy. Glands in the appendix of the ventricle (upward extension between the false

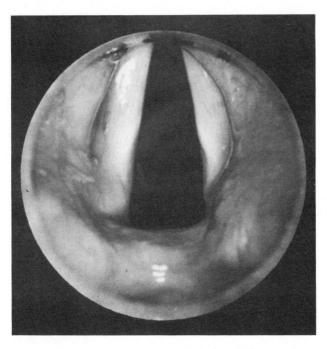

FIG. 6-2. Photograph of the larynx taken through the direct laryngoscope. Arytenoids are the mounds seen posteriorly. Anterior is above. (Courtesy Dr. Paul Holinger, Chicago, Ill.)

cord and the thyroid cartilage) secrete mucus that is said to lubricate the vocal cords.

The *glottis* is the narrowest part of the larynx. It is the space between the vocal cords anteriorly and between the arytenoid cartilages posteriorly. The glottis is somewhat larger in the male than in the female. In infants the glottic area is small. Therefore, mucosal edema (as in laryngitis) causes a much greater relative impairment of the airway in infants than in adults.

Muscles. There are intrinsic and extrinsic muscles of the larynx. The *extrinsic muscles* connect the various parts of the laryngeal framework to surrounding bones, particularly the hyoid and the sternum. The nerve supply to these muscles is chiefly through the ansa hypoglossi.

The *intrinsic muscles* (Fig. 6-3) include the cricothyroid, thyroarytenoid, cricoarytenoid, and arytenoideus. The *cricothyroid*, the only muscle supplied by the superior laryngeal nerve, joins the superior lateral surface of the cricoid cartilage and the posterior inferior surface of the thyroid cartilage. Contraction of the two cricothyroid muscles tilts the cricoid cartilage onto the thyroid cartilage. This action

stretches the vocal cords. Thus the cricothyroid muscles are known as the external tensors of the vocal cords. The *thyroarytenoid muscle* attaches anteriorly to the inside of the thyroid cartilage and posteriorly to the arytenoid base. Those fibers of the thyroarytenoid inserting into the vocal process are called the vocalis muscle. This muscle, if it acted alone, would tend to shorten the cord; but in practice it acts synergistically with the other laryngeal muscles and firms the cord. Therefore, it is called the internal tensor. The *posterior* and *lateral cricoarytenoid muscles* attach the cricoid cartilage to the arytenoid cartilage. The posterior arytenoid muscles act so as to separate the true cords (open the glottis). The lateral cricoarytenoid muscles close the glottis. The *arytenoideus* is the only unpaired laryngeal muscle. It connects the two arytenoid cartilages with each other. The muscle has transverse and oblique parts. In action, it closes the posterior part of the larynx by approximating the arytenoid cartilages. The oblique fibers continue into the aryepiglottic folds and are called the aryepiglottic muscle. Following is a list of the laryngeal muscles grouped according to their action:

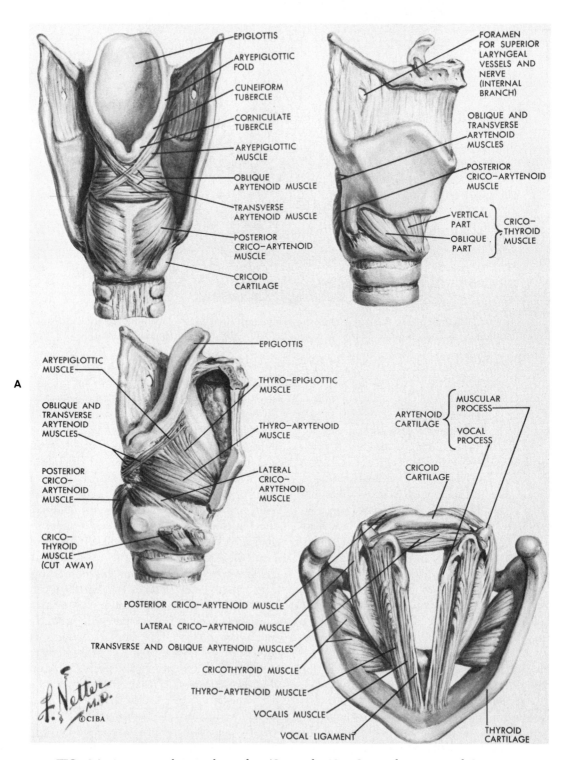

A

FIG. 6-3. **A,** Intrinsic laryngeal muscles. (Copyright 1964 CIBA Pharmaceutical Company, Division of CIBA-GEIGY Corporation. Reproduced, with permission, from the CLINICAL SYMPOSIA illustrated by Frank H. Netter, M.D. All rights reserved.)

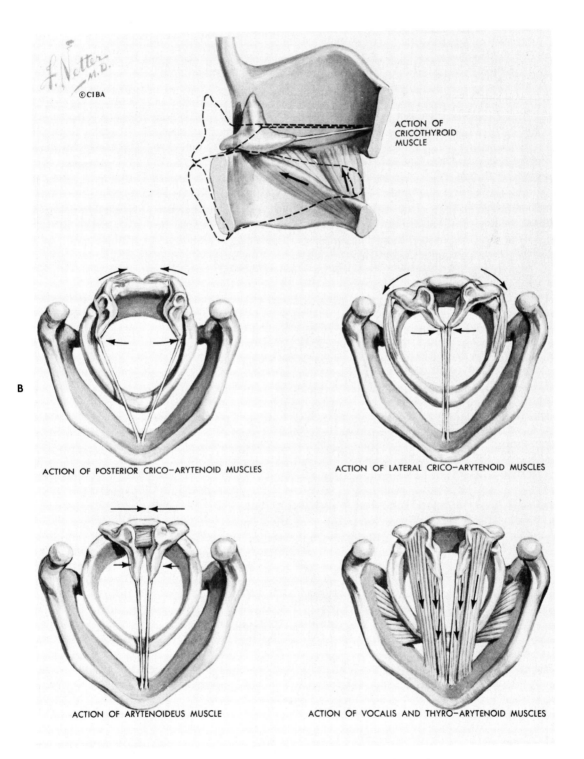

FIG. 6-3, cont'd. B, Action of intrinsic laryngeal muscles.

Constrictors
    Lateral cricoarytenoid (2)
    Thyroarytenoid (2)
    Arytenoid
        Transverse fibers
        Oblique fibers
        Aryepiglottic fibers
Dilators
    Posterior cricoarytenoid (2)
Tensors
    Cricothyroid (2)
    Thyroarytenoid (2)
        Vocalis fibers

Blood supply. The *superior and inferior thyroid arteries*, through their respective branches, the superior and inferior laryngeal arteries, provide most of the blood supply to the larynx.

Nerve supply. The entire laryngeal nerve supply (Fig. 6-4) is from the vagus. The *superior laryngeal nerve*, through its external branch,

supplies only one muscle, the cricothyroid. All the other muscles are supplied by the *recurrent laryngeal nerve*. The left recurrent nerve passes under the aorta, and the right passes under the subclavian artery. Both nerves ascend again in grooves between the trachea and the esophagus. Sometimes the recurrent nerve enters the larynx as a single trunk, or it may branch extralaryngeally into two or more divisions. The entire *sensory nerve supply* of the larynx is from the internal branch of the superior laryngeal nerve.

Lymphatic drainage. The larynx drains to lymph nodes in the middle and upper cervical chains along the internal jugular vein. The true vocal cord, where most intrainsic carcinomas develop, is said to have a sparse lymphatic supply. The arytenoid area and all parts of the extrinsic larynx have a richer lymphatic network.

As a result of either the sparse lymphatics of

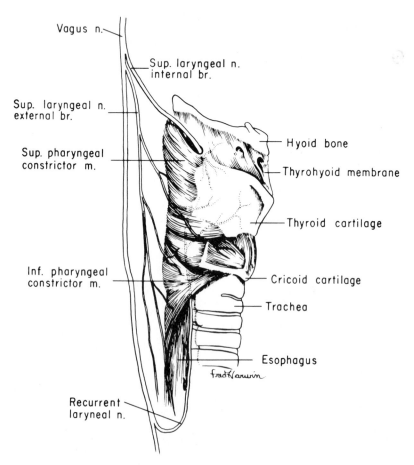

FIG. 6-4. Laryngeal nerve supply. The lowermost relationships of recurrent nerves vary on the left and right and are not drawn.

the true cord or other factors such as the type of tumor that originates there, metastases to the neck occur later in carcinoma of the true cord than in carcinoma of other parts of the larynx. In carcinoma of the pyriform recess, for example, often the first symptom is a lump in the neck.

PHYSIOLOGY

Of the several physiologic functions of the larynx, the most important is that of acting as an airway between the pharynx and the trachea. The larynx is not a simple tube like the trachea; rather it is an organ with a sphincteric action. During swallowing, for example, the aryepiglottic folds, the arytenoids, and the tubercle of the epiglottis fold inward so as to close the larynx tightly and keep food out of the trachea. Other spincteric actions (by different parts of the larynx) close the glottis when a foreign body drops into the throat and assist in coughing by helping to increase intrathoracic pressure. Also, laryngeal sphincteric action is useful in lifting and in other straining efforts, because when air is compressed within the chest, muscles of the thorax and the shoulders are given extra advantage.

The *cough reflex* is, of course, important as a protective mechanism. The laryngeal mucosa is extremely sensitive and sets off the reflex whenever a foreign body touches it. The cough reflex has been called "the watchdog of the lungs."

The *phonatory* function of the larynx is also important, but it is not the chief purpose of the larynx. During phonation, the edges of the vocal cords are firmed by a fine muscular coordination. The length of the cords can be varied at will. The tracheal air pressure increases and decreases as the edges of the vocal cords firm and relax. As the larynx moves up and down, the air columns above and below the larynx are lengthened and shortened. These, as well as other mechanisms, alter the air column and its vibrations. Finally, the tongue, the lips, and the palate (the "molds" of speech) form words from the vibrating column of air served up by the larynx.

PARALYSIS

The superior laryngeal branch of the vagus is the sensory nerve of the larynx. This nerve branches from the vagus not far outside the skull and penetrates the thyrohyoid membrane to supply mucous membranes of the larynx, the upper trachea, and the hypopharynx. It divides into two branches, *external* and *internal*. The external branch is a motor nerve and supplies one laryngeal muscle, the *cricothyroid*. The internal branch is *sensory only*.

The *entire motor supply*, except for the external branch of the superior laryngeal nerve, is provided by another branch of the vagus, the recurrent laryngeal nerve. On the left it passes under the arch of the aorta and then ascends in the groove between the esophagus and the trachea. As it approaches the larynx, it may divide into several branches or it may enter the larynx as a single trunk. On the right it passes under the subclavian artery.

Central paralysis. Laryngeal paralyses usually have peripheral causes, but it is also possible for central nervous system lesions to produce laryngeal paralysis. Each side of the larynx receives a motor supply from both sides of the cerebral cortex. However, the motor areas are so widely separated that it is very unusual to see a laryngeal paralysis caused by a cortical lesion. Such lesions would have to be massive (or exactly symmetrical) and ordinarily would be incompatible with life. On the other hand, smaller lesions at the decussation of fibers, just above the nucleus ambiguus, would be compatible with life and would cause bilateral laryngeal paralysis. A lesion in only one nucleus ambiguus would produce a unilateral paralysis.

Some textbooks describe both flaccid and spastic types of laryngeal paralysis, but it usually is not possible for the clinician to differentiate between the two. Theoretically, lesions peripheral to the nucleus ambiguus should cause a flaccid paralysis and central lesions a spastic paralysis. Multiple sclerosis, syringomyelia, brain tumor, and vascular thrombosis are some of the causes of central paralysis.

Peripheral paralysis. One need only consider the courses of the recurrent laryngeal nerves to remember the most common causes of laryngeal paralysis. On the left, as the nerve crosses under the arch of the aorta, it is subject to stretching as a result of *aneurysm* of the aorta. *Mitral stenosis*, causing enlargement of the left auricle, may also stretch the left recurrent laryngeal nerve. *Tumors* of the bronchi or lung may infiltrate or stretch the nerve. Other tumors of the mediastinum, either in the chest or in the lower part of the neck, may compress, stretch, or invade the nerve. *Tuberculous scarring* of the apex of the lung occasionally results in unilateral laryngeal paralysis.

In the neck, carcinoma of the thyroid gland may cause laryngeal paralysis. Even when there does not appear to be a tumor of the thyroid, malignant change may have taken place, making a radioactive scanning test worthwhile. If a patient has laryngeal paralysis and a goiter, malignancy of the thryoid gland should be suspected. Usually, benign thyroid enlargements do not cause laryngeal paralysis. Carcinoma of the larynx itself eventually produces fixation of one or both vocal cords, but the immobility may be the result of muscle invasion rather than nerve paralysis.

A neurofibroma of the vagus nerve, which presents as a cervical tumor, may cause laryngeal paralysis. Laryngeal paralysis also may be caused by various *neck injuries.* Recently cases have been reported in which laryngeal paralysis began after intratracheal intubation. The exact mechanism remains unexplained. Also, certain metallic poisons *(lead)* and infectious diseases *(diphtheria)* cause laryngeal paralysis by producing a neuritis.

One of the most common causes of laryngeal paralysis is *thyroidectomy.* The recurrent nerve or one of its extralaryngeal branches may be cut at the time of operation or injured later by becoming incorporated into scar tissue. Some patients with unilateral laryngeal paralysis have normal voices. To be certain of laryngeal function, mirror laryngoscopy should be done both before and after thyroidectomy. The final position of the paralyzed cord may depend on whether the entire recurrent laryngeal nerve is cut or only one or two of its branches are cut—in the case of a nerve that divides outside the larynx, as many do.

If, after thyroidectomy, there is evidence of a laryngeal paralysis (hoarseness and immobility of the vocal cord as seen by indirect laryngoscopy), immediate reexploration should be considered. A ligature used to tie a blood vessel may have included the nerve or a branch of it, or the recurrent nerve or a branch may have been severed during the procedure. By removal of the ligature, and replacment on the blood vessel only, or by careful end-to-end anastomo-

sis of a cut nerve, good function may be restored. Fortunately, *bilateral* abductor paralysis (Fig. 6-6) after thyroidectomy is rare (Fig. 6-6).

Approximately 10% of all laryngeal paralyses are unexplained. They are called idiopathic. Possibly some of them are caused by unrecognized viral infections. The vocal cord often does not remain paralyzed in patients with idiopathic paralysis. Of 29 patients observed for 3 years, only 5 had a persistent paralysis at the end of that period. Probably 80% of patients with an idiopathic paralysis of the larynx recover spontaneously. Apparently, recovery of function must begin before 6 months, or it does not take place at all.

• • •

Although a discussion of individual paralyses of the vocal cords is likely to be of interest only to the laryngologist, a few generalizations regarding laryngeal paralysis and its effect on the voice and airway are in order.

Motor paralysis. Either one or both vocal cords may be paralyzed. If one cord is paralyzed, the patient may have an entirely normal voice or a very hoarse one. The condition of the voice depends on the position and tenseness of the paralyzed cord. Sometimes the paralyzed cord is fixed in the midline and the opposite cord can approximate it, in which case a normal voice may result. On the other hand, if the cord is fixed in abduction, there is no way in which the normal cord can meet the paralyzed cord, so that the patient has a husky, air-spilling type of voice. With the paralyzed cord in the paramedian position (Fig. 6-5) and with overcompensation by the normal cord, a good or even normal voice is still possible.

Because the laryngeal airway is entirely adequate even though one cord is fixed in the midline and cannot abduct at all, there is never any dyspnea associated with unilateral cord paralysis. The good cord abducts enough for an airway.

Bilateral cord paralysis usually leaves the cords adducted; and the voice, though weak, is good. In bilateral cord paralysis it is the poor airway that incapacitates the patient. With the cords in the midline, the glottic chink is very small. The patient manages all right during bed rest or even when moving about slowly; but he is unable to walk upstairs without paus-

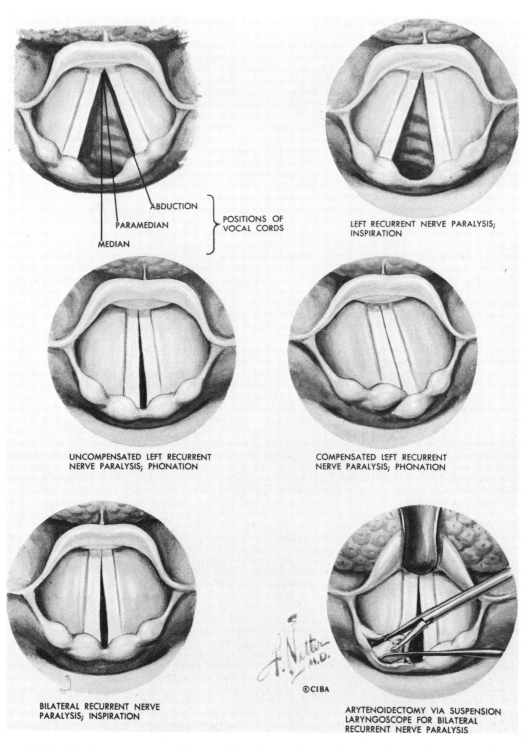

ABDUCTION

PARAMEDIAN } POSITIONS OF VOCAL CORDS

MEDIAN

LEFT RECURRENT NERVE PARALYSIS; INSPIRATION

UNCOMPENSATED LEFT RECURRENT NERVE PARALYSIS; PHONATION

COMPENSATED LEFT RECURRENT NERVE PARALYSIS; PHONATION

BILATERAL RECURRENT NERVE PARALYSIS; INSPIRATION

ARYTENOIDECTOMY VIA SUSPENSION LARYNGOSCOPE FOR BILATERAL RECURRENT NERVE PARALYSIS

©CIBA

FIG. 6-5. Various aspects of laryngeal paralyses. (Copyright 1964 CIBA Pharmaceutical Company, Division of CIBA-GEIGY Corporation. Reproduced, with permission, from the CLINICAL SYMPOSIA illustrated by Frank H. Netter, M.D. All rights reserved.)

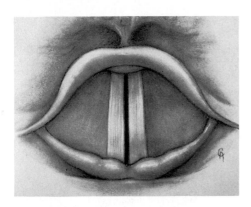

FIG. 6-6. Bilateral abductor paralysis. The voice is usually good because the cords can approximate. The airway is poor because the cords cannot abduct.

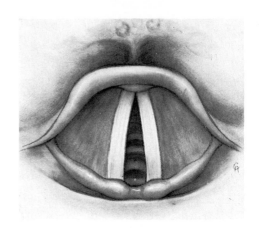

FIG. 6-7. Complete laryngeal paralysis, which is rare. Cords are halfway between abduction and adduction and do not move.

ing, and performing usual household activities is very tiring. Stridor due to exertion is common. Thus, bilateral cord paralysis affects both the voice and the airway, but it affects the airway more seriously.

Treatment for laryngeal paralysis, insofar as restoration of normal function is concerned, is useless. If only one cord is paralyzed, regardless of its position, the airway is always adequate and the patient has no symptoms other than hoarseness (and often he is not even hoarse). No treatment is needed for the airway; but if there is hoarseness, some patients are treated by injection of small amounts of Teflon substances into the shrunken musculature of the paralyzed cord. This injection is made with a special syringe that ejects measured amounts of Teflon with each "click." The procedure is carried out through a laryngoscope. The injection swells the cord and brings it nearer the midline so that the other cord can more easily approximate it. Although the result is not expected to be a perfect voice, this technique is of considerable value in patients with a breathy, air-spilling voice caused by paralysis or other conditions. However, in *bilateral abductor paralysis* (Fig. 6-6), because of the inadequate airway, an operation is indicated. Sometimes tracheotomy may be necessary as a lifesaving measure. A few patients then elect to continue with the tracheotomy rather than have a second, more definite procedure for restoring the airway. These patients, whose voice often has good quality although it may be rather weak, are afraid that a

laryngeal operation to restore the airway may sacrifice vocal quality. Sometimes it does so.

Numerous procedures to open the glottis have been devised. One of the more popular is called *arytenoidectomy.* Often the operation is done transorally through the suspension laryngoscope. After removal of one arytenoid cartilage the airway is usually sufficient to permit moderate activity. The King procedure is another operation used to improve the airway in patients with bilateral abductor paralysis. An external incision is made along the lateral area of the neck. The arytenoid cartilage is identified, and a suture is passed around the cartilage and then through the adjacent cricoid cartilage. By this means the arytenoid is rotated and fixed laterally, improving the airway. Ordinarily the operation is done only on one side, in order to conserve the voice.

Another method of relieving the problems caused by bilateral abductor paralysis is new and not yet fully accepted. It depends on reinnervation of the larynx, or at least of the abductor muscle. This is accomplished by implanting the nerve supply to the omohyoid muscle, by means of a thin muscular strip, into the chief abductor muscle of the larynx.

Complete laryngeal paralysis (Fig. 6-7) is rare.

Sensory paralysis. As mentioned previously, the entire sensory supply to the larynx is the internal branch of the superior laryngeal nerve. Because the sensory supply of one side of the larynx overlaps that of the other side, both superior laryngeal nerves must be paralyzed to produce complete anesthesia.

A diagnosis of sensory paralysis is made infrequently. One reason is that a test for anesthesia of the larynx is seldom done. Touching the vocal cords with a laryngoscopic forceps serves as a test. In some patients with a sensory paralysis, secretions flow over the cords and into the trachea without setting off a cough reflex. The patient coughs only after bronchial reflexes have been stimulated.

After local anesthesia of the larynx, as for laryngoscopy or bronchoscopy, the patient should not drink for 2 or 3 hours; otherwise, he may aspirate the liquid through the anesthetized larynx.

Larynx in senescence. In older persons there is atrophy of the muscles and mucosa of the larynx, as occurs in other parts of the body. Fatty infiltration develops, and the control of muscular action becomes less fine than it had been earlier in life, resulting in a bowing of the vocal cords that produces a hoarseness that is characteristic of the aged voice. The patient can correct this hoarseness when he tries, but only briefly. Rehabilitative measures by a speech therapist may be of some help if they are actually needed.

SELECTED READINGS

Burgess, G.E., and others: Laryngeal competence after tracheal extubation, Anesthesiology **51**(1):73-77, 1979.

Dedo, H.H., Urrea, R.D., and Lawson, L.: Intracordal injection of Teflon in the treatment of 135 patients with dysphonia, Ann. Otol. Rhinol. Laryngol. **82**(5):661, 1973.

Greene, R., and others: Trauma of the larynx and trachea, Radiol. Clin. North Am. **16**(2):309-320, 1978.

Horn, K.L., and others: Right vocal cord paralysis after open heart operation, Ann. Thorac. Surg. **27**(4):344-346, 1979.

Jackson, C., and Jackson, C.L.: Diseases and injuries of the larynx, ed. 2, New York, 1942, Macmillan, Inc.

Jordan, W.S., Graves, C.L., and Elwyn, R.A.: New therapy for postintubation laryngeal edema and tracheitis in children, J.A.M.A. **212**:585, 1970.

Levine, H.L., and others: Recurrent laryngeal secretion for spasmodic dysphonia, Ann. Otol. Rhinol. Laryngol. **88** (4, pt. 1):527-530, 1979.

Parnell, F.W., and Brandenburg, J.H.: Vocal cord paralysis; a review of 100 cases, Laryngoscope **80**:1036, 1970.

Rustad, W.H., and Morrison, L.F.: Revised anatomy of the recurrent laryngeal nerves; surgical importance based on the dissection of 100 cadavers, Laryngoscope **62**:237, 1952.

Schramm, V.L., May, M., and Lavorato, A.S.: Gelfoam paste injection for vocal cord paralysis: temporary rehabilitation of glottic incompetence, Laryngoscope **88**: 1268-1273, August, 1978.

Traff, B., and Tos, M.: Nasotracheal intubation in acute epiglottitis, Acta Otolaryngol. **68**:363, 1969.

Tucker, H.M.: Human laryngeal reinnervation: long-term experience with the nerve-muscle pedicle technique, Laryngoscope **88**:598-604, April, 1978.

Williams, J.L., Capitanio, M.S., and Turtz, M.G.: Vocal cord paralysis: radiologic observations in 21 infants and young children, Am. J. Roentgenol. Radium Ther. Nucl. Med. **128**:649-651, April, 1977.

Work, W.: Paralysis and paresis of the vocal cords, Arch. Otolaryngol. **34**:267, 1941.

7 THE LARYNX—NONNEOPLASTIC CONDITIONS

Laryngeal symptoms. Laryngeal symptoms are important because they often indicate disease processes of a vital nature. Since the larynx is easy to examine, early diagnosis of disease is possible in most patients if they report their symptoms when they occur.

HOARSENESS. Hoarseness is the most important symptom of laryngeal disease. It is common and sometimes the only early symptom. Other symptoms, such as pain and dysphagia, may cause the patient more distress but often occur at a later stage (especially in malignant diseases). Of course, not all laryngeal diseases produce hoarseness, and some diseases cause hoarseness as a late symptom rather than as an early one.

Hoarseness is caused by any condition that interferes with normal phonatory functioning of the larynx. As the vocal cords approximate for phonation, they vibrate; and air that passes through the larynx is variously affected according to the size of the glottic chink, the rapidity of the vibrations, the tenseness of the cords, and other factors. In diseases of the larynx, the cords fail to perform properly and hoarseness results. More than 50 separate causes of hoarseness are known.

Hoarseness is usually due to improper approximation of the cords. This may be the result of a tumor that holds the cords apart. Some elderly patients have tremulous voices because the laryngeal musculature is weak and the cords cannot be closed. Other causes of improper approximation, such as a foreign body caught in the larynx or the loss of cordal substance after partial laryngectomy or biopsy, are unusual.

Another cause of hoarseness is laryngeal paralysis. Some patients with vocal cord paralysis are not hoarse, because their cords still approximate during phonation. Conversely, because of loss of tension in a paralyzed cord, a patient may be hoarse even though his paralyzed cord is in a position to permit good approximation.

Any inflammation of the larynx, acute or chronic, produces changes in the mucosa of the larynx (laryngitis). If these mucosal changes affect the true vocal cords and the cords are thickened or roughened, the patient is hoarse.

Functional disturbances may also cause hoarseness. In hysterical aphonia, for example, the patient does not adduct his cords properly when speaking, but when he coughs the cords close very well. Dysphonia plicae ventricularis causes hoarseness because the ventricular bands (false cords) close over the true cords and interfere with vibrations of the air column.

Determination of the cause of hoarseness can be made only by examination of the larynx. Too often hoarseness is attributed to smoking or a "cold" without examination of the larynx, with the result that treatment of a serious disease such as a neoplasm is delayed. *Any patient who is hoarse longer than 2 weeks deserves a careful inspection of the larynx.*

DYSPNEA. Dyspnea associated with laryngeal disease is always an ominous symptom. It indicates a severe obstruction of the airway. Normally the laryngeal airway is more than adequate. Even if one vocal cord is paralyzed and cannot abduct at all, there is no dyspnea.

In children the most common cause of laryngeal dyspnea is acute laryngeal inflammation. The glottic opening is smaller in the infant or young child than in the adult. Consequently, less swelling is required to cause dyspnea. In adults (less often in children) other causes of laryngeal dyspnea are malignant growths in the larynx and hypopharynx, giant polyps and various other benign tumors in the larynx, acute angioneurotic edema, trauma (with mucosal laceration or hematoma formation), foreign bodies, and bilateral vocal cord paralysis. Occasionally patients with laryngeal dyspnea are mistakenly thought to have asthma.

Laryngeal obstruction that develops over a long period of time is much better tolerated than an equally severe sudden obstruction. Sometimes, in a patient who has had a tumor for a long time, a physician may see no airway at all. Yet this patient is more comfortable (and certainly less excited) than the patient with acute laryngeal obstruction and a better airway.

In laryngeal dyspnea, the harder a patient tries to breathe, the less air he gets. The reason is a mechanical one. The inrushing air strikes the upper surface of the true cords and forces them together. If the patient breathes slowly and quietly, he gets more air because the gently inspired air does not exert a closing effect on the cords. Expiration is no problem in a patient with laryngeal dyspnea (as it is in a patient with asthma). Laryngeal dyspnea is characterized by soft tissue retraction at the suprasternal notch, above the clavicles, and at the intercostal spaces.

In treatment, the important thing is to *look at the larynx*, estimate the amount and cause of the obstruction, and restore the airway. Restoration of the airway may require tracheotomy, although sometimes (for example, in acute laryngeal edema) one may pass an intratracheal tube and leave it in place a few hours until medical measures relieve the edema.

STRIDOR. Stridor is another ominous laryngeal symptom. It is almost always inspiratory and, like laryngeal dyspnea, is worse when the patient struggles to breathe. The inrushing air, striking the upper surface of the true cords, tends to close the glottis and worsen the stridor. In the expiratory phase the cords are separated by the outrushing air and there is less stridor or no stridor.

When stridor and dyspnea are present, a quiet approach to encourage gentle breathing and relaxation is most important. *The use of narcotics or sedatives to induce sleep is a dangerous, and sometimes even fatal, practice.* The patient with stridor and dyspnea needs his accessory muscles of respiration; and when he is asleep, these voluntary muscles are not effectively used. It is better for him to struggle for air, if necessary, than to relax, sleep, and die. Of course, long before this sequence of events occurs, a tracheotomy should be done.

DYSPHAGIA. Dysphagia is not a common symptom of laryngeal disease. Its presence indicates an obstruction of the upper esophagus or the pyriform recess. Usually a tumor of the larynx or the postcricoid region is the cause. Dysphagia may be secondary to inflammation of the larynx. Tuberculosis of the larynx used to be a common example. Pain discourages attempts to swallow. When dysphagia interferes with nutrition, nasal feedings may be used. The patient may obtain partial relief by swallowing a topical anesthetic such as lidocaine (Xylocaine Viscous), 5 ml., before meals.

PAIN. Pain is an occasional laryngeal symptom. Whereas it is an early manifestation of acute inflammatory diseases, it is usually a late symptom in neoplastic conditions. Many times pain is slight, as in mild acute laryngitis; but it may also be severe, as in tuberculous laryngitis. Narcotics are required for some patients.

In neoplasms pain is usually not present until late in the course of the disease, when there is ulceration. The patient with a tumor of the epiglottis, for example, may complain of burning in the throat when he drinks hot liquid or orange juice.

Usually, chronic inflammatory diseases of the larynx are not very painful. Some, however, such as contact ulcers of the vocal processes, produce mild pain, especially when the patient talks or swallows.

The internal division of the superior laryngeal nerve provides the sensory supply of the larynx. Neuralgia of this nerve has been reported but is unusual. *Referred pain to the ear from the larynx is common.* The nerve pathway involved (Arnold's nerve) is the same as that which induces coughing when manipulations are performed in the ear canal.

COUGH. Cough is another common laryngeal symptom. It is a part of many laryngeal and thoracic diseases, acute and chronic, inflammatory and neoplastic. Jackson called the cough reflex the "watchdog of the larynx," and so it is in the normal patient. However, in disease, the cough may lose its importance as a protective mechanism and become an aggravating factor.

Coughing is often the only symptom resulting from a minor laryngeal disorder, such as mild laryngitis caused by smoking.

Vocal nodules (singer's nodes). Misuse of the voice, as in shouting or singing above one's normal range, and especially abuse of the voice during a period of laryngitis, may produce vocal nodules. These tiny nodules are also known as "singer's nodes" or "speaker's nodes" or by similar names that indicate their prevalence in persons who use their voices a great deal. Tiny hemorrhages occur at the junction of the anterior one third with the posterior two thirds of the vocal cord. The early lesion looks red. Later, fibrous tissue replaces the hemorrhage and the nodule is white. Often there are two nodules exactly opposite one another (Fig. 7-1) that make contact during phonation. The lesions vary from no larger than a pinhead to as large as a split pea. Some nodules are so tiny that they produce no symptoms, whereas others produce hoarseness. There is no pain.

Although voice rest and speech therapy may restore a normal voice in some patients, most vocal nodules are best removed surgically. On the other hand, if the patient is not concerned with his voice, there is no urgent reason to remove the nodules. Their appearance is so characteristic that removal for routine examination is unnecessary. As in all benign laryngeal lesions, removal must be exact so that there is no injury to the substance of the cord. Otherwise, scar formation during healing produces more hoarseness. The operation may be done with the patient under local or general anesthesia and by either direct or indirect laryngoscopy. Postoperatively the patient maintains voice rest for 2 to 4 days. In some patients speech therapy may be necessary.

Vocal nodules are sometimes called "screamer's nodules" in children who constantly misuse their voices by speaking too loudly or yelling most of the time. Surgical removal of nodules in such children is not recommended unless one can be absolutely sure that the voice misuse has been corrected. Good speech therapy is the better treatment and may cause disappearance of the nodules. If it does not, surgical removal should be delayed until the child is old enough to be taught the benefits of proper voice intensity. Otherwise, the nodules will usually recur.

Laryngeal edema. Laryngeal edema may obstruct the larynx or cause hoarseness. Acute and chronic forms occur. Tumors of the neck or infections that obstruct laryngeal lymphatics, irradiation treatment of the larynx, acute angioneurotic edema, and direct injury to laryngeal structures during operative procedures or during intubation are the usual causes. Hoarseness is the first symptom and may increase until the

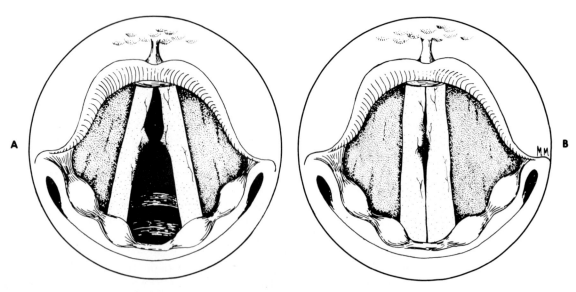

FIG. 7-1. Vocal nodules. **A,** During inspiration. **B,** During phonation. The nodules prevent complete closure of the cords, resulting in a hoarse or husky voice.

patient is barely able to speak. *Dyspnea* is a more ominous symptom. When it occurs suddenly, as it does in angioneurotic edema, the patient's airway is in grave danger. Sudden laryngeal edema is not tolerated so well as edema that develops more slowly.

Mirror laryngoscopy is usually all that is necessary for diagnosis. If it is necessary to distinguish between edema from a tumor and edema from irradiation reaction, direct laryngoscopy and biopsy may be necessary. The epiglottis and arytenoid cartilages may be so swollen that they are not recognizable (Fig. 7-2). There may be less edema of the vocal cords themselves than of the surrounding laryngeal structures.

Treatment of the patient with acute laryngeal edema, whatever the cause, is immediate restoration of the airway. Angioneurotic edema usually subsides rapidly after parenteral administration of epinephrine or corticosteroids. Nevertheless, one should not wait for these drugs to act if the patient is in impending danger of asphyxia. A tracheotomy (or sometimes the use of an oral endotracheal tube) is safer treatment.

In chronic laryngeal edema, treatment is not so urgent, since the patient has learned how to live with his difficulty. Nevertheless, tracheotomy is sometimes necessary. If a tracheotomy is done, the opening may have to remain indefinitely because correction of the underlying con-

dition, such as irradiation changes in the tissue or obstruction of the lymphatics by thyroid carcinoma, may not be possible.

Contact ulcer. The true cord attaches to the vocal process of the arytenoid cartilage. It is here that the mucosa of the larynx is the most likely to be traumatized. Vocal abuse and rough passage of intratracheal tubes are common forms of trauma. As the cords snap together during phonation, the vocal processes of the arytenoids meet forcibly. The patient who misuses his voice, especially during laryngitis, may traumatize the epithelium. An ulcerative process begins. Later, excessive granulation tissue and eventually fibrous tissue may form. Another cause of granuloma at the vocal process is injury to the mucosa during intubation for anesthesia or during bronchoscopy. Granulomas may be single or bilateral.

The chief symptoms of a contact ulcer are hoarseness and pain. The degree of hoarseness varies, depending on the amount of granulation tissue or ulceration present. Pain is present in most patients, particularly during swallowing, but is usually not severe. There may be tenderness to external palpation.

The possibility of contact ulcers and laryngeal granulomas (Fig. 7-3) should be considered in every hoarse patient, particularly if the hoarseness developed after intratracheal anesthesia.

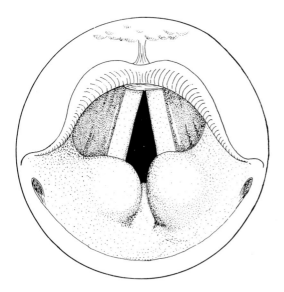

FIG. 7-2. Acute laryngeal edema with swollen arytenoids. If the edema progresses, the condition may rapidly become fatal.

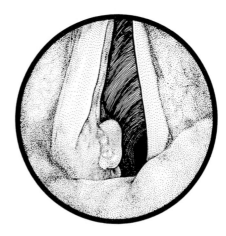

FIG. 7-3. Granuloma at the vocal process of the arytenoid.

Mirror examination demonstrates the condition readily, especially when granulation tissue is present. When contact ulcers are shallow and granulations are not present, the examiner may easily overlook the condition, because in looking at the top surface of the cords, he sees only the edge of the ulcer and not its face. Contact ulcers are usually bilateral. One ulcerated vocal process with its granulations may fit perfectly into a cup-shaped depression in its mate; the two seem to kiss.

In treatment, voice rest is valuable. If the patient talks, the contact ulcers continue to pound one another and healing is delayed. Aerosol therapy for 10 minutes several times daily, together with penicillin or another antibiotic, may be useful. Removal of the granulation tissue may be necessary.

Acute laryngitis. Acute laryngitis is common. It is often part of a general upper respiratory tract infection that involves the pharynx, larynx, and trachea; or it may occur as an isolated infection in which only the vocal cords are inflamed. Vocal abuse may also produce acute laryngitis. There is inflammation but no infection; sometimes submucosal hemorrhage occurs. Rarely, foreign bodies, inhalation of hot gases or flames, or aspiration of caustic solutions (lye) cause acute laryngitis.

The chief symptom is hoarseness, or the patient may lose his voice altogether. Cough is usually present, and the patient will say that his throat tickles or feels rough. The cough does not produce much sputum unless there is an associated tracheitis and bronchitis. Pain may also be a prominent symptom, and talking aggravates the discomfort. In patients with very severe acute laryngitis, especially in those in whom there is associated massive edema, stridor or dyspnea may be present. These symptoms are ominous.

The patient may have no fever, or his temperature may reach 104° F. As viewed in the laryngeal mirror, the true cords look red rather than white, and their edges are rounded rather than sharp. There is often hyperemia of the entire larynx, and the arytenoids may be swollen. Small pellets of secretions are seen in the trachea and sometimes on the vocal cords. In some patients there is a membrane in the larynx, which is suggestive of laryngeal diphtheria, although laryngeal diphtheria is now quite rare.

Organisms such as the streptococcus also cause membranous laryngitis. A membrane may also be seen as a slough after trauma resulting from steam, hot gases, or aspiration of a caustic. Membranous laryngitis is likely to be especially dangerous because of airway obstruction. This is particularly true in infants, in whom only a small membrane is enough to obstruct the glottis.

Most patients with acute laryngitis require no specific treatment. The laryngitis is part of a cold or other upper respiratory tract infection and subsides when the rest of the infection clears. Some patients, especially those who have fever, persistent cough, or stridor, require treatment with antibiotics, steam or aerosol therapy, and voice rest. Patients with acute laryngitis should not smoke. Throat lozenges containing a topical anesthetic, such as benzocaine, may afford relief. It is best not to recommend antibiotic lozenges, because the amount of antibiotic they contain is small and the risk of sensitization relatively great. Patients with severe acute laryngitis may require hospitalization and even tracheotomy.

Chronic laryngitis. The term *chronic laryngitis* includes many different conditions and implies long-standing inflammatory changes in the laryngeal mucosa. These conditions often blend into one another, so that exact diagnoses are not always possible by either the clinician or the pathologist.

Often the exact causes are not apparent. Probably, chronic laryngitis most often results from repeated episodes of acute laryngitis. Constant use (or misuse) of the voice such as may occur in singers and public speakers aggravates the condition or may produce it in a person with an otherwise normal larynx.

Smoking can cause chronic laryngitis. *Alcohol* contributes to chronic laryngitis, probably not because of the toxic effect of the alcohol itself but because an intoxicated person usually abuses his voice. In the past, *syphilis* of the larynx was a common cause of chronic laryngitis, but now laryngeal syphilis is very rare. Likewise, *tuberculosis* of the larynx once was much more common than now. Formerly, syphilis, tuberculosis, and cancer were known as the "laryngeal triad." These diseases were seen so frequently (sometimes combined) that it was often difficult to be sure which condition was present. Today, cancer of the larynx is the most common member of the triad. In fact, many younger otolaryngologists have never seen a patient with syphilis of the larynx.

Patients with chronic sinusitis or bronchitis have purulent drainage from above or below the larynx. The role of this drainage in the production of chronic laryngitis is often difficult to assess. Certainly, many patients with chronic sinusitis do not have laryngitis, and most patients with chronic laryngitis do not have sinusitis. Nevertheless, in certain patients, the two conditions seem to be related etiologically. Similarly, chronic inflammatory disease of the tonsils and adenoids may, at times, cause or predispose the patient to laryngitis. Other factors that may be of etiologic significance in some patients are allergy and hypometabolic states. When the cause is not apparent and usual therapeutic measures do not help, careful consideration should be given to the patient's general physical condition. Medical consultation is useful.

Hoarseness is the chief symptom of chronic laryngitis. Pain is absent or minimal. Patients often cough frequently, but unless there is an associated tracheitis or bronchitis, little or no secretion is raised. Persons who formerly could use their voices for many hours find it impossible to speak clearly for any prolonged period. The throat may ache or feel tired.

In some patients the true cords are thickened and red rather than sharp edged and white. In others the cords look polypoid and edematous. Polypoid corditis is one form of chronic laryngitis. Pearls of mucus resting on the true cords are easy to mistake for vocal nodules or other small vocal cord tumors. There is no loss of laryngeal motion in chronic laryngitis.

The false cords may also be affected in chronic laryngitis. They become thick and reddened and may be affected more than the true cords.

Taking a roentgenogram of the chest is an almost certain way of ruling out tuberculosis, because virtually all tuberculosis of the larynx is associated with far-advanced pulmonary tuberculosis. A normal blood Kahn reaction helps exclude syphilis. A tissue diagnosis may be necessary in some instances to distinguish between chronic inflammatory laryngitis and a neoplasm.

The best treatment is to remove the cause, if known. If the patient has developed chronic laryngitis because of heavy smoking, the condition will improve when he stops smoking. Often

smokers refuse to relinquish their habit, even though they complain bitterly about their symptoms. When vocal abuse causes or aggravates laryngitis, the treatment is obvious. Local treatment of the larynx is not used so much as it was in the days before antibiotics. Inhalation of unmedicated steam is of value in most patients with chronic laryngitis. However, most room steamers or vaporizers are of little value, because they are too small. A much better method is for the patient to inhale vapor as it comes from a steam kettle or to use a large commercial cold steamer in a small, closed room. Voice rest is very important. Total voice rest, which means that the patient does not speak at all, is the only practical measure. Instructions to observe partial voice rest are seldom carried out by the patient, just as most patients cannot "cut down" on cigarettes—they must stop altogether.

In general, chronic laryngitis is much more difficult to treat than acute laryngitis, because the causes are less easily removed and tissue changes may be irreversible. A biopsy may be necessary to distinguish between laryngitis and a neoplasm. Any patient with vocal cord paralysis and visible laryngeal disease probably has a malignancy rather than chronic laryngitis.

Tuberculosis. Tuberculous laryngitis is rare today, although it is still seen in sanatoriums and in an occasional private patient who consults his physician because of a weak voice, sore throat, hoarseness, or cough. *Virtually all tuberculosis of the larynx is secondary to far-advanced pulmonary tuberculosis.* The sputum infects the larynx. Laryngeal tuberculosis affects the posterior part of the larynx more than the anterior part. Carcinomas, on the other hand, tend to develop in the anterior part of the larynx.

The symptoms vary greatly, depending on the stage of the tuberculosis. Early in the disease there may be only a weak voice; hoarseness appears later. Laryngeal symptoms may be masked by the pulmonary symptoms or vice versa. In later stages of the disease there is hoarseness and often pain. The patient may lose weight simply because he refuses to swallow.

The diagnosis may be difficult, particularly if the physician is not thinking of the condition. Roentgenograms of the chest and cultures and smears of the sputum are required to confirm the diagnosis.

Use of modern antituberculosis drugs (and sometimes thoracic surgical procedures) has greatly altered the treatment and changed the prognosis in favor of more rapid arrest of the disease.

Isoniazid, para-aminosalicylic acid (PAS), and streptomycin and the drugs commonly used. Streptomycin, isolated in 1944 and the first effective antibiotic used in the treatment of tuberculosis, has the disadvantage rapid development of resistance and therefore is always used in combination with one or two other drugs. Streptomycin also possesses the disadvantage of producing a severe toxic effect on the vestibular component of the inner ear.

The modern treatment of tuberculosis has undergone great change since the days of prolonged sanitorium stay. The following excerpt, from a paper by Wallace Fox, emphasizes this change:

The first and, perhaps, the most basic concept I propose to discuss is the all important role of good regimens of chemotherapy in the cure of tuberculosis, practically to the exclusion of all other factors, provided the patient cooperates by taking drugs as prescribed.

Although by mid 1950's there was already increasing evidence of the high level of effectiveness of chemotherapy when applied to patients in sanatoria, it was still widely considered that the sanatorium stay *itself* was making an important contribution, because it offered the traditional virtues of sanatorium treatment. Since then, however, evidence from controlled clinical trials has demonstrated beyond all doubt that ambulatory treatment on an outpatient basis is highly effective in the cure of pulmonary tuberculosis even when the patients are suffering from far advanced, extensive, bilateral, cavitary disease with sputum heavily positive for tubercle bacilli, are living under very bad conditions which include gross overcrowding and inadequate diet, and are engaged in arduous occupations, which they either continue or return to after only a short interruption. . . . I would like to emphasize that the *unimportance* of rest compared with ambulation, and of treatment in sanatorium compared with treatment at home, has been established not merely in the widely quoted Madras study but in six other relevant controlled studies.*

---

*From Fox, W.: Changing concepts in the chemotherapy of pulmonary tuberculosis (The John Barnwell Lecture), Am. Rev. Resp. Dis. **97**:767, 1968.

Leukoplakia. Leukoplakia of the larynx is caused by chronic laryngeal irritation such as results from heavy smoking. Undoubtedly there are also many other causes. Leukoplakia occurs most commonly in men. A white membrane forms on one or both of the true vocal cords. The abnormality is especially marked on the anterior part of the cords. The membrane tends to be patchy and superficial and is unlike an invasive tumor. There is no cord paralysis. Except for the leukoplakic changes seen on the true vocal cords, the larynx is usually normal.

Laryngeal leukoplakia is an entirely painless disease, with hoarseness as the chief symptom. The patient may cough more than usual to remove secretions that accumulate on the cord.

The best treatment is removal of the irritant. The patient should stop smoking; a prolonged period of voice rest also may be of value. Surgical treatment consists of stripping the mucosa from the vocal cords. Care must be taken to strip off only the mucosa without causing injury to underlying muscle.

Different observers employ the term leukoplakia (white plaque) for different conditions. Some use the word to mean lesions (both in the oral cavity and in the larynx) that are frankly precancerous. A few patients with leukoplakia of the larynx do develop carcinoma of the vocal cord, but the incidence is probably lower than generally thought. Other lesions of the larynx (without a precancerous tendency) may look very much like leukoplakia (Fig. 7-4). Sometimes these lesions are described by pathologists as *hyperkeratosis*. It is impossible to differentiate clinically among the various conditions simulating leukoplakia. Also, several pathologists, looking at the same slide, may make different diagnoses. If the lesion does not appear to be invasive, and if the patient will report to the physician's office for periodic laryngeal examination, a policy of watchful waiting is safe. If there is any doubt about the diagnosis, a biopsy is necessary.

Acute epiglottiditis. Acute epiglottiditis is a syndrome characterized by the aburpt onset of rapidly progressive respiratory obstruction due to a swollen, cherry-red epiglottis. *Haemophilus influenzae*, type B, is frequently isolated from a blood culture in patients with this syndrome. The syndrome may be seen at any age but becomes a serious emergency in children between

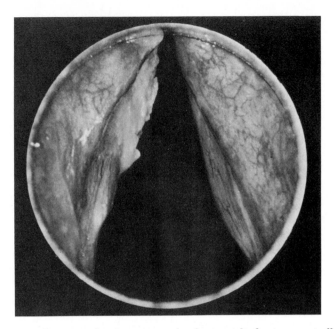

FIG. 7-4. Keratotic plaque. Such a lesion must be distinguished microscopically from leukoplakia and carcinoma. (Courtesy Dr. Paul Holinger, Chicago, Ill.)

2 and 8 years of age, since in this age group the laryngeal aperture is small. Complete airway obstruction may occur in a few hours and cause death.

The clinical course is as follows: abrupt onset of a severe sore throat; puddling of the oral secretions with drooling and dysphagia; fever between 101° and 105° F.; rapid development of dyspnea and stridor; and restlessness, cyanosis, and severe prostration, with hypoxic shock in a high percentage of patients. A white blood cell count of 18,000 to 24,000 is the rule.

Adequate treatment requires recognition of the rapidity with which obstruction may occur and the realization that the patient must be hospitalized as an emergency measure and that tracheotomy (Chapter 9) may be necessary in 50% to 70% of cases. Restlessness, stridor, cyanosis, and retraction of supraclavicular or intercostal spaces are all indications for immediate tracheotomy. A physician should be in constant attendance until airway obstruction has definitely subsided or a tracheotomy has been done. Some clinics recommend the use of a plastic endotracheal tube instead of tracheotomy. If such a tube is used, one must make certain that the tube is fixed solidly in place and that the arms are restrained so that the patient does not pull out the tube. Also, constant attendance is desirable. Ampicillin (100 to 200 mg./kg. in divided doses) is the recommended treatment. If the condition is properly treated, recovery begins in 24 to 48 hours and is usually complete. Failure to recognize the urgency of treatment may lead to death in 20% of patients.

Croup. Croup is defined as any affection of the larynx or trachea characterized by a hoarse, ringing cough and difficult breathing. Nocturnal croup in children is not uncommon. There are several causes. Because the many names and synonyms used for the condition are often confusing, it is best to classify such attacks as either inflammatory or noninflammatory.

INFLAMMATORY CROUP. Inflammatory croup is synonymous with acute laryngitis, but not all acute laryngitis produces croup. When it causes croup, acute laryngitis is usually of the subglottic type because laryngeal edema is greatest in the subglottic (conus elasticus) area. Here, where the tissue is loose, inflammation causes a swelling that looks like a red cherry (Fig. 7-5). Often the cords themselves are normal or only slightly injected. At other times the entire larynx is inflamed.

The patient with acute subglottic croup is in imminent danger of asphyxia. Hospitalization is

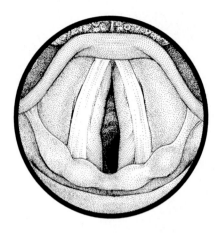

FIG. 7-5. Subglottic edema and inflammation in croup. Note the partially narrowed airway, causing stridor.

required, and patients are placed immediately in a humidified oxygen tent. The high humidity tends to soften crusts adhering to the subglottic mucosa so that they can be coughed out. If there is obvious urgent dyspnea with cyanosis on admission, a small bronchoscope or intratracheal tube is passed and a tracheotomy is performed immediately before the child is placed in the tent. For patients not undergoing tracheotomy, instruments for a tracheotomy should be available at the bedside. The use of corticosteroids may reduce greatly the need for tracheotomy. Steroids quickly reduce submucosal edema in many patients with either supraglottic or subglottic laryngitis.

NONINFLAMMATORY (SPASMODIC) CROUP. Spasmodic croup (laryngismus stridulus), a disorder of infants and young children, is often nocturnal. The child awakens out of a sound sleep with a hollow, barking cough and may shortly develop loud inspiratory stridor and dyspnea. The symptoms are often frightening to both the child and parents. In severe attacks both cyanosis and air hunger are present. Convulsions or loss of consciousness may occur. The end of the attack is as abrupt as its onset; and the child, worn out from his struggle to breathe, falls asleep. Inadequate calcium and vitamin D intake and parathyroid deficiency have been suspected as causes. However, the exact cause remains unknown.

Treatment should be conservative and expectant, since the condition is not fatal. Tracheotomy is seldom, if ever, necessary. Often the child will have repeated attacks. The parents should be reassured that recovery will occur so that they will not communicate their terror to the child. Forced inspiration always makes the symptoms worse. Steam inhalations help.

In the differential diagnosis between laryngismus stridulus and other conditions causing stridor and dyspnea, the laryngeal examination and a history of complete cessation of symptoms between attacks are important. Congenital laryngeal stridor, or laryngomalacia, for example, produces a constant inspiratory stridor. When the throat is viewed with the laryngoscope, an omega-shaped epiglottis is seen that is sucked into the airway with each inspiration. In acute laryngitis, diphtheria, and other inflammatory diseases, the temperature is elevated and the larynx looks abnormal. In contrast to these conditions, in laryngismus stridulus the larynx looks normal. Foreign bodies in the bronchus may produce a similar clinical picture and a normal larynx.

Symptoms resembling spasmodic croup occur when a sleeping child aspirates pharyngeal secretions. He starts to choke, wakes up frightened, and then coughs and gasps for air for a short time. These episodes are short lived.

Congenital laryngeal stridor. Congenital laryngeal stridor is a fairly common condition that appears shortly after birth and may last as long as 2 years. Then it disappears spontaneously. There is a laryngomalacia involving the epiglottis and the aryepiglottic folds. These structures fold in on themselves and are sucked into the airway when a deep breath is taken. Often there is an associated micrognathia and relaxation of the muscles of the neck and the floor of the mouth.

There is a loud *inspiratory* stridor that becomes worse when the child cries or breathes deeply. Except for stridor, the voice is normal. Ordinarily there is no cyanosis. The child does best when he is not crying or struggling. An equally severe stridor from any other condition would indicate impending asphyxia. Direct laryngoscopy demonstrates that the epiglottis is furled or omega shaped (Fig. 7-6) and that it becomes more so with deep inspiration. The stridor is abolished if the epiglottis is lifted with the tip of the laryngoscope. The vocal cords and trachea are always normal.

The condition is not fatal and clears sponta-

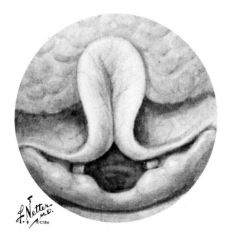

FIG. 7-6. Laryngomalacia (congenital laryngeal stridor). (Copyright 1964 CIBA Pharmaceutical Company, Division of CIBA-GEIGY Corporation. Reproduced, with permission, from the CLINICAL SYMPOSIA illustrated by Frank H. Netter, M.D. All rights reserved.)

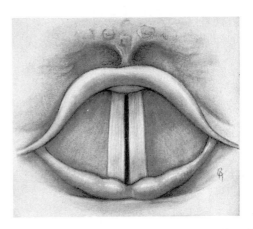

FIG. 7-7. Hysterical aphonia. The cords meet briefly and then separate slightly as the patient attempts to phonate. They actually meet when he coughs.

neously at about the age of 2 years, when the laryngeal structures become better formed. Ordinarily no treatment is necessary. Some physicians excise a V-shaped piece from the epiglottis, but this procedure hardly seems necessary merely to relieve the symptom of stridor. The parents need reassurance that the condition will correct itself.

Hysterical aphonia. Hysterical aphonia is not organic laryngeal paralysis but a functional disorder in which the patient is unable to adduct the vocal cords when attempting to speak. Sometimes, instead of complete aphonia, there is a very weak voice.

The cause is an emotional or psychogenic condition that manifests itself as aphonia. Through loss of his voice the patient hopes to be relieved of an unpleasant duty. An example is the amateur speaker who, unable to prepare his topic, develops aphonia and is thus able to cancel his speech without embarrassment. There is often a history of a similar condition months or years before. Such a patient does not look "nervous," and he may be quite calm during the examination. As he attempts to speak, no sound is made or there is only a very weak voice. Although he seems to be making a genuine effort, only a whisper results.

When the larynx is viewed during quiet respiration, no abnormality is seen. However, when the patient is asked to phonate, his cords often close briefly and then separate throughout their length just prior to phonation (Fig. 7-7). Hysterical aphonia is differentiated from organic laryngeal paralysis by having the patient cough. Usually he will cough sharply, an indication that he can adduct the vocal cords for coughing even if he cannot do so for speech.

The best treatment is psychiatric, but it is impractical in many circumstances. Strong suggestion plus intralaryngeal drops of colored water may be tried. Electric shocks to the external larynx are a strong psychic stimulus. Many times these tricks are effective and the voice is restored, at least for the time, but such measures treat the symptom rather than the cause.

Every physician must learn to treat these and other psychologic problems himself. A careful and painstaking examination will do much toward making the patient accept the strong reassurance that is needed.

Dysphonia plicae ventricularis. Dysphonia plicae ventricularis, which is common, is a cause of chronic or intermittent hoarseness. The false cords, which should rest quietly during phonation, become active and close over the true cords, causing hoarseness. Because the condition often occurs in an otherwise normal larynx, it is easily overlooked. It is also overlooked because it is an inconstant condition that may be

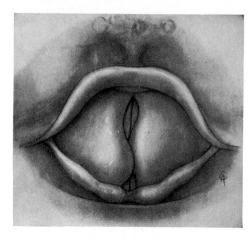

FIG. 7-8. Dysphonia plicae ventricularis. Note how the false cords close over the true cords. Sometimes the true cords are completely hidden.

present during one laryngeal examination but not during another.

Sometimes there is disease of the glottis itself (cords separated by tumor, cricoarytenoid fixation, surgical absence of one cord); and the ventricular bands (false cords), in trying to take over the function of the true cords, simply usurp their action. In other instances a psychogenic disorder is the basis for the condition.

Dysphonia plicae ventricularis causes hoarseness that varies in severity. The voice may be hoarse all the time, or it may be normal in the morning but deteriorate as the day wears on. There is an uncertainty of tone that sounds like the breaking voice of the adolescent male. This has been called "double voice."

Mirror laryngoscopy may show no abnormality whatsoever during the first few seconds of observation. Then suddenly the false cords close partially (or even completely) over the true cords (Fig. 7-8), and the voice starts to break. Sometimes the examiner may look for as long as a minute and find no abnormality in the larynx. The next day the condition may be visible.

The patient with dysphonia plicae ventricularis who has an otherwise normal larynx should be questioned about his previous vocal habits, vocal abuse, laryngeal infections, smoking, drinking, and occupation; and an attempt should be made to estimate his emotional stability. He should abstain from the use of tobacco and alcohol. A 2-week period of partial voice rest is helpful, and a change of environment may help, not so much to provide rest but temporarily relieve the patient from any aggravating home or work situations.

If a laryngeal abnormality can be corrected, an operation may be indicated. The removal of a vocal cord polyp or other tumor will restore normal laryngeal function and permit the true cords to close, thus relieving the false cords of their unaccustomed role.

Nervous cough. "Nervous" cough is more common than is generally recognized. It occurs in both children and adults and is an attention-getting mechanism that often starts when the patient has a simple laryngitis or other minor organic disorder. Frequently such patients smoke; and although they complain bitterly about their coughs, they will not relinquish the smoking habit. They often refer to the cough rather proudly as "my cough." Some patients may cough every few minutes, often loudly and deeply; but there is no hoarseness, and they raise neither blood nor sputum. Examination reveals the larynx to be normal unless the cough irritates the laryngeal or tracheal mucosa; then these parts are red.

Many times the examiner overlooks the diagnosis because he is not thinking of it. Treatment is usually unsatisfactory unless the patient obtains insight into the nature of his neurotic manifestation.

Laryngeal injuries. Because the laryngeal cartilages are relatively unprotected, one might expect the larynx to be injured easily. Actually, injuries are rare. Fracture of the larynx, inhalation of hot gases, or aspiration of caustic liquids sometimes endangers the airway.

Subcutaneous emphysema, tenderness, and discoloration of the neck are usually present after fracture. There may be crepitation as fragments of the fractured cartilage grate against one another. Mirror examination will show mucosal laceration, hematoma, or edema. Roentgenograms of the larynx are easily made and clearly demonstrate both cartilaginous and soft tissue changes. However, they usually add little information when a careful physical examination has been done.

The chief point to remember in treatment is the patient's airway. The patient's life may be saved if impending asphyxia is recognized and a tracheotomy done. If, in the healing process, scarring occurs so that there is an inadequate airway, reconstructive operations on the larynx may be done to establish more normal function.

After tracheotomy there is the problem of reconstructing the laryngeal and tracheal airway. Usually the cricoid cartilage is fractured and the mucosa of the larynx torn and swollen. Procedures used to restore the airway include resection of the fractured part and anastomosis of the thyroid cartilage to the trachea, placement of an indwelling plastic stent that will permit the mucous membrane to grow around it after several months, and skin grafting of the site of injury. Whenever possible, the tracheal stenosis is best repaired by excising the stenotic area and then approximating the two open ends. A direct anastomosis of this type may be done readily if not too much trachea must be excised. In cases in which several tracheal rings must be taken, additional relaxation of the tissues can be obtained by dividing the muscles that attach the hyoid bone to the mandible and other superior structures. This releases the hyoid and permits it and the larynx to drop downward so that the tracheal suture line is not under undue tension. Any of these methods is expected to result in a satisfactory airway, but the voice probably will always be hoarse.

Cricoarytenoid ankylosis. Not all patients with a fixed vocal cord have laryngeal paralysis. In any large series of patients with laryngeal paralysis, about 10% are said to have an "idiopathic" paralysis. Some of these so-called laryngeal paralyses are the results of cricoarytenoid ankylosis. The cause may be injury, infection, or actual arthritic changes. Rheumatoid arthritis, when generalized, may cause cricoarytenoid arthritis much more frequently than is generally suspected. Since this joint is arthrodial, it is not surprising that the pathology is similar to that found in other joints affected by rheumatoid arthritis. The symptoms are hoarseness, weak voice, and sometimes pain. Suspected cricoarytenoid ankylosis may be proved by the passive mobility test. The larynx is exposed by direct laryngoscopy and the cricoarytenoid joint probed with laryngeal forceps. Treatment of cricoarytenoid ankylosis, if any, is surgical.

Polypoid corditis. Polypoid corditis, a fairly common condition causing hoarseness, is associated with edematous changes in the true cords. The free margins of the cords are flabby and loose. Usually the entire length of one or both cords is involved. As the patient breathes, the edematous tissue flaps up and down; when he speaks, he is hoarse because the cords approximate imperfectly. The cause is not always apparent, but often it seems to be the result of vocal abuse or smoking, or both. Allergy may play a part in some patients. There is no tendency toward malignant degeneration.

Smoking should be stopped and strict voice rest practiced for 2 or 3 weeks. If the process is so far advanced that medical measures will not help, surgical treatment is indicated. With the patient under either local or general anesthesia, the mucosa is stripped from the entire length of one vocal cord and from the posterior two thirds of the opposite cord. Stripping both cords all the way to the anterior commissure is avoided because a web of scar tissue may form where the cords meet.

Hypothyroidism. When there is an insufficient amount of circulating thyroxine available for normal tissue metabolism, certain tissue changes occur in all body tissues. If the deficiency of thyroxine is severe, a state of myxedema results. One of the common manifestations of this endocrinopathy is the subcutaneous and submucosal infiltration of an edematous, viscid fluid that is different from fluid retained as a result of cardiac dysfunction, salt retention, or kidney disease. The resulting edema is more resistant and rather doughy, and it does not pit. This fluid has been shown to be composed primarily of acid mucopolysaccharides, and it distorts the tissues that it invades.

The larynx is involved in changes resulting from hypothyroidism. Huskiness of the voice or severe hoarseness is the usual symptom. It is slowly progressive if untreated. Examination of a patient with true myxedema will reveal the typical dullness, thickening, and sometimes flabbiness of the free margins of the true vocal cords. All tissues are involved, but the most striking picture in the larynx is the loss of the usual shiny, white reflection from the true vocal cords. At times the changes are so advanced that smooth, edematous polyps form on the vocal cord, or the entire cord looks like a single large, smooth, pale polyp.

The diagnosis is confirmed by basal metabolic rate determinations, determination of protein-bound iodine levels in the blood, and/or determination of the rate of radioactive iodine uptake by the thyroid gland.

Treatment is, of course, the same for laryngeal symptoms as for other systemic symptoms—thyroxine replacement with orally ad-

FIG. 7-9. Congenital web (incomplete), viewed through the laryngoscope. (Copyright 1964 CIBA Pharmaceutical Company, Division of CIBA-GEIGY Corporation. Reproduced, with permission, from the CLINICAL SYMPOSIA illustrated by Frank H. Netter, M.D. All rights reserved.)

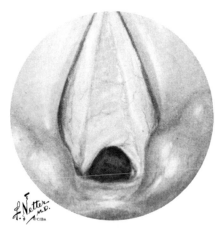

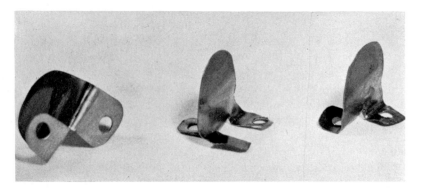

FIG. 7-10. A keel made of tantalum is placed between the vocal cords after surgical division of a laryngeal web. The operation is done through a vertical incision in the neck over the thyroid cartilage. Holes are for sutures to hold the keel in place until later removal.

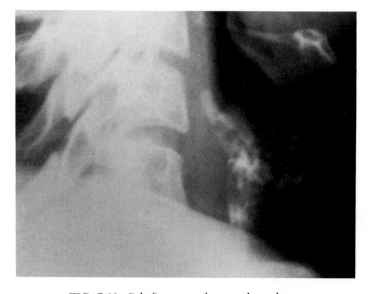

FIG. 7-11. Calcification in laryngeal cartilage.

ministered thyroid substance. This will almost always cause a reversal of the laryngeal symptoms and a return to normal of the laryngeal tissues. Sometimes, in neglected cases, it is necessary to "strip" the mucosa from the vocal cords or to remove residual polyps after thyroid replacement has been unsuccessful in producing a desirable result.

Laryngeal web. Rarely, an infant may be born with a laryngeal web. Usually such webs are partial (Fig. 7-9), but rare cases of a complete web have been reported. Since a complete web is incompatible with life, the emergency must be recognized at once; a tracheotomy must be done, or the web must be broken by passage of an endotracheal tube.

As the result of trauma or infection, a partial web may develop between the cords anteriorly and impair the voice or even produce an inadequate airway. If symptoms warrant, the web may be treated surgically. Attempts to excise the web and cauterize the raw edges meet with failure unless a temporary partition is placed in the larynx to separate the surfaces. One method is to perform a laryngofissure and then insert a very thin tantalum plate between the vocal cords (Fig. 7-10). The tantalum keel is fixed outside the larynx by bending its two flanges laterally over the edges of the split thyroid cartilage. The skin is closed over all. Later, after epithelium has lined the raw surfaces where the web was divided, the keel is removed.

Laryngeal calcification. In elderly patients calcification of the various cartilages of the larynx is expected. Occasionally, a calcification seen on x-ray film is confused with a foreign body such as a bone (Fig. 7-11).

Pulmonary hypertension and chronic upper airway obstruction. The fact that chronic upper airway obstruction can lead to pulmonary hypertension and subsequently to cor pulmonale is often overlooked, since such a chain of events is not common. Pulmonary hypertension in children is usually associated with such diseases as cystic fibrosis, bronchietasis, obesity and a pickwickian syndrome, and high-altitude habitation. Children with pulmonary hypertension are frequently severely ill; cardiomyopathy or congenital heart disease is the diagnosis usually entertained. However, the documented presence of pulmonary hypertension in the absence of any demonstrable cardiac abnormalities occasionally is the case. The most common age for such hypertension is 3 years, with a range of 2 to 9 being the most frequent. Laryngotracheolmalacia, congential tracheal web, and tonsillar and adenoidal hypertrophy are the most common causes of upper airway obstruction in children. Surgical correction of the obstruction will produce dramatic reversal of the clinical course. Thus, a thorough otolaryngologic examination is of vital importance.

SELECTED READINGS

Aminoff, M.J., Dedo, H.H., and Izdebski, K.: Clinical aspects of spasmodic dysphonia, J. Neurol. Neurosurg. Psychiatry **41**:361-365, April, 1978.

Barton, R.T.: The whispering syndrome of hysterical dysphonia, Ann. Otol. Rhinol. Laryngol. **69**:156, 1960.

Baxter, J.D., and Pashley, N.R.T.: Acute epiglottitis: twenty-five years' experience in management, the Montreal Children's Hospital, J. Laryngol. Otolaryngol. **6**:473-476, December, 1977.

Becker, W., and others: Atlas of otorhinolaryngology and bronchoesophagology, Philadelphia, 1969, W.B. Saunders Co.

Bennett, E.J., Tsuchiya, T., and Stephen, C.R.: Stridor and upper airway obstruction in infants, Anesth. Analg. **48**:75, 1969.

Cotton, R.: Management of subglottic stenosis in infancy and childhood: review of a consecutive series of cases managed by surgical reconstruction, Ann. Otol. Rhinol. Laryngol. **87**:649-657, 1978.

Davison, F.W.: Inflammatory diseases of the larynx of infants and small children, Ann. Otol. Rhinol. Laryngol. **76**:753, 1967.

Eliachar, I., and others: Combined treatment of concurrent laryngeal and tracheal stenosis, J. Laryngol. Otol. **93**(1):59-66, 1979.

Faden, H.S.: Treatment of *H. influenzae* type B epiglottitis, Pediatrics **63**(3):402-407, 1979.

Goff, W.F.: Teflon injection for vocal cord paralysis, Arch. Otolaryngol. **90**:98, 1969.

Holinger, L.D., and others: Laryngocele and saccular cysts, Ann. Otol. Rhinol. Laryngol. **87**(5, pt. 1):675-685, 1978.

Irwin, R.S., Rosen, M.J., and Braman, S.S.: Cough: comprehensive review, Arch. Intern. Med. **137**:1186-1191, September, 1977.

Kosokovic, F., and others: Contribution to therapy of dysphonia plicae ventricularis, Laryngoscope **87**:408-414, March, 1977.

Larson, D.L., and Cohn, A.M.: Management of acute laryngeal injury: critical review, J. Trauma **16**:858-862, November, 1976.

Lenney, W., and others: Treatment of acute viral croup, Arch. Dis. Child. **53**(9):704-706, 1978.

McSwiney, P.F., Cavanagh, N.P.C., and Languth, P.: Outcome in congenital stridor (laryngomalacia), Arch. Dis. Child. **52**:215-218, March, 1977.

Ogura, J.H., and Biller, H.F.: Reconstruction of the larynx following blunt trauma, Ann. Otol. Rhinol. Laryngol. **80**:492, 1971.

Pahor, A. L.: Herpes zoster of the larynx—how common? J. Laryngol. Otol. **93**(1):93-98, 1979.

Polandi, A., and Ribdri, O.: Clinical and medicolegal aspects of acute epiglottitis, J. Laryngol. **83**:141, 1969.

Raskin, N. H., and Prusiner, S.: Carotidynia, Neurology (Minneap.) **27**:43-46, January, 1977.

Saunders, W. H.: Dysphonia plicae ventricularis; an overlooked condition causing chronic hoarseness, Ann. Otol. Rhinol. Laryngol. **65**:665, 1956.

Setliff, R. C., and others: Pulmonary hypertension secondary to chronic upper airway obstruction, Laryngoscope **79**:845-856, 1969.

Shumrick, D. A.: Trauma of the larynx, Arch. Otolaryngol. **86**:691, 1967.

Taylor, H. M.: Ventricular laryngocele, Ann. Otol. Rhinol. Laryngol. **53**:536, 1944.

Wallner, L. J.: Smoker's larynx, Laryngoscope **64**:259, 1954.

Whited, R. E.: Laryngeal fracture in the multiple trauma patient, Am. J. Surg. **136**:354-355, September, 1978.

Yoder, R. L., and Merck, D. E.: Innocuous-appearing stab wounds to the neck; is exploration always indicated? South Med. J. **62**:113, 1969.

8 THE LARYNX—LARYNGEAL TUMORS

The student is advised, prior to reading this chapter, to turn to Chapter 10 and study the section on endoscopy in order to be familiar with the instruments and terminology regarding this procedure.

CARCINOMA

Carcinoma of the larynx that arises from the true vocal cords produces a very early symptom—*hoarseness*. If the patient consults a doctor soon after becoming hoarse and the doctor examines the larynx, the diagnosis can be made early. The prognosis is then excellent, and the treatment is not seriously disabling. Unfortunately, however, most patients do not consult a physician soon enough—or, sometimes, if the patient does seek medical help soon after becoming hoarse, the physician does not examine the larynx but ascribes the hoarseness to laryngitis or smoking. Reassured, the patient continues with his hoarseness. The average patient who is hoarse because of laryngeal carcinoma sees three physicians and waits 8 months before a physician finally looks at his larynx and makes a diagnosis. By then cancer is far advanced, and the prognosis is poor. *Hoarseness lasting longer than 2 weeks demands visualization of the larynx.*

Symptoms. Carcinoma may develop on the true vocal cord (*intrinsic* cancer) or in some other part of the larynx (*extrinsic* cancer). The symptoms differ, depending on the site of the lesion.

If carcinoma develops on the free edge of the vocal cord, hoarseness is an early symptom. The growth holds the cords apart, and the patient is hoarse because he cannot close the cords perfectly.

Pain is not a prominent symptom of cancer of the true vocal cords. Dyspnea is a late symptom. Metastases from neoplasms of the true cords occur later than do metastases from neoplasms of the extrinsic larynx. At least one reason is that the lymphatics in the true cord are sparse.

In contrast to intrinsic tumors of the larynx, growths of the extrinsic larynx do not produce early symptoms, because small neoplasms of the extrinsic larynx do not interfere with the voice. A tumor of the epiglottis, for example, can become quite large before causing symptoms. The earliest symptom is often pain caused by ulceration. Many patients say that the throat burns when they drink hot liquids or orange juice. Still later, dysphagia and dyspnea may develop. Hoarseness, another late symptom in extrinsic carcinoma of the larynx, may be due to interference with movement of the base of the tongue rather than to fixation of the cord. A muffled tone, known as the "hot potato voice," is heard. Additional late symptoms include weight loss, foul breath, and general debility. Metastases to the neck occur relatively early from primary lesions in the extrinsic larynx. In fact, a lump in the neck may be the first symptom.

Recently, laryngeal tumors have been broadly classified as arising in the supraglottic, glottic, transglottic, and subglottic zones. The supraglottic region is made up of the posterior surface of the epiglottis, the aryepiglottic folds, the arytenoids, the ventricular bands (false cords), and the ventricular cavities. Glottic tumors arise on the vocal cords and on the anterior and posterior commissure areas. The term transglottic applies to present tumors both above and below the ventricle. Primary subglottic tumors are rare, but subglottic extension of a lesion from the vocal cord is common. Accurate appreciation of the site of the tumor is important because the spread of laryngeal cancer (both locally and by metastasis) depends on its location and also because postoperative functioning of the larynx is related directly to the type of operation required to remove a particular tumor.

Examination. The most valuable examination is made with the *laryngeal mirror*. In intrinsic lesions, an irregular, constructive process is seen on one or both vocal cords (Fig. 8-1). The cords seem to be infiltrated. The growth usually begins on the anterior half of one cord. Eventually it extends across the anterior commissure to the opposite cord or posteriorly to the arytenoid of the same cord. Fixation of one or both cords, either by infiltration of the cord or involvement of the nerve supply, is common. At times the cord is only partially fixed. Occasionally it is difficult to assess completeness of movement because of the size of the tumor mass. Besides infiltrating the true cords and growing into the glottic chink, the neoplasm may also extend subglottically (under the cord, Fig. 8-2) or upward into the ventricle and false cord. The arytenoid cartilage (to which the cord attaches posteriorly) is frequently involved in patients with advanced disease. This posterior extension reduces the likelihood of a cure, because the lymphatics are abundant in this area.

In extrinsic lesions, especially those of the epiglottis, the tumors are often fungating; these lesions ulcerate more easily than do lesions of the cord. Often, when the patient is first seen, the normal appearance of the larynx is greatly distorted by a massive, ulcerated lesion that has eroded the epiglottis and other extrinsic laryngeal structures. Usually the true cords are unaffected in patients with supraglottic growths. Malignant tumors often bleed readily if palpated, and carcinomas of the larynx are no exception. However, bleeding is seldom profuse. Neck metastases are usually single and remain movable until very late in the disease. The most common metastasis is high in the neck, at the level of the carotid bifurcation (digastric or tonsillar node). However, any node in the neck can be involved. Most of the nodes are under the sternocleidomastoid muscle, where they may be easily overlooked unless the neck is palpated

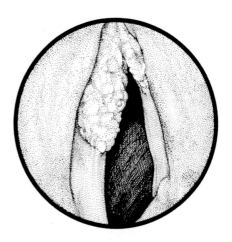

FIG. 8-1. Squamous cell carcinoma. Note extension across the anterior commissure. Carcinoma spreads by continuity.

carefully. Distant metastases, although unusual, do occur. In the normal patient, a definite crepitation can be produced by rocking the larynx vigorously from side to side. When there is a carcinoma of the pyriform recess (Fig. 8-3) or of the postcricoid region, normal crepitation may be lacking on one or both sides. Crepitation is caused by the rocking of the laryngeal cartilages across the vertebral bodies; it is absent (and replaced by a rubber cushion effect) when a neoplasm displaces the larynx away from the spine.

Diagnosis. The easiest way to diagnose carcinoma of the larynx is by mirror laryngoscopy. Also, direct laryngoscopy is necessary because tumors in the laryngeal ventricle, in the immediate subglottic area, and deep in the pyriform recess are not well seen by mirror examination. Even in patients with obvious carcinomas that can be diagnosed readily by mirror laryngoscopy, direct examination with the laryngoscope is desirable to obtain any possible additional information.

In some patients, especially those with lesions of the extrinsic larynx, roentgenographic techniques may aid in defining the limits of the tumor. In making a laryngogram, the examiner anesthetizes the larynx and then instills a radiopaque dye that outlines the various structures of the larynx and makes tumors clearly visible (Fig. 8-4). Laminography also is useful, as well as the routine esophagogram, which helps in delineating lesions of the pyriform recess and postcricoid areas.

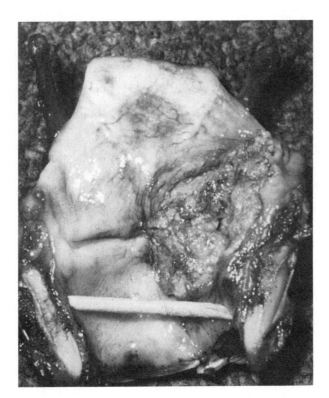

FIG. 8-2. Advanced carcinoma. Note the subglottic extension. A radical neck dissection should be done in continuity with laryngectomy for this type of lesion. The larynx has been split vertically. The false cord and the true cord can be clearly seen on the left side, with the epiglottis above.

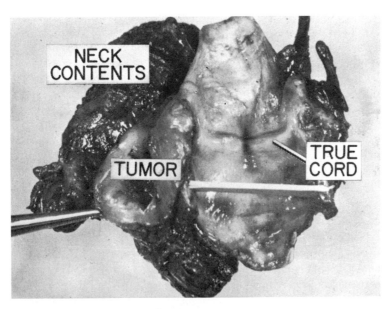

FIG. 8-3. Carcinoma of the pyriform recess. Note the normal vocal cords. Neck dissection was done in continuity with laryngectomy; of 20 nodes examined, 2 were positive.

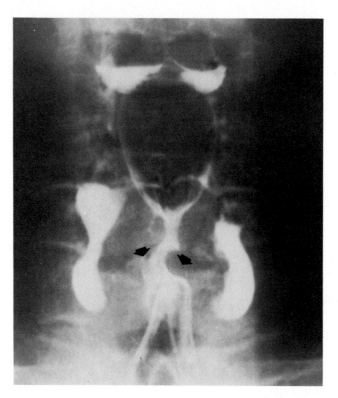

FIG. 8-4. Laryngogram. Left arrow indicates the eroded area (filled by dye). Right arrow points to normal true and false cords.

More and more, laryngologists are coming to use the Zeiss operating microscope to examine the larynx, in conjunction with a suspension laryngoscope (Fig. 10-1, *B*). The suspension laryngoscope provides binocular vision, which is not possible through most other laryngoscopes. Also, when the suspension laryngoscope is used, the examiner need not hold the laryngoscope with one hand; thus he has two free hands for aiding the examination.

A *biopsy* may be done using either indirect (mirror) laryngoscopy (Fig. 8-5) or direct laryngoscopy. The patient may be given either a local or a general anesthetic. The size of the biopsy specimen removed varies with the site of the lesion. In patients with carcinoma of the epiglottis, for example, a large piece of tissue may safely be removed. In patients with lesions of the true cord, a smaller piece should be taken; if the patient does not have a malignancy, removal of a large piece of tissue could produce permanent damage to the vocal cord.

Pathology. The great majority of laryngeal malignancies consists of squamous cell carcinomas. The degree of differentiation varies widely. In fact, the pathologist is sometimes greatly taxed to differentiate between leukoplakia and carcinoma in situ or between carcinoma in situ and early invasive carcinoma. Likewise, poorly differentiated tumors are difficult to classify. Adenocarcinoma, sarcoma, and other malignant tumors also occur. Metastases to the larynx from other organs have been reported but are very rare.

Prognosis. When malignancy involves only the true vocal cord but not the arytenoid, the prognosis is excellent. An 85% to 90% 5-year survival rate is expected following proper treatment. The prognosis may be equally good if the tumor has extended only a little across the anterior commissure. However, depending on the degree of bilateral extension present, the patient may lose his entire larynx rather than half of it.

If the posterior part of the intrinsic larynx or any part of the extrinsic larynx is involved, or if extension occurs beneath the true cord, the prognosis for 5-year survival drops precipitous-

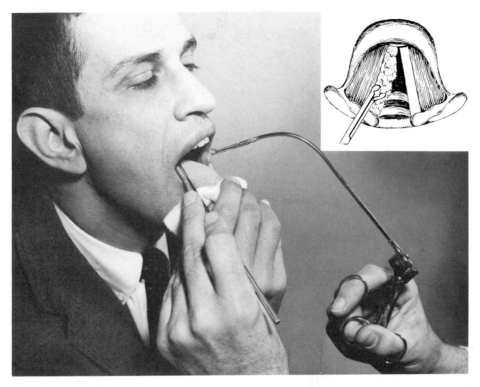

FIG. 8-5. Biopsy by indirect laryngoscopy. With practice, a very delicate intralaryngeal technique can be developed.

ly. Instead of an 85% survival rate, the usual figure of 70% is more applicable; and if neck metastases are present, the prognosis is still worse.

Surgical treatment. In general, there are four types of operations for carcinoma of the larynx: (1) excision using suspension laryngoscopy, (2) laryngofissure with partial laryngectomy, (3) total laryngectomy, and (4) supraglottic laryngectomy. Radical neck dissection often is combined with the second and third procedures but not with the laryngofissure procedure. The best prognosis is associated with partial laryngectomy, because this operation is reserved for patients with early lesions and for patients with cordal lesions, which seldom have early metastases.

EXCISION USING SUSPENSION LARYNGOSCOPY. In carcinoma in situ and other minimally invasive lesions, surgical treatment may be carried out by means of *suspension laryngoscopy* and magnification with the operating microscope (Fig. 10-3). This method provides an excellent view of the larynx and gives the surgeon free-

dom of both hands. He can, for example, grasp the vocal cord with small forceps and use scissors or a knife to cut away the diseased portion. Careful work will leave a substantial part of the vocalis muscle so that postoperatively the voice may be essentially normal. Obviously, this technique must be reserved for very early cases.

PARTIAL LARYNGECTOMY—LARYNGOFISSURE APPROACH. In partial laryngectomy, in which a laryngofissure splits the larynx in the anterior midline very much as one would open a clamshell, the amount of tissue removed depends on the extent of the disease. Surgeons use the general term partial laryngectomy to refer to several different operations. However, the name of the operation has little significance to the patient. Of importance to him is the knowledge that he will still be able to talk and will have a normal airway. A high cure rate is associated with partial laryngectomy (Fig. 8-6).

INDICATIONS. Ideally, the patient should have an early lesion confined to one cord or at least to the anterior part of the larynx (Fig. 8-7, A). Some surgeons extend the indications to in-

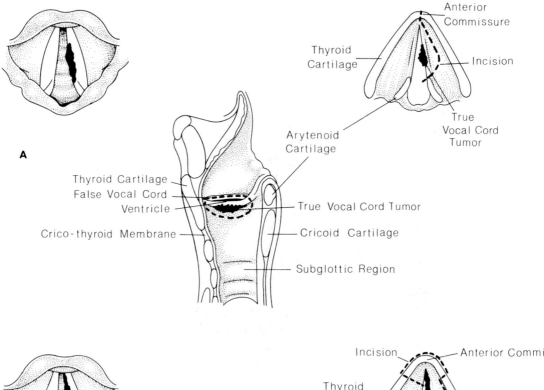

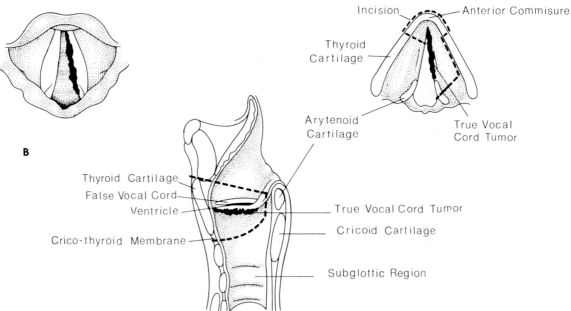

FIG. 8-6. A, Laryngofissure approach with partial laryngectomy. Only the true cord is excised. **B,** Extended partial laryngectomy (frontolateral). Note that excision includes the anterior commissure, the true cord, the false cord, and part of the arytenoid.

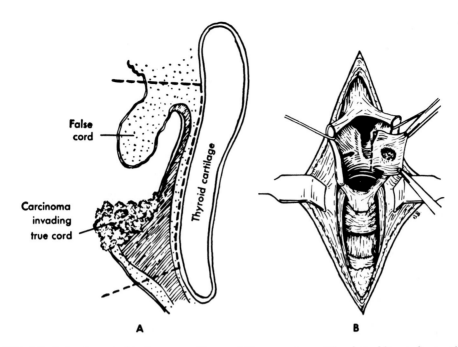

False cord

Carcinoma invading true cord

Thyroid cartilage

A   **B**

FIG. 8-7. A, Lesion suitable for removal by partial laryngectomy. The dotted line indicates the wide margin of normal tissue removed along with the tumor. In this case, since the false cord obviously is not involved, it would not have to be excised. If one is certain of the limits of the tumor, the false cord may not have to be excised. **B,** Partial laryngectomy. The incision into the larynx is from the thyroid notch above to the cricoid below. The drawing shows excision of a lesion on the true cord along with a wide margin of normal tissue.

clude a larynx in which the involved vocal cord is fixed, but such a case is much less likely to have a favorable result than cases in which the cord still moves.

CONTRAINDICATIONS. If major portions of both cords are affected, total laryngectomy ordinarily is required, but even here some surgeons have removed most of both cords and then used adjacent structures to reconstruct the larynx. Also, if the lesion has extended subglottically, even though only on one side, total laryngectomy is usually indicated. As noted above, fixation of a vocal cord has long been considered a contraindication for partial laryngectomy. Lesions extending superiorly from the true cord to involve the ventricle and false cord also can be removed by hemilaryngectomy, but the additional extension beyond the limits of the true cord lowers the cure rate. Involvement of the arytenoid cartilage makes the procedure even more risky but may not preclude it. Neck metastases usually necessitate laryngectomy and radical neck dissection in continuity.

OPERATIVE TECHNIQUE. With the patient under either local or general anesthesia, the larynx is split open in the midline (Fig. 8-7, *B*). All malignant tissue and a good margin of normal tissue are removed. This may mean only a cordectomy, or it may mean removal of the true cord, ventricle, and false cord. Sometimes a true hemilaryngectomy, involving excision of half of the thyroid cartilage along with the soft tissue on the inside of the larynx, is done.

POSTOPERATIVE RESULT. A tracheotomy tube ensures an airway during the immediate postoperative period. After healing, the airway is entirely adequate.

Scar tissue forms on the side that was operated on and provides a cushion against which the normal cord can work. Usually there is a serviceable voice.

TOTAL LARYNGECTOMY. Total laryngectomy is indicated in patients with far-advanced lesions. Many patients who must have a total laryngectomy could have been spared the loss of voice that accompanies this operation if they

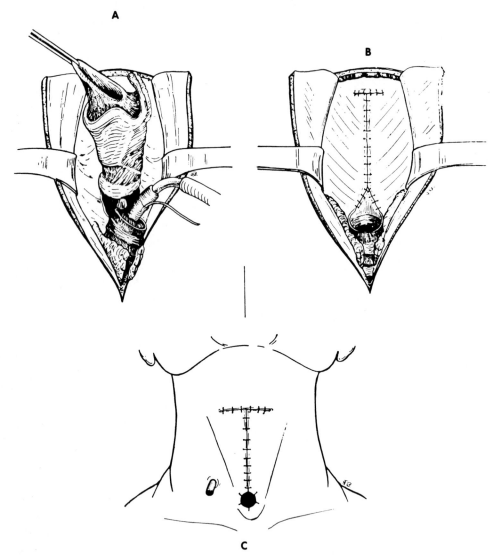

FIG. 8-8. Total laryngectomy. **A,** Usually one or two tracheal rings *and the hyoid bone* are included with the specimen. **B,** The mucous membrane and muscles of the pharynx are closed in layers. **C,** Tracheostomy—the trachea is sutured to the skin.

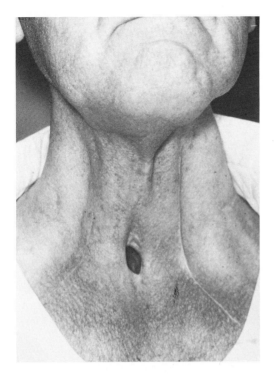

FIG. 8-9. After laryngectomy. Note the scars of bilateral radical neck dissections. The patient also had a pneumonectomy for a pulmonary metastasis.

had consulted a physician as soon as hoarseness developed.

INDICATIONS. Total laryngectomy is indicated in patients in whom a partial or supraglottic laryngectomy will not suffice.

CONTRAINDICATIONS. Total laryngectomy is contraindicated in patients with distant metastases and in those with local lesions that are not resectable.

OPERATIVE TECHNIQUE. The entire larynx is removed. In the "wide field" operation now in general use, the hyoid bone, the preepiglottic space, the strap muscles, and one or more tracheal rings are removed with the larynx (Fig. 8-8). If the neoplasm is large and predominantly one-sided, and especially if it involves the pyriform recess or extrinsic larynx, a radical neck dissection (Fig. 8-9) is done in continuity with laryngectomy. Finally, a constant, closed suction-type drainage system is installed (Fig. 8-10).

POSTOPERATIVE RESULT. After total laryngectomy there is a permanent opening into the trachea through the neck. Because no air can enter the nose, there is no sense of smell. One might think that the incidence of pneumonia or other lower respiratory tract disease would be high in patients who must breathe through a tracheostomy, but such is not the case. As long as such patients remain free of cancer, the incidence of other diseases is not increased. A great problem is loss of voice. Since total aphonia is a serious psychologic problem to the patient, it should be explained to him preoperatively that he will lose his voice as a result of the operation but that his voice is very poor anyway and is certain to become worse. It should also be explained to him that many patients learn to speak again by using a so-called esophageal voice.

SUPRAGLOTTIC LARYNGECTOMY. In addition to the surgical techniques generally called partial laryngectomy (through the laryngofissure approach) and total laryngectomy, another method recently popularized is *horizontal*, or *supraglottic, laryngectomy.* In this technique, which is used in certain extrinsic tumors, enough normal larynx remains after adequate resection for functioning. A carcinoma of the epiglottis, for example, could be excised just beneath both false cords (through the ventricles). This leaves the true cords intact. Usually a radical neck dissection is done simultaneously on the involved side. Patients have some difficulty swallowing for a week or two after the operation, but eventually most of them get along quite well. The great advantage of supraglottic laryngectomy, as compared to total laryngectomy, is that it preserves the voice. Great care must be taken, however, to choose suitable cases, since if there is local recurrence, additional therapy is compromised. Laryngograms are especially valuable in diagnosis, since these lesions are bulky and neither mirror nor direct laryngoscopy is as accurate as in a small cordal lesion.

Most patients who now have a supraglottic laryngectomy formerly would have had a total laryngectomy and would have lost their voices. Supraglottic laryngectomy probably is indicated more often than total laryngectomy. Cure rates are the same for supraglottic lesions whether the patient has a supraglottic ("conservation") laryngectomy or a total laryngectomy.

SUPERIOR MEDIASTINAL DISSECTION. Excision of the manubrium and the clavicular heads or the resection of the medial one third of the

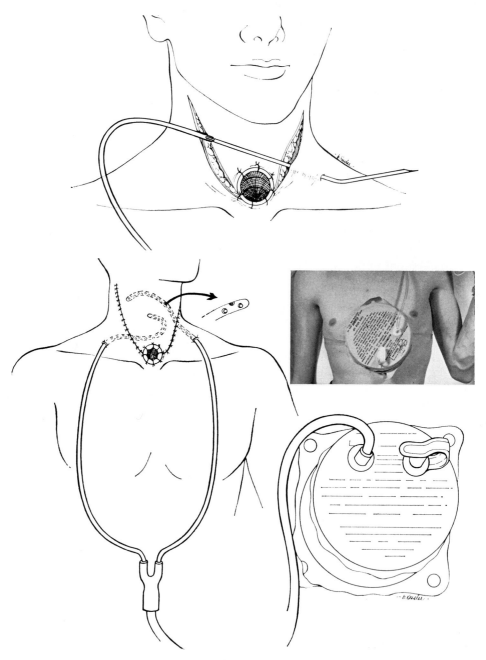

FIG. 8-10. Hemovac apparatus for constant closed suction. In this system of wound drainage, suction is maintained by means of a plastic container with a spring inside that tries to force apart the lids and thereby produces suction that is transmitted through the plastic tubing. The neck skin is pulled down tight, and no external dressing is required. The container serves as both suction source and receptacle for blood. It is emptied as required, and the drainage tubes are left in the neck for 3 days.

clavicular heads is necessary for removal of superior mediastinal disease (uncommon). These surgical techniques are particularly useful for exposure of the great vessels in removal of subglottic extension of malignancies. Stomal recurrence, cervical esophageal disease, substernal thyroid neoplasia, and metastatic disease to mediastinal nodes are also indications for mediastinal dissection. Direct surgery under visualization is necessary for adequate resection and protection of the great vessels and for avoidance of pneumothorax, which blunt dissection often can cause.

COMPLICATIONS. Several postoperative complications may follow total or conservation laryngectomy. *Fistula formation* from the reconstructed hypopharynx to the skin is one of the more common ones. These fistulas almost always heal spontaneously, but some take weeks and even months to close. They may also be closed surgically, but usually they are left to close spontaneously. *Rupture or blowout of the carotid artery* is a very fearsome complication that may follow radical neck dissection and laryngectomy. It is especially likely to occur in a patient who has received preoperative irradiation therapy. The only immediate treatment is for the nurse or relative who may be at hand to compress the neck wound and stop the bleeding until the patient can be transported to the operating room and the common carotid ligated below the point of rupture. This complication is almost always seen in patients who have fistulas with oral secretions bathing the carotid artery. *Stenosis of the tracheostomy* weeks or months after laryngectomy is fairly common. The tracheostomy becomes too small to function adequately, and the patient is constantly short of breath. A surgical revision of the tracheostomy is done in order to enlarge it, or the patient is fitted with successively larger tracheotomy tubes until a large one can be inserted; it is then left in place for months or even permanently. Also available, and somewhat more pleasant for the patient to wear, are small plastic tracheostomy buttons; these are hollow in the center with a flange on each end to anchor the device just at the surface of the neck.

Irradiation therapy. Although operative removal of the larynx is the treatment generally used, irradiation therapy is effective in certain cases. It gives the best results in patients with early carcinomas that involve only one cord and in patients without cord fixation or extralaryngeal extension. The cure rate in *early* carcinoma of the cord is about the same whether the patient is treated by roentgenotherapy or partial laryngectomy. Irradiation therapy does least good in patients with far-advanced carcinoma, subglottic extensions, and neck metastases. There is an advantage to irradiation therapy in that it leaves the patient with a better voice than does an operation, even partial laryngectomy. Irradiation therapy must be administered carefully and the larynx observed frequently during treatment if serious complications are to be avoided.

Hypopharyngeal lesions. Carcinomas of the hypopharynx may occur separately from the general laryngeal structure. Thus a lesion of the pyriform recess (Fig. 8-3) may require total laryngectomy, or a more conservative procedure may suffice if the lesion is small and the laryngeal and arytenoid surfaces of the pyriform recess are free of disease. Carcinoma of the base of the tongue may extend to the epiglottis or vice versa, and total laryngectomy or supraglottic laryngectomy may be required to manage such a lesion.

Verrucous carcinoma. Verrucous carcinoma is a special type of carcinoma that seldom metastasizes and that readily may be confused with hyperkeratosis. The clinical appearance is that of an exophytic, warty tumor with multiple filiform projections. If viewed microscopically, the tumor shows club-shaped papillomatous folds of well-differentiated keratinizing epithelium. There may be great difficulty in recognizing cytologic abnormalities required for a diagnosis of malignancy. The tumor tends to be of the pushing type rather than a tumor with an infiltrating margin.

Irradiation therapy is contraindicated in these tumors, since it tends to convert them into a more aggressive and infiltrating type of carcinoma. The best treatment is surgical excision, and this may well mean total laryngectomy.

Methods of compensating for loss of voice. Care should be given to the preoperative and postoperative education of the laryngectomy patient. His psychological adjustment depends upon a proper understanding of the loss of voice and an ability to compensate by means of esophageal speech, an electrical prosthetic device, or another method. A useful booklet is *A Handbook for the Laryngectomee*, by Robert L. Keith, available from the Interstate Printers and Publishers, Inc., Danville, Illinois 61832.

Most patients with voice loss after laryngectomy learn to speak by learning "esophageal speech." In effect, these patients swallow air and then hold it in the upper esophagus. By controlling the flow of air, they are able to pronounce as many as six to ten words or more before pausing to reswallow air. The voice is deep, but it is loud and entirely servicable when the technique is mastered.

Not all patients learn to use the esophageal voice effectively, and some fail altogether. For these patients mechanical and electrical devices are available. With one such device the patient holds the end of a speaking tube in his mouth and forms words; with another he presses an electric vibrator firmly against the side of the neck while he speaks. The tone produced is monotonous and artificial, but it is better than no speech (Fig. 8-11).

The *Assai procedure* (and related techniques) is another method of providing the postlaryngectomy patient with serviceable speech. A subcutaneous skin-lined tube is constructed in the anterior midline of the neck so that the upper end of the tube is sutured to mucosa in the hypopharynx, whereas the lower end opens into the tracheostomy. By occluding the tracheostomy with his thumb, the patient can direct air upward through the subcutaneous tube into the pharynx and speak. Retrograde aspiration of liquids sometimes produces a problem. The technique, excellent when it works, is not uniformly successful.

A similar result can be obtained by making a surgical opening between the upper trachea and the esophagus and inserting a specially designed plastic tube that extends outward to the tracheal stoma in the anterior neck. The tube has a

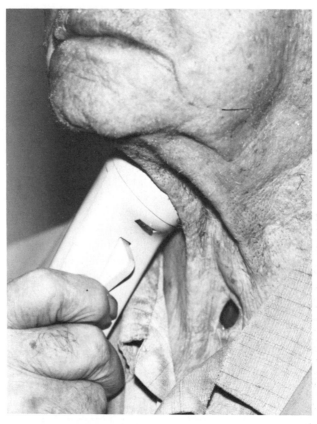

FIG. 8-11. Electric larynx applied to the neck of a patient who has not developed an effective esophageal voice after laryngectomy.

flanged outer end that is fixed with tape. The tube is removed daily, cleaned, and replaced by the patient. The special design allows air to flow from the trachea to the esophagus, but the one-way valve does not allow reverse flow of air. As in the Assai procedure, the stoma must be closed off with a finger in order to allow the tracheal air to enter the tube.

BENIGN TUMORS

Most benign laryngeal tumors are not true neoplasms but are the result of infection, trauma, or developmental anomalies. For example, juvenile papilloma is believed to be caused by a virus, whereas vocal nodules, or "singer's nodes," are commonly the result of vocal trauma. Laryngoceles and some cysts are congenital anomalies. Other benign tumors are true neoplasms.

The most common symptom of benign laryngeal tumors is *hoarseness.* Not all laryngeal tumors cause hoarseness, and some do so only intermittently. Certain very large tumors may cause dyspnea; and, rarely, death has been attributed to a large pedunculated tumor lodging in the glottis. Pain is rarely present. By definition, metastases do not occur, although some tumors are locally recurrent.

It is important to remember that the diagnosis is made by *looking at the larynx.* Unless the laryngeal lesion is easily recognized as benign (for example, vocal nodules), the tumor must be removed for examination by the pathologist.

Treatment for most benign tumors is surgical excision, which is done through a laryngoscope while the patient is under either local or general anesthesia. Care must be taken, particularly in patients with small growths on the true cord, not to remove more tissue than is necessary. Removal of any appreciable amount of cordal substance will result in postoperative scarring that may leave the patient permanently hoarse. Sometimes excision of the tumor by laryngofissure is necessary. Occasionally, indirect laryngoscopy suffices.

Recently there has been a strong trend toward the use of suspension laryngoscopy in the treatment of benign laryngeal conditions. A suspension attachment holds the laryngoscope in place, enabling the surgeon to use both hands. It also makes possible the use of the operating microscope for magnification (Fig. 10-3).

Juvenile papillomas. Juvenile papillomas (Fig. 8-12) are believed to be caused by a viral infection. They occur in young boys and tend to re-

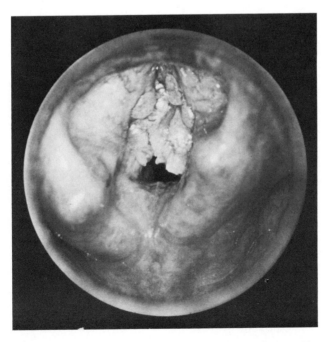

FIG. 8-12. Juvenile papillomatosis. (Courtesy Dr. Paul Holinger, Chicago, Ill.)

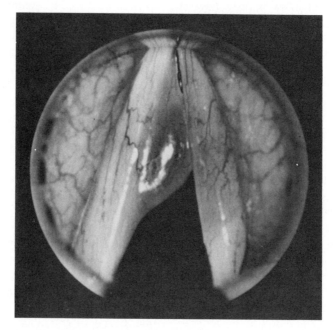

FIG. 8-13. Sessile laryngeal polyp. (Courtesy Dr. Paul Holinger, Chicago, Ill.)

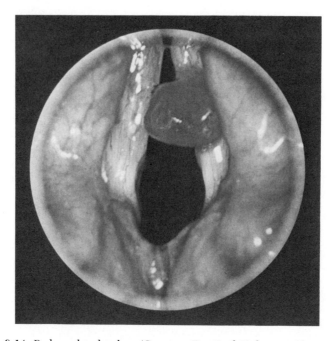

FIG. 8-14. Pedunculated polyp. (Courtesy Dr. Paul Holinger, Chicago, Ill.)

gress after puberty. Often there are multiple lesions in the larynx. The true cord, false cord, arytenoid, epiglottis, and even the trachea may be the sites of wartlike growths that bleed when removed. Symptoms are hoarseness or even almost total loss of voice, and more ominously, air hunger and stridor. Traditional treatment is removal of the growths by direct laryngoscopy with the patient under general anesthesia. Unfortunately, the growths often recur. They may need to be removed several times over a period of years. Repeated removal causes repeated trauma, and the end result may be severe scarring of the larynx and a poor voice. Some patients with severe papillomatosis may require a tracheotomy on one or several occasions.

A newer and apparently effective treatment is the use of ultrasonic irradiation directed to the larynx through a laryngoscope and a pencillike sound probe. Several treatments may be necessary until the papillomas regress and an essentially normal larynx results.

Other papillomas. Single papillomas, usually pedunculated, may occur in any part of the larynx of a patient of any age. These lesions are usually small and easily removed. As in all benign lesions, great care must be taken not to bite into substance of the true cord or permanent hoarseness may result.

Fibroma. Laryngeal fibroma may occur as a true neoplasm, but usually the so-called fibroma is scar tissue organization in a hematoma or similar change in a polyp. The tumors are removed by direct laryngoscopy with laryngeal forceps. Rarely, laryngofissure may be required.

Angioma. Most angiomas are not true neoplasms but result from inflammation or trauma. For example, many vocal nodules begin as red nodules that may be called angiomas. Later, they undergo fibrous changes and look white and firm.

Laryngeal polyps. Polyps are attached by a sessile base (Fig. 8-13) or a small stalk to one vocal cord (Fig. 8-14). They are not true neoplasms and vary in their histologic appearance. The cause is often not known; but, as in many benign laryngeal lesions, polyps may arise during periods of vocal abuse or in response to irritative factors. The only symptom produced, except in the case of giant polyps, is hoarseness. Sometimes the hoarseness is inconstant because

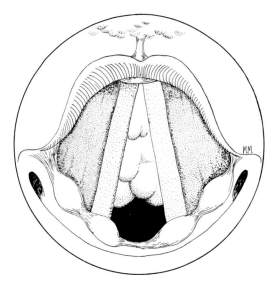

FIG. 8-15. Subglottic polyp. This type of polyp can be single and smooth or lobulated as shown.

if the polyp drops beneath the cords momentarily, the voice is normal. Rarely, when a huge polyp almost fills the glottis, dyspnea and stridor are present (Fig. 8-15). The physician may not be certain whether a laryngeal polyp is benign or malignant. Laryngeal polyps should be removed for examination.

Hyperkeratosis. Some patients with chronic hoarseness and large fungating lesions of the vocal cords do not have carcinoma. They have hyperkeratosis. The history is likely to describe hoarseness lasting for months or years. Mirror laryngoscopy shows movement of both cords if the hyperkeratotic mass is not so great as to obstruct action of the cords. The results of a biopsy often surprise the physician who has suspected the lesion to be malignant. In fact, malignancy may be present in another part of the specimen. Also, later change from a benign to a malignant condition is not impossible. The condition, therefore, is always potentially hazardous. If the hyperkeratotic mass is not too large, it can be excised from one or both cords through the conventional laryngoscope or through the suspension laryngoscope. Sometimes, however, it is necessary to perform a laryngofissure in order to excise the lesion adequately. There is a tendency toward local recurrence, which is more likely if the patient does not stop smoking.

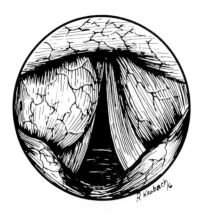

FIG. 8-16. Cystic enlargement of the right false vocal cord.

Other laryngeal "tumors." Cysts of various types (Fig. 8-16), amyloid deposits, prolapse of the mucosa of the ventricle, chondromas, chemodectomas, neurofibromas, lipomas, and other benign tumors have been described in the literature. Most of these tumors are quite rare. A congenital anomaly, the *laryngocele,* is an air sac connected to the laryngeal ventricle. When a patient with a laryngocele coughs or strains, the sac dilates and may bulge externally.

Saccular cysts are supraglottic lesions located in the anatomic plane of the saccule; they ap-appear to result from cystic distension of the laryngeal appendage. According to this interpretation, a laryngocele differs from a saccular cyst only in that it contains air, whereas the cyst contains mucus. A laryngopyocele is an infected air cyst. *Ductal cysts* may be found at any site within the larynx and may result from retention of mucus in the collecting ducts of submucosal glands.

LASER SURGERY

The word "laser" is an acronym for "light amplification by stimulated emission of radiation." Basically, when an electron drops from a high energy level (in a molecule) to a lower energy level, light is emitted. This light is a photon, which, when dropped to a second lower level, releases a second photon with the same wavelength, direction, and phase as the initiating photon. A chain reaction (photon cascade) builds up as the light bounces back and forth between mirrors. A mirror at the end of a focusing chamber has a small aperture that allows the escape of only some light beams traveling parallel to the long axis of the chamber. Such laser light leaves the source in a narrow, parallel bundle, with a narrow band and with waveforms in phase.

Such a beam can be easily focused with a lens, which increases the power. Various types of lasers can be constructed to destroy tissue in varying widths or depths by means of proper control of the beam.

Ruby lasers (developed in 1960) emit short bursts of high energy. Such bursts—when hitting tissue—cause miniature explosions and scattering of the tissue. Carbon dioxide lasers and argon lasers scar the tissue without explosion of tissue. The energy produced by these types of lasers is converted to heat in the tissue, vaporizes the cellular water, and ignites the remaining flammable tissue—leaving a shallow, charred crater. Heat damage at the sides of the crater reduces or eliminates bleeding from capillaries and other small blood vessels. Vessels larger than 0.5 mm. in diameter may bleed, and the laser is not effective in sealing them, since the energy is dissipated by the bleeding and thus cannot cause coagulation. Wound healing, following laser resection, is excellent.

The advantages of laser surgery (where applicable) are (1) ease of application, (2) decreased capillary bleeding, (3) greater accuracy in tissue removal, and (4) decreased morbidity. The laser can be (and is in otolaryngology) used in conjunction with an operating microscope. The active laser light must be *exactly* focused on the tissue to be destroyed. Various "sighting" and "focusing" methods are used in the several laser instruments now manufactured, but, in each, the focusing must be exact so that only the tissue in question is removed and damage to the surrounding normal tissue is minimized. An exact focus can be obtained by manipulating a focusing mirror attached to a "joystick." When focused, the laser beam is activated for the second or fraction of a second necessary to vaporize a small portion of tissue. By means of repeated short bursts (usually generated with a foot pedal) a sizable tumor can be carefully peeled away from normal tissue, leaving a shallow, charred crater. The only residues are vapor and smoke, which are removed, almost continuously, with suction, providing constant visibility of the operative field.

The carbon dioxide laser is the most commonly used laser in otolaryngology. It has been used most successfully in the treatment of laryngeal papillomas in children (p. 123). The ability to remove the papillomas discretely results in less damage to normal tissue, less edema, a shorter period of hospitalization, less scarring, and less likelihood that repeated removals will be necessary, when compared to forceps removal. This type of laser surgery is equally applicable to other benign laryngeal lesions and to some early, well-localized neoplasms.

The eradication of various oral lesions is an obvious use for laser surgery. Experimentally the laser has been successfully used for myringotomy (Chapter 23) and for stapedectomy (Chapter 25). Laryngeal polyps, leukoplakia, laryngeal webs, and certain laryngeal cysts have been treated with the carbon dioxide laser. Nasal lesions such as granulomas, papillomas, and small hemangiomas have been similarly removed. Cutaneous lesions such as port wine hemangiomas and tatoos have been effectively managed.

As in any medical or surgical treatment, complications can occur. The intense laser energy can cut through or vaporize plastic intratracheal tubes, some cardiac arrythmias may occur, normal tissue can be injured, and some postoperative pulmonary problems may be produced. The carbon dioxide light can scatter, damaging the eyes of the patient or those of the members of the surgical team. For this reason *all personnel* in the operating room *must* wear protective glasses while the laser is in use, and the patient's eyes must be properly protected.

The future application of laser surgery will be limited only by the feasibility and pace of technical improvements, such as reduction in the size and complexity of present instruments and the addition of safeguards to prevent complications.

SELECTED READINGS

Apfelberg, D., and others: Argon laser treatment of decorative tattoos, Br. J. Plast. Surg. **32:**141-144, 1979.

Bakamjian, V.Y.: Total reconstruction of pharynx with medially based deltopectoral skin flap, N.Y. J. Med. **68:**2771, 1968.

Baker, D.C., and Weissman, B.: Postirradiation carcinoma of the larynx, Ann. Otol. Rhinol. Laryngol. **80:**634, 1971.

Ben-Bassat, M., and others: Treatment of hereditary haemorrhagic telangectasia of the nasal mucosa with the carbon dioxide laser, Br. J. Plast. Surg. **31:**157-158, 1978.

Biller, H.F., Ogura, J.H., and Pratt, L.L.: Hemilaryngectomy for T2 glottic cancers, Arch. Otolaryngol. **93:**238, 1971.

Biller, H.F., and others: Hemilaryngectomy following radiation failure for carcinoma of the vocal cords, Laryngoscope **80:**249, 1970.

Birt, B.D.: The management of malignant tracheal neoplasms, J. Laryngol. Otol. **84:**723, 1970.

Bocca, E., Pignataro, O., and Mosciaro, O.: Supraglottic surgery of the larynx, Ann. Otol. Rhinol. Laryngol. **77:**1005, 1968.

Bridger, G.P., and Nassar, V.H.: Cancer spread in the larynx, Arch. Otolaryngol. **95:**497, 1972.

Bryce, D.P., and Rider, W.D.: Pre-operative irradiation in the treatment of advanced laryngeal carcinoma, Laryngoscope **81:**1481, 1971.

DeSanto, L.W., Devine, K.D., and Weiland, L.H.: Cyst of the larynx; classification, Laryngoscope **80:**145, 1970.

Doyle, P.J., Flores, A., and Bell, D.R.: Glottic squamous cell carcinoma (T_2): retrospective study, Ann. Otol. Rhinol. Laryngol. **86:**719-723, 1977.

Holinger, L.D., and others: Laryngocele and saccular cysts, Ann. Otol. Rhinol. Laryngol. **87:**675-685, 1978.

Holinger, P.H., Schild, J.A., and Weprin, L.: Pediatric laryngology, Otolaryngol. Clin. North Am. **3:**625, 1970.

Kirchner, J.A.: One hundred laryngeal cancers studied by serial section, Ann. Otol. Rhinol. Laryngol. **78:**689, 1969.

Kirchner, J.A., and Som, M.L.: Clinical and histological observations on supraglottic cancer, Ann. Otol. Rhinol. Laryngol. **80:**638, 1971.

Kirchner, J.A., and Som, M.L.: Clinical significance of fixed vocal cord, Laryngoscope **81:**1029, 1971.

Klos, J.: Clinical causes of laryngeal papillomatosis in children, Ann. Otol. Rhinol. Laryngol. **79:**1132, 1970.

Lederman, M.: Radiotherapy of cancer of the larynx, J. Laryngol. Otol. **84:**867, 1970.

LeJeune, F., Jr.: Intralaryngeal surgery 1977, Laryngoscope **87:**1815-1819, 1977.

McNeilis, F.L., and Esparza, A.R.: Carcinoma-in-situ of the larynx, Laryngoscope **81:**924, 1971.

Meyers, A., and Kuzela, D.: Dose response characteristics of the human larynx with carbon dioxide laser radiation, Am. J. Otolaryngol.—(2):136-140, 1980.

Mihaski, S., and others: Laser surgery in otolaryngology: interaction of CO_2 laser and soft tissue, Ann. N.Y. Acad. Sci. **267:**254-262, 1976.

Miller, A.H., and Fisher, H.R.: Clues to the life history of carcinoma in situ of the larynx, Laryngoscope **81:**1475, 1971.

Nave, C., and Nave, B.: Physics for the health sciences, Philadelphia, 1975, W.B. Saunders Co., pp. 250-265.

Norris, C.M., and others: A correlation of clinical staging, pathological findings and five year end results in surgically treated cancer of the larynx, Ann. Otol. Rhinol. Laryngol. **79:**1033, 1970.

Norton, M.: New endotracheal tube for laser surgery of the larynx, Ann. Otolaryngol. **37:**554-557, 1978.

Ogura, J.H.: Selection of patients for conservation surgery of the larynx and pharynx, Trans. Am. Acad. Ophthalmol. Otolaryngol. **76:**741, 1972.

Ogura, J.H., Biller, H.F., and Wette, R.: Elective neck dissection for pharyngeal and laryngeal cancers, Ann. Otol. Rhinol. Laryngol. **80:**646, 1971.

Olofsson, J., and others: Anterior commissure carcinoma; primary treatment with radiotherapy in 57 patients, Arch. Otolaryngol. **95**:230, 1972.

Reed, G.F., and Miller, W.A.: Elective neck dissection, Laryngoscope **80**:1292, 1970.

Saunders, W.H.: The larynx, Clin. Symp. **16**:67, 1964.

Strong, M., and Jako, G.: Laser surgery in the larynx, Ann. Otolaryngol. **81**:791-98, 1972.

Strong, M.S., Vaughan, C.W., and Incze, J.: Toluidine blue in diagnosis of cancer of the larynx, Arch. Otolaryngol. **91**:515, 1970.

Strong, S., and others: Transoral management of localized carcinoma of the oral cavity using the CO_2 laser, Laryngoscope **89**:897-905, 1979.

Stutsman, A.C., and McGavran, M.H.: Ultraconservative management of superficially invasive epidermoid carcinoma of the true vocal cord, Ann. Otol. Rhinol. Laryngol. **80**:507, 1971.

Tucker, G.F., Jr., Alonso, W.A., and Speiden, L.M.: Comparative application of revised (1971 "T") classification, pathological findings, and five-year results in surgically treated cancer of the larynx, Larynscope **81**:1512, 1971.

Vaughan, C.W., Strong, M.S., and Jako, G.J.: Laryngeal carcinoma: transoral treatment utilizing the CO_2 laser, Am. J. Surg. **136**:490-493, October, 1978.

9 TRACHEOTOMY

Tracheotomy is done to form a temporary opening in the trachea. *Tracheostomy*, in which the trachea is brought to the skin and sewed in place, provides a permanent opening. Usually a tracheostomy is done in connection with laryngectomy.

Basically there are two groups of patients requiring tracheotomy. Occasionally a tracheotomy is done in other patients for somewhat special reasons—for example, to reduce the dead air space in a patient with chronic pulmonary disease or to provide a convenient and safe method of administering positive-pressure ventilation in a comatose or unconscious patient.

Patients in the first group have *an obstruction* at or above the level of the larynx. The obstruction is caused by such conditions as carcinoma of the larynx (Fig. 9-1); the presence of foreign bodies in the larynx; angioneurotic edema of the larynx; severe infections of the neck, larynx, and oral cavity; and trauma to the mandible or tongue. Patients with tracheal stenosis or tracheoesophageal fistula may also require tracheotomy. These patients are in danger of asphyxia. All that is needed to restore an airway is the provision of an opening into the trachea below the point of obstruction. *Symptoms of laryngeal obstruction* are often ominous. They include *dyspnea* and *inspiratory stridor*. Use of the accessory muscles of respiration causes characteristic *retraction*, which is most noticeable at the suprasternal fossa but is also present at the intercostal spaces and above the clavicles. In children the sternum and epigastrium may be sucked in. If laryngeal obstruction is severe, and particularly if it is both severe and of recent onset, the patient may become ashen. *Restlessness* is especially prominent in children, and misguided efforts to re-duce apprehension by giving sedatives or narcotics have resulted in death. The diagnosis is not difficult if one remembers to *look at the larynx*. In adults and in many children this can be done using the laryngeal mirror, but if necessary the direct laryngoscope can be used.

Patients in the second group have no actual obstruction in the airway but for some reason *cannot raise secretions* from the chest. Such patients may virtually drown in their own secretions. Tracheotomy provides an easy way to aspirate secretions from the chest as often as required. Left to themselves, unconscious or moribund patients fail to cough. As secretions accumulate, anoxia occurs, and the patient may die.

Patients with poliomyelitis or meningitis cannot cough because of paralysis of the chest muscles and diaphragm. Other patients who need a tracheotomy are those with head injuries who do not cough, because they are unconscious; narcotized patients (in cases of drug poisoning); patients with fractured ribs who will not cough, because of pain; and some patients with pneumonia. *Tracheotomy in these and similar patients is becoming more and more common.*

Members of either group of patients requiring tracheotomy may develop serious alterations in the respiratory center as the result of progressive hypercapnia, acidemia, and anoxemia. Early in anoxia, there is stimulation to the respiratory center; but as ventilatory obstruction persists, there is depression. Normally about 500 ml. of air is moved with each respiration. In respiratory depression and in patients with chronic pulmonary disease who have reduced vital capacity, only 200 ml. may be moved with each respiration. The result is that only 50 ml. of inspired air is available for gaseous exchange in the alveoli, whereas 150 ml.

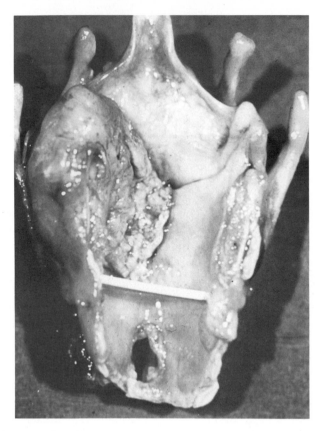

FIG. 9-1. Tracheotomy done for carcinoma of the larynx. If the stick were removed, the larynx would afford no airway. Here the tracheotomy was done through the first ring so as to interfere less with a subsequent tracheostomy formed at the time of laryngectomy.

occupies the "dead space" of the mouth, hypopharynx, and trachea. Tracheotomy helps to reduce this dead space so that more oxygen becomes available to the lungs. After chest trauma it is possible for a patient to have pink color in an oxygen tent and yet still retain enough carbon dioxide to cause respiratory acidosis, which causes a vicious circle of decreasing ventilation and further acidosis, and eventual coma and death. Tracheotomy and insertion of a cuffed tube will permit positive-pressure ventilation, which will correct the situation (Fig. 9-9).

Other means of suctioning the tracheobronchial passages (besides tracheotomy) are also available. However, when a patient requires repeated suctioning (sometimes as often as every 15 to 30 minutes) over a period of several days, there is no substitute for tracheotomy. Bronchoscopic suctioning is a good method for the patient who requires only an occasional

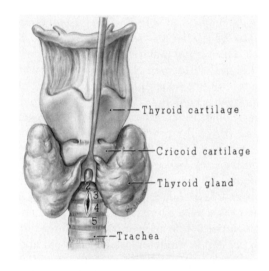

FIG. 9-2. Proper level for tracheotomy. Note that the first tracheal ring should not be cut. Note also that the thyroid isthmus must often be retracted upward. If necessary, it can be divided. (From Jacob, S.W., and Francone, C.A.: Structure and function in man, ed. 2, Philadelphia, 1970, W.B. Saunders Co.)

aspiration. The passage of a nasotracheal tube for aspiration is another method.

There are two types of tracheotomy procedures—the orderly, or routine, tracheotomy and the emergency tracheotomy (Fig. 9-2).

Orderly, or routine, tracheotomy. In the routine tracheotomy, the one of choice, the patient is brought to the operating room and a sterile field is prepared as for any surgical operation. A folded sheet is placed under the patient's shoulders to extend the neck. There is no hurry, and presumably every necessary surgical instrument is available, as well as two surgical assistants, a scrub nurse, and a circulating nurse. The anesthetist stands by to give oxygen if necessary.

ANESTHESIA. Lidocaine (Xylocaine), 2%, or procaine, with or without epinephrine, is infiltrated into the subcutaneous tissue of the anterior part of the neck from about the level of the thyroid cartilage to the suprasternal notch. Additional, deeper injections may be made alongside the trachea. A total of 10 to 15 ml. of solution should suffice. Sometimes an intratracheal tube is passed before the operation starts, to assure that the airway will remain adequate during the operation. In infants an intratracheal tube also makes the trachea easier to palpate.

The operation is seldom done under general anesthesia. Cooperation of the patient is gained by a preliminary explanation in his room and quiet reassurance just before and during the operation. In all operations performed with the patient under local anesthesia, and particularly in tracheotomy, the operative team should be careful to talk as little as possible and to avoid the use of words such as "knife," "scissors," or "needle," which might frighten the patient. Similarly, efforts at retraction of tissue and repositioning of the patient must be more gentle than when the patient is asleep.

OPERATIVE TECHNIQUE. A *vertical incision* is made in the midline of the neck, from the level of the lower border of the thyroid cartilage to one or two fingerbreadths above the suprasternal notch. The incision should not be unnecessarily long, but an incision that is too long is greatly preferable to one that is too short. The experienced surgeon can work through a smaller incision than can the novice; and, even more important, he knows when to lengthen his incision if more room is needed.

There is no objection to the use of a collar incision rather than a vertical one, except that the former cuts through more blood vessels; its supposed advantage, a smaller scar, is a fallacy. It is not the incision that causes the scar, but the tracheotomy tube. The tube is the same in either instance.

After the initial incision the wound is deepened by sharp or blunt dissection, usually both, and care is taken *not to dissect widely* into the planes of the neck. When the isthmus of the thyroid is seen, it is divided between clamps or retracted upward (Fig. 9-3, *A*) after incision of the pretracheal fascia, which binds the isthmus to the trachea. The latter technique is usually easier and causes less bleeding.

Once the thyroid has been retracted or cut, the rings of the trachea are seen. The trachea is incised vertically, usually through the third and fourth rings (Fig. 9-3, *C*). A cross incision may be made to make the opening larger, or a small section of trachea may be removed.

When the trachea is incised, the patient usually coughs up accumulated secretions. Secretions are also aspirated by a catheter placed on the end of a metal suction tube. A topical anesthetic such as 2% Xylocaine, 5% cocaine, or 1% tetracaine (Pontocaine) may be instilled into the trachea to reduce coughing after the trachea has been opened. The same medication may be injected into the tracheal airway before the tracheal incision is made. Neither practice is always necessary.

A previously selected tracheotomy tube (Fig. 9-4 to 9-6) is then inserted into the tracheal opening. The metal or plastic pilot is quickly removed and replaced with the inner tracheotomy tube. Absolute hemostasis is advisable; and if the wound is not already bloodless, it should be made so at this point because postoperative hemorrhage can be severe and is serious if blood runs into the airway. The wound is *not closed tightly*, since tight closure leads to subcutaneous and mediastinal emphysema. During the suturing of the wound, it is important that an assistant hold one finger on the flange of the outer tube so that it is not coughed out. Cloth tapes hold the tube in place.

POSTOPERATIVE CARE. After tracheotomy the patient is returned to his room. There is a definite program of postoperative care. First, if at all possible, it is desirable to have a special nurse. If this is not possible, the patient should

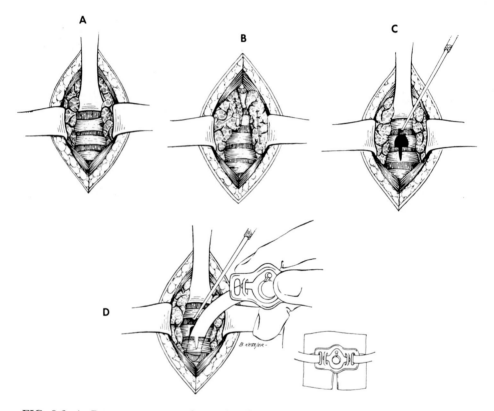

FIG. 9-3. **A,** Retractor exposing the trachea by drawing the isthmus of the thyroid upward. **B,** Alternate method to that shown in **A,** in which the isthmus of the thyroid is divided to expose the trachea. **C,** Two tracheal rings are cut, and the upper ring is partially resected. A tracheal hook pulls the trachea from the depth of the wound nearer to the surface. **D,** Insertion of the tracheotomy tube with the pilot in place. *Inset,* Tube in place and ties about neck.

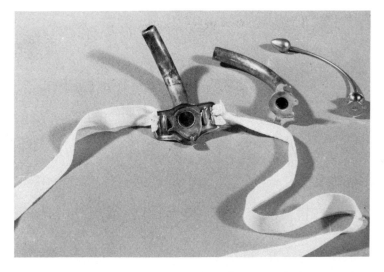

FIG. 9-4. Parts of a tracheotomy tube: outer tube with ties attached, inner tube, and pilot.

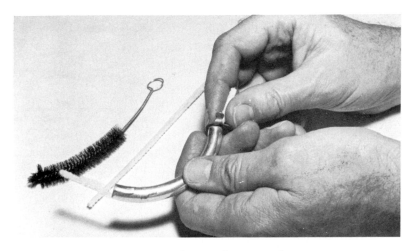

FIG. 9-5. Cleaning the inner tube.

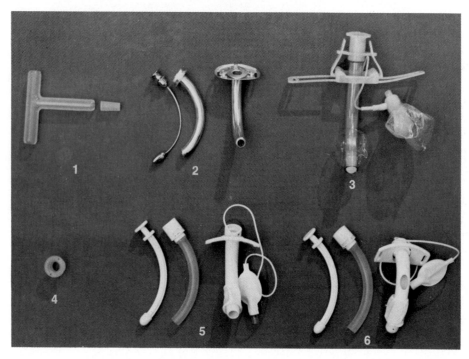

FIG. 9-6. *1,* Montgomery T-tube. *2,* Jackson silver tracheal tube. *3,* Lanz low-pressure, cuffed tracheal tube. *4,* Tracheal stomal button. *5,* Shiley cuffed tracheal tube. *6,* Shiley fenestrated tracheal tube.

be in a room directly across from the nursing station. Second, since the patient who has had a tracheotomy cannot speak, or at least not loudly, he must have a bell or other means of calling for help. Third, the inner tube must be cleaned regularly. The nurse removes the inner tube and uses a pipe cleaner or small flexible brush to clear dried secretions and blood (Fig. 9-5). In some patients the inner tube must be cleaned every 30 minutes; in others, it is necessary only a few times each day. The outer tube may be removed for cleaning after the tracheotomy channel is well formed—usually 48 hours.

Suctioning of the trachea is very important. The catheter used to provide suction through the cannula should have only one orifice, and it should be a blunt-nosed, firm soft rubber or plastic catheter large enough to aspirate thick secretions and blood clots. The catheter is passed with the finger off the thumbhole that controls the suction—in other words, there is no suction at the tip of the catheter as it is introduced. Then, when the thumbhole is occluded, strong suction clears the trachea as the catheter is slowly withdrawn. How often suctioning is done depends on the secretions. Generally, in an unconscious patient or in a patient with bulbar poliomyelitis, suctioning is needed oftener than in a patient with laryngeal obstruction. Usually it is done every 10 to 15 minutes at first and then less often as the secretions no longer accumulate.

Humidification of air is important for most patients after tracheotomy. It is especially important for infants in whom the trachea is very small and therefore easy to plug with secretions. The need for humidification varies also with the reason for which the tracheotomy was done. Patients with laryngotracheobronchitis, for example, are going to form more tenacious secretions that must be coughed up or aspirated than are patients who have had a tracheotomy for a condition not associated with infection. Steam tents are used, as are small cupolas over the cannula (Fig. 9-7), to deliver oxygen and moisture directly to the tracheotomy site.

Granulation tissue (Fig. 9-8) may form about the stoma and should be removed with biting forceps. The bleeding base should then be cauterized with a silver nitrate stick.

When the time comes to close the opening, a circumstance that depends on the condition for which the tracheotomy was done, it is usually best to block the tube with a rubber cork for 24 hours. During this time the cork should not be removed or the trachea suctioned. If the tracheotomy was done for laryngeal edema, for example, and mirror examination shows that the edema has completely subsided, a trial with the cork may not be necessary. The tube is removed, and tape is applied so as to fold the skin inward. Most tracheotomy openings heal in a few days or a week; rarely, a secondary operative closure is necessary. The neck heals very well, and there is rarely a cosmetic deformity.

COMMON ERRORS. Following are the common errors associated with routine tracheotomy:

1. The patient is not properly prepared psychologically for the procedure. A few minutes spent in explanation makes the entire procedure much smoother.
2. The operator begins the procedure hurriedly and without adequate assistance.
3. An intratracheal tube should have been passed but was not. This is especially important in cyanotic, poor-risk patients and in small children.
4. Bleeding vessels are not ligated before the trachea is opened, causing the blood to run into the patient's airway.
5. The assistant fails to guard against the patient's coughing out the tube.
6. The wound is closed too tightly, and emphysema results.

Emergency tracheotomy. Emergency tracheotomy is required less commonly than orderly, or routine, tracheotomy. It may be necessary to perform an emergency tracheotomy in the hospital emergency room, on the street, or even in the operating room if there should not be time to perform a routine procedure. Emergency tracheotomy is more difficult and more hazardous than routine tracheotomy. Complications are more frequent.

OPERATIVE TECHNIQUE. There are two ways to do an emergency tracheotomy. The *first* method is to follow the procedure for an orderly, or routine, tracheotomy but to omit the local anesthesia and work without assistants (and usually without adequate instruments), attempting to condense a 30-minute procedure into 30 seconds. When the tracheotomy is done low in the neck and the thyroid isthmus is cut,

Text continued on p. 141.

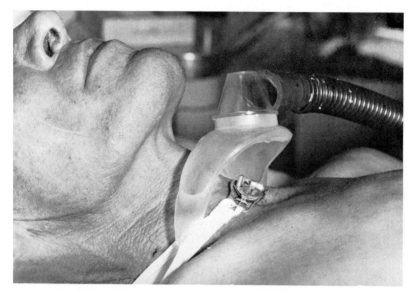

FIG. 9-7. Humidifier for tracheotomy. Here the cupola is lifted to show the tracheotomy tube in place.

FIG. 9-8. Granulation tissue may form around the tracheotomy stoma and needs to be removed. The base of the wound should be cauterized.

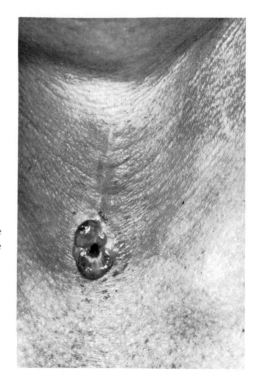

Tracheotomy Care

This information is to help you learn about your tracheotomy care.

These might be answers to some of your questions.

A tracheotomy is an artificial opening to the air passages (trachea) through the neck.

A tracheotomy tube (a short curved silver or plastic tube) is inserted into this opening.

The tracheotomy tube is composed of two parts: the outer and inner cannula.

Moist vapor mixed with oxygen will be administered through a mask positioned over your tracheotomy opening. This will keep the secretions in the air passages from drying. The mask should fit securely over the tracheotomy tube without pulling on the tube.

Moist vapor should be present on the inside of the mask and should be cool.

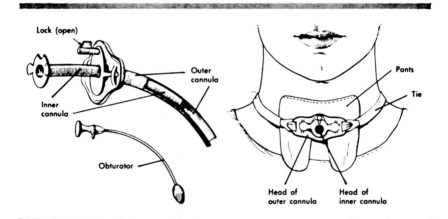

In case your tracheotomy tube becomes dislocated, the obturator tacked to the head of your bed will be used to correct the position of the tube.

Tracheotomy ties, pants and dressings are changed by the doctor unless he orders such in writing for the nurse. Additional dressings may be placed below the tracheotomy tube to collect secretions.

A pad and pencil will be left for you at your bedside to be used instead of speaking. Your doctor will tell you when you are ready to use your voice.

From Work, W. P., and Smith, M. F. W.: Postgrad. Med. 34:479, 1963.

Suctioning

1. CATHETERS

a. It is necessary to keep your air passages free of mucus or secretions.

b. Two sterile suction catheters will be provided. One is for suctioning the tracheotomy tube and one is for suctioning through the nose and mouth.

c. The use of two catheters is to protect against infection and therefore they should be kept separate.

2. CATHETER CARE

a. Bottles of solution are used for storing the catheters separately and for rinsing them.

b. The solutions and their placement in the bottle rack are arranged to keep them separate in order to prevent infection.

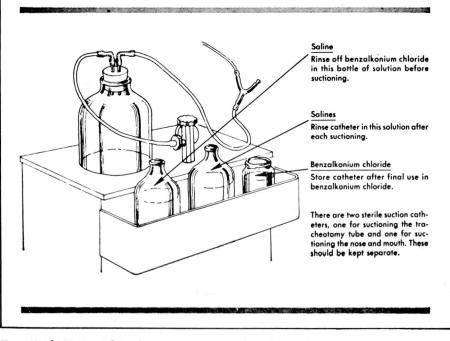

Saline
Rinse off benzalkonium chloride in this bottle of solution before suctioning.

Salines
Rinse catheter in this solution after each suctioning.

Benzalkonium chloride
Store catheter after final use in benzalkonium chloride.

There are two sterile suction catheters, one for suctioning the tracheotomy tube and one for suctioning the nose and mouth. These should be kept separate.

From Work, W. P., and Smith, M. F. W.: Postgrad. Med. 34:479, 1963.

Three Points to Remember About Suctioning

1. Wash hands before suctioning
2. Keep nasal catheter and tracheal catheter separate
3. Be gentle, very gentle, in suctioning

PROCEDURE:

1. Position the mirror so that you can see your tracheotomy.
2. Release lock on outer cannula in order to withdraw the inner cannula. (Plastic tracheotomy tubes do not have locks for the inner cannula. The inner cannula on this tube would just be withdrawn.)
   a. The inner cannula should not be left out for more than five minutes, as secretions will collect in outer cannula.

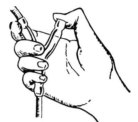

Step number 5

3. Suction the passageway of the outer cannula by passing the catheter to the end of the tube.
4. Begin suctioning only when the catheter is down.
5. After suction machine is turned on, place thumb over open end of glass tube to create suction.
6. Slowly withdraw the catheter, completely turning it, while at the same time suctioning the passageway.
7. The catheter should not be left in the trachea more than 20 seconds.
8. Repeat suction until passageway seems clear of mucus.
9. Cover bottles of solution with a towel when not in use.

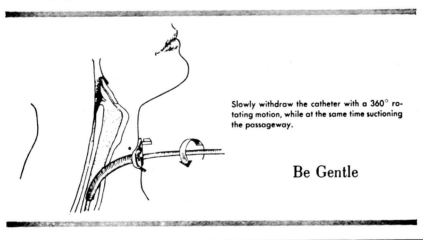

Slowly withdraw the catheter with a 360° rotating motion, while at the same time suctioning the passageway.

Be Gentle

From Work, W. P., and Smith, M. F. W.: Postgrad. Med. 34:479, 1963.

Cleaning the Inner Cannula of the Tracheotomy Tube

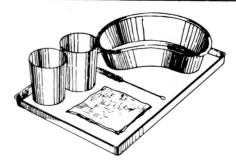

1. The inner cannula may be removed and placed into a cup of half hydrogen peroxide and half saline solution.
2. Place the cannula in emesis basin and, using this solution, scrub with a brush.
3. Rinse the inner cannula with normal saline.
4. Inspect the opening of the tube to see if the mucus is removed.
5. Shake to remove excess moisture. Gauze sponges may be used to remove excess secretions and solution after cleansing.
6. Inspect the opening of the tube once again to see that it is clear before it is inserted.
7. Reinsert into outer cannula. Fasten lock if you have a silver tracheotomy tube.

Home Care

Your doctor will tell you if you need to continue suctioning after your discharge from the hospital. If you do, this information may be helpful to you.

PROCEDURE:

1. The procedure for suctioning your trachea remains much the same as you have been doing in the hospital.
2. Saline is the only solution you will need at home. You should continue to rinse your catheter in this after each suctioning.
3. After final use, the catheter should be rinsed in cold water, then washed in warm water and soap. It should be kept clean for the next use.

EQUIPMENT:

1. A bottle of saline will be given to you. Saline is salt solution, and if more is needed you may make the solution by adding 2 teaspoonfuls salt to 1 qt. of boiled water. In order to keep the solution clean, it may be placed in the original saline bottle.
2. Suction machines may be obtained at a drugstore.
3. Funds to cover the cost of suction machines are available for some patients. Social Service maintains a list of agencies which provide funds. Among these is the American Cancer Society. Your physician may be consulted if you are eligible for this.

From Work, W. P., and Smith, M. F. W.: Postgrad. Med. 34:479, 1963.

there may be severe bleeding; also, there may be difficulty in finding the trachea, even in an adult.

The *second* method, which is better because there are clear landmarks above and below the incision site and relatively few blood vessels, is to make a midline stab incision *directly above the cricoid cartilage* (Fig. 9-2). This incision cuts through skin and the cricothyroid membrane. Immediately beneath the membrane is the airway.

This incision is actually above the trachea, but it is well under the level of the vocal cords, so that any laryngeal obstruction is bypassed. The incision may be a stab wound or a short transverse incision. Tissues are held apart with the fingers until an instrument such as a hemostat or a knife blade can be inserted and twisted sideways.

Later, with the airway established, the patient is removed to a hospital, where a routine tracheotomy can be done and the emergency incision closed. A tracheotomy tube is not left for an extended period through the cricothyroid membrane, because laryngeal stenosis may result. There is no aftereffect, however, if a tube is left in place for only 12 to 24 hours.

This procedure is known as cricothyrotomy. Recently this procedure has been used in non-emergency situations as a substitute for elective tracheotomy. Like tracheotomy, it is done with local anesthesia and usually with an endotracheal tube in place. There are now available several instruments for performing an *emergency* cricothyrotomy. These range from a large-bore, quarter-turn needle with an attached syringe to a specially designed "cricostat." The proper use of these instruments should be learned before working with them is attempted.

Complications of tracheotomy. Many complications are associated with tracheotomy, both in the actual performance of the operation and in the postoperative management. The operation is especially difficult in small children, and the complication rate is much greater in them than in adults. It is essential that the operation be done promptly when the indications develop. Undue delay on the surgeon's part increases both mortality and morbidity. The preliminary placement of an intratracheal tube may do as much as any one measure to reduce mortality during and immediately after the operation.

Among the operative complications are hemorrhage, pneumothorax, mediastinal emphysema, laceration of the esophagus, and death from asphyxia before the airway can be established. Probably all these complications can be avoided in almost every instance if a meticulous surgical technique is observed that includes absolute hemostasis, exact identification of all structures, and minimal dissection into tissue planes.

Postoperative complications are frequent. Subcutaneous emphysema is usually caused by excessively tight closure of the skin incision, but ordinarily this is not a serious matter. Plugged tubes can account for death, especially in infants and small children, in whom only a small tube can be placed. Atelectasis, pneumonitis, tracheal granuloma and stricture, hemorrhage, and wound infection have all been reported as causing death after a tracheotomy. In infants and children the cannula should be removed as soon as possible to help avoid the many problems encountered in late decannulations.

Removal of secretions, reduction in the ventilatory dead space, and circumvention of laryngeal and supraglottic obstruction all combine to wash out accumulated carbon dioxide. Sometimes there is profound and abrupt reversal of respiratory acidosis, resulting in arterial hypotension and arrythmias. The use of a cuffed tracheotomy tube (Fig. 9-9) will permit positive-pressure ventilation with oxygen and corrects the situation.

A serious, late complication of tracheotomy is tracheal stenosis. Fortunately this complication is becoming less frequent since the advent of plastic tubes with large, soft cuffs. The usual form of stenosis is firm scar tissue at the site of the tracheotomy tube. Treatment by means of repeated dilations may sometimes be successful, but it may require surgical resection of the stenosis and reanastamosis of the transected trachea.

THE CUFFED TUBE. Inflating a cuff about a tracheotomy tube has become a popular way of controlling secretions that trickle down the trachea and of affording an easy method of positive-pressure breathing. Unfortunately, numerous complications can result from the use of an inflated cuff—such as erosion of the tracheal mucosa (sometimes to the point of producing a tracheoesophageal fistula), stenosis, and infection. Mechanical complications include slippage

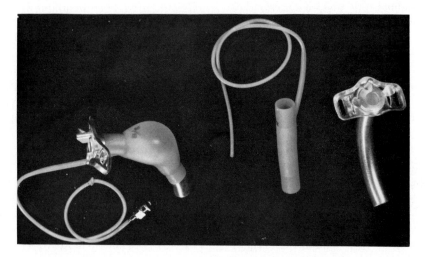

FIG. 9-9. Cuffed tracheotomy tube permits positive-pressure ventilation.

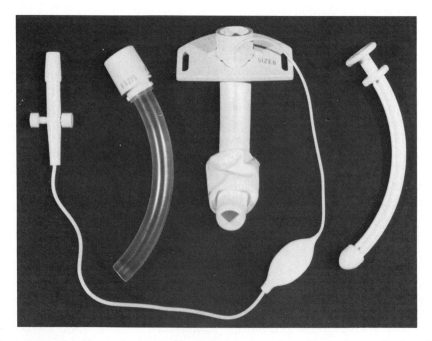

FIG. 9-10. Disposable tracheotomy tube with low-pressure cuff to reduce risk of tracheal stenosis due to local ischemia.

of the cuff over the end of the tube and narrowing of the tube during inflation. The cuff, which should be deflated at regular intervals, should be used only when definitely needed. A low-pressure cuff may be used to reduce the risk of some complications (Fig. 9-10).

Instruction of patients. A simple explanation of tracheotomy and its care that can be given to patients is presented on pp. 137 to 140. This material was prepared by Walter P. Work, M.D., and Mansfield F.W. Smith, M.D., University Hospital, Ann Arbor, Michigan.

SELECTED READINGS

Baker, D.G., Jr., and Savetsky, L.: Decannulations problems in infants, Ann. Otol. Rhinol. Laryngol. **81:**555, 1972.

Bass, J.W.: Routine tracheotomy for epiglottitis; what are the odds? J. Pediatr. **83:**510, 1973.

Brantigan, C.O.: Delayed major vessel hemorrhage following tracheostomy, J. Trauma **13:**235, 1973.

Chew, J.Y., and Cantrell, R.W.: Tracheostomy; complications and their management, Arch. Otolaryngol. **96:**538, 1972.

Cohen, S.R., and Chai, J.: Epiglottitis: twenty-year study with tracheotomy, Ann. Otol. Rhinol. Laryngol. **87:**461-467, July-August, 1978.

Gaudet, P.T., and others: Pediatric tracheostomy and associated complications, Laryngoscope **88:**1633-1641, October, 1978.

Haller, A.J., Jr., and Talbert, J.L.: Clinical evaluation of a new Silastic tracheostomy tube for respiratory support of infants and young children, Ann. Surg. **171:**915, 1970.

Hardy, K.L.: Tracheostomy; indications, technics, and tubes, Am. J. Surg. **126:**300, 1973.

Magovern, G.J., and others: The clinical and experimental evaluation of a controlled-pressure intratracheal cuff, J. Thorac. Cardiovasc. Surg. **64:**747, 1972.

Margolis, C.Z., Ingram, D.L., and Meyer, J.H.: Routine tracheotomy in Hemophilus influenzae type B epiglottitis, J. Pediatr. **81:**1150, 1972.

Pickard, R.E., and Oropeza, G.: Tracheotomy in premature infants, Laryngoscope **81:**418, 1971.

Rabuzzi, D.D., and Reed, G.F.: Intrathoracic complications following tracheotomy in children. Laryngoscope **81:**939, 1971.

Snow, J.B., Jr., and Preston, W.J.: Dry, aseptic method of tracheotomy care, Arch. Otolaryngol. **92:**191, 1970.

Toremalm, N.G.: The pathophysiology of tracheotomy, Laryngoscope **82:**265, 1972.

Utley, J.R., and others: Definitive management of innominate artery hemorrhage complicating tracheostomy, J.A.M.A. **220:**577, 1972.

Westgate, H.D., and Roux, K.L., Jr.: Tracheal stenosis following tracheostomy; incidence and predisposing factors, Anesth. Analg. **49:**393, 1970.

10 ENDOSCOPY, DIAGNOSTIC PROBLEMS, AND FOREIGN BODIES OF THE TRACHEA AND BRONCHI

ENDOSCOPY

Symptoms and signs often requiring diagnosis by endoscopy are hoarseness, persistent cough, hemoptysis, unexplained chest lesions demonstrated by roentgenograms, atelectasis, recurrent asthma, dysphagia, and upper gastrointestinal bleeding with hematemesis. Conditions requiring treatment by endoscopy include benign neoplasms, ulcers, strictures, chronic infection, and foreign bodies.

After the history has been taken, the physical examination has been completed, and roentgenograms have been made, there are many patients in whom the exact diagnosis cannot be established or in whom there is a justifiable doubt as to which of two or three conditions may be the cause of symptoms. In such patients the most accurate information can usually be obtained by direct visualization of the larynx, trachea, bronchi, or esophagus. Direct visualization of these structures is given the general designation of "endoscopy" or "peroral endoscopy." The individual examination is referred to by the particular structure it visualizes—that is, bronchoscopy, esophagoscopy, or direct laryngoscopy.

Although the instruments for the various examinations differ somewhat, all are designed to meet basic requirements. Each is a hollow metal tube with a distal light source that illuminates the area just beyond the end of the instrument. The instruments are of various sizes and shapes (round, oval, short, long) to accommodate the specific orifice to be entered and the size of the patient (Figs. 10-1 and 10-2). For example, a bronchoscope used for infants may

have a diameter of only 3 mm., whereas an esophagoscope for adults may be 10 to 15 mm. in its widest diameter. The length of the instruments varies from 20 to 50 cm.

In recent years several new diagnostic endoscopes have been developed. The use of fiberoptic illumination makes possible visualization around corners and through small-diameter endoscopes of various kinds. The flexible bronchoscope, inserted through the nose and guided into the trachea, has become a valuable diagnostic instrument. Similarly, the flexible gastroscope allows the physician to examine and see the esophagus, stomach, duodenum and upper gastrointestinal tract. Biopsies and other specimens can be obtained for culture and for tissue examination.

Either local or general anesthesia may be used for endoscopic examination. Except in special situations, endoscopy is performed with the patient under local anesthesia (in adults) or under general anesthesia (in children).

Regardless of the method of anesthesia, the patient to be examined is usually placed in the supine position with the head beyond the end of the examining table. The head is supported by an assistant, who flexes, extends, or rotates it into various positions during the examination. A second assistant handles suction apparatus and other instruments, which are passed to the examining endoscopist as needed. The endoscopist is able to visualize strictures, tumors, ulcers, foreign bodies, and other abnormalities. He may collect secretions for study with special suction tubes. He may remove tissue for biopsy. Or he may completely remove benign lesions

144

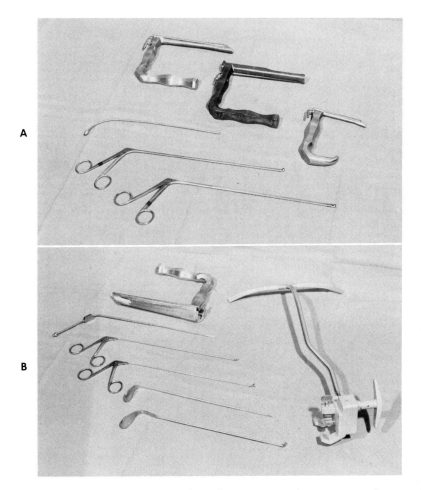

FIG. 10-1. A, Standard instruments for direct laryngoscopy. Three types are shown, including an infant size. Suction and biopsy forceps are shown below the laryngoscopes. **B,** Instruments for suspension laryngoscopy. *Upper left,* Jako laryngoscope. *Right,* Laryngoscope self-retainer. This instrument allows the operating surgeon to use both hands for instrumentation. *Lower left,* Microlaryngoscopic instruments.

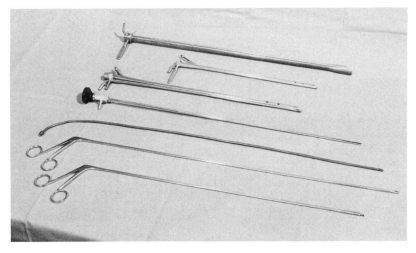

FIG. 10-2. Instruments for bronchoscopy and esophagoscopy. *Top to bottom,* Esophagoscope, small bronchoscope, adult-size bronchoscope, telescope, metal suction tube, cup biting or biopsy forceps, and square-ended basket biopsy forceps.

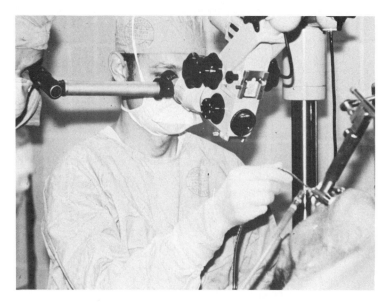

FIG. 10-3. Laryngoscopy using the operating microscope to provide both illumination and magnification. The laryngoscope is self-retaining.

or foreign bodies. Specially designed instruments are available to aid in all these procedures.

The instruments are used not only to obtain diagnostic information but also to carry out therapeutic measures in certain conditions.

Another method of direct laryngoscopy is by use of the so-called *suspension laryngoscope.* The patient is positioned supine as for any direct laryngoscopy, but an attachment is placed to hold the laryngoscope and thus free both of the examiner's hands. More and more popular in conjunction with suspension laryngoscopy is the use of the operating microscope to provide magnification and binocular vision (Fig. 10-3).

Anatomy. The trachea is a hollow tube supported by cartilaginous rings that are incomplete posteriorly. It is lined by ciliated respiratory epithelium. The superior opening is protected by the glottis (vocal cords, Fig. 10-4). The posterior wall is a "party" wall contiguous with the anterior wall of the esophagus. At the bifurcation of the trachea is a ridge, known as the carina, which separates the orifices of the right and left main bronchi. The carina forms a lanamark for the endoscopist when he is examining the trachea and bronchi (Fig. 10-5).

The right and left main bronchi are approximately of the same diameter. The right main

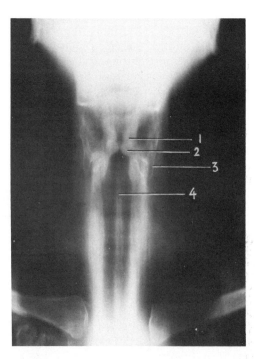

FIG. 10-4. Normal laminagram. *1,* False cord. *2,* True cord. *3,* Thyroid cartilage. *4,* Tracheal air column.

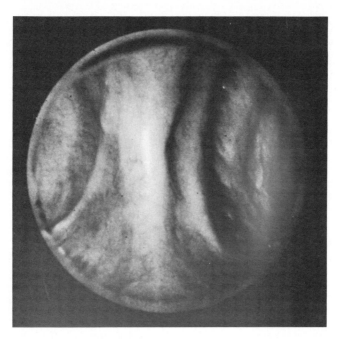

FIG. 10-5. Normal carina as seen through a bronchoscope. (Courtesy Dr. Paul Holinger, Chicago, Ill.)

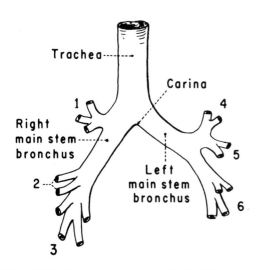

FIG. 10-6. Trachea and bronchi. *1,* Right upper lobe secondary bronchi. *2,* Right middle lobe secondary bronchi. *3,* Right lower lobe secondary bronchi. *4,* Left upper lobe apical bronchi. *5,* Left upper lingular bronchi. *6,* Left lower lobe secondary bronchi.

bronchus leaves the trachea at an obtuse angle, and the left main bronchus forms a less obtuse angle with the trachea (Fig. 10-6). For this reason aspirated secretions or foreign bodies more easily enter the right main bronchus than the left main bronchus.

Both the right and left lower lobe bronchi leave their respective main bronchi in almost a straight line. The right middle lobe bronchus is directed almost horizontally across the chest. Both upper lobe bronchi leave their respective main bronchi at a sharp angle. This anatomic relationship makes examination of the lower lobe bronchi and the right middle lobe bronchus easier than examination of the upper lobe bronchi.

In adults the diameters of the trachea and of the right and left main bronchi are large enough to permit examination with a bronchoscope up to 9 mm. in diameter. In infants and small children instruments as small as 3 mm. in diameter may be required.

Anesthesia. Intratracheal anesthesia by means of any accepted anesthetic agent can be used for esophagoscopy but obviously cannot be used for bronchoscopy. A combination of thiopental (Pentothal) sodium, topical anesthetic, and drugs producing temporary paralysis of muscles may be used. This combination is most

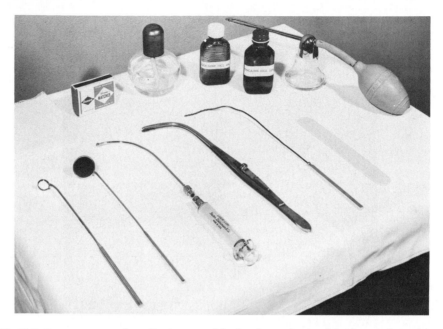

FIG. 10-7. Instruments and medications used for local anesthesia of the larynx, bronchi, and esophagus. *Top row,* Gauze to hold tongue, matches, alcohol burner, cocaine, and spray bottle. *Bottom row,* Small and large laryngeal mirrors, syringe and curved cannula, curved forceps for cotton, curved cotton carrier, and tongue blade.

often employed in patients undergoing procedures that require only a few moments (such as removal of a single polyp from the larynx). However, the use of this combination for prolonged endoscopic procedures can be dangerous.

Local anesthesia is used for diagnostic endoscopic procedures and also for therapeutic procedures when possible. Local anesthesia is accomplished as follows (Fig. 10-7):

1. The patient is first given a barbiturate, a narcotic, and atropine.
2. The throat is sprayed with a 4% to 5% cocaine solution or with a 0.5% to 1% tetracaine (Pontocaine) solution. Cocaine has the wider margin of safety. In either instance, the patient is warned not to swallow the solution but, instead, to hold it in the throat for a few moments and then spit it out. This may be repeated three to five times or until the throat begins to feel numb.
3. With curved forceps or a curved cotton carrier, a stronger solution (usually 10% cocaine) is painted over the surface of the hypopharynx, the base of the tongue, and the epiglottis. A similar cotton applicator,

moistened in the anesthetic solution, is placed in the pyriform fossa (Fig. 10-8) on each side of the larynx and held in place for a minute. The topical anesthetic is absorbed through the mucosa of the pyriform fossa and blocks the superior laryngeal nerve as it passes just beneath the mucosa in this area. Another excellent topical anesthetic is 10% lidocaine (Xylocaine), available as a dental preparation in a spray bottle.

4. If bronchoscopy is to be done, a few drops of topical anesthetic are instilled through the vocal cords by means of a curved cannula. The patient is told to suppress his cough at first and then to cough out the residual anesthetic.

The procedure outlined produces good anesthesia, abolishes the gag reflex, and allows inspection of the esophagus, larynx, or bronchi with minimal or no coughing. The anesthesia will last 30 to 60 minutes, after which time normal sensation returns.

Another method of obtaining anesthesia of the larynx is by the injection of 1% Xylocaine through the skin of the neck, laterally, at the level of the thyrohyoid space (Fig. 10-9). It is

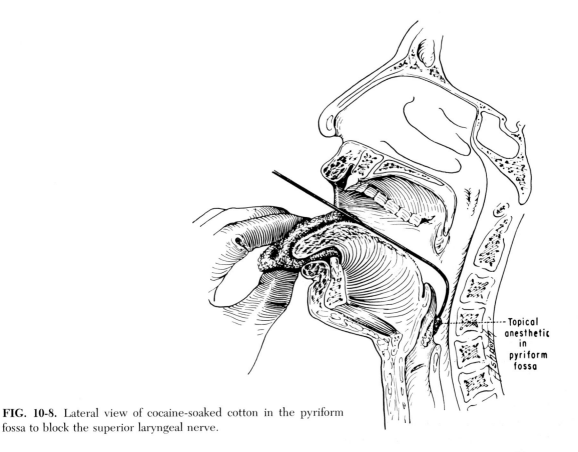

FIG. 10-8. Lateral view of cocaine-soaked cotton in the pyriform fossa to block the superior laryngeal nerve.

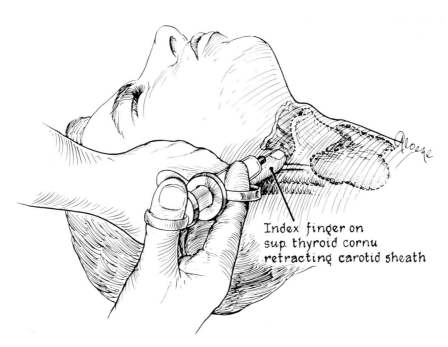

FIG. 10-9. One method of inducing laryngeal anesthesia: external block of the superior laryngeal nerve by injection through the thyrohyoid membrane. (From Gaskill, J.R., and Gillies, D.R.: Arch. Otolaryngol. **84:**654, 1966.)

here that the superior laryngeal nerve enters the larynx. This injection, done bilaterally, combined with a spray of cocaine or Pontocaine in the throat, produces excellent anesthesia.

After adequate anesthesia has been produced, direct examination of the larynx, bronchi, or esophagus should be done carefully and without haste.

Direct laryngoscopy. To make a direct examination of the larynx, the endoscopist stands above the head of the supine patient. A laryngoscope is introduced into the patient's mouth over the tongue. The tongue is raised with the instrument, the patient's neck is slowly extended, and the laryngoscope is passed carefully over the posterior face of the epiglottis and raised to expose the vocal cords.

Bronchoscopy. For examination of the trachea and bronchi a brochoscope can be inserted directly, or the bronchoscope can be introduced through a previously placed laryngoscope, which is removed after the bronchoscope has been introduced. Gentle pressure with the tip of the bronchoscope will slip it past the vocal cords and into the trachea. After examination of the trachea the bronchoscope is passed downward to the carina (Fig. 10-10). Each main bronchus and the secondary bronchi are then examined. Suction is used when necessary, and secretions or tissue is removed for study. When carcinoma is suspected but is not visible, secretions can be collected and stained by the Papnicolaou method. Positive diagnosis can be made by this technique in about 30% of patients.

Within the past few years a fiberoptic bronchoscope has been introduced. The flexibility of the tip of this bronchoscope makes it possible to visualize more adequately the second- and third-order bronchi. Biopsy specimens can be obtained from areas previously inaccessible. Bronchial brushing with a firm fiber brush on a flexible handle may also increase diagnostic accuracy by removing small amounts of surface tissue for pathologic study.

Bronchoscopy is usually done with the patient in the supine position. There are patients, however, who find it difficult to breathe while lying down. Bronchoscopy may then be done with the patient sitting up, and may even be done as a bedside procedure in exceptional cases.

Esophagoscopy. The esophagus is examined with an esophagoscope. This instrument is usu-

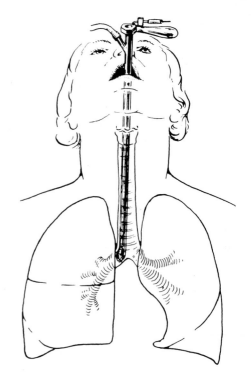

FIG. 10-10. Bronchoscope in place just beyond the carina in the right main bronchus.

ally somewhat larger in diameter than a bronchoscope and has rounded distal edges that prevent trauma to the esophageal mucosa. The esophagoscope is passed carefully beyond the epiglottis and then past the posterior margin of the larynx. The larynx is firmly raised to visualize the constriction of the esophageal inlet formed by the cricopharyngeus muscle. The esophagoscope is then pressed gently against this constriction, and when relaxation of the cricopharyngeus muscle occurs (usually with inspiration), the esophagoscope is passed into the esophagus. The entire length of the esophagus is examined; and when possible, the stomach is entered. Experience and gentleness are necessary during examination of the esophagus, since the procedure is inherently a dangerous one. Spasm of the inlet should not be forced, since perforation of the esophagus may result from improper introduction of the instrument, particularly when elderly or debilitated patients are examined.

Bronchography. Adequate diagnosis of pulmonary and tracheobronchial disease requires proper interpretation of all diagnostic findings. History, physical examination of the chest, and

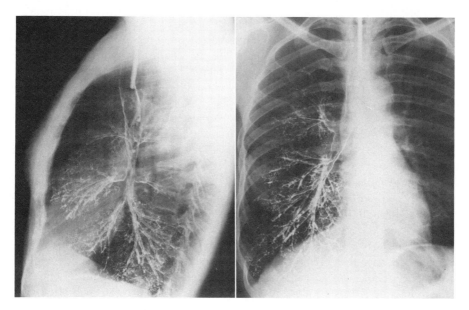

FIG. 10-11. Normal bronchogram of the right lung, lateral and anteroposterior views. Note the tube in the trachea for the instillation of the opaque medium.

roentgenography are the common means used in making the diagnosis. Ordinary roentgenograms of the chest are valuable because of the information they give regarding the parenchyma of the lungs. However, they do not visualize lesions of the bronchi very well. Bronchoscopic examination may reveal additional necessary information. If additional information is needed, radiopaque oil can be introduced into the trachea to outline the walls of the trachea and bronchi. This technique, called bronchography, outlines the smallest bronchioles. It aids in determining the extent of dilation of the bronchi in bronchiectasis and helps in locating bronchial tumors. The procedure is done as follows:

1. The pharynx, larynx, trachea, and bronchi are anesthetized with a local anesthetic as described previously in this chapter, in the discussion of endoscopy.

2. A rubber catheter is inserted through the nose, passed into the pharynx, and guided between the vocal cords into the trachea.

3. Under fluoroscopic guidance, radiopaque oil, such as Lipiodol, is injected through the catheter.

4. When adequate filling of one or both bronchial systems has been accomplished, roentgenograms are taken (Fig. 10-11).

DIAGNOSTIC PROBLEMS

Conditions such as hemoptysis, bronchogenic carcinoma, bronchial adenoma, bronchiectasis, atelectasis and chronic suppurative bronchitis present diagnostic problems.

Hemoptysis. Bleeding from the trachea, bronchi, or alveoli of the lung often presents a diagnostic problem. It is not always clear whether blood appearing in the mouth is coughed up or whether it comes from some part of the upper respiratory tract. It is essential for the physician to determine the exact source of bleeding, if possible. Even when roentgenograms reveal an obvious tumor or tuberculosis, the extent of the disease or the precise cause of the bleeding cannot be determined until bronchoscopy is done. Definitive treatment may depend on knowledge of the extent of the involvement of the mucosal surface of the tracheobronchial tree, regardless of the extent of the parenchymal involvement demonstrated by the roentgenogram. Bronchoscopy is therefore desirable in all patients with hemoptysis.

Bronchogenic carcinoma. The alarming increase in malignancy of the lung or bronchi in the past 35 years has magnified the importance of early and adequate diagnostic measures. Often a roentgenogram of the chest taken for other reasons shows a shadow in the lung that cannot be explained without further examination. Such unexplained shadows require further investigation of the tracheobronchial system by bronchoscopy. A small tumor of a bronchus may be visualized and the diagnosis established by biopsy in time to allow successful removal of the involved lobe or of the entire lung. The likelihood of cure of carcinoma of the lung or bronchus depends on the size and location of the lesion.

If direct visualization of the bronchi with the rigid bronchoscope does not reveal a lesion when one is suspected, a *bronchoscopic telescope* is inserted through the bronchoscope. The telescope is made like an elongated cystoscope and has a lens system that allows visualization at angles. Lesions that are not visible through the bronchoscope can sometimes be seen with the telescope. Also of value in this situation is use of the flexible fiberoptic bronchoscope, discussed earlier.

If none of these instruments discloses a suspected lesion, washing of the bronchi with saline solution may dislodge tumor cells. The solution containing the cells can be centrifuged and the sediment examined after staining. By this method the number of early diagnoses is increased, and the percentage of cures is raised.

Bronchial adenoma. The differentiation between bronchogenic carcinoma and bronchial adenoma is important. When detected early, bronchial adenoma is potentially benign and can sometimes be cured by removal through the bronchoscope. Lobectomy or pneumonectomy may be necessary to remove an adenoma, but the choice of procedure must be made after bronchoscopic examination.

Bronchiectasis. Bronchiectasis of one or more lobes of the lung causes chronic debility that is difficult to treat adequately without mechanical or surgical measures. Recurring segmental atelectasis is common in bronchiestasis and, when not relieved, contributes to the spread of bronchiectasis. Purulent secretions that cannot be raised by voluntary coughing or by postural drainage can be removed through the bronchoscope, a procedure that improves aeration of the lung. As a result, medication introduced into the bronchi directly through the bronchoscope or by inhalation becomes more effective.

Atelectasis. Major or minor bronchi can become plugged with mucus or partially obstructed by swelling of the bronchial mucosa. After upper abdominal operations the motion of the diaphragm can be restricted because of pain. This may cause stasis of the normal bronchial secretions, which then plug a bronchus. Any of these obstructions, as well as foreign bodies, may produce atelectasis of one lobe of the lung or of the entire right or left lung, depending on which bronchus is plugged (Fig. 10-12).

When atelectasis is present, the classical signs of dull percussion, absent breath sounds, and sometimes mediastinal shift are present. If the atelectasis involves the entire lung or more than one lobe, the patient is often apprehensive, perspires freely, and has a sharp rise in fever. The most important finding, however, is tachycardia. The pulse rate will often remain at 120 to 140 beats per second.

If forced coughing or tracheal suction does not relieve the atelectasis, such patients should undergo bronchoscopy for removal of the obstructing plug. Relief is often dramatic.

Chronic suppurative bronchitis. Chronic purulent infection of the tracheobronchial tree, with or without bronchiectasis, requires both antibacterial therapy and good drainage. Control of infection reduces edema and congestion and therefore enhances drainage. Cultures of bronchial secretions are necessary but do not always reveal all pathogens. Both aerobic and anaerobic techniques should be used. Eosinophils in clumps, which are characteristic of allergy, may appear to be pus cells. Consequently, Wright's stain must be used to identify the eosinophils.

Penicillin usually is the drug of choice for treatment. It has predictable effectiveness against *Diplococcus pneumoniae* and certain of the important anaerobes. In high concentration it is also effective against *Haemophilus influenzae*. Most important, however, selection of an antibiotic should be based on careful culture and sensitivity studies.

Effective bactericidal blood levels cannot always be maintained with the use of oral or procaine penicillin. Intravenous administration of penicillin is more reliable. *Aerosol* penicillin is less likely to give an effective bactericidal blood level and is more likely to produce penicillin sensitivity than either the procaine or the aqueous varieties. A combination of peni-

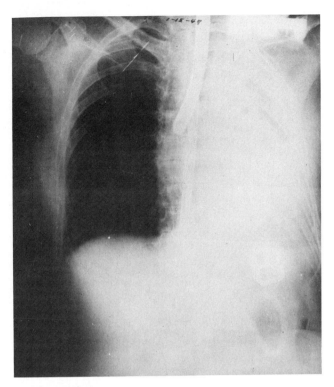

FIG. 10-12. Atelectasis of the left lung caused by an intratracheal anesthetic tube inserted too far. The tube is in the right main bronchus, blocking the left. Atelectasis was relieved by bronchoscopic aspiration.

cillin and tetracycline may be necessary for control of the infection. Sulfonamides may be used when indicated.

Chloramphenicol and streptomycin therapy may be used in resistant infections (after bacterial sensitivity tests). These drugs have toxic side effects, however, and should be reserved for patients with resistant infections.

Tetracycline drugs may be used in prophylactic doses in some instances to prevent recurrences. Most people will tolerate prolonged low dosage of tetracycline without overgrowth of resistant bacteria or of fungi.

In the past few years it has been recognized that there are several antibody-deficiency syndromes and that these conditions predispose the patient to frequent upper and lower respiratory tract infection. If a child has either congenital or acquired hypogammaglobulinemia and is not treated, he may develop progressive bronchiectasis and may die later of pulmonary complications even if he survives multiple acute infections. Many such children are

also atopic and need careful attention to possible allergic sensitizers as well as control of infection.

Whenever chronic or frequently recurrent upper and lower respiratory system disease is encountered, the physician should be constantly aware of the possibility of a systemic defect—in particular, antibody deficiency, cystic fibrosis, metabolic insufficiency, or allergy.

FOREIGN BODIES

Foreign bodies of many kinds can enter the trachea or bronchi. Aspiration of stomach contents during anesthesia or when the protective cough reflex is dulled by alcoholic stupor may lead to immediate asphyxiation or atelectasis. Large foreign bodies may cause complete obstruction of the trachea, usually leading to death.

Most cases involving foreign bodies in the bronchi occur in children who suddenly inspire when they have foreign bodies in their mouths. Vegetable foreign bodies, such as beans, peanuts, carrots, or corn, may be aspirated and

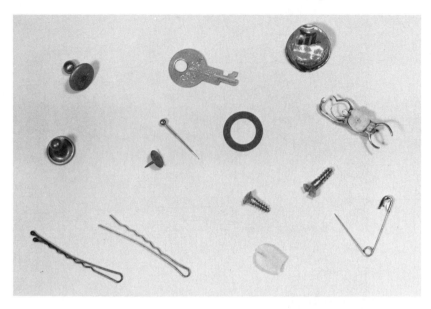

FIG. 10-13. Various foreign bodies removed from the bronchi and esophagus. At lower right is half a peanut, a common and serious foreign body found in children.

lodge in a main or secondary bronchus. Peanuts are so dangerous as foreign bodies that they should never be given to young children. During removal they tend to crumble or split, and a case that started as a single foreign body suddenly becomes one of multiple foreign bodies. Other commonly aspirated foreign bodies are nails, bobby pins, screws, thumbtacks, and other small metallic objects (Fig. 10-13).

The characteristic symptoms of a foreign body in the bronchus are (1) recurrent spasmodic cough with periods of quiescence between spasms; (2) an audible wheeze, usually heard during both inspiration and expiration; and (3) increasing dyspnea. Often the characteristic wheeze can be heard by listening to the breath sounds with the unaided ear held against the chest or in front of the open lips. The wheeze is loud when the chest is examined with a stethoscope.

In almost every patient a careful history will elicit an account of the episode of *sudden coughing and choking* that marked the moment of aspiration. After such an episode there is often a delay of several hours and sometimes of several days before the typical triad of symptoms becomes evident. Some small metallic foreign bodies may remain in the bronchus for months or years and cause only a small area of asymptomatic atelectasis. They may be seen incidentally when a roentgenogram of the chest is taken for some other reason or when there is a mild recurrent cough.

In addition to the usual signs of increased rate of respiration and an audible wheeze, characteristic signs are elicited by auscultation and percussion of the chest. The chest findings vary according to the type of bronchial obstruction present. If the foreign body has caused complete blockage of a main or lobular bronchus, *atelectasis* is produced. In this situation there will be decreased or absent breath tones and dullness to percussion over the involved lung area. If the atelectasis involves an entire lung, there will be a mediastinal shift toward the obstructed side. In many instances of partial obstruction from a vegetable foreign body, air can enter the bronchus but is prevented from leaving it by the ball-valve action of the foreign body. This produces *obstructive emphysema* of the involved lung segment; breath sounds are distant or may be absent. Percussion shows hyperresonance on the affected side and a mediastinal shift to the opposite side (Fig. 10-14).

When a ball-valve blockage in a main bronchus produces obstructive emphysema, signs of dyspnea begin early and may require prompt

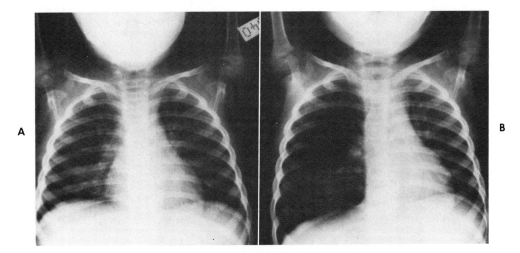

FIG. 10-14. Roentgenograms, made during inspiration and expiration, typical of obstructive emphysema of the right lung. **A,** Film made during inspiration. Note that this is almost normal, with a nonopaque foreign body. **B,** Film made during expiration. Note overaeration of the right lung, depression of the right diaphragm, and mediastinal shift to the left.

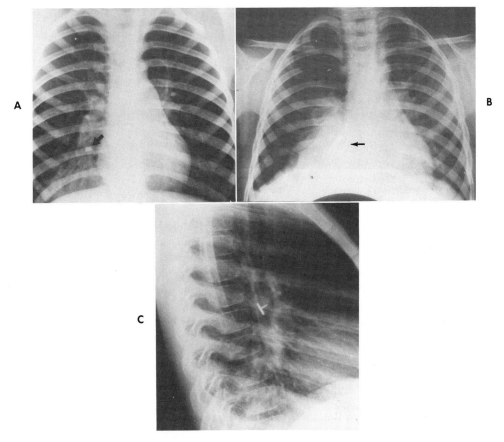

FIG. 10-15. Opaque foreign bodies in the bronchi. **A,** Arrow points to a tooth in the right main stem bronchus. **B,** A screw in the right main stem bronchus, partially obscured by surrounding inflammatory response. **C,** Lateral view of a thumbtack in the bronchus.

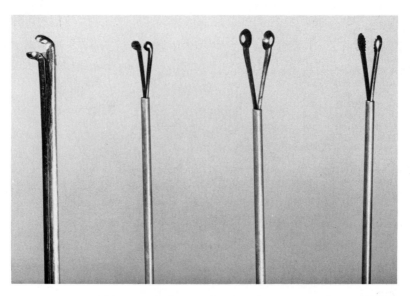

FIG. 10-16. Various tips of forceps used to remove foreign bodies. Refer to Fig. 10-2 for a full view of forceps and other instruments for bronchoscopy and esophagoscopy.

treatment to prevent death from asphyxia. The emphysematous lung is underaerated, and the mediastinal shift to the opposite side may compress the uninvolved lung enough to cause cyanosis and even death. Cyanosis is always a grave sign and demands prompt treatment.

Opaque foreign bodies are visible in chest roentgenograms in most instances (Fig. 10-15). When atelectasis is present, the cardinal sign in the roentgenogram is clouding of the atelectatic segment. If an entire lung is atelectatic, narrowing of the interspaces between the ribs and an elevated diaphragm on the involved side are additional signs. The mediastinum is shifted to the involved side. When an obstructive emphysema is present, the involved lung is overaerated and the mediastinum is shifted to the opposite side. Mediastinal shift, regardless of its direction, can often be seen more easily by fluoroscopy than in a single roentgenogram. For this reason it is best to request that *roentgenograms* be taken during both *inspiration* and *expiration* when a foreign body in the bronchus is suspected. In atelectasis the mediastinal shift is seen in the *inspiratory* view, when the uninvolved lung is full of air. In obstructive emphysema the shift is toward the uninvolved side during the *expiratory* phase, when the lung is partially empty.

Foreign bodies of the bronchi must be removed through a bronchoscope. In infants and small children bronchoscopy is done without anesthesia if unusual respiratory embrarrassment is already present. Oxygen must always be available, since the instrumentation necessary may cause further reduction of the airway. Many specially designed instruments are available for the removal of different types of foreign bodies (Fig. 10-16).

During bronchoscopy in a small child it is necessary to observe the child's general condition closely. When there has been underaeration of the lung for any length of time, an extra burden is put on the heart. The pulse rate is high. Cardiac collapse can occur if too much additional cardiac effort is needed. On occasion it is necessary to discontinue attempts to remove a foreign body when the procedure is prolonged. A later attempt, made after the child has been given a period of rest to compensate for lack of oxygen, may ensure a safer procedure.

After months or years sharp metallic foreign bodies may erode a bronchus and enter the lung parenchyma to produce a lung abscess. When this occurs, the abscess must be drained and the foreign body removed by a transthoracic approach.

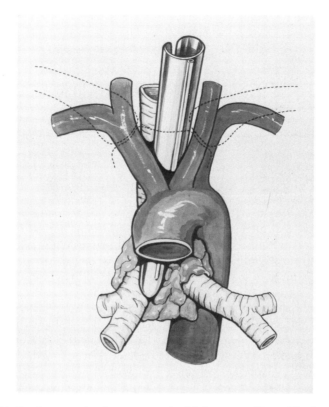

FIG. 10-17. Mediastinoscope in place near tracheal bifurcation. (From Ward, P., Stephenson, S., Jr., and Harris, P.: Ann. Otol. Rhinol. Laryngol. **75:**368, 1966.)

MEDIASTINOSCOPY

The superior mediastinum may be inspected rather easily and material obtained for examination by the pathologist through the technique of mediastinoscopy (Fig. 10-17). An instrument like a laryngoscope is inserted through an incision in the skin immediately above the sternum and advanced along a previously dissected tract made by blunt dissection downward to the level of the tracheal bifurcation.

The technique is safe when done correctly. One must be careful that the dissection downward into the mediastinum stays always on the anterior wall of the trachea; and before a biopsy is made, aspiration should always be done to make certain that the tissue to be sampled is not the wall of a major vessel. Mediastinoscopy will obviate the need for open biopsy of the chest, at least in some cases.

SELECTED READINGS

Davison, F.W.: Chronic sinus and bronchopulmonary disease, Minn. Med. **50:**855, 1967.

Heroy, J.H., and others: Airway management in the premature infant, Ann. Otol. Rhinol. Laryngol. **87:**53-59, 1978.

Jackson, C.L., and Diamond, S.: Haemorrhage from the trachea, bronchi, and lungs of nontuberculous origin, Ann. Rev. Tuberc. **46:**126, 1942.

Lundgren, J., and others: Toluidine blue: an aid in microlaryngoscopic diagnosis of glottic lesions? Arch. Otolaryngol. **105**(4):169-174, 1979.

March, B.R., and others: Flexible fiberoptic bronchoscopy; its place in the search for lung cancer, Ann. Otol. Rhinol. Laryngol. **82:**757, 1973.

Montgomery, W.W.: Endoscopy and surgery of the larynx and trachea, Radiol. Clin. North Am. **16**(2):219-226, 1978.

Norris, C.M.: Early clinical features of bronchogenic carcinoma, Dis. Chest. **14:**198, 1948.

Richards, L.G.: Vegetal foreign bodies in the bronchi, Ann. Otol. Rhinol. Laryngol. **50:**860, 1941.

Teirstein, A.S., and others: Flexible bronchoscopy in nonvisualized carcinoma of the lung, Ann. Otol. Rhinol. Laryngol. **87:**318-321, 1978.

Weaver, A., and others: Triple endoscopy: a neglected essential in head and neck cancer, Surgery **86**(3):493-496, 1979.

11 DISEASES OF THE ESOPHAGUS

Esophageal disease is indicated by one or more of the following symptoms: *dysphagia, pain during swallowing, regurgitation of undigested food, complete inability to swallow*, and *hematemesis*. Often, in the early stages of esophageal disease the patient complains only of a vague feeling of a "lump in the throat" with no pain or dysphagia. Although this symptom can be caused by tension or emotional upset, it must be investigated thoroughly to rule out organic esophageal disease. (See the discussion of globus hystericus, p. 163.)

When a history is obtained that raises suspicion of esophageal disease, proper roentgenograms must be taken prior to endoscopy. In addition to intrinsic disease of the esophagus, older patients may have sharp osteophytes of the cervical spine that can complicate the procedure of esophagoscopy, and preoperative knowledge of their presence is helpful. The roentgenograms required are anteroposterior and lateral views of the chest, a lateral view of the soft tissue of the cervical region with the head in hyperextension, and fluoroscopic views of the esophagus. Fluoroscopic examination is important because the rate and method of advance of the contrast medium can be followed. Often such an examination demonstrates a disturbance that may not show on the roentgenogram after the contrast medium has passed. Thin barium is most often used as a contrast medium. When the presence of a foreign body is suspected, it may be helpful to have the patient swallow small pieces of cotton coated with barium. If the cotton hesitates at some point in the esophagus, a foreign body may be detected that would otherwise be invisible. Whenever there is danger of aspiration, and almost always in children, Lipiodol should be used as the contrast medium. Lipiodol is easily coughed up from the lungs if it is aspirated, whereas barium cannot be coughed up from the tracheobronchial tree and may cause irreparable damage or even death.

The use of the cinefluoroscope in recent years has made it possible to obtain a moving picture of normal and abnormal swallowing with or without contrast media. Filmstrips can be developed that are much superior to single-spot films in many conditions. In addition, the use of an image intensifier gives excellent contrast as well as some magnification of specific areas of the esophagus, and it can be used to visualize more adequately the passage of contrast media throughout the entire esophagus.

After the roentgenograms have been studied, esophagoscopy is usually indicated to complete the diagnostic study.

Congenital abnormalities. Like other parts of the body, the esophagus may be abnormal at birth. Atresia of the esophagus and web formation are such anomalies.

ESOPHAGEAL ATRESIA. Infants may be born with an atretic esophagus that may or may not be associated with a tracheoesophageal fistula. When the upper esophagus ends in a blind pouch, the infant regurgitates all food, chokes, becomes dyspneic, and may die in a few days if atresia is not suspected. Any infant with these symptoms in the first few days of life should be examined immediately for the possibility of atresia.

An attempt to pass a tube into the stomach will be unsuccessful in the infant with esophageal atresia. If there is no tracheoesophageal *fistula*, there will be no air in the stomach when a roentgenogram of the abdomen is obtained. When a fistula is present (Fig. 11-1), ingested

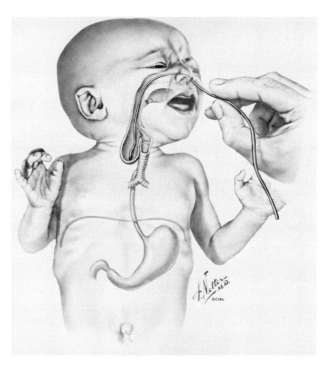

FIG. 11-1. Congenital atresia of the esophagus with a tracheoesophageal fistula. Note the catheter in the pouch. (Copyright 1964 CIBA Pharmaceutical Co., Division of CIBA-GEIGY Corporation. Reproduced, with permission, from the CLINICAL SYMPOSIA illustrated by Frank H. Netter, M.D. All rights reserved.)

fluids may be immediately coughed up and the coughing may be accompanied by struggling, choking, and cyanosis.

Injection of Lipiodol through a tube placed in the upper esophagus will demonstrate the atresia on fluoroscopic examination or after inspection of the roentgenograms. If a fistula is present, it may also be demonstrated. When the diagnosis is established, early surgical correction must be performed to maintain life. Closure of the fistula and anastomosis of the esophagus or esophagogastrostomy must be done. Postoperative dilation of the esophagus may be necessary to prevent later stricture.

Tracheoesophageal fistula without atresia should be suspected when an infant has recurrent bouts of pneumonitis during the first few weeks or months of life. Often careful examination, including bronchoscopy or esophagoscopy or both, will confirm that the cause is aspiration rather than infection.

CONGENITAL WEBS. Some infants are born with webs of fibrous tissue across, or partially across, the esophageal lumen. Regurgitation and choking are the usual symptoms. Simple webs can easily be broken and dilated through an esophagoscope or by simply passing a stomach tube. Thicker, more fibrous webs may require several dilations.

Cardiovascular anomalies. Sometimes the symptoms of choking, recurrent cyanosis, and dysphagia in the infant may be due to "vascular rings." These rings are abnormalities of the great vessels of the mediastinum, usually anomalous arteries, that compress the esophagus, the trachea, or a bronchus. Roentgenograms made following the injection of Lipiodol as the contrast medium may demonstrate a typical compression opposite the aortic arch. Confirmation by esophagoscopy or bronchoscopy will establish the diagnosis in most cases. Treatment is surgical, and the operation is performed by the transthoracic route.

Strictures of the esophagus. Strictures of the esophagus may be caused by chemical burns, injury from ingested foreign bodies, or operations on the esophagus. Chemical burns in children are most often the result of accidental ingestion of caustic lye, bleaches, or acids used in the home for cleaning. There is usually little doubt about the diagnosis, because the parent brings the child in for emergency treatment and gives a history of the accident.

When a known caustic has been ingested, particularly lye, gastric lavage may be a dangerous procedure. Toxicity is severe in some patients. Care should be taken *not to judge the severity of the esophageal injury by the amount of visible burning of the mouth, lips, and tongue.* Often minimal damage to the oral cavity is accompanied by severe esophageal damage.

Immediate treatment consists of supportive measures. No food or fluids are given by mouth for 2 or 3 days. Fluids by intravenous injection and antibiotics are indicated to assure adequate hydration and to prevent infection of the mediastinum. Cortisone, used in full dosage for the patient's size and weight, is helpful in reducing inflammatory reaction and in maintaining the patient during the first several days of tissue shock. Cortisone also is of value because of its action in preventing or delaying fibrosis while permitting mucous membrane to heal. Thus the drug may be used for 2 weeks as prophylaxis against stricture formation.

There is a difference of opinion concerning the value of esophageal dilation in connection with fresh esophageal burns. Before cortisone was available, dilation was always used as the treatment of choice. If dilation is used, early and gentle passage of the Hurst mercury-filled bougies should be started within 24 to 48 hours after the burn and continued daily during the subsidence of the acute tissue reaction. Early dilation is an accepted preventive measure against later stricture formation.

Esophagoscopy may be delayed 7 to 10 days while the immediate inflammatory reaction subsides the tissue repair begins. It must be done, however, and sometimes immediately (within 48 hours) to assess the amount of damage, the areas of greatest injury, and possible perforations.

When severe esophageal burns have *not* been treated during the acute phase, the patient has a period of 10 to 14 days of dysphagia, fever, and pain, followed by a period of relief with nearly normal swallowing ability for 1 to 12 months. Slow dysphagia may then occur and indicates a developing stricture that may require dilation

from above or by the retrograde method for months or years. Some strictures caused by lye are so extensive that a partial esophageal resection with end-to-end anastomosis or an esophagogastrostomy must be done.

Strictures caused by injury to the wall of the esophagus by sharp foreign bodies that have been swallowed or strictures following an operation on the esophagus should be dilated as soon after the trauma has occurred as is consistent with early healing of soft tissue. An interval of 2 to 3 weeks following injury or operation is sufficient time to wait before gentle dilation is started. When dilation is carried out soon after trauma, good results are expected. If too much time intervenes between the injury and dilation, heavy scar tissue may form and contract, making dilation more difficult and giving less satisfactory results.

Cardiospasm (achalasia of the esophagus). Achalasia of the esophagus, or cardiospasm, is a common condition. The cause is not known. Microscopic examination of the esophagus after the death of patients known to have had this condition shows degeneration of the ganglion cells in Auerbach's plexus and in Meissner's plexus, atrophy of the esophageal mucosa and muscle fibers of the esophageal wall, and thickening and fibrosis of the muscle and soft tissue of the cardiac portion of the esophagus. This pathologic picture is the result of slow stretching of the esophagus and enlargement of its lumen.

The primary symptom of cardiospasm is intermittent dysphagia that is slowly progressive. Since food remains in the esophagus for long periods after meals, it may be necessary for the patient to drink large amounts of water to force it into the stomach. Often substernal pressure is so annoying that the patient voluntarily induces vomiting to empty the esophagus and then tries again to eat. The subjective feeling is one of pressure. Frequently liquids are less well tolerated than solid food. Sometimes a patient will learn to swallow air to force the food through the tight cardiac end of the esophagus. When dilation of the esophagus is greatest, pressure on the trachea causes annoying cough.

The diagnosis of cardiospasm is established by roentgenograms and esophagoscopy. The roentgen picture is typical. When cardiospasm is present and barium is swallowed, fluoroscopic

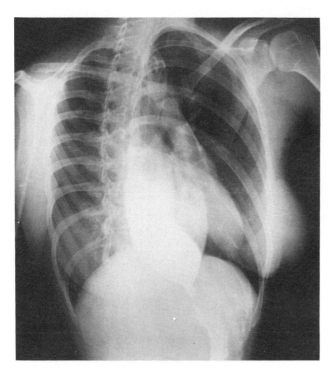

FIG. 11-2. Roentgenogram showing cardiospasm (achalasia). Note the tapered lower end and dilation of the upper esophagus.

examination demonstrates absence of peristalsis of the esophagus and dilation throughout the entire esophagus. The cardiac end of the esophagus is tight. The roentgenogram shows a smooth narrowing that comes to a point at the esophagogastric junction (Fig. 11-2). Barium spills into the stomach slowly. Examination through an esophagoscope demonstrates the dilation, pale atrophic esophageal mucosa, and spasm at the lower end of the esophagus.

Treatment should be conservative. Dilation of the esophagus with Hurst mercury-filled bougies is the treatment of choice. An attempt is made to pass the largest bougie possible through the cardia so that the spastic and fibrotic cardia will be stretched. Dilation may have to be done at intervals for years. Often a successful dilation will control symptoms for 6 to 12 months. If ulceration is present at the lower end of the esophagus, diet and medication similar to that used in the treatment of gastric ulcer are necessary. When the patient with cardiospasm does not respond to sedation, antispasmodics, dietary control, and dilation, operative repair (Heller procedure) can be done. The

operation is designed to split the fibrotic tissue around the cardia and repair it in a manner similar to pyloroplasty. Other surgical procedures, such as excision of the lower esophagus or anastomosis to the stomach, are also done.

Esophageal varices. Cirrhosis of the liver, Banti's disease, and other disturbances of the portal circulation may cause esophageal varices. Massive hematemesis is the only symptom. At times it is abrupt and massive enough to cause death. Usually the bouts of hematemesis are recurrent and severe. Examination of the esophagus by roentgenography and by esophagoscopy will demonstrate large varicosities in the lower third of the esophagus (Fig. 11-3).

In the past, attempts have been made to sclerose the dilated veins by injecting them with sodium morrhuate introduced through the esophagoscope. In some instances this procedure has been lifesaving. However, it is usually not effective, because the varices may be so numerous that effective sclerosis of all of them is impossible. Splenectomy and portacaval shunt operations have been done with varying degrees of success. Most effective has been re-

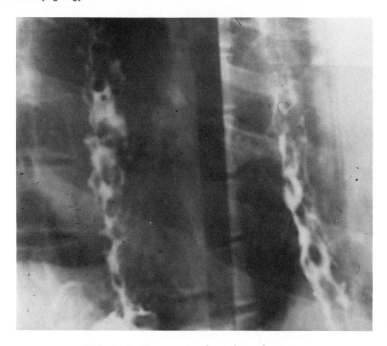

FIG. 11-3. Two views of esophageal varices.

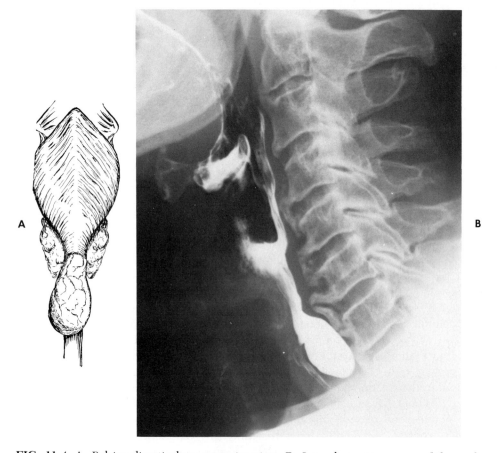

FIG. 11-4. **A,** Pulsion diverticulum, posterior view. **B,** Lateral roentgenogram of the neck showing pulsion diverticulum. Note that barium outlines the valleculae and pyriform fossa and fills the diverticulum.

section of the lower portion of the esophagus with its varices, resection of the cardia of the stomach, and esophagogastrostomy.

Pulsion (Zenker's) diverticulum. Diverticulum of the upper posterior portion of the esophagus (Fig. 11-4) is believed to result from a weakness (perhaps congenital) of the esophageal wall at the junction of the inferior constrictor and the cricopharyngeus muscles. The symptoms, which vary with the size of the diverticulum, usually are dysphagia and intermittent regurgitation of undigested food that may have been eaten several hours previously. The regurgitation occurs without vomiting. Sometimes a feeling of fullness in the neck occurs at the time of eating and is relieved only when the patient voluntarily regurgitates to empty the sac. A large diverticulum causes some compression of the trachea when it is full and may initiate a hacking, dry cough. When liquids are present in the diverticulum, the patient feels a gurgling sensation in the neck at or just above the level of the clavicle. This problem may occur only at night when the patient is lying down. Pain is not present.

Findings of the physical examination may be entirely normal. Mirror examination of the larynx and hypopharynx usually reveals them to be normal. It may reveal pooling of saliva in the pyriform recesses. Palpation of the neck just above the clavicle may produce a gurgling sound similar to the sound of air and fluid expressed together from a bag. Roentgenograms show the characteristic picture of a sac filled with the contrast medium and protruding from the posterior part of the esophagus just above the level of the clavicle. Esophagoscopy demonstrates the opening into the diverticulum from the esophageal lumen. Sometimes the orifice of the diverticulum is larger than the normal esophageal lumen.

Excision of the diverticulum is the accepted treatment. An incision is made along the anterior border of the sternocleidomastoid muscle. This muscle and the carotid sheath are retracted laterally. The thyroid gland and trachea are retracted medially. Incision through the alar fascia between the carotid sheath and the thyroid gland exposes the diverticulum. It is dissected to its neck and then resected. The esophagus is closed with inverted sutures in the same manner that the bowel or stomach is closed. This

procedure results in cure in almost all patients. Recurrence is rare. Occasionally a closure that is too tight will make several dilations of the esophagus necessary during the postoperative period.

Prior to the use of antibiotics, mediastinitis was a potential complication of surgical excision. Because of this danger, a two-stage procedure for resection was done. Today the excision is usually done in one stage.

A pulsion diverticulum can be successfully managed by incision of the cricopharyngeus muscle through an esophagoscope. A specially designed slotted esophagoscope can be placed in such a way that the anterior half rests in the esophagus and the posterior half rests in the diverticulum. The common wall between the esophagus and the diverticulum is divided with a cutting current after cauterizing has been done along each side. Although the dilated portion of the diverticulum remains, it is no longer a blind pouch and does not collect food or saliva. Regurgitation and possible aspiration are prevented.

This method of treatment of a pulsion diverticulum is valuable in the elderly, poor-risk patient. It can be done quickly, and there are few postoperative complications.

Traction diverticulum. Inflammatory disease in the chest that produces periesophageal lymphadenopathy may also cause scar tissue to form. Sometimes contraction of inflammatory tissue will produce a diverticulum of the lower esophagus (Fig. 11-5). There are no characteristic symptoms of traction diverticulum. Usually it is seen incidentally on fluoroscopic examination of the stomach after the administration of barium. As a rule the orifice from the esophagus to the diverticulum is small, and it may not be seen during esophagoscopy. Most traction diverticula do not require treatment. If a diverticulum is large, excision by the transthoracic route may be necessary.

Globus hystericus. Globus hystericus is a common syndrome seen particularly in women. The typical complaint is a vague sensation of a lump low in the throat and a desire to swallow so as to dislodge the lump. This symptom appears and disappears. Usually it is present when the patient is nervous, tired, or worried. Characteristically, it is not present when food or fluids are ingested, an important difference between the

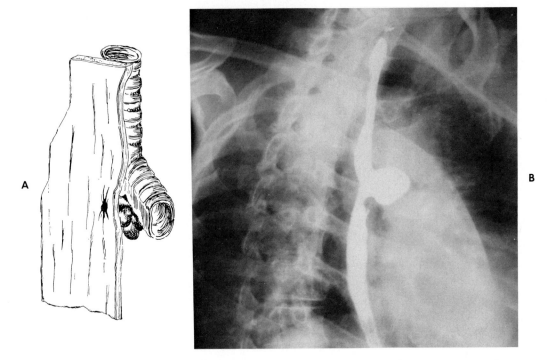

FIG. 11-5. A, Traction diverticulum. **B,** Traction diverticulum, asymptomatic. (**A,** After Netter.)

functional condition and organic causes of similar symptoms. Although the complaint is of a feeling of obstruction to swallowing, there is no actual obstruction.

The cause is not known. However, hypertonicity of the cricopharyngeus muscle may be the responsible factor. Recent electromyographic studies show a greater action potential in the cricopharyngeus muscle of patients with this complaint than in the same muscle of normal persons used as controls. It is possible that autonomic imbalance is the basic disturbance.

Findings of the physical examination are entirely normal. Roentgenographic examination should reveal the esophagus and neck to be normal, but more and more, patients with so-called globus hystericus are found to have abnormalities when an esophagram is done. For example, hiatal hernia is not uncommonly reported. Esophagoscopy, although usually unnecessary, reveals no abnormality.

Treatment consists of strong reassurance, because many patients with this complaint are afraid they have cancer of the throat. A thorough, painstaking examination, including roentgenograms of the esophagus, will make reassurance more effective. Occasionally, mild sedation will help. A search for some environmental stress, such as marital difficulties or financial problems, may be necessary. Drugs that relax smooth muscle may be beneficial.

Cricopharyngeal achalasia. So-called cricopharyngeal achalasia (failure to open) can cause a total or severe esophageal obstruction. The condition may be associated with central nervous system disease such as a stroke, or its cause may be undetermined. One treatment is surgical division of the fibers of the cricopharyngeus muscle.

Osteophytic lesion. Rarely, an osteophytic lesion of the cervical region may be the cause of dysphagia. The lesion is related to degeneration of an intervertebral disk, an indication of osteoarthritis or cervical spondylosis. In addition to dysphagia there may be complaints of a sensation of a foreign body in the throat, pain on swallowing, or hoarseness.

In advanced cases an osteophytic mass may be seen protruding into the pharynx or hypopharynx. The mass is very firm and may be large enough to prevent a clear view of the larynx with a mirror. Usually the diagnosis is made

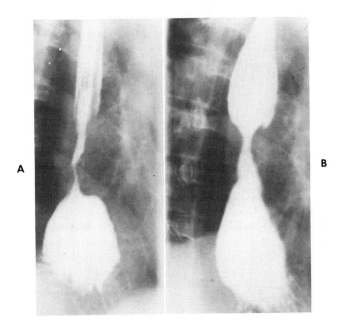

FIG. 11-6. A, Stricture of the midportion of the esophagus. **B,** Hiatal hernia, with the stomach coming up through the diaphragm.

from a lateral roentgenogram of the cervical area. The osteophytes can be seen projecting from the anterior surface of one or more vertebrae. The fifth and sixth cervical vertebrae are the ones most often affected, but any of the cervical vertebrae can show osteophytes. It is important to prove the presence of osteophytes of any size, if they are suspected; esophagoscopy may be more hazardous when they are present, because of the possibility of an esophageal tear. Surgical removal may rarely be indicated when osteophytes are large and if the dysphagia is disabling.

Esophagitis and peptic ulceration. When the sphincter action of the cardiac portion of the esophagus (esophagogastric junction) is inadequate, reflux of hydrochloric acid from the stomach can cause inflammation and peptic ulceration of the lower esophagus. This condition usually occurs in persons who have an enlarged diaphragmatic hiatus that allows herniation of the stomach into the mediastinum. Rarely, the condition results from a congenitally short esophagus in which there is no true narrowing at the cardia (Fig. 11-6).

The symptoms produced are similar to those

of gastric ulcer. Burning and pain are present in the epigastrium or behind the manubrium. The pain may be referred to the back. Rough or highly seasoned foods cause additional discomfort. The discomfort is less severe after eating. Symptoms are usually more severe at night when the patient is recumbent, because then the stomach is most likely to herniate through the diaphragm. Later in the course of this disease, if repeated ulceration and inflammation have produced scar tissue, symptoms of partial obstruction of the lower esophagus may occur.

Roentgenograms usually show some narrowing of the lower esophageal segment, roughness of the usual smooth esophageal mucosal pattern, and ulcer craters (if they are present). Esophagoscopy reveals a fragile, inflamed mucosa in the lower esophagus that bleeds easily.

Treatment is the same as for gastrc ulcer. It consists of bland diet, interval feedings, antacids, and avoidance of stress. Sometimes gentle dilation of the esophagus with Hurst bougies is necessary. Often repair of the hiatal hernia will stop further regurgitation of acid and allow the area to heal. If medical management fails or there is recurrent bleeding from the ulcerated

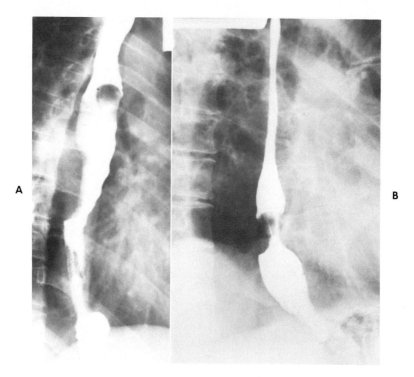

FIG. 11-7. **A,** Leiomyoma of the esophagus. Note the smooth, filling defect in the upper third of the roentgenogram. **B,** Barium esophagram showing carcinoma. Note the overhanging edges.

area, partial resection of the esophagus and vagotomy may be necessary.

Scleroderma. Scleroderma is a chronic disease of unknown origin affecting women three times as often as men. It occurs in two forms—localized (morphea) and systemic (progressive systemic sclerosis). The histopathology is that of chronic progressive sclerosis of the connective tissue of the skin and mucous membranes. The collagen fibers of these tissues become dense and hypertrophic. Scleroderma most commonly occurs in the third to fourth decade of life. Dermal manifestations begin with induration and stiffness of the skin and progress to an atrophic state characterized by tensing, smoothing, and hardening of the dermis. The face becomes masklike because of loss of expression and tightening of the lips. Tightening of the skin over the dorsum of the nose also occurs.

Mucous membrane involvement causes induration and pain of the gingiva and tongue. Dysphagia results from diminished or absent peristalsis, especially in the distal third of the esophagus. The patient tends to regurgitate

and has difficulty getting food "all the way down." A barium esophagram and fluoroscopy will usually show a characteristic picture of confused esophageal motility with a reflux pattern. Treatment is administration of steroids and dilation for esophageal stenosis, which must be done with care to prevent esophageal perforations.

Tumors. Tumors of the esophagus can be benign or malignant. Both are relatively rare, and both occur at any site along the esophagus. Malignant tumors are more common in the lower half of the esophagus.

BENIGN TUMORS. Benign tumors may produce mild dysphagia, substernal pressure, vague epigastric distress, or anorexia. Often they are asymptomatic. The most common benign tumor is leiomyoma (Fig. 11-7, *A*). It may be pedunculated or intramural. Fibromas and lipomas occur less often. Benign tumors produce a smooth, rounded filling defect on roentgenograms made after barium ingestion. Unless such a tumor is large or produces obstruction, treatment may not be necessary. When removal is indicated, it can be done through an esophagoscope if the tumor is pedunculated.

MALIGNANT TUMORS. The most common malignant tumor of the esophagus is squamous cell carcinoma. The usual symptoms are progressive dysphagia (first for solid food, later for soft food, and finally for liquids), weight loss, and substernal pressure and pain.

The next most frequent malignant tumor is adenocarcinoma of the cardia of the stomach, which extends upward into the esophagus. This is often a submucosal extension that produces only mild dysphagia and mild epigastric discomfort without ulceration of the esophageal mucosa.

Roentgenographic examination of patients with carcinoma of the esophagus reveals an irregular narrowing of the esophageal lumen. There is usually a filling defect of the lumen, with a sharp border (Fig. 11-7, *B*). The diagnosis is established by esophagoscopy and biopsy. On esophagoscopy the lesion has the appearance of an ulcerated, fungating, friable mass. It bleeds easily when manipulated or when tissue is removed for biopsy.

Treatment of malignant tumors of the esophagus consists of resection of the involved area and esophagogastrostomy. The stomach is mobilized and brought as high as the arch of the aorta. Segments of the large bowel have been used to replace resected segments of the esophagus. Irradiation therapy is palliative only, and the prognosis is poor. Patients live for approximately 2 years from the time of diagnosis unless complete resection is possible.

Foreign bodies. Almost anything taken into the mouth and swallowed can become lodged in the esophagus. Partial obstruction of the esophagus usually follows. Sometimes, however, the esophagus is completely obstructed, so that the patient cannot even swallow his own saliva. As a consequence, saliva drools from the mouth, and choking and gagging ensue.

Any condition that reduces the size of the esophageal lumen may stop the downward progress of poorly masticated food. In patients with esophageal strictures, further complications frequently occur when foods such as peas, corn, or meat cannot pass. The first symptom of carcinoma of the esophagus may be sudden obstruction from a foreign body.

Upper dentures do not allow tactile sensation in the palate and thus they prevent detection of a bone before it is swallowed. Also, patients with dentures often chew their food inadequately. Consequently they swallow *large pieces of meat*, sometimes containing a bone that will not pass through the esophagus. *Pork chop* and *chicken bones* are the most common offenders.

Children put foreign objects such as *marbles, coins,* and *safety pins* in their mouths and swallow them inadvertently. Psychotic persons may also try to swallow a foreign object, sometimes in an attempt at suicide.

In children the only symptom may be gagging or inability to swallow food normally. Infants become irritable, refuse to eat, or regurgitate food or formula after a few swallows. A sharp foreign body will cause some pain. Often the parent is aware of the child's having swallowed something either because the child says so or because he was seen putting something in his mouth.

Adults almost always know when they have swallowed a foreign body because they immediately have symptoms from partial or complete obstruction. Most often they can accurately localize the level of pain or irritation. Small bones, such as thin, sharp chicken bones or fish bones, may lodge in the base of the tongue or the aryepiglottic fold without entering the esophagus. The patient has pain high in the neck; if asked to point one finger toward the painful area, he will indicate a spot high under the angle of the jaw (Fig. 11-8). The subjective sensation is similar to that produced by being stuck with a sharp needle and occurs with each act of swallowing.

When a patient complains of discomfort high in the throat and there is a history of possible foreign body ingestion, a careful examination of the larynx, hypopharynx, and base of the tongue is essential. It can be done adequately only with a laryngeal mirror and a head mirror. Usually in such instances the small, sharp bone (or other foreign object) can be seen and removed with long, curved forceps. It may be necessary to spray the throat with cocaine to abolish the gag reflex. A careful examination will often make it unnecessary to obtain roentgenograms or to consider esophagoscopy.

A foreign body in the esophagus most commonly lodges at the level of the cricopharyngeus muscle. This is the esophageal inlet just below and behind the larynx. When a foreign body

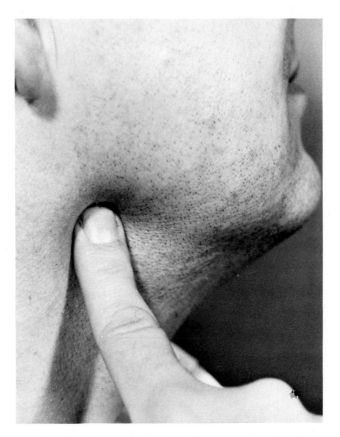

FIG. 11-8. Patient indicating a foreign body in the throat—at the valleculae, the pyriform recess, or the base of the tongue. Small, sharp fish bones are often found in these locations.

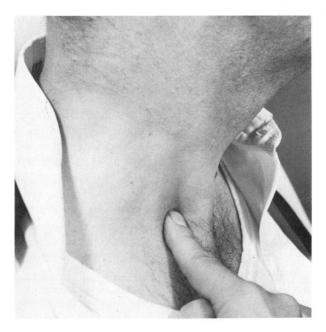

FIG. 11-9. Patient indicating a foreign body in the cervical esophagus—lodged at the narrowing of the cricopharyngeus muscle.

remains at this level, the patient locates the discomfort or obstruction at a spot just above the clavicle and to the right or left of the trachea (Fig. 11-9). Attempts to swallow cause pain and varying degrees of obstruction, depending on the size of the foreign body. In most instances if the foreign body remains for several hours or a day, the symptoms of discomfort increase and obstruction progresses, often to total occlusion. This is caused by edema and irritation of the esophagus as a result of pressure from the foreign body.

If a sharp foreign body penetrates the esophageal wall, it may cause mediastinitis and produce progressive pain, fever, chills, and prostration.

Some sharp foreign bodies scratch the surface of the tongue, pyriform fossa, or esophagus and pass on into the stomach. Yet the patient may still complain of a sharp, sticking sensation each time he swallows saliva. This discomfort may last several hours or several days. A situation of this kind presents two problems. If no foreign body is present, unnecessary esophagoscopy must be avoided. If a small foreign body is present, it must not be overlooked. Occasionally there will be tenderness low in the neck, which should cause the examiner to be suspicious of actual or impending perforation.

When the presence of a foreign body is suspected in the hypopharynx or esophagus, thorough examination of the mouth, throat, nasopharynx, larynx, hypopharynx, and neck is necessary. This requires the use of the laryngeal mirror. Unless the foreign body is visible, the only finding may be a collection of saliva in the pyriform fossa that will not disappear after swallowing. Rarely, a large foreign body stuck at the esophageal introitus can be seen behind the larynx with a mirror.

Examination by means of fluoroscopy and roentgenograms is important. Fluoroscopic examination will reveal all opaque foreign bodies, including *metallic objects, most plastic objects,* and *large bones* (Fig. 11-10). Nonopaque foreign bodies and small slivers of bone are not well seen with the fluoroscope. Thin barium is used as a contrast medium if no foreign body is visible on fluoroscopy. Pooling of the barium or obstruction of its normal flow toward the stomach may indicate the presence of a nonopaque foreign body. The barium may coat the foreign body, or residual traces of barium may indicate where the foreign body is lodged. When the foreign body is not demonstrated by these means, the following procedure may be helpful. The patient is asked to swallow small pieces of cotton that have been soaked in thin barium. The passage of the cotton down the esophagus is then watched under the fluroscope. The cotton may catch on the foreign body and remain for several minutes, whereas thin barium alone may pass on without hesitation.

In addition to fluoroscopy, roentgenograms must be taken. Anteroposterior and lateral views of the chest and of the soft tissue of the neck are necessary. It is essential that the lateral view of the neck be taken with the patient's head in hyperextension. With the patient in the normal erect position, the esophageal inlet, which is the most common site of foreign bodies, is hidden by the shadow of the clavicle. Small bony foreign bodies may not be seen if the head is held in the erect position. When the head and neck are extended, the larynx and upper esophagus are raised so that the esophageal inlet can be seen in the lateral view (Fig. 11-11).

When the presence of a foreign body of the esophagus has been established, it must be removed through an esophagoscope. General anesthesia is required in all children and in most adults. This allows relaxation of the cricopharyngeus muscle, abolishes the gag reflex, and permits removal of the foreign body with minimum trauma to the mucosa and wall of the esophagus. Esophageal perforation can lead to fatal mediastinitis even when a tear is small. Occasionally, smooth foreign bodies, such as coins, can be removed in adults under local anesthesia (Fig. 11-12).

Removal of open safety pins from the esophagus can be hazardous. Safety pins invariably lodge in the esophagus with the spring end down—the dangerous position. The point of the pin, often hidden in the wall of the esophagus, must be found and brought into the esophagoscope before removal is attempted. Sometimes it is necessary to push the pin into the stomach, turn it, and remove it with the spring end up and the point trailing.

In rare instances sharp foreign bodies will perforate the esophagus and require removal from the mediastinum by a transthoracic approach. If a foreign body passes the esophagus

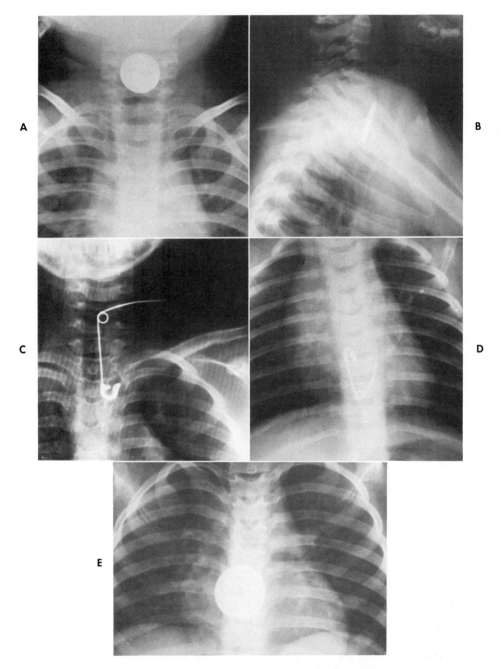

FIG. 11-10. Various metallic foreign bodies in the esophagus. **A** and **B**, Anterior and lateral views showing a coin at the cricopharyngeus. **C**, Safety pin (large) at the cricopharyngeus has perforated into the neck. **D**, Open safety pin in the midesophagus—in the usual position, spring down, **E**, Large metal washer in the midesophagus.

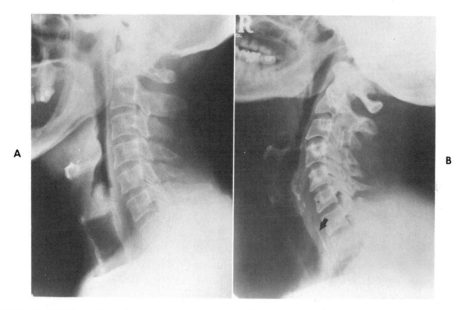

FIG. 11-11. The value of hyperextension. **A,** Head erect. **B,** With the head held in extension, 1 to 2 inches more of the esophagus is visible. Arrow indicates bone. Note calcification in the cricoid cartilage above arrow on the anterior wall. This is normal and should not be mistaken for a foreign body.

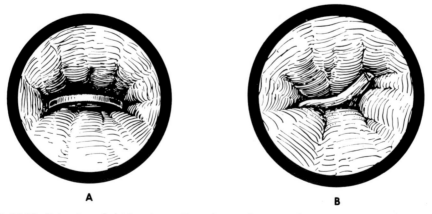

FIG. 11-12. Coin, **A,** and chicken bone, **B,** in the esophagus as they appear through the esophagoscope.

at its upper end, it may lodge at the cardia. Again, removal is necessary by means of the esophagoscope. If the foreign body passes both the esophageal inlet and the cardia, it will continue through the gastrointestinal tract and be eliminated in the stool. Occasionally in infants a foreign body will pass the cardia and remain in the duodenum. If it does, removal through an abdominal incision may be required. A conservative approach is desirable. In the absence of abdominal symptoms, nothing should be done for several days. Daily fluoroscopic examination of the abdomen will enable the physician to follow the progress of the foreign body.

COMPLICATIONS. Except for mediastinitis, there are few complications following removal or foreign bodies in the esophagus if they are promptly removed. *Attempts to force a foreign body through the esophagus by means of bougies or other instruments are dangerous and should never be made. The use of protein digestants, in the hope of dissolving a large bolus of meat, is also dangerous. Such chemicals may cause perforation of the esophagus.*

When the esophagus is known to be perforated, either by a foreign body or by the instrumentation necessary to remove it, localized or generalized mediastinitis frequently follows. Because of this probability, antibiotics should be given immediately following perforation. Since the infection may be caused by any of the several bacteria always present in the mouth, a combination of antibiotics is desirable. For several days no food or fluids are allowed by mouth. Fluids are given intravenously until danger of spreading mediastinal infection has passed.

If treatment is instituted early, mediastinitis will not develop in most patients and recovery will be complete. If spread of infection occurs in spite of preventive measures, or if no treatment has been given, a mediastinal abscess may develop. If mediastinitis is well developed prior to any treatment, early drainage to the mediastinum may prevent abscess formation or death. When perforation occurs high in the mediastinum, the infected periesophageal space can be drained through the neck. If the perforation is low in the esophagus, drainage is best accomplished through a posterior thoracic approach.

Spontaneous esophageal rupture. Violent vomiting is the most common cause of spontaneous rupture of the esophagus. It has also occurred during weight lifting, epileptic seizures, and childbirth. The rent in the esophagus is almost always longitudinal and usually occurs in the left posterolateral area of the distal esophagus.

When the stomach contents enter the mediastinum, a virulent chemical and bacterial inflammation often breaks through the pleura into the right or left chest cavity. The presenting symptoms may suggest acute abdominal signs or, more commonly, chest signs. Subcutaneous emphysema in the neck, severe substernal pain, dyspnea, cyanosis, and shock are common.

Pneumothorax, or pleural effusion, may be temporarily treated by open or closed thoracotomy. However, recovery depends on repair of the esophageal tear through the chest cavity. In cases in which the tear remains unrecognized for 48 hours or more, the mortality is high.

Esophageal dilation. Even though a liquid diet can maintain nutrition when a normal esophageal lumen is not present, such a diet is troublesome to prepare and disturbing to a patient's morale. Therefore, whenever the esophageal lumen is inadequate, it should be dilated to provide enought space for the passage of soft food and, preferably, some solid food. Dilation of the esophageal lumen is not always possible, but it can be accomplished in a high percentage of patients. In cases in which dilation provides an inadequate lumen, resection of the structure and primary restoration is indicated.

In some conditions causing narrowing of the esophageal lumen, dilation is contraindicated. The most serious of these conditions is carcinoma of the esophagus. In carcinoma, dilation gives only temporary relief. Consequently, when malignancy is suspected or proved, relief from dilation not only gives the physician a false sense of security but delays surgical intervention, which may save the life of the patient with an early lesion. Other conditions causing narrowing of the esophageal lumen can be managed by dilation. Those most frequently encountered are congenital stenoses, strictures, and cardiospasm.

There are four commonly used esophageal dilators: the olive-tipped bougie, the Jackson flexible-tipped bougie, the Hurst mercury-filled dilator, and the retrograde dilator (Fig. 11-13). Each has some advantage that makes it more suitable than the others for management of a particular condition.

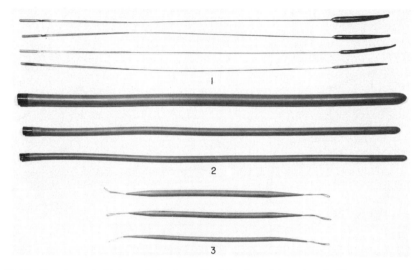

FIG. 11-13. Esophageal dilators. *1*, Jackson flexible-tipped bougies. *2*, Hurst mercury-filled dilators. *3*, Retrograde dilators.

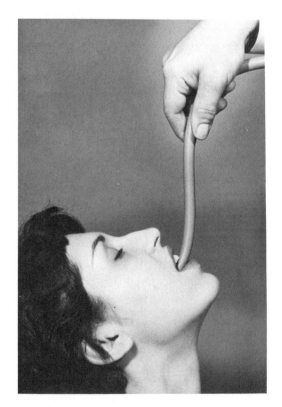

FIG. 11-14. Patient swallowing a Hurst dilator. The physician guides the dilator into the esophagus. The dilator is kept in place briefly after it passes the cardia.

1. The olive-tipped bougie is perforated. Hence, a swallowed string threaded through the perforation aids in guiding the bougie through a tortuous stenosis.
2. The Jackson flexible-tipped bougie can be inserted easily into an esophagoscope, but the lumen of the esophagoscope limits the size of the bougie that can be used. The flexible-tipped bougie is more dangerous to use than the olive-tipped bougie when dilation is being done without an esophagoscope.
3. The Hurst mercury-filled dilator is safest for direct dilation. Furthermore, the patient can be taught to use it at home (Fig. 11-14). In many instances this allows more frequent dilation and reduces the patient's expenses.
4. The retrograde dilator may be required when repeated difficult dilation is necessary over a long period of time, as in the management of some strictures caused by corrosives. Several dilators in graduated sizes are strung together like links of sausages and pulled into a gastrostomy opening, up the esophagus, and out the mouth (Figs. 11-13, *3*, and 11-15).

Dilation of the esophagus should never be attempted until esophagoscopy has been carried out to establish or confirm a diagnosis suggested by the history and roentgen study. To attempt bouginage without esophagoscopy is to invite

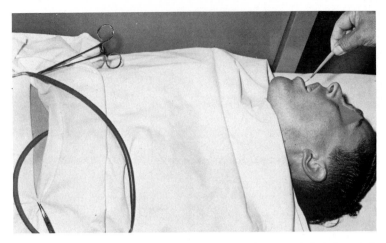

FIG. 11-15. Use of retrograde dilators. Each cigar-shaped dilator is slightly larger than the one used previously. As each is pulled out of the throat, the following dilator is fed into the gastrostomy.

disaster. In most instances of injury to the esophagus with resultant mediastinitis, the cause has been blind bouginage. Once the exact pathologic condition has been established by esophagoscopy, it may be permissible—and is sometimes desirable—to continue dilation without further esophagoscopy. This is particularly true in the management of patients with cardiospasm and short benign strictures.

Many severe burns of the esophagus require weekly dilations for several years. Under these circumstances, retrograde dilation may be the procedure of choice, particularly when dilation was not started early.

When retrograde dilation is contemplated, the type of gastrostomy performed is important. For dilation it is necessary to have the direction of the opening cephalad. An opening created for feedings and directed toward the pylorus makes dilation difficult and sometimes impossible. The opening necessary for retrograde dilation can also be used for feeding until a useful lumen is established. Perforation of the esophagus during retrograde dilation is not likely.

In many cases it is necessary for the patient to have a string in the esophagus continuously until a lumen of small size has been permanently established. One end of the string can be brought out through the nose, carried backward over the ear, and brought down to the abdomen to be attached to the opposite end of the string by means of a continuous loop through the gastrostomy opening. As soon as the string can be

swallowed easily, the patient should be asked to begin swallowing it the day before returning for subsequent dilation. It can then be picked up in the stomach through the gastrostomy opening, and the retrograde dilation can be performed. At times it is necessary to pick up the lower end of the string through a bronchoscope or cystoscope introduced into the gastrostomy opening.

Occasionally it is impossible to find a lumen above, particularly in patients with neglected corrosive burns. In such cases it is sometimes possible for a urologist to catheterize the lower end of the esophagus with a urethral catheter in a cystoscope in the gastrostomy opening. The catheter can be seen from above through an esophagoscope and can be pulled upward. When this procedure has been accomplished, it is possible to place a string in the esophagus.

No set rule can be made as to frequency or extent of dilation for each successive attempt. In general, it is wise not to force a dilator beyond that size which passes the constriction with slight resistance. If a dilator must be forced because it is too large, there may be trauma to, and splitting of, the lumen with subsequent scarring and loss in the caliber of the lumen.

The Hurst mercury-filled bougies have been most satisfactory for the treatment of cardiospasm. In most cases it is possible to use a No. 60 French bougie. When it passes the cardia, it assures enough stretching of the fibers to provide relief. The only difficulty in passing a bougie of this size is that encountered in getting it

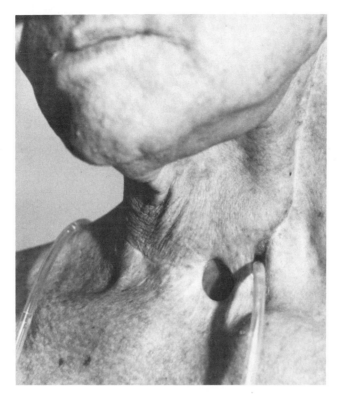

FIG. 11-16. Cervical esophagostomy adjacent to a tracheostomy in a laryngectomy patient with a recurrent tumor in the hypophyarynx, precluding a nasogastric tube.

past the larynx. A No. 46 French bougie is sometimes the largest size that can be used when the patient is of small stature and has a correspondingly small esophageal introitus. However, in such a patient a bougie of this size will give adequate dilation. Dilation with the Hurst bougies can be carried out easily in the office.

Cervical esophagostomy provides an alternative to gastrostomy for feeding a patient who suffers from an obstruction of the hypopharynx or who is aspirating food and liquid and in whom a nasogastric feeding tube, for one reason or another, is impractical. The mucosa of the pyriform recess or of the cervical esophagus is easily pressed externally (by an instrument held in the hypophyarynx) until it is almost subcutaneous. Then it is a simple matter to incise the skin of the neck laterally and join mucosa to skin, thus forming a permanent fistula through which a feeding tube may be introduced. This arrangement is generally preferable to gastrostomy (Fig. 11-16) If there is irritation of the skin ad-

jacent to the stoma, a protective ointment such as Silicote or aluminum paste may be applied.

SELECTED READINGS

Ahmed, N.: Fish-bone impaction of the throat, Aust. New Zeal. J. Surg. **38**:231, 1969.

Bikhazi, H.B., and Shumrick, D.: Caustic ingestions; current status, Arch. Otolaryngol. **89**:770, 1969.

Cardona, J.C., and Daly, J.F.: Current management of corrosive esophagitis; and evaluation of results in 239 cases, Ann. Otol. Rhinol. Laryngol. **80**:521, 1971.

Celerier, M., Kaswin, R., and Dubost, C.: Early surgical management of severe corrosive burns of the esophagus, Ann. Otolaryngol. Chir. Cervicofac. **95**:379-388, June, 1978.

Chodosh, Paul L.: Gastroesophagopharyngeal reflux, Laryngoscope **87**:1418-1427, September, 1977.

Fischer, R.A., and others: Esophageal motility in neuromuscular disorders, Ann. Intern. Med. **63**:229, 1965.

Holinger, P.H., and Schild, J.A.: Zenker's (hypopharyngeal) diverticulum, Ann. Otol. Rhinol. Laryngol. **78**:679, 1969.

Kirsh, M.M., and others: Treatment of caustic injuries of the esophagus: ten-year experience, Ann. Surg. **188**:675-678, November, 1978.

Kuhn, F.A., Sessions, D.G., and Ogura, J.H.: Hypopharyngeal diverticulum, Laryngoscope **87**:147-153, February, 1977.

Mansour, K.A., Hatcher, C.R., and Haun, C.L.: Benign tumors of the esophagus: experience with 20 cases, South Med. J. **70**:461-464, April, 1977.

Middelkamp, J.N., and others: Management and problems of caustic burns in children, J. Thorac. Cardiovasc. Surg. **57**:341, 1969.

Price, S., and Castell, D.O.: Esophageal mythology, J.A.M.A. **240**:44-46, July 7, 1978.

Sandrasagra, F.A., English, T.A.H., and Milstein, B.B.: Management and prognosis of esophageal perforation, Br. J. Surg. **65**:629-632, September, 1978.

Saunders, W.H.: Cervical osteophytes and dysphagia, Ann. Otol. Rhinol. Laryngol. **79**:1091, 1970.

Scher, L.A., and Maull, K.I.: Emergency management and sequelae of acid ingestion, J. Am. Council Emerg. Physicians **7**:206-208, May, 1978.

Triggiani, E., and Belsey, R.: Esophageal trauma: incidence, diagnosis and management, Thorax **32**:241-249, June, 1977.

Weisman, R.A., and Calcaterra, T.C.: Head and neck manifestations of scleroderma, Ann. Otol. Rhinol. Laryngol. **87**:332-339, 1978.

Welsh, J.J., and Welsh, L.W.: Endoscopic examination of corrosive injuries of the upper gastrointestinal tract, Laryngoscope **88**:1300-1309, August, 1978.

Wychulis, A.R., Fontana, R.S., and Payne, W.S.: Instrumental perforations of esophagus, Dis. Chest **55**:184, March, 1969.

12 THE NOSE AND PARANASAL SINUSES

ANATOMY

External nose (Fig. 12-1). Terms commonly used to describe the external nose are the tip or apex, the base (which includes the nares), the root (where the nasal bones join the skull above), the dorsum (between the root and the tip), and the bridge (the upper part of the dorsum).

The two nasal *bones* vary in size and sometimes are even absent. They join each other in the midline and articulate above with the frontal bone and laterally with the frontonasal processes of the maxillary bones.

Only the upper third of the external nose is bony. The lower two thirds are cartilaginous. Variations in the size and shape of the nose are due in large part to differences in the cartilages. The *lower lateral (major alar) cartilages* form the rim and the flaring curve of the ala. There is a lateral crus and a medial crus. The major alar cartilages form most of the tip of the nose. The *upper lateral (lateral nasal) cartilages* lie in the middle third of the nose, between the nasal bones above and the lower lateral cartilages below. These cartilages account for the shape of the middle third of the nose. There are several *sesamoid* and *minor alar cartilages* lateral to the two large cartilages of the external nose. Also contributing to the shape of the ala and middle third of the nose is fibroadipose tissue.

The *nasal septum*, discussed in detail in the section on the internal nose (which follows), forms part of the dorsum as it extends upward between the two upper lateral cartilages and between the medial crura of the lower lateral cartilages.

Muscles of the external nose are rather rudimentary in humans. The *procerus muscle* extends between the nasal bones and the frontalis muscle; the *depressor septi muscle* and certain fibers that cause dilation of the nasal alae are also recognized.

Internal nose. One each side of the nose are anterior and posterior openings called the nares. The posterior nares are also called the *choanae*. The *vestibule* is the anterior, skin-lined part of the nasal cavity that contains the vibrissae, or nasal hairs, the follicles of which often become infected. A *recess* of the vestibule reaches upward into the tip. The junction of the skin and nasal mucous membrane occurs at a variable distance inside the nose. Usually the junction is clearly defined because of the difference in color between skin and mucosa.

The *nasal septum* (Fig. 12-2) divides the nose into the two nasal fossae. It is cartilaginous in front and bony behind. The septum is straight at birth and in early life but becomes deviated or deformed in almost every adult. Only the posterior end, separating the posterior nares, remains constantly in the midline. Anteriorly the *quadrilateral*, or *septal*, *cartilage* is frequently dislocated into one nasal vestibule. Posteriorly the septal cartilage joins the perpendicular plate of the ethmoid above and the vomer below. The other bony parts of the septum (the palate bone, crest of the maxilla, and rostrum of the sphenoid) are small.

The lateral wall of the nose (Fig. 12-3) is a complicated area anatomically and a very important area clinically. There are four nasal turbinates, or conchae. Named from below upward, they are the inferior, middle, superior, and supreme turbinates. The *supreme turbinate* is very small and is not seen during clinical examination; the *superior turbinate* is so placed that usually it can be seen only with a postnasal mirror.

The *inferior turbinate* is a separate bone, whereas the other turbinates are parts of the

177

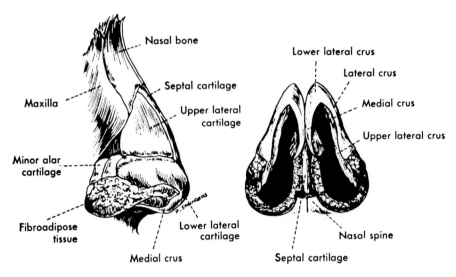

FIG. 12-1. External nose.

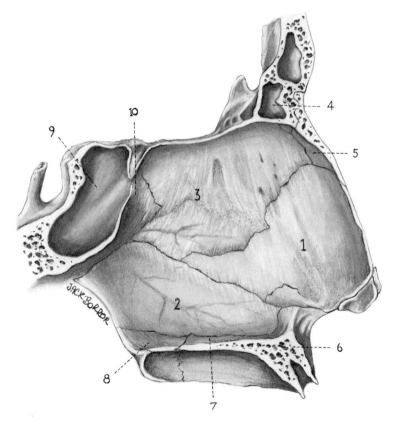

FIG. 12-2. Nasal septum. *1*, Septal cartilage. *2*, Vomer. *3*, Perpendicular plate. *4*, Frontal sinus. *5*, Nasal bone. *6*, Maxilla. *7*, Maxillary crest. *8*, Palate. *9*, Sphenoid sinus. *10*, Rostrum of the sphenoid.

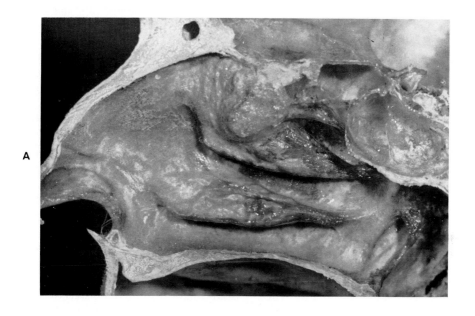

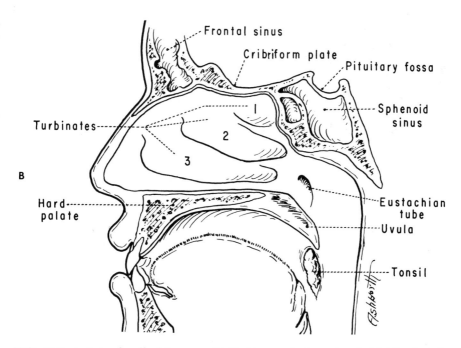

FIG. 12-3. A, Lateral wall of the nose. **B,** Turbinates. *1*, Superior. *2*, Middle. *3*, Inferior.

ethmoid bone. The mucous membrane of the inferior turbinate is very rich in blood vessels and is semierectile. It is this structure that vasoconstrictors affect most. Sometimes the bony part of the inferior turbinate lies close to the lateral nasal wall, but at other times it juts out prominently into the airway and causes nasal obstruction. Often the mucosa of the inferior turbinate touches the septum.

The *middle turbinate* is somewhat smaller than the inferior turbinate because it is shorter. It often contains an air cell; sometimes the air cell dilates the turbinate enough to produce nasal obstruction.

The several nasal meatuses are named according to the turbinates that overlie them. Thus the inferior meatus lies under the inferior turbinate, and the middle meatus under the middle turbinate. Above the superior and supreme turbinates is the *sphenoethmoid recess*, into which the sphenoid sinus opens.

The *inferior meatus* may be large or small, depending on the position of the inferior turbinate and its state of vascular engorgement. The only channel opening into the inferior meatus is the *nasolacrimal duct* (which opens toward its anterior end). Posteriorly there are large blood vessels (sphenopalatine branches) under the mucosa of the lateral wall of the inferior meatus. They may bleed severely.

The *middle meatus* contains the drainage sites of the maxillary, frontal, and anterior ethmoid sinuses. About midway along the meatus, the ethmoid bulla (an air cell) bulges from the lateral wall of the nose into the meatus. Just anterior to the bulla is a groove, the *infundibulum*, which curves from above downward and then posteriorly around the bulla. This area is very important clinically because it is into the upper end of the infundibulum that the *nasofrontal duct* drains, whereas the maxillary sinus drains into the posterior and lower part of the infundibulum. The anterior ethmoid cells drain, along with the frontal sinus, anteriorly and superiorly. By knowing the general sites of sinus drainage, the clinician, looking at a stream of pus, is better able to differentiate between maxillary and frontal (or anterior ethmoid) sinusitis. The actual ostia of the sinuses, except rarely the sphenoid, are not seen during clinical examination.

The posterior ethmoid cells drain into the *superior meatus*. Pus from the sphenoethmois recess and the superior meatus is usually best seen with the postnasal mirror. As seen anteriorly (with the nasal speculum), pus from the frontal, anterior ethmoid, and maxillary sinuses drains under the middle turbinate (into the middle meatus), but pus from the posterior sinuses drains medial to the middle turbinate (between it and the septum) (Fig. 16-2).

The *olfactory* area is a 2.5-cm. area located high in the nose in a narrow niche formed by the superior turbinate, the upper septum, and the cribriform plate. The olfactory epithelium consists of three types of cells: receptor, supporting, and basal cells. The supporting cells serve a secretory and nutritional function and provide firm attachment between cells. The unmyelinated axons of the receptor cells ascend through the cribriform plate and eventually reach the rhinencephalon, the uncus, the hippocampus, the mamillary bodies, and the amygdaloid nucleus. Unlike other senses, olfaction is not relayed through the thalamus.

Blood supply of the nose (Figs. 12-4 and 12-5). Both the *external* and the *internal carotid systems* provide a blood supply to the nose. The external carotid does so chiefly through one of its terminal divisions, the internal maxillary artery, and to a limited extent through nasal branches of the facial artery. The internal maxillary artery, and more particularly its terminal branch, the sphenopalatine, has been called the rhinologist's artery because it supplies so much of the nose. The sphenopalatine artery supplies most of the posterior part of the nasal septum and most of the lateral wall of the nose, especially posteriorly.

The *anterior* and *posterior ethmoidal arteries*, branches of the ophthalmic artery, derive their blood from the internal carotid system. The anterior ethmoidal artery is the second largest vessel supplying the internal nose. It gives blood to both the anterior-superior part of the septum and the lateral wall of the nose.

The *external nose* receives blood from approximately the same arteries as does the internal nose. The venous drainage is of importance because part of it, through the angular vein, leads into the inferior ophthalmic vein and eventually to the cavernous sinus. Most of the venous drainage, however, is downward through the anterior facial vein.

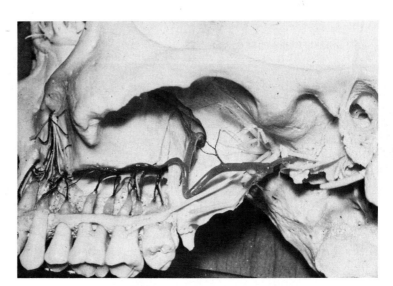

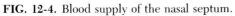

FIG. 12-4. Blood supply of the nasal septum.

FIG. 12-5. A, Internal maxillary artery. B, Blood supply of the lateral nasal wall. Coming from above are the anterior and posterior ethmoid arteries and, posteriorly, branches of the sphenopalatine artery.

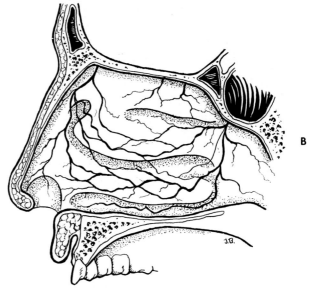

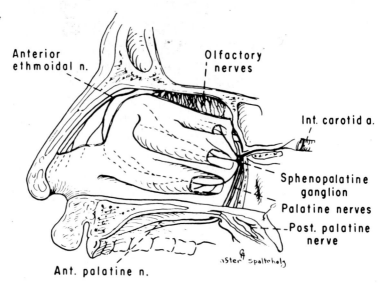

FIG. 12-6. Nerve supply of the lateral wall of the nose.

Lymphatics of the nose. Lymphatic drainage of the nose is extensive and parallels the venous drainage. Lymphatics along the anterior facial vein terminate in submaxillary lymph nodes.

Nerve supply of the nose (Figs. 12-6 and 12-7). The muscles of the *external nose* are supplied by the seventh cranial nerve; the skin receives its sensory supply from the first and second divisions of the fifth nerve.

The *internal nose* has a more complicated nerve supply. The olfactory nerves have been mentioned. Their cell bodies (in the mucous membrane) send fibers upward through the cribriform plate. These fibers enter the olfactory bulb. Olfaction is disturbed or lost when there is enough nasal obstruction to keep air currents from the olfactory mucosa (as in nasal polyposis). Anosmia also results from fractures through the cribriform plate, tumors of the frontal lobe, or meninges, and some viral infections.

The general sensory nerve supply to the internal nose comes from the first and second divisions of the fifth cranial nerve. The *nasociliary*, or *anterior ethmoidal*, *nerve* is a branch of the ophthalmic (first) division and supplies some of the superior and anterior part of the septum and lateral nasal wall. *Sphenopalatine* branches of the maxillary division supply most of the posterior part of the nose.

Parasympathetic fibers with cell bodies in the sphenopalatine ganglion are distributed to the

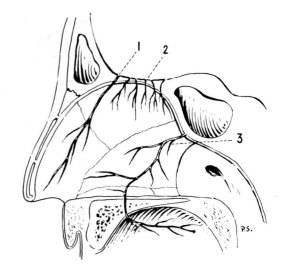

FIG. 12-7. Nerve supply of the nasal septum. *1*, Anterior ethmoidal or nasociliary nerve (septal branch). *2*, Olfactory nerves penetrating the cribriform plate. *3*, Nasopalatine nerve (septal branch).

nasal mucosa. *Sympathetic fibers* that reach the nose come from fibers around the carotid plexus. These carotid fibers join and form the deep petrosal nerve, which joins the greater superficial petrosal nerve (branch of the facial nerve) to form the vidian nerve. The vidian nerve thus carries preganglionic parasympathetic fibers and postganglionic sympathetic fibers to the

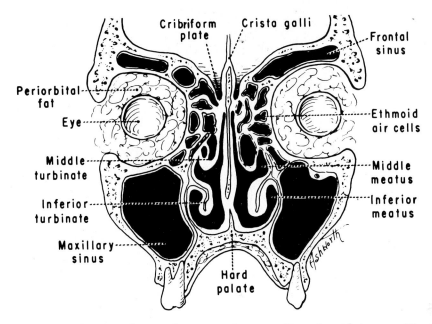

FIG. 12-8. Frontal section showing the paranasal sinuses. For sphenoid sinus see Fig. 12-3.

sphenopalatine ganglion. Here the parasympathetic fibers synapse.

It is sometimes thought that the general sensory nerve supply of the nose is from branches of the sphenopalatine ganglion, but actually the ganglion is parasympathetic; the maxillary fibers merely branch off at this level. Other *parasympathetic* ganglia of the head are the *otic*, associated with the parotid gland; the *submaxillary*, associated with the tongue and submandibular salivary gland; and the *ciliary*, associated with the eye. The *sphenopalatine ganglion*, besides supplying the nose, also supplies the lacrimal gland and palate.

The *mucous membrane* of the nose is described in detail in the discussion of the physiology of the nose (p. 187).

The paranasal sinuses (Fig. 12-8). There are four paranasal sinuses (air-filled spaces lined by mucous membrane) on each side of the head. The *ethmoid sinus* is often called the ethmoid labyrinth because of its many cellular divisions. The others are the *maxillary* (or antrum of Highmore), the *frontal* (Fig. 12-9), and the *sphenoid sinuses*. The sinuses develop as outpocketings of nasal mucous membrane. At birth only the maxillary and ethmoid sinuses are present. The frontal sinus develops from one of the anterior ethmoid cells but does not start to pneumatize the frontal bone until the first or

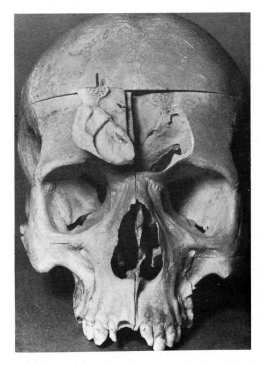

FIG. 12-9. Prepared skull showing the frontal sinus opened. Note that the floor of the frontal sinus is the roof of the orbit. The ethmoid sinuses are between the nose and the medial wall of the orbit.

second year of life. Similarly, the sphenoid sinus begins to invade bone about the third year of life.

Practical considerations. There are fewer glands in the mucosa of the nasal sinuses than in the mucosa of the nose. Most nasal discharge of a mucoid type is produced by nasal glands and does not come from the sinuses. The walls of the sinuses are less sensitive to pain than are their ostia or most parts of the nasal mucosa. *A great deal of the head pain and mucoid nasal discharge ordinarily attributed to chronic sinusitis is in reality caused by other disease.*

Sometimes one frontal sinus is missing; at other times there are more than two frontal sinuses, each with a separate drainage canal into the nose. When disease of the frontal sinus occurs, the orbit and the anterior cranial fossa are the places in which complications are most likely to occur.

The relationship of the maxillary sinus to the upper teeth is important because of the frequency with which pain from dental abscess is confused with pain from sinusitis, and also because tooth extraction may result in loss of a root tip (or even a whole tooth) into the maxillary sinus.

The ethmoid air cells pneumatize not only the ethmoid bone but also parts of adjacent bones. The lamina papyracea is a thin plate of bone separating the ethmoid labyrinth from the orbit. This "paper plate," often incomplete, is a common place for infection from the sinuses to enter the orbit.

The sphenoid is the most deeply placed of the sinuses. The two sphenoids are seldom of the same size and are sometimes very small. Directly above the sphenoid sinus is the sella turcica. From here, pituitary tumors may erode downward and fill the sphenoid. Located laterally there is the cavernous sinus, with the third, fourth, fifth, and sixth cranial nerves. The brain stem is located posteriorly.

PHYSIOLOGY

Functions of the nose. Since the nose is exposed to constant differences in temperature and relative humidity, as well as to particles present in the atmosphere, it must be able to perform a variety of functions. These functions are aided by the turbinates. Projecting into the nasal cavity, the turbinates produce a broad surface covered by mucosa that supports a specialized epithelium.

Nasal obstruction, produced by a great variety of conditions (see Chapter 15), usually seems worse to a patient when he is lying down. This is because tissue fluids and blood tend to pool in the head more when he is recumbent than when he is standing. This phenomenon is analogous to the swelling of the feet and lower extremities that some patients notice toward the end of a long day's standing and the relief that follows when they are able to elevate the lower extremities. Patients also commonly complain that at night when they lie on one side, the dependent side of the nose becomes obstructed and they find it necessary to roll over in bed to make that side open. Then the other side becomes obstructed, and they roll over again.

OLFACTION. The olfactory area is located high in the nasal vault above the superior turbinate. Sensory hairs extend from the surface of the olfactory area to the cells that lie deep in the mucosa. The central axons of the cells penetrate the cribriform plate and travel to the olfactory area of the cortex through the first cranial nerves. These nerves lie under the frontal lobes of the brain and on top of the cribriform plate.

In human beings the sense of smell is much less important than it is in other mammals. A wild animal may depend on the sense of smell to warn him of an impending attack or to locate a source of food. Man's use of the olfactory sense is primarily for pleasure. With training, his sense of smell can be developed to a high degree of sensitivity, as is done by persons who are engaged in the testing of wine, cheese, or perfumes.

Under ordinary conditions the human being is aware only of odors that are pleasant or unpleasant. When the sense of smell is poor or absent, the only immediate discomfort is a change in taste. The taste of food is recognized and enjoyed through simultaneous stimulation of the taste buds of the tongue and the olfactory cells of the nose. When odors cannot reach the olfactory area, or when the sense of smell is absent (anosmia), food tastes flat and unpalatable. Alteration of the taste of food is a common complaint of the patient with a blocked nose caused by acute infection or, more often, by nasal allergy associated with nasal polyps. When the sense of smell is absent for a long time, the sensitivity of the taste buds apparently increases.

Anosmia may be the result of simple nasal obstruction—for example, nasal polyposis—that prevents air currents from reaching the olfactory area high in the nose. Some patients with anosmia, however, have no nasal obstruction whatsoever, but a neural defect. The onset of anosmia is often sudden. A patient may have a normal sense of smell one day but will be able to smell nothing the next. He may remember a severe upper respiratory infection, or he may have had perfect health when he lost his sense of smell.

A multitude of conditions, including drug toxicity, skull fracture, tumor, congenital defects, and viral infections, can be responsible for anosmia in patients in whom intranasal appearances are normal.

Inflammation and edema, as seen in acute rhinitis, sinusitis, allergic rhinitis, nasal polyps, or atrophic rhinitis, may be accompanied by anosmia (see Chapter 15). This type of anosmia is usually transient, with the sense of smell returning as infection and swelling subside.

Anosmia may occur after nasal surgery or nasal trauma. Again, the sense of smell almost always returns as the tissues heal.

Trauma to the head, with injury to the olfactory nerves as they pass through the cribriform plate, may cause anosmia. Anosmia may occur in 2% to as many as 20% of such cases, depending on the severity of the injury. If the sense of smell is going to be recovered, return of function should be expected in the first few weeks following the injury.

Patients in whom the larynx has been removed (usually because of cancer) have anosmia. The most obvious explanation is the lack of airflow through the nose, since they must breathe through a tracheostomy (see Chapter 9). There is evidence of probable neural feedback between the vagus nerve and the olfactory system, which may be the true mechanism of this type of anosmia.

Intracranial tumors, most commonly olfactory meningiomas, may cause anosmia. Frontal lobe tumors may give rise to a syndrome of anosmia, ipsilateral optic atrophy, and contralateral papilledema (Foster Kennedy syndrome).

Agenesis of the olfactory bulb, an X-linked recessive combination of anosmia and hypogonadism (Kallmann's syndrome) may rarely be seen.

Viral infections, often unsuspected, are the *most common* cause of anosmia. Symptoms include, in addition to the loss of the sense of smell, dryness of the nose and decreased quality and quantity of nasal discharge. Examination reveals only that less than normal moisture is present in the nose. Viral hepatitis may also involve anosmia or hyposmia as an associated complaint.

Treatment of anosmia has been unsatisfactory. Vitamin A, given orally or by injection, has been used with partial success in some patients.

Testing of olfactory function may be done in several ways. Various familiar odors, such as those of coffee, chocolate, tobacco, and perfume, may be used to test each side of the nose separately, with the eyes closed. Water or mineral oil, which have no odor, can be used as controls. A method for testing when malingering is suspected is to use coffee and ammonia. The anosmic patient will not recognize the coffee but will react to the ammonia, since it will stimulate the trigeminal nerve rather than the olfactory nerves. The malingerer will deny smelling either one. Other, more exact and quantitative tests may be used. Most of them require closely controlled laboratory conditions.

Parosmia is an alteration of the sense of smell in which a person may smell odors that do not exist or may interpret existing odors incorrectly. Such persons often complain of smelling disgusting odors such as burning chicken feathers of decaying garbage, and they are likely to be more annoyed by their symptoms than are persons with complete anosmia. The explanation for parosmia is not clear, but the disorder often occurs after a preliminary period of anosmia. It may be that after destruction by a viral infection, for example, regenerating nerve fibers find their way along unaccustomed pathways. An analogous situation is thought to be present in some patients who recover from Bell's palsy. In them, regenerating fibers of the facial nerve apparently do not reach the same muscles that they originally reached, resulting in uncontrolled "mass motion" of the face.

AIR CONDITIONING. The primary function of the nose is to condition the inspired air for its entrance into the trachea, bronchi, and lungs. The atmosphere varies in temperature, relative humidity, and cleanliness. Whether the outside air is 100° "in the shade" or 40° below zero, the temperature of the inspired air is changed to approximate body temperature during its brief passage through the nose.

The relative humidity of atmospheric air may vary from less then 1% to more than 90%. The nose can add moisture to the inspired air or remove moisture from it, so that the air that reaches the pharynx is of almost constant relative humidity.

The air around us is never gaseous alone. At all times it contains particles of smoke, dust, pollens, and bacteria, as well as products of combustion. The nose attempts to remove these particles before the air reaches the pharynx and the lungs.

When the nose is functioning normally, it accomplishes these tasks efficiently.

TEMPERATURE CONTROL. Air entering the nose travels primarily through the space between the turbinates and the nasal septum. It also passes over the broad surface of the turbinates. Numerous capillaries make the blood supply of the turbinate tissue as rich as that in any other area of the body. These capillaries are associated with erectile tissue that contains large spaces filled with rapidly circulating blood. The erectile tissue enables the blood spaces to enlarge or contract rapidly, as is necessary for temperature alteration. Because of this ability to change size, the blood spaces have been called "swell spaces."

Cold air causes blood to fill the "swell spaces." This induces swelling of the turbinates.

Their resultant enlarged surface area allows greater transfer of heat from the blood to the incoming air. The process is reversed when air warmer than body temperature enters the nose.

Air reaches the nasopharynx approximately ¼ second after it enters the nose. During this time the air is warmed or cooled to the proper temperature, regardless of its temperature prior to entering the nose. The nasopharyngeal temperature ranges from 96.8° to 98.6° F.

HUMIDITY CONTROL. The surface of the nasal mucosa is covered with a blanket of mucus and serum. This is supplied by the mucous and serous glands of the respiratory mucosa of the nose (Fig. 12-10). Air reaching the nasopharynx has a constant relative humidity of 75% to 80%. When the outside air is cold and dry, large amounts of water must be transferred to the inspired air during its passage through the nose. When relative humidity is high, little, if any, fluid is lost from the mucous membrane.

It is estimated that as much as 1,000 ml. of moisture can be evaporated from the nose during normal breathing in a 24-hour period. The actual amount of fluid lost varies with the relative humidity of the inspired air. As the air absorbs water from the mucosa, the submucosal glands replenish the supply. Unless the epithelium of the nose is damaged, the mucosal surface rarely becomes dry.

Extensive surgical removal of intranasal tissue may produce a nasal cavity in which the air space is large and the moist surface small. Dryness and crusting inside the nose can then be-

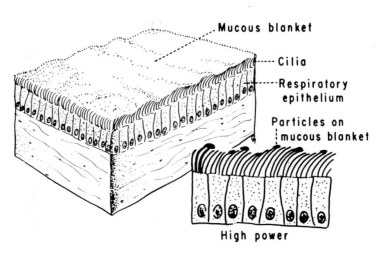

FIG. 12-10. Respiratory mucosa.

come a distressing symptom. Atrophy of the nasal mucosa and turbinates may so alter the normal surface that dryness and crusting develop.

PARTICLE CONTROL (CLEANING). As previously stated, the entire lining of the nose is covered with a thin blanket of moisture. This is known as the mucous blanket of the nose. A similar blanket of moisture covers the mucosa of the sinuses, the eustachian tube, the trachea, the bronchi, and the bronchioles.

The mucous blanket rests on top of the cilia of the respiratory epithelium (Fig. 12-10). On this blanket are deposited bacteria and other particles present in the inspired air. Constant ciliary action carries these particles to the nasopharynx and pharynx, after which they are swallowed and disposed of in the stomach. The nose empties itself and replaces the mucous blanket by a continuous process simulating a moving belt.

Respiratory epithelium and the mucous blanket.
The respiratory tract, with the exception of the pharynx, is lined by specialized respiratory epithelium. This epithelium is pseudostratified columnar in type and is ciliated. Beneath the surface cells three or four layers of replacement cells lie on a submucosa that is thickest in the most exposed areas of the nose and thin in the paranasal sinuses. The same epithelium lines the paranasal sinuses and the eustachian tube. In the anterior third of the nose the cell type differs; the epithelium is squamous in character and has no cilia. The epithelial cells are less columnar, and the entire epithelium is thinner inside the sinuses.

Beneath the submucosa are found both tubular and racemose glands that supply both serous and mucous secretions. Goblet cells, intermixed with the columnar epithelial cells, are numerous and add to the secretion of the respiratory epithelium.

CILIA AND CILIARY MOVEMENT. Each surface cell of respiratory epithelium has 25 to 30 cilia. The cilia are 5 to 7 mμ in length. The cilia seem to work automatically, and contractions continue in a rhythmic manner even after a cell has been artificially broken into small pieces. The cilia beat in such a way that anything carried on their surface is propelled in the direction of the cilicary motion. This is accomplished by a rapid beat in the direction of the flow and a slower recovery phase in the opposite direction.

During the recovery phase the cilia are bent and the motion is slower than during the active phase, when the cilia are straight. In humans the cilia beat approximately 250 times per minute.

THE MUCOUS BLANKET. The submucosal glands and the goblet cells of the respiratory epithelium supply a continuous flow of secretion that forms a viscid blanket. This mucous blanket is continuous throughout the nose, the sinuses, the pharynx, and the tracheobronchial tree. Its surface promptly collects any particle that comes into contact with it. Dust, bacteria, pollens, and other airborne particles cling to it on contact.

The pH of the secretion remains fairly constant near 7. The secretion contains lysozyme, an enzyme that destroys most bacteria. Lysozyme effectively causes disintegration of bacteria on contact. Ciliary action and lysozyme activity are most effective at pH 7. Serious alteration of the pH of the nasal secretion, whether by disease or medication instilled into the nose, can slow or stop ciliary action and inhibit the action of lysozyme.

Secretion is continuously produced from the epithelium of the sinuses, the nose, and the tracheobronchial tree. Ciliary action carries the blanket with its contained particles toward the pharynx, where it is swallowed. In the stomach the gastric juice and hydrochloric acid destroy residual bacteria. The mucous blanket in the nose travels approximately 5 to 10 mm. per minute. It is somewhat faster near the ostia of the paranasal sinuses. The secretion is replaced about every 20 minutes. Its volume approximates 600 to 700 ml. every 24 hours.

The protective action of the mucous blanket is obvious. When this action is altered by trauma, drying, irritating chemicals, or any other factor, the nose, sinuses, and lower respiratory tract become more susceptible to infection.

SELECTED READINGS

Batsakis, J.G.: Mucous gland tumors of the nose and paranasal sinuses, Ann. Otol. Rhinol. Laryngol. **79:**557, 1970.

Davidson, F.W.: Hyperplastic rhinosinusitis, Ann. Otol. Rhinol. Laryngol. **82:**703, 1973.

Doty, R.L., and others: Factors influencing intranasal trigeminal detection of chemical vapors by humans, Trans. Am. Acad. Ophthalmol. Otolaryngol. **82**(2): 261-262, 1976.

Griffith, I.P.: Abnormalities of smell and taste, Practitioner **217**(1302):907-913, 1976.

Hasegawa, M., and others: Dynamic changes of nasal resistance, Ann. Otol. Rhinol. Laryngol. **88**(1, pt. 1):66-71, 1979.

Henkin, R.I., Larson, A.L., and Powell, R.D.: Hypogeusia, dysgeusia, hyposmia, and dysosmia following influenza-like infection, Ann. Otol. Rhinol. Laryngol. **84** (5, pt. 1):672-682, 1975.

Hyams, V.J.: Papillomas of the nasal cavity and paranasal sinuses, Ann. Otol. Rhinol. Laryngol. **80**(2):192, 1971.

Pinching, A.J.: Clinical testing of olfaction reassessed, Brain **100**(2):377-388, 1977.

Proetz, A.W.: Essays on applied physiology of the nose, ed. 2, St. Louis, 1953, Annals Publishing Co.

Schechter, P.J., and Henkin, R.I.: Abnormalities of taste and smell after head trauma, J. Neurol. Neurosurg. Psychiatry **37**(7):802-810, 1974.

Tremble, G.E.: A few highlights concerning respiratory cilia, Ann. Otol. Rhinol. Laryngol. **64**:1146, 1955.

13 NOSEBLEED

Causes. The most common cause of nosebleed is *trauma*. In some instances the type of trauma may be quite obvious, as when a crust has been picked off the nasal septum or when there is excessive drying of the nasal mucosa. In other instances the cause may be less obvious—for example, when there is a defect intrinsic in the blood vessel. Nosebleeds are more common in patients who have hypertension or sclerotic blood vessels. Certain diseases such as rheumatic fever, purpura, and leukemia may be the underlying cause of epistaxis. Patients with these diseases represent a small percentage of the total number suffering from nosebleed. Even in such patients, however, trauma may be the precipitating cause.

Often the cause of epistaxis may be obscure. The patient's nose simply starts to bleed spontaneously. Dry air causes the nasal septum to crust. As the crusts are removed by blowing or picking, the mucosa is torn and small vessels are opened.

Bleeding from the posterior half of the nose is not likely to be caused by external trauma. Instead, it results from splitting of a sclerotic blood vessel. The defect is intrinsic in the vessel and is made worse if the patient is hypertensive.

Certain conditions commonly thought to cause nosebleeds have been overemphasized. For example, a disturbance in the blood-clotting mechanism is often considered to be a common cause of nosebleed. But alterations in the vitamin C or K level, changes in the prothrombin time, or changes in bleeding and clotting are not commonly associated with epistaxis. If these conditions were the cause of epistaxis, the patient would bleed from other mucous membranes and into the skin and viscera rather than only from the nose. *A patient who is not bleeding from any other part of the body rarely has nosebleed resulting from a hematologic disorder.*

The distinction between nosebleed caused by trauma and nosebleed resulting from a generalized systemic disorder is important in treatment. In many instances a patient's nose is not packed accurately and the bleeding continues. Then, instead of replacing the packing, the physician ascribes the bleeding to a hematologic disorder and prescribes various medications designed to promote coagulation. The rent in the vessel wall remains, however, and the patient continues to bleed.

Sites that bleed. The proper management of nosebleeds depends on the physician's ability to look into the nose and discover the exact bleeding site.

ANTERIOR PART OF THE NOSE. Most nosebleeds in the anterior part of the nose start from the vascular network in the anterior part of the nasal septum (Kiesselbach's plexus, Fig. 13-1). Occasionally bleeding occurs from the anterior end of the inferior turbinate. Most of the blood that supplies the anterior part of the nasal septum comes from the external carotid system.

POSTERIOR PART OF THE NOSE. In the posterior part of the nose the bleeding vessels may be derived from either the external carotid system or the internal carotid system. They are large vessels, and bleeding is usually severe. A very common site for hemorrhage from the posterior part of the nose is from under the posterior half of the inferior turbinate (in the *inferior meatus*). Vessels in this area are branches of the internal maxillary artery (external carotid). The *anterior ethmoid artery*, a branch of the ophthalmic artery (internal carotid system), supplies the upper portion of the posterior part of the nose. Bleeding from this artery usually

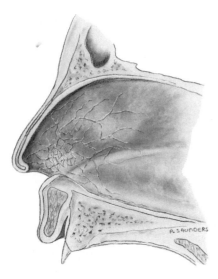

FIG. 13-1. Kiesselbach's plexus—the site of most nosebleeds.

is seen high in the nose between the nasal septum and the middle turbinate.

OTHER SITES. Sometimes blood oozes from the anterior end of the middle or inferior turbinate. Blood may come from the paranasal sinuses following severe head injury or in the presence of a neoplasm. When a patient has hereditary hemorrhagic telangiectasia or a blood dyscrasia, virtually all of the nasal mucosa may bleed. However, patients with blood dyscrasias do not bleed only from the nose; they also have skin petechiae, ecchymoses, hematuria, or other manifestations of a generalized hematologic disturbance.

The nose is expected to bleed from only one place at a time. Frequently, when bleeding is serious, blood passes behind the nasal septum and appears in the unaffected, as well as the affected, side of the nose. This seems to represent an instance of bilateral nosebleed. Actually, bilateral nosebleed is uncommon except in nasal fractures or after instrumentation in the nonbleeding side. Some patients with blood dyscrasias bleed from both sides. Except for these special situations, *bleeding is expected to be from one side only* and then usually from only one spot.

Diagnosis of the site of bleeding. Before treatment is instituted, the exact site of bleeding must be determined. Obviously, effective treatment for bleeding from Kiesselbach's plexus will not control bleeding from the posterior part of the nose. A satisfactory approach for determining the site of bleeding is as follows:

1. The patient and the examiner are gowned.
2. The patient is seated in a chair. He should not be examined in the recumbent position unless he is weak or in shock.
3. Any blood clots are sucked from the nose with an angulated sucker and a strong suction pump. If suction apparatus is unavailable, the patient is instructed to blow his nose to clear it of blood clots.
4. With a *bright* light (either a head mirror or head lamp), the anterior part of the nose is inspected. If a bleeding spot is seen on the nasal septum, the search has ended.
5. If the blood does not seem to come from the anterior part of the nasal septum and the patient continues to swallow blood as it trickles down the back part of his throat, it may reasonably be assumed that the bleeding is from the posterior part of the nose. It may be from a vessel in the inferior meatus or from the ethmoid artery.

It is not uncommon to see a patient bleeding from Kiesselbach's plexus whose nose has been packed with yards of petrolatum gauze pushed back so far that the bleeding vessel is not compressed. Conversely, it is not uncommon to see a patient bleeding from the posterior part of the nose whose nose is packed anteriorly only. In both situations the packing merely acts as a wick for the blood. The patient continues to bleed.

Nosebleed from the anterior part of the nose (Fig. 13-1). The easiest nosebleeds to treat are those from Kiesselbach's plexus. Here, epistaxis is easy to control because the anterior part of the nasal septum is readily accessible and the bleeding vessels are relatively small. After the exact site of the nosebleed has been determined, the following procedure will usually stop the bleeding:

1. With the use of strong suction, blood clots and fresh blood are aspirated from the nose (Fig. 13-3, *A*).
2. Aqueous epinephrine, 1:1000, is applied to a cotton ball, which is inserted into the bleeding nostril (Fig. 13-3, *B*).
3. Strong pressure is applied for several minutes against the ala so as to compress the cotton ball against the septum (Fig. 13-3, *C*).

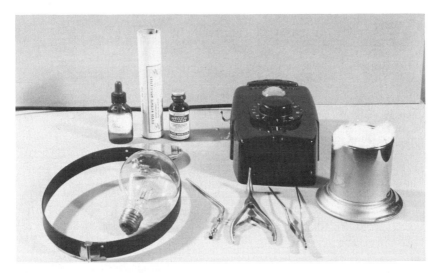

FIG. 13-2. Instruments needed for control of nosebleeds from the anterior part of the nose. One bottle contains 5% cocaine and the other contains 1:1000 epinephrine. Silver nitrate applicators are in the third container.

4. The cotton ball is removed and the bleeding point cauterized with a silver nitrate stick, trichloroacetic acid, or an electric cautery (Fig. 13-3, *D* and *E*). The septum should be dried after chemical cautery so that the medication does not spread over the mucous membrane excessively. Cocaine, 5%, or 2% tetracaine (Pontocaine) provides sufficient anesthesia for intranasal cautery. In adults chemical cautery may be used without anesthesia. Young children who will not voluntarily submit to nasal cautery and who have recurrent severe nosebleeds may have to be given a general anesthetic.

After the bleeding has been controlled, the patient is warned not to pick or blow his nose. After a week it may be desirable to prescribe petrolatum or mineral oil to be applied to the nasal septum. It should not be necessary to pack the nose after the bleeding point has been adequately cauterized.

INTRACTABLE NOSE PICKING. Some patients who will not stop picking their noses may actually cause septal ulceration or even septal perforation. Nose picking may be a habit, or it may be done of necessity to remove crusts from around an ulceration or a perforation that was already present. In either case healing of the mucous membrane can be accomplished, if usual methods fail, by prolonged packing of both sides of the nose with cotton greased with either Neosporin or oxytetracycline (Terramycin) antibiotic ointment. The cotton balls used as packing are left in place 7 to 10 days, with the nose carefully taped shut (Fig. 13-4). Although this treatment annoys the patient because it forces him to breathe through his mouth, it is effective both in healing the mucosa and in discouraging his nose picking.

If packing is needed in the anterior or upper parts of the nose (more than a greased cotton ball at Kiesselbach's area), special nasal packs of folded petrolatum gauze or a long, continuous strip of ½-inch-wide petrolatum gauze can be used. The packing must be placed under direct vision, obtained by use of a nasal speculum and bright light reflected from the head mirror. It should be placed in layers, one over the other, somewhat like the folds of an accordion, until all available space in the bleeding side of the nose is filled. To prevent odor, the petrolatum gauze can be impregnated with an antibiotic ointment such as Neosporin or Terramycin. A preliminary spray of cocaine solution, 5%, or Pontocaine, 1%, makes the procedure less unpleasant.

Complete packing of this type may be done in conjunction with a postnasal pack. It is also used in some patients who bleed from the *ethmoidal artery*. In such cases, however, a small piece of greased packing should be wedged

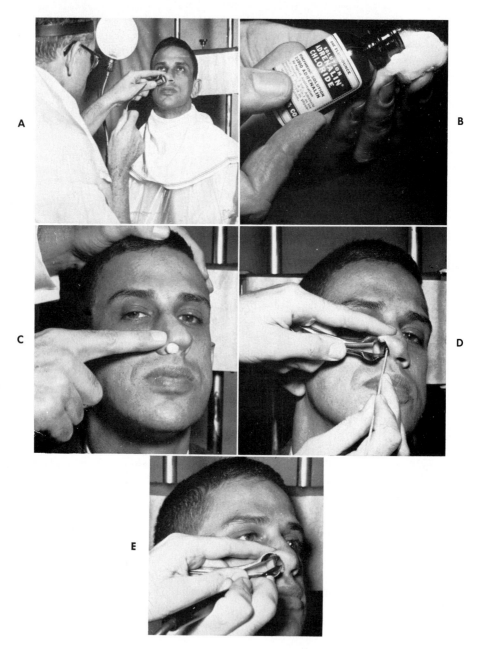

FIG. 13-3. Treatment of nosebleeds from the anterior part of the nose. **A,** First step—suction of clots, and blood from the nose. Note gowns on both the patient and the physician. **B,** Second step—application of epinephrine to a cotton ball. **C,** Third step—compression of the cotton for several minutes against the bleeding septum. **D,** Fourth step—cautery of the bleeding vessel with a silver nitrate stick. **E,** Same as **D** but using an electric cautery instead of silver nitrate.

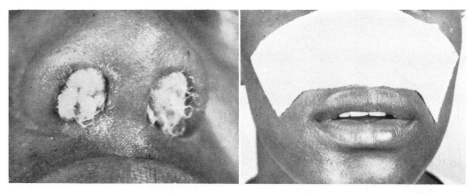

FIG. 13-4. Treatment for intractable nose picking. Cotton impregnated with antibiotic ointment is placed in the nose anteriorly, and the nose is taped shut for a week.

tightly into the space between the septum and the middle turbinate to obtain more discrete pressure at the bleeding site.

OPERATIVE PROCEDURES. Sometimes, when projecting parts of the septum are traumatized by the drying effect of inspired air, a submucous resection of the nasal septum is performed to straighten the nasal septum. Usually, however, operative procedures on the nasal septum are not required for the control of nosebleeds. In many instances the use of a lubricant such as petrolatum or mineral oil permits healing and an operation is unnecessary.

Nosebleed from the posterior part of the nose.

Epistaxis from vessels in the posterior part of the nose is often profuse. Both because of the severe bleeding and because the posterior part of the nose is hard to see, treatment is difficult. If it were technically possible, the same principles of treatment that apply to nosebleed of the anterior part of the nose would apply to bleeding from the posterior part—namely, excellent illumination, accurate suction, and point cautery. Practically, however, it is often impossible to see the exact bleeding site in the posterior part of the nose.

FINDING THE SITE. The patient should be seated rather than in the supine position, because when he is on his back, blood runs down his throat and chokes him. By using suction and clearing blood as the suction tip advances, the physician eventually reaches the spot at which the nose fills with blood when the suction tip is passed farther. This is the site of the bleeding. Usually the bleeding vessel itself cannot be seen. It may be well back in the inferior meatus (under cover of the inferior turbinate) or high

above the middle turbinate. The nose fills with blood rapidly even when strong suction is used.

The use of cautery in the posterior part of the inferior meatus is impractical because of the difficulty in reaching the bleeding spot and because of the quantity of blood.

METHODS OF POSTNASAL PACKING. Since cauterization cannot be carried out effectively in the posterior part of the nose, bleeding must be controlled by compression of the bleeding vessel. Packing must be placed so that it will remain in place and provide enough pressure to stop the bleeding.

LOCAL PACKING. Otolaryngologists sometimes use a small piece of petrolatum gauze or a small cotton ball soaked in epinephrine, wedged firmly into the inferior meatus at the approximate bleeding point (Fig. 13-5). This localized pack is placed with either a small hemostat or bayonet forceps. The pack should be left in place a day or two and then removed with forceps. In localizing and treating the bleeding point, it may be helpful for the physician to fracture the inferior turbinate medially (toward the nasal septum) to gain a better view of the inferior meatus. In comparison with a postnasal pack that obstructs the nose completely on one or both sides, the great advantage of a local pack is the comfort of the patient. The disadvantage of local packing of this sort is that it may slip and not maintain proper pressure, necessitating a conventional postnasal pack.

CONVENTIONAL POSTNASAL PACK. Treatment of postnasal hemorrhage may require the use of a postnasal pack. The pack is made of gauze in which stout silk sutures or umbilical tape is sewn to give it shape and to provide a means of

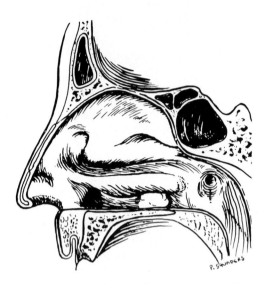

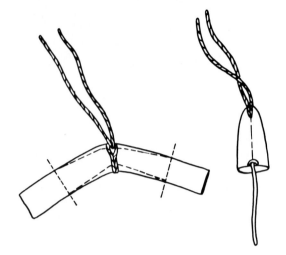

FIG. 13-5. Local packing under the inferior turbinate for control of hemorrhage from the posterior part of the nose.

FIG. 13-6. Construction of a postnasal pack from a vaginal tampon.

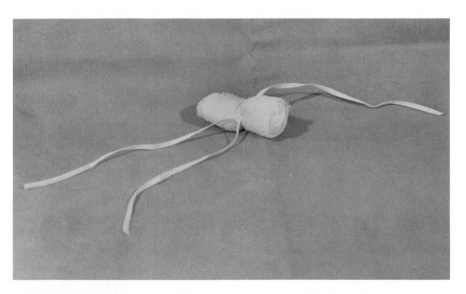

FIG. 13-7. Postnasal pack made from fine mesh gauze and umbilical tape. Note that two tape ends come through nose and the third hangs down in nasopharynx to assist in later removal of the pack.

traction (Fig. 13-7). It is then impregnated with petrolatum (or an antibiotic ointment). A pack can easily be constructed by cutting a large-size vaginal tampon in half, adjusting the tampon so that the two string are again in the center, and sewing a third string to the opposite end (to be used in withdrawing the pack) (Figs. 13-6 and 13-7).

Postnasal packs are often so large that they occlude both choanae instead of only one. Then the patient has no nasal airway. Large packs also compress the eustachian tube and cause ear symptoms. The physician should look at the patient's eardrum every day to see if the pack is causing otitis media or hemotympanum. Post-

nasal packs are unpleasant to the patient at the time they are placed and for as long as they are in place.

The pack is removed in 48 to 96 hours. If the patient bleeds seriously after it is removed, it should be replaced.

For the *placement of a postnasal pack* (Fig. 13-8), a rubber catheter is passed through the bleeding side of the nose and pulled out through the mouth with a hemostat. One end of a suture or string is tied to the catheter, and the other end is attached to the two strings on the anterior end of the pack. The catheter is then pulled out of the nose. This maneuver pulls the postnasal pack into the mouth and up be-

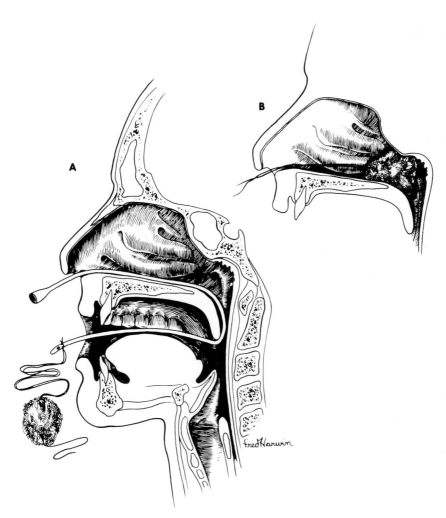

FIG. 13-8. Postnasal packing. **A,** First step. **B,** Second step. Anterior packing with ½-inch petrolatum gauze is then placed.

hind the soft palate into the nasopharynx. A finger inserted above the soft palate helps to seat the pack. After the postnasal pack is in place, the anterior part of the nose (on one side only) is packed with a long strip of petrolatum gauze. Finally, the two strings brought out of the same side of the nose are tied tightly around the gauze.

Another type of postnasal pack can be devised using a Foley catheter with the balloon blown up in the nasopharynx. Although this device does not in itself create pressure against the bleeding site, which is not in the nasopharynx but in the nose, it does provide a posterior buttress against which additional anterior packing can be forced. It also has the advantage of easier availability and probably is easier for the inexperienced physician to place.

Patient's position. Bleeding tends to be less if the patient is kept in a sitting position. Also, in this position blood does not drip into his throat and gag him. Many times merely elevating the head of the bed eliminates oozing of blood in the packed nose. Paradoxically, removing the nasal packing may also stop bleeding. It occasionally does so in the patient with oozing blood around nasal packing that has been in place for several days.

Arterial ligation. There are many reports in the literature concerning treatment of epistaxis by *ligation* of either the external carotid artery or the anterior ethmoidal artery (blood derived from the internal carotid artery). Arterial ligation is occasionally required, but in most patients more efficient packing would probably serve better. When a serious nosebleed is uncontrolled even after proper packing, arterial ligation is necessary. Some authorities believe that the discomfort to the patient is much less with ligation than with prolonged packing, and they begin with ligation rather than first using packing.

A common error is to assume, without careful search, that the source of bleeding is the *external carotid* system. Most of the blood supply to the nose is from this system, but when bleeding is from high in the nose posteriorly, the bleeding is from the internal carotid system through the *anterior ethmoidal artery.* The internal carotid artery cannot be ligated safely, but it is safe to ligate the anterior ethmoidal artery. With the patient under local anesthesia,

an incision made along the side of the nose near the inner canthus of the eye can be used to expose the artery. The periosteum (periorbitum) is elevated carefully, and the artery is identified as it crosses from the orbit to the interior of the nose. A silver clip makes a convenient ligator. If the surgeon decides to ligate the external carotid artery, he must bear in mind the only certain way to distinguish the external carotid from the internal carotid: the external carotid has branches; the *internal carotid has no branches in the neck.* To make doubly sure, the surgeon should identify two branches before ligating.

An alternative to ligating the external carotid artery in the neck is ligation of one of its terminal branches, the *internal maxillary artery.* Because this artery supplies so much blood to the nose, it has been called the "rhinologist's artery." The approach to the internal maxillary artery is by way of an incision made under the upper lip, as for the Caldwell-Luc operation (Figs. 13-9 and 16-12). After an opening has been made through the anterior wall of the normal maxillary sinus, the operating microscope is brought into use and the posterior wall of the maxillary sinus is removed. It is here that the internal maxillary artery can be isolated and ligated. Proponents of early ligation of the internal maxillary artery say that this procedure is less uncomfortable for the patient than several days of suffering with a postnasal pack.

Other means of control. Another method of controlling epistaxis from the internal maxillary artery is by transpalatal injection of saline solution into the greater palatine foramen. When this simple measure works, it is an easy one, but often the control of epistaxis is only temporary.

When a patient has bled enough to be in shock, immediate *transfusion* is required. However, most patients do not require transfusion. Since hemoglobin determinations made immediately after a nosebleed may not represent the patient's true condition because of hemoconcentration, the hemoglobin values should be rechecked when fluid balance has been restored.

Patients with epistaxis often become pale and may be in shock but rarely die. (Some authorities state that death may occur from coronary insufficiency resulting from severe nosebleed, but such instances must be extremely unusual.)

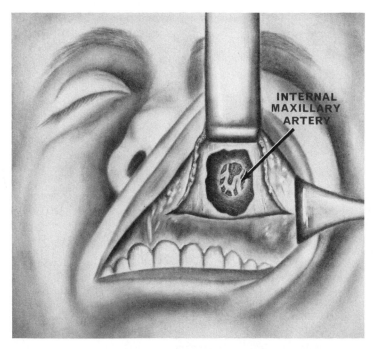

FIG. 13-9. Caldwell-Luc approach to the maxillary sinus and removal of the posterior bony wall of the sinus to expose the internal maxillary artery. One or more clips on this vessel will be used to control posterior epistaxis. (From Chandler, J.R., and Serrins, A.J.: Laryngoscope **75:** 1151, 1965.)

When a patient bleeds enough to go into shock, his blood pressure falls and bleeding almost always stops. Thus there tends to be a check on the amount of blood a patient can lose from epistaxis at any one time.

Hemorrhagic hereditary telangiectasia (Rendu-Osler-Weber disease) is an unusual cause of recurrent and severe nosebleeds (Fig. 13-10, *A*). The disorder affects most organs and epithelial surfaces, but usually the patient bleeds only from the nose or gastrointestinal tract. We know of one patient who required 6,000 transfusions during her lifetime. Several others have had 2,000 transfusions, and a history of 50 is common.

Septal dermoplasty is an effective operation to control bleeding in these patients. The principle of this operation is the fact that although these patients have telangiectases on the skin and oral mucosa, lesions covered by squamous epithelium rarely bleed because squamous epithelium is tough and resists trauma. Nasal mucosa, on the other hand, is exceptionally fragile.

A graft of split-thickness skin from the thigh is placed in the nose to cover the anterior parts of the septum and the floor and lateral walls of the nose *anteriorly*. A raw surface for grafting is created by scraping of the mucous membrane but *not the perichondrium* (Fig. 13-10, *B*). The grafts are held in place 5 days by appropriate nasal packing. Usually there is great reduction in the severity and frequency of epistaxis after septal dermoplasty. Some patients never bleed again.

Medical treatment. Every few years a new drug is offered to the medical profession for the control of epistaxis. However, there is danger in the routine use of drug therapy in the treatment of nosebleed. *It may cause a physician to rely on medical treatment for a surgical condition.* For instance, he may administer drugs instead of removing a poorly placed pack and correctly repacking the bleeding site. Instances in which the use of drugs seems to be effective in the treatment of epistaxis should be reevaluated. It must be remembered that time is a factor in nosebleeds, and, given enough time (whether or not medicines are being used), most nosebleeds will stop spontaneously.

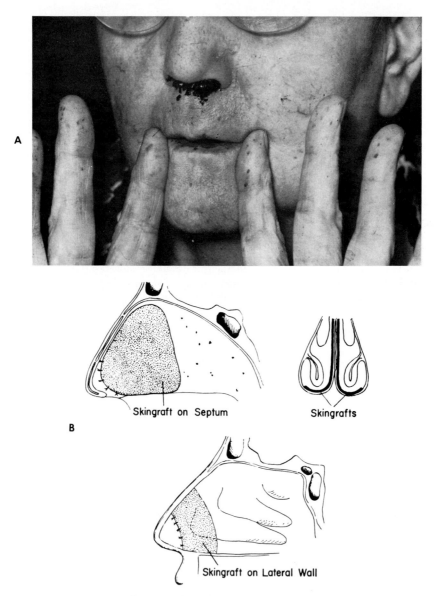

FIG. 13-10. A, Severe nasal crusting like this is common in patients with hereditary hemorrhagic telangiectasia. Note also telangiectases on the lips, fingertips, and face—all common sites. **B,** Septal dermoplasty operation. The skin grafts can be considered posterior extensions of the normal vestibular skin. (From Saunders, W.H.: Arch. Otolaryngol. **76:**245, 1962.)

SELECTED READINGS

Chandler, J.R., and Serrins, A.J.: Transantral ligation of the internal maxillary artery for epistaxis, Laryngoscope **75:**1151, 1965.

Ibrashi, F., and others: Effects of atherosclerosis and hypertension in arterial epistaxis, J. Laryngol. Otol. **92:**877.

Kuhn, A.J., and Hallberg, O.E.: Complications of postnasal packing for epistaxis, Ann. Otol. Rhinol. Laryngol. **62:**62, 1955.

McCaffrey, T.V., Kern, E.B., and Lake, C.F.: Management of epistaxis in hereditary hemorrhagic telangiectasia: review of 80 cases, Arch. Otolaryngol. **103:**627, 1977.

Petruson, B., Rudin, R., and Svardsudd, K.: Is high blood an etiologic factor in epistaxis? O.R.L. **39:**155, 1977.

Roberson, G.H., and others: Angiography and embolization of the internal maxillary artery for posterior epistaxis, Arch. Otolaryngol. **105:**333, 1979.

Saunders, W.H.: Practical management of nosebleeds, G.P. **17:**100, 1958.

Saunders, W.H.: Hereditary hemorrhagic telangiectasia; its familial patterns, clinical characteristics, and surgical treatment, Arch. Otolaryngol. **76:**245, 1962.

14 THE NASAL SEPTUM; MAXILLARY AND NASAL FRACTURES

THE NASAL SEPTUM

Deviated septum. At birth the nasal septum normally is straight, and it remains straight and thin during infancy and early childhood. However, as age progresses, there is a tendency for the septum to become deviated to one side or the other or for an irregular projection to develop (called a septal spur, shelf, or hump, depending on the shape). Often there is no history of injury to account for the irregular septum. In some persons the nasal septum seems to lose its midline position during the growth process rather than as the result of injury. Few adults have a septum that is altogether in the midline.

Sometimes the septum is bent as a result of birth trauma, so that the infant's nose is twisted. Usually there is no bleeding. Often the nose will right itself after a few days (the injury is of the greenstick type), but sometimes the deformity persists. It is worthwhile to reduce the deformity when it is first seen. Correction is usually simple and can be made by lightly pressing the thumb on the convex side of the nose or by tweaking the tip between the thumb and index finger to pull the nose back to the midline. No packing or splint is required.

When trauma causes a septal injury during childhood or adult life, similar maneuvers may suffice to correct the deformity. However, more forceful manipulation with the patient under local or general anesthesia may be necessary.

Physicians do not always agree on the symptoms that may be caused by a deviated septum, but one symptom, *nasal obstruction*, is recognized by patients and physicians alike. However, there are many other causes of nasal obstruction, and a deviated septum may be the least important of several causes. A septum that appears severely obstructive may not, in fact, cause the patient any discomfort at all. In a group of patients with the same apparent degree of obstruction, it will be found that some have no complaint whereas others are in distress. Except for nasal obstruction, other symptoms resulting from septal malformations are less well defined. *Headache* is frequently attributed to a septal spur impinging on the inferior turbinate or to a septal deviation when it causes nasal obstruction. Yet, many patients seen with these conditions have no headache. The possibility of coincidence in patients who have both head pain and a septal deformity is great. Great care must be taken before a causal relation is suggested. *Sinusitis* may be influenced by a deviated septum that occludes a sinus ostium, but such a relationship is rare. The physician should be careful not to promise that a septal operation will cure sinusitis. The reputation of nasal surgery suffers when a patient fails to obtain relief after an operation; the patient blames the operation, whereas the fault was in the diagnosis. Sometimes *nosebleeds* are produced as a result of air currents drying the mucosa that covers a deflected septum. As the mucosa is traumatized, crusts form and bleeding results when they are picked off or come loose. Such trauma is confined to the anterior part of the nose. Occasionally a patient may feel a septal irregularity just inside the nasal vestibule and be inclined to pick at it.

On inspection the septum is seen to be inclined or bent to one side (sometimes an S curve blocks both sides) and the airway is greatly reduced. The obstruction may be anterior (cartilaginous) or posterior (bony). Sometimes the anterior (caudal) end of the septal cartilage

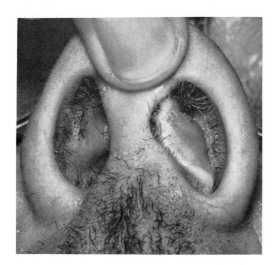

FIG. 14-1. Dislocation of the columellar end of the septal cartilage.

is dislocated into one nasal vestibule (Fig. 14-1). In such conditions, if the patient complains, an operation called a submucous resection (or nasal septal reconstruction) is performed to relieve the nasal obstruction. *It is dangerous, however, to suggest to the patient who has a deviated septum that an operation to straighten the septum will do anything more than improve his nasal septum. The operation is not intended to correct headache (usually incidental) or reduce mucous discharge (postnasal drip).*

Submucous resection (nasal septal reconstruction). Many different procedures are used to straighten and thin the septum. In the most common procedure (the Killian) an incision is made through the mucosa and perichondrium (on one side only) just behind the mucocutaneous junction. Then the mucoperichondrium and mucoperiosteum are elevated on one side, and the cartilage is cut through at the site of the original incision (great care must be taken not to cut through the opposite mucoperichondrium). The soft tissue on the opposite side is elevated until the septal cartilage and bones are freed of all soft tissue attachments, and pieces of cartilage or bone or both are removed or placed in a better position.

In one technique almost all the framework of the septum (except for a strut at the top and in front) is removed (Fig. 14-2). In other techniques an effort is made to excise as little framework as possible but to shave off thick

places, break the "spring" of the cartilage, and leave as much rigid septum as possible (thinned and straightened) (Fig. 14-3). In another approach an incision cuts through the entire membranous columella just in front of the cartilage, affording an end-on view of the free edge of the cartilage. This approach is especially useful when the caudal edge of the cartilage is dislocated and appears in one vestibule rather than in the midline (Fig. 14-1).

Great care must be taken to avoid two opposing incisions (or tears) in the mucoperichondrial flaps. A perforation of the septum may result. Also, care should be taken to leave sufficient support for the nose so that the bridge does not fall or become pulled down by scar contracture (saddle deformity) (Fig. 14-4).

Septal perforations. The most frequent causes of nasal septal perforations are chronic infections caused by repeated trauma (picking the nose) and operative procedures. Perforations resulting from syphilis and tuberculosis, once quite common, are now seldom seen. Carcinoma may also cause septal perforations, but rarely. Other causes of septal perforation are Wegener's granulomatosis, cocaine addiction, and inhalation of acid fumes. Septal perforations do not always cause symptoms. When they do, recurrent nosebleeds and nasal crusting are the common symptoms. Small perforations may produce a whistle when the patient breathes.

A septal perforation (Fig. 14-5) is usually obvious but may be overlooked when the septum is crusted. There is a tendency to look through a *large* septal perforation and see the normal mucosa of the opposite side of the nose without realizing which mucosa is being seen. Perforations are usually in the cartilaginous septum (anteriorly) but may also involve the bony septum.

Surgical closure of septal perforations is possible, but operations are not always successful. In general, discomfort can be kept at a minimum if the patient avoids picking the nose, uses bland ointment such as petrolatum to control crusting, and treats symptoms as they occur. Bleeding from the margins of the perforation may require packing or cautery.

Septal abscess. Although unusual, a septal abscess is important because it is painful and because serious consequences may result. The

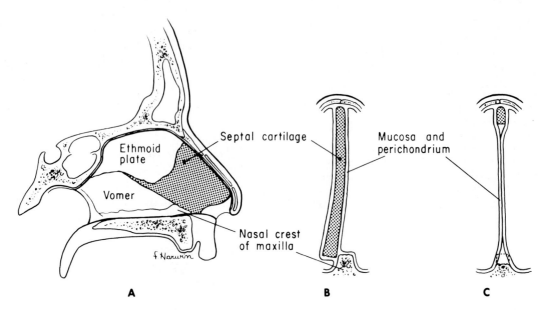

FIG. 14-2. A, Chief components of the septum. **B,** Septum with a deviated cartilabe and spur at the junction of the nasal crest and septal cartilage. **C,** Part of the cartilage and bone have been resected, allowing the mucoperichondrium of the two sides to grow together in the midline.

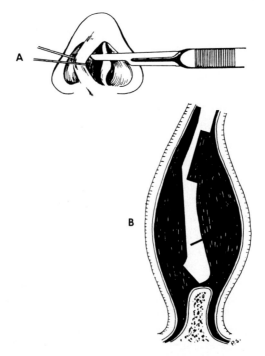

FIG. 14-3. Another type of septal operation. **A,** Complete transfixation of the membranous portion of the columella just in front of the septal cartilage. **B,** The cartilage is shaved down, and cuts are made to break the spring, but very little is resected.

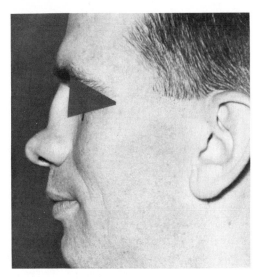

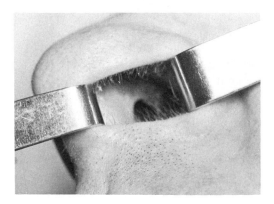

FIG. 14-5. Septal perforation.

FIG. 14-4. Saddle deformity of the nose caused by depression of the septal cartilage.

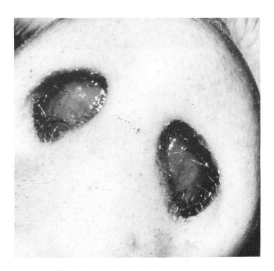

FIG. 14-6. Septal abscess.

septum balloons out on both sides and is red (Fig. 14-6). The widening begins just behind the columella and extends a variable distance posteriorly. Pressure with a probe or bayonet forceps causes pitting of the swollen area and increases pain. Incision releases pus.

Pus, which is between the cartilage and its perichondrium, cuts off the blood supply from the cartilage. Necrosis of the cartilage may result, and after the infection heals, the dorsum of the nose may fall (Fig. 14-4). Thrombosis of the cavernous sinus may occur. Infections about the nose drain through the angular vein, to the inferior ophthalmic vein, and thus to the cavernous sinus. Thrombosis of the cavernous sinus, in spite of modern therapy, is dangerous and can cause death in a few days.

A septal abscess should be incised and drained. Through-and-through drainage is contraindicated because a septal perforation may result. Systemic antibiotics are prescribed in full dosage.

Septal hematoma. After injury, or sometimes after a nasal operation, a hematoma may develop in the septum. The intranasal appearance may be similar to that of a septal abscess, but instead of pus there is blood between the cartilage and perichondrium. The proper treatment is incision and drainage, although often the drainage incision heals so quickly that blood reaccumulates. Packing the nose helps to pre-

vent additional bleeding. Treatment with antibiotics is customary to prevent a septal abscess, even if no infection is present.

FRACTURES

Cervical fractures. After head and neck trauma great attention must be given to the possibility of an associated fracture of the cervical spine. If such a fracture is present, manipulation of the head, as occurs during laryngoscopy, could easily cause an injury to the cervical spine that might have been avoided had the fracture been detected. Therefore x-ray films of the cervical spine in the anteroposterior and lateral projections are required.

Maxillary fractures. Fractures of the maxilla usually result from severe direct trauma, such as a blow with the fist, a fall, or an automobile accident. Auto accidents often produce a very severe injury, the so-called middle third or Le Fort III fracture, in which both maxillae are fractured in several places and the entire middle third of the face (including the nose) is driven backward. The resulting deformity is a very flat face, with the mandibular teeth protruding beyond the maxillary teeth, so that normal occlusion is impossible. The entire maxilla can be rocked back and forth if the examiner takes hold of the upper teeth and palate and moves these parts. This "middle third" fracture (also known as the "guest passenger" accident) usually occurs when an auto is stopped suddenly. The passenger in the right front seat is thrown forward, and his face strikes the hard dashboard. The driver is usually protected by the wheel and steering column. Padded dashboards and seat belts help to prevent this particular accident. Other maxillary fractures are less severe but more common.

Roentgenograms are an indispensable aid in diagnosis. Several views should be taken, including the Waters, Caldwell, and lateral views. Because maxillary fractures are sometimes associated with unrecognized mandibular fractures, roentgenograms of the mandible should be made if there is any doubt.

The physical examination is very important. Palpation along the superior rim of the maxilla (the inferior orbital area) may reveal a steplike segment where a piece of the orbital rim is displaced downward into the maxillary sinus (Fig. 14-8). In the patient with a severe middle third fracture, the entire upper jaw is loose and the examiner can move it in and out readily. The teeth should occlude properly. If they do not, either the maxilla is pushed posteriorly or the mandible is fractured.

When the entire upper jaw is loose and can be moved back and forth, there is great difficulty in maintaining reduction. If the patient has maxillary and mandibular teeth that can be wired together, the problem is greatly simplified. When the patient is edentulous, other means must be used to maintain reduction. Kirschner wires can be used to fix the upper jaw to a solid zygoma, or the maxilla can be suspended by a subcutaneous wire attached to the outer orbital rim. Also, temporary dentures attached to the palate and mandible by wires

can be wired to each other to maintain reduction.

Small local fractures of the orbital rim may be reduced by elevating them through a Caldwell-Luc type of antrotomy. Gauze packing placed in the maxillary sinus will hold the fragments in place. Also, an incision can be made directly over the fracture to wire one large loose piece in place. Even when several fragments are present, wiring is still possible.

Fractures of the nasal bones are often associated with more severe facial fractures. The tendency is not so much to overlook fractures of the nasal bones in the presence of known maxillary fractures, as the reverse.

In all cases of severe facial injury, it is important to determine whether there has been any intracranial or cervical damage before correcting a major facial fracture. Immediate reduction of any of the facial bones is not imperative; results just as satisfactory can be obtained 2 or 3 days later.

Blowout fractures. The so-called blowout fracture results when blunt trauma to the orbit suddenly raises the intraorbital pressure and drives orbital fat and muscles through a fracture in the bony floor of the orbit. This means that the orbital contents are hanging into the maxillary sinus. Sometimes there is not a significant depression of the bony fragment, yet double vision may result from incarceration of extraocular muscles in the fracture site (Fig. 14-9). Surgical exploration using either an orbital or a transsinal approach, or both, is required if the posttraumatic symptom of diplopia (double vision) is to be corrected.

Zygomatic fractures. The zygoma (malar bone) is also frequently injured when the maxilla is fracture, or it may be fractured independently of the maxilla (Fig. 14-10). The zygomatic arch, composed of parts of the malar and temporal bones, is often depressed, so that its normal convexity is lost. An x-ray film made in the mentovertical diameter usually shows this deformity best.

In reducing fractures of the zygomatic arch, a good technique is to make an incision above the fracture (and above the hairline) to insert an elevator under the temporalis fascia and pry the depressed fragment upward. Sometimes, using a towel clip, the physician can grasp the depressed bone through the skin and then pull

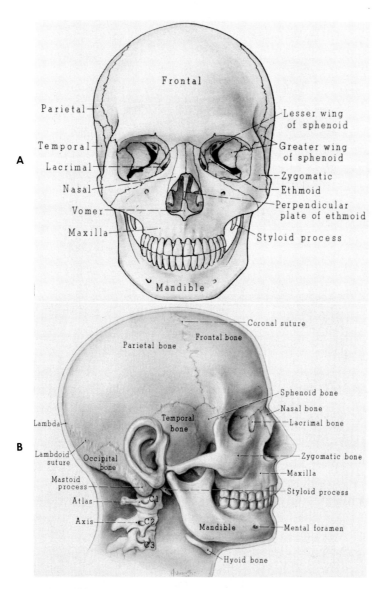

FIG. 14-7. A, Frontal view of the bony structure of the face and skull, **B,** Lateral view of the
bony structure of the face and head. Note relation of the zygoma to the maxilla and to the orbit.
(From Jacob, S.W., and Francone, C.A.: Structure and function in man, ed. 2, Philadelphia,
1970, W.B. Saunders Co.)

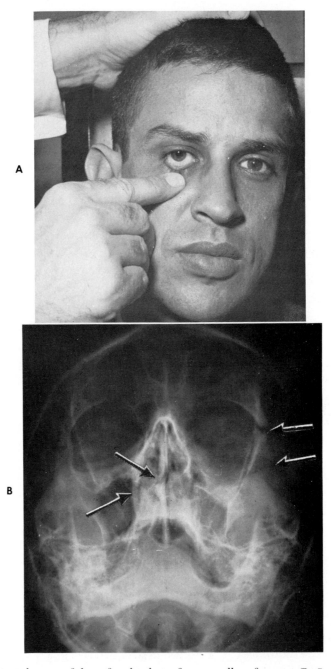

FIG. 14-8. A, Palpation of the infraorbital rim for a maxillary fracture. **B,** Severe zygomatic and maxillary fracture. Note depression of the infraorbital plate and rotation of the zygoma into the maxillary sinus.

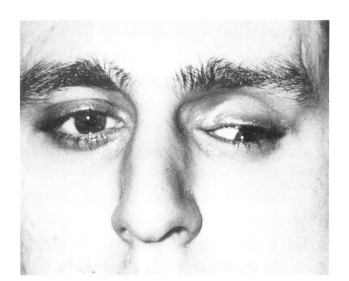

FIG. 14-9. Permanent deformity after untreated fracture of the inferior orbital rim and "blowout" fracture.

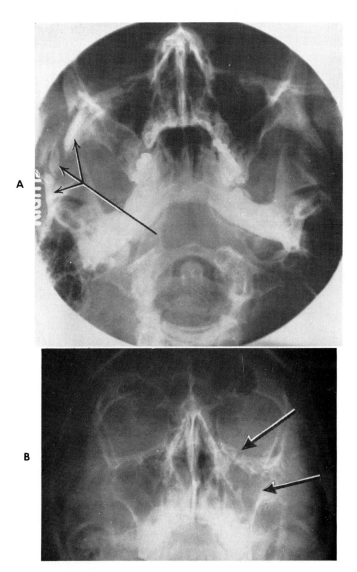

FIG. 14-10. A, Comminuted zygomatic fracture. **B,** Palpable steplike fracture of the infraorbital rim. Note clouding of the maxillary sinus caused by blood.

it forward; or a Caldwell-Luc incision and transantral approach may work best. Generally, once a simple depressed fracture of the zygomatic arch is reduced, additional fixation is unnecessary.

Mandibular fractures. Mandibular fractures are diagnosed on the basis of abnormal occlusion, abnormal mobility with irregularity of the dental arch, and pain when the jaws are clenched at the site of the fractures. Careful intraoral inspection and palpation are important. Fractures of the coronoid and condylar processes often must be diagnosed from a palpable localized hematoma or point tenderness. Bimanual examination of the retrotonsillar fossa offers further information about the ramus of the mandible. Roentgenograms are invaluable and serve not only as diagnostic aids but also as permanent records of the injury.

Treatment of most mandibular fractures is not difficult if there are teeth in the upper and lower jaws. Then interdental wiring can be used to stabilize the fractured segments until union occurs (Figs. 14-11 and 14-12). In the absence of teeth, fixation may have to be achieved by open reduction and wiring of the fragments or by use of Kirschner wires or a metal plate. Generally, the best results are obtained by using the simplest methods because elaborate, complicated appliances may themselves cause complications.

Nasal fractures. Nasal fractures are quite common. Occasionally during birth the nose is fractured in the birth canal. Such fractures are usually of the greenstick type, and the nose inclines a little to one side. Treatment is simple. The nose can be straightened by merely grasping its tip and pulling it toward the midline or pushing slightly on the convex side.

In adult life nasal fractures commonly result from a "right cross," which smashes both nasal bones to one side; from a frontal blow, which depresses the nasal bones; or from various other injuries that cause misalignment of the septum with or without nasal bone injuries. Facial fractures, particularly of the inferior orbital rim or zygoma, may be associated with severe nasal fractures.

If the external nose is lacerated, a compound fracture may exist. Usually, however, nasal frac-

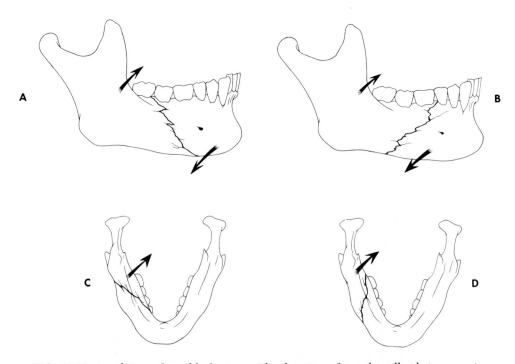

FIG. 14-11. A and **D** are favorable fractures. The direction of muscle pull aids in approximation of the fragments. **B** and **C** are unfavorable. The muscle pull tends to separate the fragments. Open reduction and wiring are required.

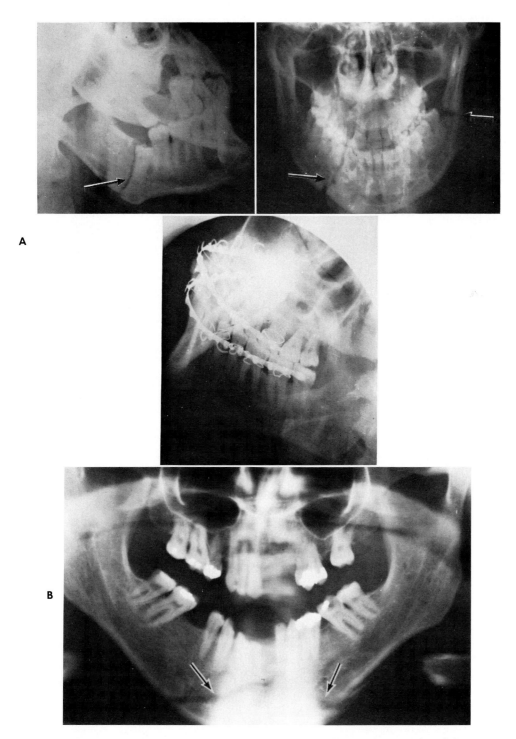

FIG. 14-12. A, Examples of mandibular fractures and interdental wiring with arch bars—one method of fixation. **B,** Panorex view of the mandible showing fracture.

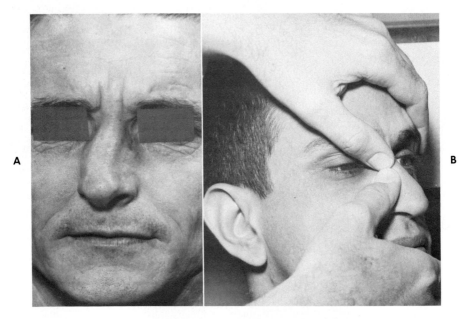

FIG. 14-13. A, Typical nasal deformity from a right cross. Prompt treatment would have restored alignment. Now a rhinoplasty is needed. **B,** One method of reducing a fresh fracture.

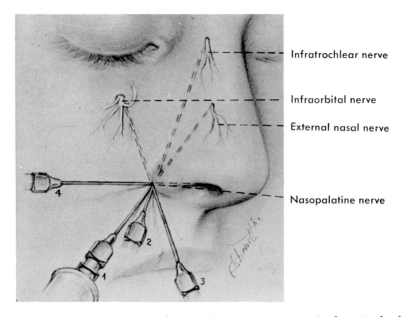

FIG. 14-14. Anesthesia of the external nose. (Courtesy Dr. Lewis Jordan, Portland, Ore.)

tures are simple, or comminuted, rather than compound. If the cartilage of the septum is injured but not the nasal bones, the tip of the nose may deviate to one side while the upper bony part of the nose remains straight. The opposite may also occur, or both the septum and the nasal bones may be twisted. Occasionally the tip is injured independently of the rest of the nose, in which case there is usually a hematoma of the upper lateral cartilage and the swelling pushes one side of the nasal tip outward.

Treatment of most fractured noses is not difficult. The aims of reduction are to *obtain a satisfactory airway and to restore the original appearance of the nose.*

In the *lateral type of fracture* (Fig. 14-13, *A*), in which one nasal bone is smashed inward and the other outward, simple thumb pressure on the convex side is often enough to push the bones back (Fig. 14-13, *B*). The nasal septum may also be displaced, but it returns to normal position when the nasal bones are repositioned. Ordinarily no anesthesia is required. The lateral type of fracture is the most common.

Depressed fractures are more difficult to reduce than fractures of the lateral type. Generally, reduction must be done with the patient under either local or general anesthesia. When a general anesthetic is necessary, the patient should be hospitalized so that the anesthetic can be administered by a qualified anesthetist.

When a local anesthetic is to be used, the patient should be given preliminary medication with a barbiturate drug such as pentobarbital (Nembutal), 0.1 gm., 30 minutes before the operation. Either cocaine, 5% or 10%, or 2% tetracaine (Pontocaine) is used to induce local anesthesia. It is sprayed into the nose, and the nose is packed with gauze strips, ¼-inch wide, moistened with the same solution. Spraying the nose should be done with a hand spray (atomizer) rather than a power spray because of the danger of spraying too much solution.

Even better anesthesia can be obtained by placing two applicators on each side of the nose, one high in the nose adjacent to the septum to block the anterior ethmoidal nerve and the other far back at the end of the middle turbinate for the so-called sphenopalatine ganglion block (Fig. 15-6). The applicators are soaked in 10% cocaine or in cocaine crystals (5 grains) and

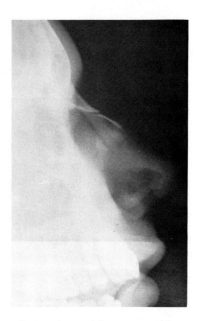

FIG. 14-15. Simple nasal fracture. Much more information is gained from clinical examination than from x-ray films.

enough epinephrine to make a thick syrup ("cocaine mud").

Additional anesthesia for the external nose (Fig. 14-14) is obtained by the injection of 1% procaine or lidocaine (Xylocaine) near the infratrochlear and infraorbital nerves. Usually about 5 ml. should suffice for both sides.

An elevator or a hemostat covered with a thin rubber tubing is used to pry up the nasal bones.

In the occasional difficult case, wiring, packing, or splinting is required. In most instances, however, the replaced bones stay in position without packing or splinting. A new injury will disturb the fragments, but with only reasonable care the patient is safe.

COMMON ERRORS. Following are some common errors associated with treatment of nasal fractures:

1. The physician attempts to set a nose that was fractured many years previously. In such instances the patient becomes aware of the deformity only when a new trauma calls his attention to his nose.

2. X-ray films reveal no fracture, but actually there is one. In general, roentgenograms are of little practical value in the management of nasal fractures (Fig. 14-15). The physician's clinical judgment is much

more important. However, x-ray films are of great value in the management of associated fractures, especially those of the zygoma and inferior orbital rim.

3. The physician regards an easy-to-reduce fracture too seriously (gives general anesthesia) or a severe fracture too lightly (treats it in his office rather than in a hospital).

4. The physician waits too long to reduce the fracture. If treated within 5 or 6 days after injury, a nasal fracture can be reduced easily. Thereafter, reduction may be difficult.

SELECTED READINGS

Bailey, B.J., and Goskill, J.R.: Management of fractures of the mandible, Laryngoscope **77**:1137, 1967.

Bernstein, L., and McClurg, F.L.: Mandibular fractures: review of 156 consecutive cases, Laryngoscope **87**:957, 1977.

Dingman, R.O., and Natvig, P.: Surgery of facial fractures, Philadelphia, 1964, W.B. Saunders Co., pp. 133-209.

Facer, G.W.: Nonsurgical closure of nasal septal perforations, Arch. Otolaryngol. **105**:6, 1979.

Hayes, H.: Immediate management of severe facial injuries, Am. J. Surg. **110**:845, 1965.

Hilger, J.A.: The open reduction of nasal fractures, Laryngoscope **71**:292, 1961.

Klein, J.C.: Intraoral open reduction, Arch. Otolaryngol. **103**:645, 1977.

Lewis, J.R.: Management of soft-tissue injuries of face, J. Int. Coll. Surg. **44**:441, 1965.

Marciani, R.D., and others: Treatment of the fractured edentulous mandible, J. Oral Surg. **37**:569, 1979.

May, M.: Nasofrontal-ethmoidal injuries, Laryngoscope **87**:948, 1977.

Olsen, K.D., and others: Nasal septal trauma in children, Pediatrics **64**:32, 1979.

Soll, D.B., and Poley, B.J.: Trap-door variety of blowout fracture of the orbital floor, Am. J. Ophthalmol. **60**:269, 1965.

Tardy, M.E.: Sublabial mucosal flap: repair of septal perforations, Laryngoscope **87**:275, 1977.

Turvey, T.A.: Mid-facial fracture: a retrospective analysis of 593 cases, J. Oral Surg. **35**:887, 1978.

15 ACUTE AND CHRONIC DISEASES OF THE NOSE

Inflammation of the tissues of the nose may be localized or diffuse. Inflammation involving the vestibule is localized and does not ordinarily extend to the mucosa of the nasal cavity. Inflammation of the mucous membranes of the nose is usually diffuse, but it does not produce concomitant inflammation of the skin of the vestibule.

When the nose is partially or completely blocked, even for a short time, most people complain. Obstruction to the normal free passage of air through the nose gives rise to a sensation of fullness in the face, shortness of breath, and often headache. Nasal obstruction may be temporary or fixed. It may be caused by changes in the tissue of the nasal cavity (septum or turbinates), disease of the nasal vestibule, or tumors of the nasal cavity. Most conditions that cause nasal obstruction can be treated successfully.

DISEASES OF THE NASAL VESTIBULE

Vestibulitis (folliculitis). The vestibule of the nose contains numerous hair follicles, which can become infected. The typical complaint is recurrent crusting inside the vestibule and recurrent tenderness of the nasal tip or alae. The symptoms vary in severity and seem to disappear after several days, only to recur a few weeks or months later. Examination shows mild imflammation at the base of one or several hair follicles. The infection spreads from one group of hair follicles to another.

Unless treated, this mild but annoying infection sometimes lasts indefinitely. The usual treatment consists of rubbing ointment into the skin of the nasal vestibule two or three times a day. Ointments containing antibiotics with or without cortisone are frequently used and are effective. Ammoniated mercury ointment, 5%, is also very effective. Treatment should be continued for 2 to 3 weeks after symptoms disappear. If it is discontinued as soon as tenderness and crusting have stopped, recurrences are more frequent.

Warning: Ammoniated mercury ointment should not be used off and on over a period of several months. Indiscriminate use of this drug over long periods of time can lead to chronic mercury poisoning.

Furunculosis. Furunculosis of the nasal vestibule is common. Usually trauma from picking the nose or from blowing the nose vigorously causes a break in the skin, which allows the entrance of staphylococcal or streptococcal organisms into the subcutaneous tissue. The nose becomes tender as the infection develops, and the entire tip of the nose, the alae, and the upper lip may become swollen and red. There is mild fever. Often signs of systemic toxicity appear. After 2 to 3 days the furuncle localizes and can be seen inside the nasal vestibule (Fig. 15-2).

Sometimes the infection remains diffuse and a spreading cellulitis develops as a result of attempts to squeeze the furuncle or to incise it before pus has localized. This area, as well as the area of the upper lip, has direct venous drainage through the angular vein to the cavernous sinus. Attempts to express pus from a furuncle or to incise it in an area in which there is cellulitis may cause the infection to spread to the cavernous sinus and death to occur in a few days. The triangle formed by lines drawn from the corners of the mouth upward to the glabella is referred to as the danger triangle. Infections

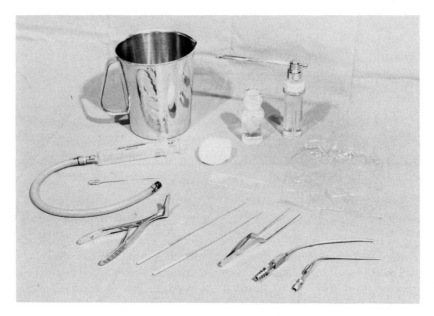

FIG. 15-1. Instruments necessary for adequate examination of the nose and sinuses. *Upper left*, Cannister, syringe with rubber tubing, and antral trochar (needle). *Upper right*, Cotton, glass slide (for nasal smears), cocaine bottle, atomizer of vasoconstrictor (ephedrine 2%), and cellophane square. *Bottom*, Nasal speculum, cotton carriers, bayonet forceps, and suction tips.

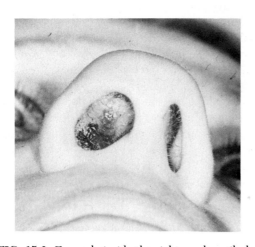

FIG. 15-2. Furuncle inside the right nasal vestibule.

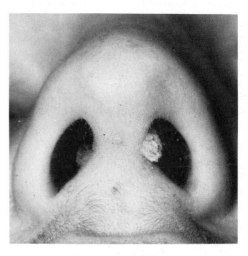

FIG. 15-3. Squamous papilloma of the columella of the left nasal vestibule.

of the skin in this area (including the vestibule of the nose) should be treated *without mechanical manipulation* to avoid cavernous sinus thrombosis.

The treatment consists of adequate doses of appropriate antibiotics, hot wet packs, and analgesics or narcotics for relief of pain. *There*

should be a hands-off policy regarding any surgical treatment until the surrounding inflammation has subsided and the furuncle has localized. Then, with sterile technique, it can be incised safely.

Fissures. Small breaks in the skin of the vestibule often occur at the junction of the skin and the mucous membrane. A crust forms that the patient removes from time to time. Under the crust is a painful fissure. Fissures are not dangerous and rarely become infected. Superficial cautery of the fissure with silver nitrate, followed by application of ammoniated mercury or antibiotic ointment, is usually satisfactory treatment.

Squamous papilloma. Small wartlike growths may develop in the squamous epithelium of the vestibule. The cause of these papillomas is unknown, although a virus is suspected. Malignant degeneration of this type of papilloma has not been reported.

These benign papillomas usually occur singly (Fig. 15-3), and some of them regress spontaneously. However, because patients tend to pick at them, spontaneous regression often is prevented and excision is required.

Simple excision at the base of the lesion will not prevent recurrence. The effective removal of the lesion requires a small incision. Some of the surrounding normal tissue is included in the excised tissue.

DISEASES OF THE NASAL CAVITY

Acute rhinitis (the common cold). The most common cause of acute rhinitis is the common cold. The symptoms are familiar to both physician and patient.

It has been proved by experiments on both humans and monkeys that the common cold is caused by a filtrable virus. The disease can be transmitted after as many as 80 transfer subcultures. It is probably the most common infectious disease in humans. Children under 5 years of age are the most susceptible; susceptibility is progressively less from the age of 5 to 18 or 20 years. Thereafter it remains constant. On the average, a child or an adolescent may have three to five colds a year, depending on contacts and certain environmental changes.

The disease is spread by droplet contact from sneezing. Chilling of the body, fatigue, and crowded living quarters are predisposing factors. Immunity lasts approximately 1 month and then is lost. So far, it has not been possible to develop vaccines to increase the length of immunity.

The typical symptoms are well known. The onset is usually manifested by a feeling of irritation and a burning sensation in the nasopharynx.

Sneezing and copious nasal discharge soon follow. Mild fever and malaise are usually present. As the disease progresses, the nose becomes more obstructed and the discharge becomes purulent. Headache is a common symptom during the first 2 days. Sore throat is not a characteristic complaint of the patient with a common cold. Any significant pain should make the physician wary of a complication. When uncomplicated, the common cold is self-limited. Most symptoms subside in 4 or 5 days, and the nose returns to normal in 6 or 7 days. However, when the condition is complicated by a secondary invasion of virulent bacteria, the symptoms persist and become worse. Then there may be symptoms and signs of *sinusitis*, otitis media, bronchitis, or pneumonia.

Treatment of the common cold is symptomatic. There is no specific remedy. Rest, preferably in bed, plus adequate fluids and a regular diet are as effective as any known medication. Overheating and chilling should be avoided. Aspirin may help the general feeling of malaise. On occasion the use of antihistaminics during the first day of the disease will alleviate some of the symptoms, but antihistaminics are not curative. There is no indication for the use of antibiotics during an uncomplicated cold. Nose drops may be prescribed but should be used infrequently and only to allay prolonged nasal obstruction. *There is a great tendency for some patients to continue the use of nose drops longer than necessary and thereby to addict the nasal mucosa to their use (rhinitis medicamentosa).* Some investigators believe that closure of the nose during the acute symptoms may be a protective mechanism and that use of nose drops may cause infection to spread.

Whenever possible, isolation of the patient is advisable. Usually the symptoms are not so severe that the patient will stop work during the contagious first 2 or 3 days of the disease. If isolation could be accomplished, the incidence of the common cold in the general population might be lowered appreciably.

Allergic rhinitis. Often called hay fever, allergic rhinitis may be acute and seasonal or it may be chronic and perennial. The usual symptoms are obstruction of the nose, sneezing, and recurrent thin nasal discharge. Itching of the nose and eyes and tearing are common. Frontal headache is not unusual.

Not infrequently the patient with perennial allergic rhinitis will complain that he has frequent colds. However, a carefully taken history will reveal that his symptoms are those of allergic rhinitis rather than the acute symptoms of the common cold. The final diagnosis may depend on examination of the nose during an attack and microscopic study of the nasal secretions. The discharge from the nose in allergic rhinitis usually contains large numbers of eosinophils, whereas that in the common cold contains desquamated cells, lymphocytes, and large numbers of polymorphonuclear leukocytes.

Seasonal allergic rhinitis is usually caused by pollens from trees, grasses, or flowers. It lasts several weeks, disappears, and recurs the following year. Perennial allergic rhinitis may occur intermittently for years with no pattern, or it may be present constantly. This type of allergic rhinitis is usually caused by sensitivity to house dust, newspaper, wool, feathers, foods, tobacco, or other contacts constantly present in our environment. The symptoms of perennial allergic rhinitis are usually less severe than those of acute hay fever, but they present a greater problem in therapy because identification of the offending allergen is difficult. Perennial allergic rhinitis is often associated with allergic sinusitis (see p. 232).

Often the nasal mucosa in patients with allergic rhinitis exhibits a characteristic appearance. The typical finding is *edema* and *pallor* of the turbinates, especially the inferior turbinates. The surface of the mucosa is smooth and glistening, and the turbinates fill the air space and press against the nasal septum. Not infrequently, rather than being pale, the turbinates look violaceous or almost blue. At other times, the membranes may be inflamed and look dull red rather than pale. The mere fact that the typical pale appearance is not present does not rule out allergic rhinitis.

Examination of the nasopharynx often reveals the posterior ends of the inferior turbinates to be so enlarged that they protrude into the nasopharynx. They are pale or bluish. When they are pitted and bluish, they are called mulberry turbinates. However, not all mulberry turbinates are associated with allergic rhinitis.

Microscopic examination of the nasal secretion often provides a useful clue to diagnosis when characteristic intranasal appearances are not present. Nasal secretions can be obtained with a cotton swab or by gentle suction. When suction is used, a small glass trap can be placed between the suction tip and the tubing attached to it or the secretion can be blown out of the suction tip onto a slide. A still easier method is to have the patient blow his nose into a square of cellophane. The secretion, even though scanty, is smeared on a glass slide and stained. A special stain, called Hansel's stain,* is used after the specimen has dried. With this stain the red cytoplasmic granules in eosinophils stand out sharply. The normal nasal secretion contains few or no eosinophils. In allergic rhinitis, the number of eosinophils may be as high as 90%. More than 3% or 4% in a nasal smear suggests that allergy may be the underlying cause of a patient's nasal complaint.

The best treatment for allergic rhinitis is finding the allergen and then eliminating it, but it is not always possible to do so. Another approach is desensitizing the patient to his allergen. Often a very carefully taken history will give a clue to the allergen. If it does not, extensive tests will be required. However, even after these tests it is often not possible to discover the allergen. This is more true in patients with perennial allergic rhinitis than in those with seasonal allergic rhinitis. When skin tests are refused or cannot be performed, the following practical measures may make the symptoms less troublesome: (1) covering the pillow and mattress with plastic, (2) eliminating chocolate, milk, and eggs from the diet or limiting their use, (3) removing domestic animals from the home, (4) covering overstuffed furniture (mohair is a common allergen), (5) using nonallergenic cosmetics, (6) eliminating the use of wool bedding, (7) air conditioning the home, and (8) using antihistaminics.

Hypertrophied turbinates. The combination of long-standing allergic rhinitis and low-grade inflammation may produce permanent enlargement of the turbinates, particularly the inferior turbinate. When this occurs, the turbinate loses most of its normal ability to expand and to shrink. The result is continuous nasal obstruction. Nose drops, antihistaminics, and allergic desensitization do not relieve the obstruction.

In some instances injection of a sclerosing

---

*Devised by Dr. French K. Hansel, St. Louis, Mo.

solution beneath the mucosa of the turbinate will reduce its size. In others careful submucosal electrocoagulation gives similar results. In still other instances successful treatment is possible only by submucous resection of the turbinate itself.

Submucous resection is performed with the patient under local anesthesia. The mucosa and submucosa along the free margin of the turbinate are incised. Some or all of the bones of the inferior turbinate is removed, and the mucosa is reapproximated. Packs are left in the nose longer than they are after the routine submucous resection operation (nasal septum) because of a tendency toward postoperative bleeding. After healing, the turbinate is smaller but the functioning mucosa remains.

Nasal polyps (Figs. 15-4 and 15-5). Nasal polyps are most often seen in patients with allergic rhinitis. A nasal polyp forms gradually from recurrent localized swelling of the sinus mucosa or from the nasal mucosa. At first the polyp is small. With each succeeding increase in submucosal edema, it becomes larger until, when fully developed, it appears as a smooth, pale tumor. The base is pedunculated but is not seen. In most instances nasal polyps are mul-

tiple. They can be moved back and forth. Turbinates, with which nasal polyps are often confused, cannot move freely, and they are tender when probed. Polyps cause symptoms because they protrude into the airway. They may be large or numerous enough to occlude the nose completely. If untreated for years, they may cause gradual spreading of the nasal bones and widening of the nasal bridge.

Sometimes cortisone, used systemically or injected locally, will cause nasal polyps to disappear. However, when the cortisone is discontinued they usually reappear. For the most part, nasal polyps require operative removal. This is performed with the patient under local anesthesia, using 10% cocaine. Two cotton applicators, moistened with the cocaine, are used. One is placed between the posterior end of the middle turbinate and the septum (sphenopalatine block), and the other is placed high in the anterior part of the nose to block the anterior ethmoidal nerve (Fig. 15-6). Each polyp is avulsed with a wire snare. Often, because the underlying allergy cannot be well controlled, the polyps tend to recur.

Many nasal polyps actually arise from the paranasal sinuses, and one should not be sur-

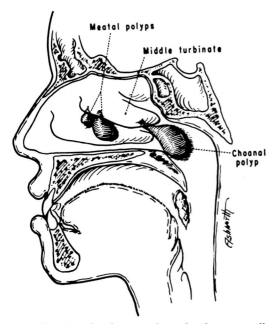

FIG. 15-4. Nasal polyps. A choanal polyp is usually single and originates in the maxillary sinus. Most polyps are found in the middle meatus.

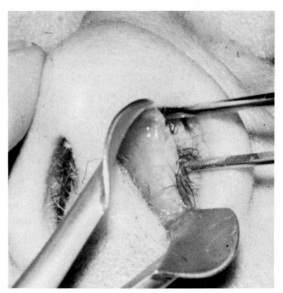

FIG. 15-5. Typical nasal polyp—soft, pale gray, nontender, and mobile.

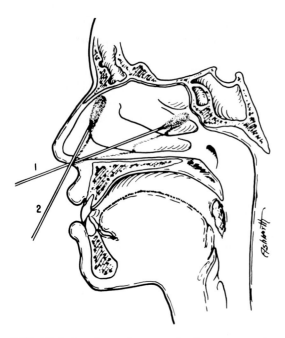

FIG. 15-6. Local anesthesia inside the nose. Applicator No. 1 is placed between the posterior end of the middle turbinate and the nasal septum. Applicator No. 2 is placed opposite the junction of the nasal bone and cartilage high in the nasal vault.

prised to see changes in the sinuses on roentgenograms. Intranasal polypectomy may have to be repeated at intervals of months or years. In patients in whom the condition is severe, a more extensive operation, such as intranasal ethmoidectomy and sphenoidectomy and the Caldwell-Luc procedure, will be needed to prevent recurrence.

In an asthmatic patient the presence of nasal polyps suggests aspirin hypersensitivity. Although authorities tend to disagree on the subject, many surgeons believe that in such a patient polypectomy may precipitate a severe asthmatic attack even though the patient is not given aspirin.

Nonallergic vasomotor rhinitis. Many patients complain of chronic, intermittent nasal obstruction or nasal stuffiness. The obstruction may be accompanied by increased nasal discharge, either thin or viscid. These symptoms are often considered by the patient (and sometimes by the physician) to be allergic, even when there is no good proof of nasal allergy.

Sometimes nervous, tense persons complain about normal postnasal discharge. The 500 to 700 ml. of nasal mucus that normally must be

swallowed daily is distasteful to some patients. Reassurance and careful explanation of nasal physiology will satisfy some of these patients. Treatment with nose drops or other medication is rarely helpful and should be avoided. Overuse of nose drops may cause nasal stuffiness (*rhinitis medicamentosa*), which becomes worse with each successive dose. Since the state of engorgement of the turbinates is controlled by the autonomic nervous system, and since vasoconstrictors stimulate the sympathetic nerves, there tends to be a compensatory relaxation of the turbinal vessels after the effect of the nose drops has stopped. Thus, after temporary relief, the nose becomes more stuffy than it was originally. To be cured of the condition, the patient must tolerate a blocked nose for 2 to 3 weeks without recourse to vasoconstrictors of any type. Then normal reflexes return, and the nose may function properly again.

Nasal stuffiness may also result from certain endocrine disturbances that cause the turbinates to become boggy and edematous. The most important of these is hypothyroidism, or hypometabolism. When no obvious cause can be found for a chronic nasal obstruction, hypometabolism should be suspected. In many patients thyroid extract or triiodothyronine (Cytomel) will alleviate the condition. Most of these patients do not have typical myxedema but are regarded as having a subclinical hypothyroidism. In patients with true myxedema, a pale, boggy mucosa and chronic nasal obstruction are characteristic.

Recently allergic and immunologic studies have indicted aspirin as the sensitizing substance in some patients who have a history of intermittent asthmatic attacks and progressive, bilateral nasal obstruction with recurrent, multiple bilateral nasal polyps. Therefore aspirin must be added to a list of drugs that can give rise to submucosal edema and polyp formation in the nose.

Occasionally, severe nasal obstruction develops during pregnancy. The complaint usually begins near the end of the first trimester. The mucosa is pale, and the turbinates are swollen. They press against the nasal septum and completely obstruct the nose. Treatment is ineffective. The nose resumes its normal appearance and function shortly after delivery.

Some patients react to any stress by the de-

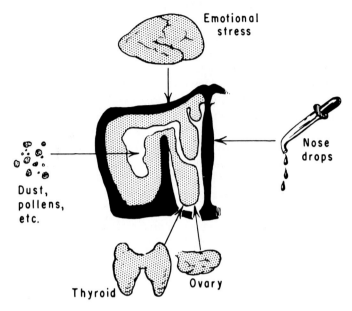

FIG. 15-7. Allergic and nonallergic causes of stuffy nose. Note edema of the nasal and sinus mucosa.

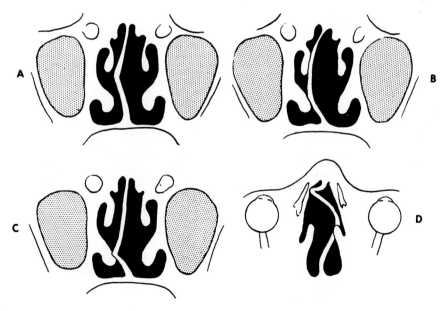

FIG. 15-8. Various types of septal deviations. **A,** Mild, sharp angle. **B,** Smooth curve touching both the middle and inferior turbinates. **C,** Sharp angle impinging on the inferior turbinate. **D,** S-shaped deviation, seen from above, causing bilateral obstruction.

velopment of nasal symptoms. Emotional, sexual, and financial problems may give rise to stuffiness or dryness of the nose or increased nasal discharge. These patients are often diagnostic enigmas. They may need psychiatric consultation.

A very common cause of nasal obstruction is deviation of the nasal septum (Figs. 14-1 to 14-3, and 15-8). If symptoms are mild and intermittent, treatment may not be necessary. However, if the obstruction is constant, whether unilateral or bilateral, submucous resection of the nasal septum is indicated.

Rhinitis medicamentosa is an important cause of nasal obstruction because it is so common. This condition develops in patients who are habitual users of nose drops or nose sprays, and the nasal mucosa often becomes fiery red. They can breathe for an hour or two after using nose drops, but the nose then becomes obstructed again; this cycle of medication and obstruction may continue for months or even years. *Any patient who complains of nasal obstruction and in whom there is no obvious cause for his obstruction should be asked if he is a longtime user of nose drops.* The treatment is simply to have the patient throw away all intranasal medications and to give him a sedative to help him sleep and an orally administered antihistaminic. He will recover in 2 or 3 weeks.

Atrophic rhinitis. The cause of atrophic rhinitis is unknown. Fortunately, it seems to be a disappearing disease. Symptoms begin near the age of puberty, and women are affected more often than men. When the atrophy is well established, the nose is dry and often filled with crusts. Paradoxically, even though the nasal airway is more open than it is normally, the patient with atrophic rhinitis complains of nasal stuffiness. The condition is painless. Often a foul or fetid odor called ozena accompanies the crusting of the nose and may be the most disturbing symptom.

Examination reveals yellow or green crusts associated with some surface purulent exudate. After removal of the crusts, the nose is wide open and the nasopharynx can usually be clearly seen. The turbinates are thin and atrophic. These changes are usually present on both sides of the nose. Rarely, atrophic rhinitis is unilateral. The nasopharynx and pharynx frequently

appear smooth, dry, and shiny rather than pink and moist, as they do normally.

Atrophic rhinitis is resistant to most forms of treatment. In the past nasal sprays of oily solutions containing estrogens were used. Cortisone has been tried in recent years. All antibiotics have been used. None appears to be effective. In most instances gentle, daily irrigation of the nose with isotonic saline solution provides as much symptomatic relief as any known medical treatment.

Some patients have subjective improvement when ordinary confectioner's (powdered) sugar is blown into the nose with a powder blower once or twice daily. In these patients the appearance of the nasal mucosa may also show improvement.

Surgical procedures designed to narrow the airway have been effective in some patients. Bone chips from the crest of the ilium can be implanted in a subperiosteal pocket in the lateral wall of the nose. This procedure narrows the airway and may cause cessation of odor and crusting.

Septal abscess. See Chapter 14, p. 213, for a discussion of septal abscess.

Erysipelas. Erysipelas of the face, as shown in Fig. 15-9, can be seen following streptococcal skin infections of the nose or nasal vestibule. It can also occur spontaneously without any appar-

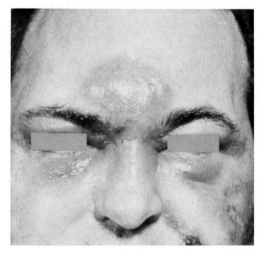

FIG. 15-9. Erysipelas of the face and forehead. Note the "butterfly" pattern over the face and the sharply demarcated, raised border.

ent skin infection. It is characterized by high fever, toxicity, and a red, spreading lesion that has raised borders. The discrete margin of this advancing inflammation can be felt by gently passing the finger from the normal skin to the lesion.

UNILATERAL NASAL DISCHARGE

Infectious, allergic, and degenerative changes in the nose usually cause bilateral symptoms. When discharge comes from one side of the nose only, the physician should be alert to certain special conditions.

Choanal atresia. Some infants are born with atresia of the posterior choana of the nose. When the atresia is bilateral, symptoms of choking, inability to nurse, and bouts of cyanosis usually lead to early diagnosis. When the atresia is unilateral, the infant may nurse and breathe normally but has a unilateral nasal discharge. The discharge is thick and viscid but rarely infected. In making a diagnosis, the physician should attempt to pass a small rubber catheter through the nose into the pharynx. Normally such a catheter can be passed without difficulty, but in an infant with choanal atresia it fails to enter the pharynx when it is inserted into the obstructed side of the nose. Roentgenograms taken after Lipiodol has been instilled into the nose will demonstrate a posterior blockage.

The atresia may be bony or membranous. The treatment is by operative removal of the obstructing partition, usually through a transpalatal approach.

Foreign bodies (Fig. 15-10). Children often put foreign bodies in the nose, just as they do in the ear. Rubber erasers, paper wads, pebbles, beads, and beans are the most common objects. The cardinal symptom is unilateral purulent nasal discharge. Usually there is no pain or other symptoms. The parents usually have no knowledge of the foreign body. It is easy to make an erroneous diagnosis of sinusitis if the nose is not carefully cleaned of secretions before it is examined.

In removing the foreign body, one must have good visualization of the object and the proper instruments. Often the child must be restrained. General anesthesia may be necessary at times. After shrinking of the nose with a vasoconstrictor, the foreign body is removed with grasping forceps.

Rarely, a foreign body will remain in the nose for many years and calcium will become deposited around it. After the surrounding purulent secretion has been removed, a chalky white foreign body called a *rhinolith* is found.

Malignancies. Unilateral bloody discharge from the nose should always make the physician think of a neoplasm of the nose or sinuses. This type of discharge tends to be scanty and intermittently blood tinged. Sometimes, chronic sinusitis with granulation tissue can also cause a bloody nasal discharge. This type of bleeding should not be confused with the fresh, brisk bleeding or ordinary epistaxis. (See also Chapter 17.)

Cerebrospinal rhinorrhea. Occasionally, unilateral nasal discharge will be sparkling clear. Such discharge may occur spontaneously, or it may follow a head injury or a tumor. When clear fluid flows from one side of the nose in any significant amount, and particularly when the symptom recurs, cerebrospinal rhinorrhea should be suspected. Lowering the head or compressing the jugular veins may increase the

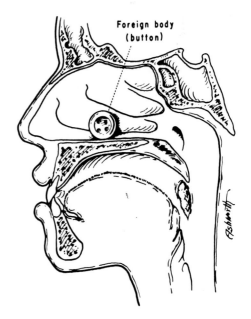

FIG. 15-10. Foreign bodies in the nose usually lodge in the anterior or middle third of the nose and rest on its floor.

flow. The mucosa of the nose looks normal. When cerebrospinal rhinorrhea is suspected, a sample of the discharge should be collected. A simple test for the presence of glucose will enable one to make the diagnosis.

Treatment may require surgical closure of the defect, usually near the cribriform plate. The operation is performed by either an otolaryngologist or a neurosurgeon.

SELECTED READINGS

Becker, W., and others: Atlas of otorhinolaryngology and bronchoesophagology, Philadelphia, 1969, W.B. Saunders Co.

Cramblett, H.G.: Viral respiratory illnesses of infants and children, Bacteriol. Rev. **28:**431, 1964.

Davison, F.W.: The antibody deficiency syndrome, Laryngoscope **76:**1254, 1966.

Delaney, P., and others: Olfactory sarcoidosis: report of five cases and review of the literature, Arch. Otolaryngol. **103:**717, 1977.

Eggston, A., and Wolff, D.: Histopathology of the ear, nose and throat, Baltimore, 1947, The Williams & Wilkins Co.

Frederick, J., and Braude, A.I.: Anaerobic infection of the paranasal sinuses, N. Engl. J. Med. **290:**135, 1974.

Gorbach, S.L., and Bartlett, J.G.: Anaerobic infections. II, N. Engl. J. Med. **290:**1237, 1974.

Hansel, F.K.: Allergy and immunity in otolaryngology, Rochester, Minn., 1975, American Academy of Otolaryngy.

Ritter, F.N.: The effects of hypothyroidism upon the ear, nose and throat, Laryngoscope **77:**1427, 1967.

Roth, R.P., and others: Nasal decongestant activity of pseudoephedrine, Ann. Otol. Rhinol. Laryngol. **86:**235, 1977.

Shapiro, R.S.: Nasal septal abscess, Can. Med. Assoc. J. **119:**1321, 1978.

Saunders, W.H.: Atrophic rhinitis, Arch. Otolaryngol. **68:**342, 1958.

Singleton, G.T., and Hardcastle, B.: Congenital choanal atresia, Arch. Otolaryngol. **87:**620, 1968.

Williams, H.L.: The relationship of allergy to chronic sinusitis, Ann. Allergy **24:**521, 1966.

Wilson, W.H.: Hypersensitivity to foods: adaptation phenomenon, Laryngoscope **87:**657, 1977.

16 ACUTE AND CHRONIC SINUSITIS

For many years nonmalignant disease of the paranasal sinuses has been poorly understood by the medical student, the general physician, and the laity. Too often the paranasal sinuses have been indicted as the underlying cause of nasal obstruction, headaches, fever of unknown origin, chronic sore throat, chronic fatigue, recurrent cough, chronic dyspepsia, and almost any symptom of the upper respiratory or upper gastrointestinal tracts.

The misconceptions regarding sinusitis are common among lay persons, and they are unwittingly fostered by the physician. The laity use the term "sinus" rather than sinusitis, and the physician may speak of "sinus trouble." Such thinking has become so common that many headaches and most nasal symptoms are referred to as sinus trouble. Frequently the lay person thinks that a simple intranasal operation for relief of nasal obstruction is a sinus operation. Acute hay fever and chronic allergic rhinitis are erroneously called sinus infection. The normal postnasal discharge resulting from the physiologic cleansing function of the mucous blanket has been attributed to sinus disease. Sinusitis has been improperly blamed for the ill effects of tobacco, alcohol, and drugs. The student will benefit from a review of the causes of nasal obstruction and vasomotor rhinitis, as well as of headache, before studying sinusitis.

As the suffix "itis" indicates, sinusitis means an inflammatory change in the mucosa of a sinus. When such a pathologic change occurs, definite signs and symptoms are produced. Most of the signs can be seen on physical examination of the nose or can be demonstrated by roentgenograms or other special diagnostic procedures. If the symptoms and signs are not present, many other local or systemic conditions may need to be investigated to discover the

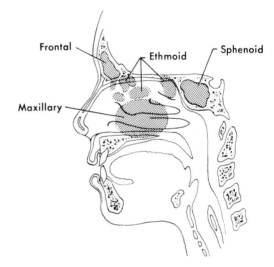

FIG. 16-1. Lateral wall of the nose. The relative positions of the various paranasal sinuses are indicated.

cause of nasal symptoms. Of every 100 patients who consult an otolaryngologist because of "sinus trouble," fewer than 10 have sinusitis.

Sinusitis may be conveniently classified as acute, subacute, and chronic suppurative sinusitis; allergic sinusitis; and hyperplastic sinusitis.

Acute suppurative sinusitis. Acute suppurative sinusitis most often accompanies or follows the common cold. It sometimes occurs endemically from a specific organism when there has been a sudden drop in temperature. It may also occur by infected water being forced into the nose when the patient is swimming or diving. The bacteria most often responsible for acute suppurative sinusitis are the gram-positive cocci—streptococci, staphylococci, and pneumococci. Other bacteria may cause acute sinusitis but much less frequently than the cocci. *Haemophilus influenzae* may give rise to serious complications.

223

The onset of acute sinusitis is not abrupt *except when it occurs after the patient has been swimming or diving*. The first symptom is usually a stuffy feeling in the nose, followed by slowly developing pressure over the involved sinus. There are mild general malaise and toxicity, and headache may be present. The temperature is only slightly elevated (99° to 99.5° F.), or it may be subnormal throughout the course of the disease. The white blood cell count remains normal in most patients. Leukopenia (5,000 to 6,000 cells/mm³) is common. If the temperature is high and the blood cell count is elevated, another disease should be suspected.

Symptoms progress over 48 to 72 hours until there is severe localized pain and tenderness over the involved sinus. In maxillary sinusitis, the pain is over the cheek and the upper teeth. The patient frequently attributes the pain to an ulcerated tooth. The pain involves all or several teeth in one upper alveolus rather than a single tooth. In ethmoid sinusitis, the pain is medial and deep to the eye, or it may seem to be in the eye. In frontal sinusitis, the pain is in the forehead, above the eyebrow. In infection of the sphenoid sinus, the pain is deep behind the eye, in the occiput, and sometimes is referred to the vertex of the skull. In acute frontal and maxillary sinusitis, pain is typically not present in the early morning after a night of rest. It usually appears 1 or 2 hours after the patient arises, increases for 3 or 4 hours, and becomes less severe in the late afternoon and evening.

Discharge from the nose may be bloody or blood tinged in the first 24 to 48 hours of the disease. It rapidly becomes purulent and copious. The nose becomes more blocked, and the throat may become inflamed and sore on one side as a result of the purulent postnasal discharge.

The nasal mucosa on the involved side is hyperemic and edematous. The turbinates are enlarged. They fill the air space of the nose and usually press against the nasal septum. In most patients purulent discharge is visible in the nose (Fig. 16-2). When only swelling and redness are seen, pus can be demonstrated after a vasoconstrictor is applied to shrink the turbinates and afford visualization of the posterior middle meatus. Ciliary action directs the pus toward the nasopharynx, where it can be seen with the nasopharyngeal mirror in the middle or superior meatus or in both. Localized tenderness over the involved sinus is a constant finding. The tenderness is easily demonstrated and is sharply localized to the anatomic boundaries of the involved sinus (Fig. 16-3). On transillumination the involved maxillary or frontal sinus is dark because it will not transmit light (Fig. 1-30). It is not possible to transilluminate the ethmoid or sphenoid sinuses.

Roentgenographic examination shows the involved sinus to be clouded, and sometimes a fluid level is visible (Fig. 16-4). However, roentgenograms are usually not necessary to establish the diagnosis (Fig. 16-5).

Treatment of acute suppurative sinusitis is medical, *not surgical*. The only exception to this rule occurs when the natural ostium of the sinus is completely blocked, resulting in empyema. Pain becomes unbearable, and extension of the infection outside the walls of the sinus may occur.

Treatment is directed at relief of pain, shrinkage of the nasal mucosa, and control of infection. Codeine or occasionally morphine or meperidine (Demerol) will control the pain. Aspirin is not enough. It may be necessary for the patient to take codeine every 2 or 3 hours for several days. The application of heat is therapeutic and also affords symptomatic relief. Wet heat often gives more relief than dry heat. Hot wet packs applied to the face over the involved sinus either continuously or for 2 hours at a time, four times a day, will hasten resolution of the inflammation.

The nose should be kept open as well as possible. This can be accomplished by the use of nose drops or a nasal spray containing a vasoconstrictor such as 2% ephedrine, 0.25% phenylephrine (Neo-Synephrine), or other, longer-acting shrinking solutions. Solutions containing antibiotics or corticosteroids neither hasten the resolution of the infection nor make the patient more comfortable.

Antibiotics may be prescribed, but they are not mandatory in acute sinusitis. The typical patient will have discomfort and copious purulent discharge for 3 or 4 days, after which there is slow resolution of the infection. Complete resolution normally occurs in 10 to 14 days. If purulent discharge persists, or if pain, fever, and the white blood cell count are out of proportion to the expected course of the disease, antibiotics should be prescribed in full dosage. Pen-

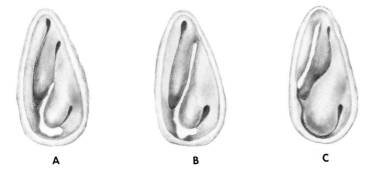

FIG. 16-2. Sites of purulent discharge. **A,** Maxillary sinusitis (low in the middle meatus). Actually, pus from the maxillary sinus is best seen in the nasopharyngeal mirror as it runs over the posterior tip of the inferior turbinate. **B,** Frontal sinusitis. **C,** Sphenoid or posterior ethmoid sinusitis (superior meatus).

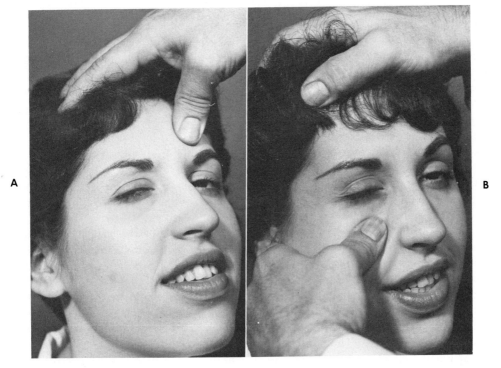

FIG. 16-3. Pressure over the frontal sinus, **A,** or the maxillary sinus, **B,** elicits pain in *acute* sinusitis.

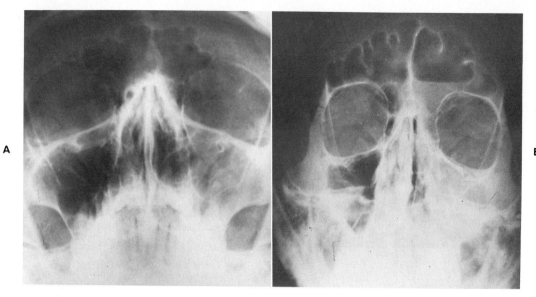

FIG. 16-4. A, Waters view showing clouding of the left maxillary sinus. **B,** Caldwell view showing clouding of the left maxillary sinus and a fluid level in the left frontal sinus.

icillin is the drug of choice for empirical selection, but cultures often show organisms not sensitive to penicillin, and anaerobic infections are not uncommon. When antibiotics are required, treatment should continue 4 or 5 days beyond the time of apparent complete resolution of the infection.

As previously mentioned, in some patients the natural ostium of the involved sinus is completely occluded by edema or the viscosity of the purulent discharge. The frontal sinus is the most frequent site, but occlusion may occur in the maxillary sinus. In the presence of virulent infection, blocking of the ostium of the frontal sinus may lead to an early spread of infection through the posterior wall of the sinus. The immediate threat is meningitis, epidural abscess, or abscess of the frontal lobe.

When pain is out of proportion to the usual picture, and when pus fails to drain into the nose after the usual treatment (local application of heat and nasal shrinkage), it may be necessary to drain the involved sinus. The operative procedure can be performed with the patient under local or general anesthesia. A small incision is made just under the eyebrow. The periosteum is retracted, a small opening is made into the floor of the frontal sinus, and a drain is placed into the cavity of the sinus. Occasionally it is necessary to puncture the medial wall of the maxillary sinus when drainage cannot be established by conservative means (see discussion of antral puncture, in section on subacute suppurative sinusitis). Both of these procedures are reserved for unusual situations. *Ordinarily, any surgical procedure involving the bony walls of the sinus is contraindicated during the acute phase of sinusitis.* Osteomyelitis of the facial bones or of the skull may occur as the result of ill-advised puncture during acute sinusitis.

A single episode of acute sinusitis does not necessarily predispose the patient to chronic sinusitis. It can do so, however, if the acute sinusitis is neglected or is complicated by another disturbance in nasal physiology, such as allergy.

Subacute suppurative sinusitis. More than 90% of patients with acute suppurative sinusitis are cured by conservative treatment. In the remainder the condition persists as a subacute infection. During this stage of infection persistent purulent nasal discharge is the only constant symptom. The nose may remain stuffy. Although localized tenderness is no longer present, there may be vague intermittent discomfort over the involved sinus or the face. There may

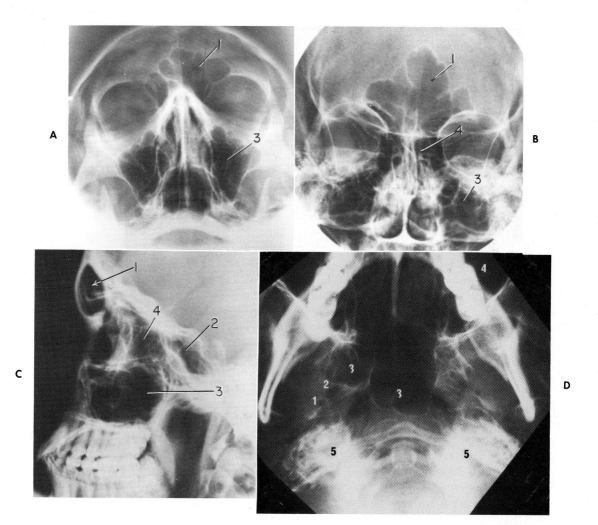

FIG. 16-5. Usual views used in making roentgenograms of the paranasal sinuses. **A,** Waters view. The orbits, the frontal and maxillary sinuses, and the nasal septum can be seen clearly. **B,** Caldwell view. The frontal sinuses can be seen clearly. Ethmoid air cells show between each orbit and the nasal septum. The petrous portion of the temporal bone can be seen in the lower part of the orbits. **C,** Lateral view. This view is particularly valuable for the sphenoid sinus and the posterior wall of the frontal sinuses. Additional views from below and from oblique angles are taken when necessary. *1,* Frontal sinuses. *2,* Sphenoid sinus. *3,* Maxillary sinus. *4,* Ethmoid sinuses. **D,** Roentgenogram of normal base of skull. *1,* Foramen spinosum. *2,* Foramen ovale. *3,* Sphenoid sinuses. *4,* Maxillary sinus. *5,* Petrous bones.

be a feeling of fatigue or of tiring more easily than usual. A nonproductive cough may become annoying.

The chief physical sign is persistence of pus in the nose. Pus present in the nose more than 3 weeks after the acute stage of infection requires treatment. If the frontal or maxillary sinus is involved, transillumination still fails.

Roentgenograms are indicated during the subacute phase of the infection to determine whether more than one sinus is involved. *A culture of the nasal discharge should be made.* Since it is unusual for the disease to persist, the causative organism may be an unusual one. One should also keep in mind that many instances of sinusitis are caused by anaerobes, so that special culture techniques are needed if the organism is to be demonstrated. It is desirable to know to which antibiotic the organism is sensitive in the event that it is necessary to prescribe antibiotics. *Neisseria catarrhalis* (a common non-pathogen of the upper respiratory tract) may cause a low-grade, continuing nasal discharge for weeks when it involves the maxillary or ethmoid sinuses. A culture revealing this organism should not be disregarded. Treatment requires systemic sulfonamide therapy, since the bacterium is not sensitive to penicillin or tetracycline therapy.

The possibility that the patient has an allergy should be considered. Patients with an allergy often have a persistent sinus infection. Early recognition of allergy as an underlying factor will aid the therapeutic program.

During the subacute stage, treatment can be more vigorous than during the acute phase without the danger of spreading the infection to bone. No medication is necessary to relieve pain. Nasal shrinkage should be continued. Heat may be beneficial and is often better supplied by infrared rays or diathermy than by simple surface heat from a hot-water bottle or a heating pad. Irrigation of the involved sinus may afford some relief. In some patients the frontal sinus can be irrigated through the natural ostium by means of specially designed cannulas. If irrigation cannot be accomplished easily, it should not be performed. Trauma to the natural ostium should be avoided because it may produce adhesions and narrowing. Obstruction to normal drainage of the sinus hinders

successful treatment and may lead to future difficulties.

Irrigation of the maxillary sinus (antrum) can be performed through the natural ostium in the middle meatus or through the thin bone of the medial wall of the sinus under the inferior turbinate. Some otolaryngologists prefer the former, and others the latter. When the route of the natural ostium is used, a special cannula is employed. As in attempted irrigation of the naso-frontal duct, trauma to the natural ostium should be avoided. If the ostium cannot be entered without trauma to its margin, infra-meatal antral puncture is the better procedure.

Antral puncture is not a difficult, painful, or dangerous procedure. It is probably the most beneficial method of treatment in subacute and early chronic suppurative sinusitis. It can be repeated many times without permanent damage to the nose or the maxillary sinus. The puncture is performed as follows.

A cotton-tipped applicator, moistened in 5% to 10% cocaine solution, is placed high under the inferior turbinate against the lateral wall of the nose (Fig. 16-6). The applicator should be placed immediately under the attachment of the inferior turbinate. After 5 to 10 minutes a large needle (16 to 18 gauge) is inserted under the turbinate, and firm, controlled pressure is applied until the needle pierces the medial wall of the antrum and enters the cavity of the sinus. Then a glass syringe is attached to the needle either directly or with a rubber or plastic tube. Suction backward on the syringe will bring purulent material or air into the syringe to prove its presence in the cavity of the antrum. This is an essential part of the procedure. No solution should be irrigated through the needle until the open tip of the needle is in the cavity of the sinus. Injection of air or solution into any surrounding soft tissue may spread infection or produce an air embolism. When proper placement of the needle is proved, the sinus is washed out with saline solution. The fluid enters through the needle and flows into the nose through the natural ostium of the antrum (Fig. 16-7). The patient leans over a basin, into which the fluid and pus drain (Fig. 16-8).

Another method, which is coming to be more and more preferred, is to puncture the anterior wall of the maxillary sinus, anesthetizing under

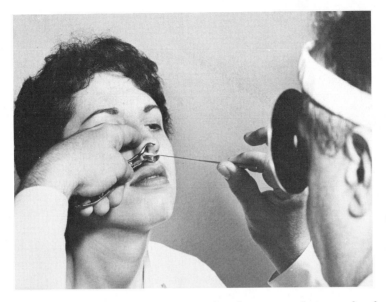

FIG. 16-6. Placing a cotton applicator moistened with cocaine solution under the inferior turbinate.

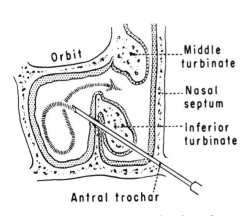

FIG. 16-7. Trochar inserted under the inferior turbinate (through the medial wall of the antrum). Contents of the sinus are washed into the nose through the natural ostium.

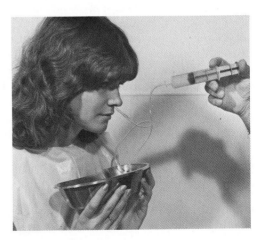

FIG. 16-8. Irrigation of the maxillary sinus. With the head tipped forward, solution returns via the natural ostium and out the anterior nose for examination and/or culture.

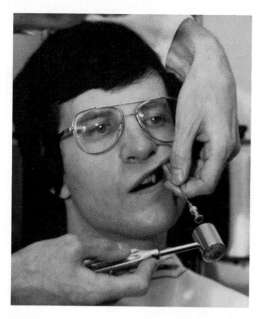

FIG. 16-9. Tapping a trochar with stylet (16 gauge) through anterior wall of maxillary sinus for irrigation. Local anesthesia is used.

the upper lip and then tapping a 16-gauge needle (with stylet in place) through the soft tissue and bone (Fig. 16-9). This approach has the advantage of being the most direct and *may well be the method of choice.*

Many solutions have been used to irrigate the maxillary sinus for treatment of subacute or chronic infection. Antibiotics can be used. However, the mechanical cleansing of the sinus is more important than the solution used. The ciliated epithelium of the lining of the maxillary sinus has remarkable powers of recovery. Return of normal ciliary activity can occur a few hours after irrigation. Then further clearing of the purulent material may occur spontaneously. During the subacute stage of infection, one irrigation will often suffice. More than two or three irrigations are required only rarely.

Antral puncture is used for diagnosis as well as for treatment. When the maxillary sinus fails to transmit light and the roentgenogram shows clouding, pus *may* be present. The change from normal may, however, be due to a thickening of the lining mucosa produced by allergy or by antecedent disease of the sinus that is no longer active. Puncture and washing of the antrum will demonstrate whether active infection is present or absent.

Whereas the maxillary sinuses can be directly irrigated, it is not possible to irrigate the ethmoid sinuses directly. Infection of the sphenoid sinus is usually associated with infection of the posterior ethmoid cells or of all the ethmoid cells. Isolated sphenoid sinusitis rarely occurs. To control subacute or chronic sinus infection adequately, it is necessary to deliver retained purulent material from the ethmoid and sphenoid sinuses. This can be satisfactorily accomplished by the *Proetz displacement method,** now used much less frequently than in the pre-antibiotic era. Although it is most effective when disease is present in the small and inaccessible ethmoid air cells, some material from the maxillary sinus is also displaced when this method is used.

The principle of gravity displacement of one fluid by another is well known. If thick, purulent secretions in a sinus can be partially suctioned into the nose, and if a thinner fluid is introduced into the sinus faster than the thick material can reenter, the thin fluid will replace the thick fluid. The displacement is accomplished as follows.

The patient is placed in a supine position on a flat surface, usually an examining table. His head is lowered over the end of the table, or his shoulders are elevated with a pillow (Fig. 16-10). While the patient breathes through the mouth and does not swallow or talk, isotonic saline solution containing a vasoconstrictor is introduced into the nose. Enough solution is used to fill the nose or at least to cover the ostia of the sinuses. Gentle intermittent suction is then applied to one nostril while the other nostril is occluded by the physician. During the suction the patient is asked to repeat rhythmically 10 to 15 times the letter "k" or the word "hook." Suction is applied during the time the letter or word is spoken and is released between words. Each time the letter "k" or the word "hook" is repeated, the soft palate closes over the nasopharynx. There is a closed system with negative pressure in the nose. Without the sealing of the nasopharynx, the solution would merely be suctioned out of the nose and would not create temporary negative pressure. Each return to normal pressure allows the saline solution placed in the nose to enter the sinus faster

---

*Devised by Dr. Arthur Proetz, St. Louis, Mo.

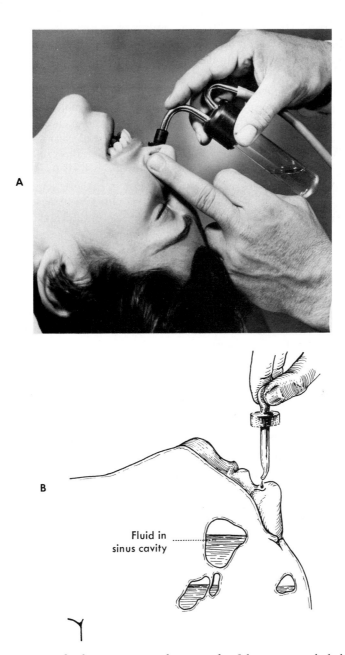

FIG. 16-10. A, Proetz displacement. Note that one side of the nose is occluded. The finger of the physician's right hand closes a hole in the curved metal tube to alternately create and release vacuum. **B,** After displacement, thin fluid replaces pus in the sinuses. This is also an ideal position for instilling nose drops.

than the thick mucopurulent secretion. The thick retained secretions are thus displaced into the nose and removed by suction.

This treatment is effective and can be repeated daily if necessary. Drugs other than saline solution and vasoconstrictors can be used during this procedure, just as after antral puncture. *Displacement therapy should not be used in cases of acute suppurative sinusitis*, because it may spread the sinus infection to other areas.

Along with antral puncture or displacement, general systemic medication may be necessary to cure subacute sinus infection. Systemic antibiotics are sometimes beneficial. Antihistaminics are often effective because persistence of infection is common in patients with an allergy. Systemic administration of corticosteroids for short intervals (3 to 5 days) may help because of their anti-inflammatory and anti-allergic effects. One or all of the methods of treatment described may be necessary to clear the infection.

Proper treatment of subacute sinusitis is the best means of preventing chronic purulent sinusitis.

Chronic suppurative sinusitis. When suppurative sinusitis is neglected during the acute or subacute phase, or when recurrent attacks damage the mucosa, permanent change may take place. It has been proved conclusively that bacteria can invade the tissue of the sinuses, become walled off, and produce chronic inflammation. At some time during any prolonged infection of soft tissue, pathologic change may become irreversible. The term *chronic* suppurative sinusitis indicates that the physician believes irreversible tissue changes have occurred in the lining membrane of one or more of the paranasal sinuses.

Symptoms of *uncomplicated* chronic suppurative sinusitis are similar to those of the subacute process. Purulent nasal discharge is the most constant symptom. If is often the only symptom. Contrary to popular belief, chronic infection of the paranasal sinuses is not a common cause of recurrent headache. Although low-grade headache can be a symptom, it is rarely due to the sinus infection. A far more common cause of headache in the frontal region or between the eyes is allergic rhinitis. Swelling of the nasal tissue, which creates increased intranasal pressure, is also a common cause of headache. The mere presence of pus in a sinus, *without accom-panying positive or negative pressure*, does not usually produce pain. When persistent pain occurs in a patient with known chronic sinus infection, the physician should be alert to the probability of an *impeding complication* or of the presence of *unsuspected neoplasm.* Symptoms of allergy are common in patients who have chronic sinusitis. The combination of allergic change and infection is discussed in the section on hyperplastic sinusitis (p. 216).

Since purulent nasal discharge is the one common sign of chronic suppurative sinus disease, proof of the presence or absence of pus in a sinus is essential to diagnosis. Visible pus in the nose in the absence of acute respiratory disease should be considered to come from one of the sinuses until proved otherwise. If pus cannot be seen in the nose but a purulent nasal discharge is suspected because of the case history, further examination should be performed to prove or disprove the presence of pus in a sinus. Transillumination, roentgenography, antral puncture, and displacement should be used to establish the diagnosis or refute the suspicion of chronic suppurative sinusitis.

There is not always a good correlation between the information obtained from transillumination, roentgenograms, and irrigation or displacement. Sinuses that appear dark when transilluminated or clouded on the roentgenogram may have no active infection. Sinuses that appear dark to transillumination and clear on the roentgenogram may contain pus. Sinuses that are clear by transillumination and either clouded or clear on the roentgenogram may contain pus. Therefore all methods must be used. Of the diagnostic examinations performed, antral puncture and displacement are the most valuable, and it is on the results of these procedures that a final opinion must be based.

Treatment of chronic suppurative sinusitis is primarily surgical. In a small percentage of patients repeated irrigation or displacement and antihistaminics or antibiotics as indicated may result in a cure of the disease. In most patients, however, an operation is necessary.

The physician must remember to investigate general systemic conditions that adversely affect the ability of the body to overcome infection. Allergy has been mentioned. Hypometabolism, lowered plasma gamma globulin, anemia, and

FIG. 16-11. Frontal section through the maxillary sinus after a Caldwell-Luc operation.

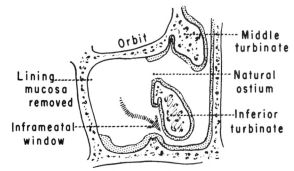

malnutrition are others. These conditions may require treatment before either medical or surgical treatment of chronic inflammatory disease will be successful.

Sound operative treatment of chronic suppurative sinusitis requires removal of all diseased soft tissue and bone, adequate postoperative drainage, and obliteration of the preexisting sinus cavity when possible. A specific technique is used for each sinus. The aim of each operation is to eradicate the infection but to leave contiguous structures normal. Half measures are of no value. Partial removal of involved tissue with the hope that the body will then resolve what it has been unable to manage for months or years is untenable.

When subacute infection of the maxillary sinus will not respond to systemic treatment, nasal shrinkage, and antral washing, it is necessary to provide drainage. This can be accomplished by making a window, called the *antral window*, through the lateral wall of the nose under the inferior turbinate. Local anesthesia is used. The operation is performed through the nose by fracturing the inferior turbinate medially or by removing a portion of its anterior end. The bony wall between the nose and atrum is removed widely, producing a permanent window. This window allows retained pus to drain into the nose by gravity and may cure the sinusitis. In some patients early chronic maxillary sinusitis can be treated in this manner. Most chronic suppuration requires a more radical operation.

The *Caldwell-Luc operation*, named after two surgeons, is the most generally accepted operative procedure for chronic maxillary sinusitis. It is also referred to as a radical antrum operation. Either local anesthesia or general anesthesia may be used. Local anesthesia is preferred.

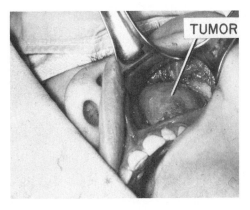

FIG. 16-12. Method of approach to the antrum in the Caldwell-Luc procedure. In this case a tumor was present. The bone of the anterior wall of the antrum has already been removed.

Anesthesia inside the nose is accomplished by the use of cocaine applied topically (Fig. 15-6). A local injection into the soft tissue over the maxillary sinus and blocking of the infraorbital nerve complete the anesthesia.

The maxillary sinus is entered through an incision under the upper lip and above the level of the roots of the maxillary teeth. Part of the anterior bony wall of the antrum is removed. Through this window in the bone all of the diseased mucosa and periosteum is removed. The bone of the lateral wall of the nose in the inferior meatus, which divides the nose from the antrum, is removed. The mucous membrane and periosteum of the lateral wall of the nose are preserved, fashioned into a hinged flap with the base down, and turned from the nasal cavity into the floor of the antrum (Figs. 16-11 and 16-12). The incision over the upper alveolus is closed with sutures.

The antrum may be packed with gauze to con-

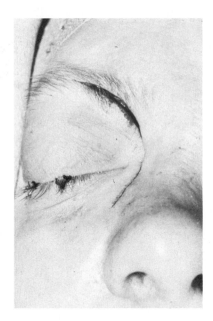

FIG. 16-13. Incision to expose the ethmoid and frontal sinuses. Almost no visible scar results.

trol bleeding. However, bleeding from the exposed bone is often so slight that no packing is required. When general anesthesia is used, an intratracheal tube should be employed to prevent blood from draining into the nasopharynx and pharynx during the operative procedure. Also, when general anesthesia is used, it is advisable to pack the antrum following the operation. However, 24 to 48 hours after the operation the packing should be removed through the nose and the nasoantral window that has been created. During the postoperative period the maxillary sinus heals. The exposed bone is covered by mucosa that grows into the cavity from the nose.

Exenteration of the ethmoid air cells can be accomplished by an operation (*ethmoidectomy*) through the nose or through an incision around the inner canthus of the eye. The external approach is recommended because it affords greater visibility, making possible a more thorough removal of tissue. The incision heals well and does not result in any cosmetic deformity (Fig. 16-13).

Intranasal ethmoidectomy is most often performed with the tissue anesthetized by local injection and topical cocaine. The middle turbinate is fractured medially toward the nasal septum. The turbinate may be partially re-

moved to gain access to the ethmoid sinuses. The ethmoid air cells and all infected tissue are removed to, or including, the medial wall of the orbit, and the nose is packed. If the nasofrontal duct is threatened by infection or is already involved, the floor of the frontal sinus is removed to provide an adequate opening into the nose for future normal discharge of mucus from the frontal sinus.

External ethmoidectomy can be performed with the patient under either local or general anesthesia. After the skin, subcutaneous tissue, and periosteum have been incised, with a curved incision around the inner canthus, soft tissue is dissected subperiosteally to expose the lateral bony wall of the ethmoid area. This is the common bony wall separating the ethmoid sinuses from the periorbital fascia, which encloses the eye and eye muscles. The ethmoid air cells, all infected tissue, and the lateral wall of the nose medial to the ethmoid area are removed. If the sphenoid sinus is involved, its anterior face and lining mucous membrane are removed. The operative area is packed, and one end of the packing is brought into the nose. The skin and soft tissues are closed with sutures. The packing is removed through the nose during the postoperative period.

The floor and anterior wall of the frontal sinus can be exposed by extending the incision used for external ethmoidectomy into the eyebrow and carrying it to the lateral limit of the eyebrow (*frontoethmoidectomy*). The floor of the frontal sinus, or its anterior wall above the supraorbital ridge, can be removed in order to remove *all* the lining mucosa of the frontal sinus. The extent of bony removal necessary depends on the size of the frontal sinus and the accessibility of its superior recess through the incision into the eyebrow. The ethmoid cells are always removed when the frontal sinus is exenterated to provide adequate drainage into the nose while healing takes place. The cavity created during the operation is packed. The packing is brought into the nose and is later removed through the nose. The external soft tissues are closed with sutures.

When possible, it is advantageous to create a hinged flap from the mucosa of the lateral wall of the nose, with the hinge superior. Such a flap can be turned up into the cavity and used to line the medial wall of the frontal sinus. It will prevent obstruction to drainage later.

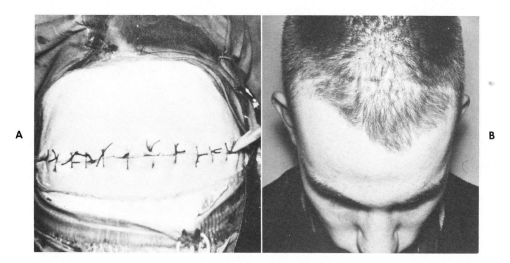

FIG. 16-14. A, Incision behind the hairline across the skull to expose both frontal sinuses (coronal incision). Sutures in place after operation. **B,** Healing hairline incision (3 weeks postoperatively).

When infection is present in both frontal sinuses, or when a frontal sinuses is pneumatized high into the frontal bone (approaching the hairline), an incision through the scalp just posterior to the hairline may be used. The incision extends from temple to temple and is carried through the full thickness of the scalp. The soft tissue of the forehead is turned forward and downward to expose the anterior wall of both frontal sinuses. Through such an incision, both frontal sinuses and the ethmoid air cells on both sides can be exenterated. Often the ethmoid sinuses cannot be completely removed from above and must be treated through the inner canthus incision after the frontal sinus disease has been removed. When osteomyelitis of the frontal bone occurs as a complication of purulent sinusitis, this operative approach is the best (Fig. 16-14).

An *osteoplastic flap* operation also is used on the frontal sinus. This means that after an incision is made through the skin and subcutaneous tissue (scalp) either in the eyebrow area or above the hairline (coronal incision), a vibrating bone saw is used to cut into the frontal sinus above and on each side. Then, with the lower or eyebrow margin left uncut, the bone is fractured from above downward so as to leave a hinged attachment inferiorly. This opens the sinus wide and permits removal of all mucosa and then drilling of the bony walls themselves to doubly ensure that all mucous membrane is removed. Then a plug of fat taken from the abdominal wall is placed in the cavity, and the osteoplastic flap (anterior wall of the frontal sinus) is replaced. With no mucous membrane to regenerate, there is little likelihood that a mucocele will form postoperatively—one of the complications after frontal sinus operations.

Allergic sinusitis. Allergic sinusitis does not occur without allergic rhinitis. In allergic sinusitis the sinus mucosa exhibits the same changes as seen in the nose in allergic rhinitis. The symptoms are the same—stuffiness of the nose, itching and burning of the nose, frequent attacks of sneezing, recurrent frontal headache, and thin nasal discharge. The nasal discharge may be mucoid and sticky or, more often, thin and copious. Acute hay fever is the typical example of this symptomatology.

It is probable that patients with allergic rhinitis never have rhinitis alone but also have allergic sinusitis, with the lining of all the sinuses undergoing the same changes as occur in the mucosa of the nose. Polyps are common in allergic rhinitis (see Figs. 3-16 and 15-4). Similarly, polypoid change in the lining of the sinuses is common in allergic sinusitis.

Headache, usually located in the frontal region or between the eyes, is a frequent symptom. Edema, which causes swelling within the soft tissue, is a far more common cause of headache than is pus in the sinuses.

In the absence of secondary infection, allergic

sinusitis is treated in conjunction with the allergic rhinitis that it accompanies. Extensive tests for allergy and management by diet or vaccines, as indicated by the results of such tests, may be required. Antihistaminics are beneficial in controlling symptoms for temporary periods. Occasionally the corticosteroids may be used, but their use over long periods of time is unjustified.

Hyperplastic sinusitis. The term "hyperplastic sinusitis" is used to describe inflammation of the sinuses caused by purulent sinusitis superimposed on allergic rhinitis and sinusitis. The underlying diseased tissue reacts to infection in greater degree than does normal tissue. Tissue edema is severe. There is a tendency for mucosal polyps to develop and to recur again and again even after apparently adequate surgical removal. Chronic thickening of the mucosa and submucosa lining the sinuses and the formation of polyps cause blocking of the natural ostia and make drainage of purulent secretion difficult. Recurrent episodes of acute infection lead to chronic purulent infection that does not respond to conservative treatment. The nose may remain more or less plugged most of the time. The nasal tissue responds poorly to shrinking solutions. Low-grade frontal headache is common and difficult to relieve. Complications are more common than in purulent sinusitis without hyperplastic changes.

Treatment of hyperplastic sinusitis most often is by an operation. An operation on more than one of the sinuses may be necessary. The pathologic change in the tissues is diffuse and tends to involve all the sinuses on one or both sides. Treatment of the allergy is necessary if the infection is to be controlled successfully. Even with adequate management of the allergy and proper surgical removal of diseased tissue, some nasal symptoms and nasal discharge remain for years. Further surgery may be necessary at a later date if acute infection is again superimposed on the allergic base.

Rhinocerebral phycomycosis. Rhinocerebral phycomycosis is a rapidly progressive infection caused by fungi of the group Phycomycetes. Mucormycosis is a similar fungal infection caused by fungi of the order Mucorales, with *Rhizopus* being the most common infecting organism. The phycomycetes are saprophytic fungi found in soil, manure, decaying fruits, starchy foods, and dust. Infections with these organisms commonly begin in the nose and spread to the sinuses and orbit and finally intracranially. Death by arterial thrombosis is the usual result in untreated cases.

Frequent manifestations are diabetic ketoacidosis, blepharoptosis, ophthalmoplegia, "black" turbinate, clouding of the sinus on x-ray study, meningoencephalitis, cerebrovascular thrombosis, and unilateral blindness. The typical patient is debilitated with uncontrolled diabetes or leukemia. The diagnosis is made on the basis of history, physical examination, and biopsy specimen showing typical broad-branching, nonseptate hyphae. The differential diagnosis includes malignancy, suppurative sinusitis, lethal midline granuloma, tuberculosis, cavernous sinus thrombosis, and rhinoscleroma. The treatment is by surgical debridement and administration of amphotericin B.

Antral cyst. Frequently, on looking at a Waters view of the maxillary sinuses, the physician may see a smooth, rounded density in the lower aspect of one maxillary sinus. Such a swelling ordinarily need not be investigated surgically if the surrounding bony walls are intact. It represents a cyst containing clear fluid.

SELECTED READINGS

Alford, B.R., Gorman, G.N., and Mersol, V.F.: Osteoplastic surgery of frontal sinus, Laryngoscope **75:**1139, 1965.

Carenfelt, C.: Pathogenesis of sinus emphyema, Ann. Otol. Rhinol. Laryngol. **88:**16, 1979.

Davison, F.W.: Chronic sinus disease; differential diagnosis, Laryngoscope **78:**1738, 1968.

Eisenberg, L., Wood, T., and Boles, R.: Mucormycosis, Laryngoscope **87:**347, 1977.

Evans, F.O., and others: Sinusitis of the maxillary antrum, N. Engl. J. Med. **293:**735, 1975.

Goode, R.L.: Surgery of the turbinates, J. Otolaryngol. **7:**262, 1978.

Hamory, B.H., and others: Etiology and antimicrobial therapy of acute maxillary sinusitis, J. Infect. Dis. **139:**197, 1978.

Hawkins, D.B., and others: Orbital involvement in acute sinusitis: lessons from 24 childhood patients, Clin. Pediatr. **16:**464, 1977.

Karma, P., and others: Bacteria in chronic maxillary sinusitis, Arch. Otolaryngol. **105:**386, 1979.

McCaffrey, T.V., and others: Clinical evaluation of nasal obstruction: a study of 1000 patients, Arch. Otolaryngol. **105:**542, 1979.

Meyers, B.R., and others: Rhinocerebral mucormycosis: prevention, diagnosis, and therapy, Arch. Intern. Med. **139:**557, 1979.

Proetz, A.W.: The displacement method, St. Louis, 1941, Annals Publishing Co.

Rachelefsky, G.S., and others: Sinus disease in children with respiratory allergy, J. Allergy Clin. Immunol. **61:** 310, 1978.

Ritter, F.N.: A clinical and anatomical study of the various techniques of irrigation of the maxillary sinus, Laryngoscope **87:**215, 1977.

Stevens, M.H.: Aspergillosis of the frontal sinus, Arch. Otolarygnol. **104:**153, 1978.

Yanagisawa, I., and others: Rhinocerebral phycomycosis, Laryngoscope **87:**1319, 1977.

Zonis, R.D., Montgomery, W.W., and Goodale, R.L.: Frontal sinus disease; 100 cases treated by osteoplastic operation, Laryngoscope **76:**1816, 1966.

17 COMPLICATIONS OF ACUTE AND CHRONIC SINUSITIS; TUMORS OF THE NOSE AND SINUSES

COMPLICATIONS OF ACUTE AND CHRONIC SINUSITIS

As long as infection remains localized within the paranasal sinuses, the symptoms remain localized. However, when it extends beyond the limits of the sinuses, usually new symptoms and signs appear that are no longer localized to the anatomic region of the involved sinus. Many of these symptoms and signs indicate spread of the infection to vital structures. Infection of the ethmoid and frontal sinuses is particularly dangerous because these sinuses are intimately associated with the orbit, the optic nerve, and the dura covering the frontal lobe of the brain (Fig. 17-1). Complications of maxillary sinusitis are less common, and, except for osteomyelitis of the superior maxilla, they are less dangerous.

Complications of sinusitis usually follow the acute stage of the disease or occur during an acute exacerbation of a chronic infection. They are most frequently caused by inadequate therapy during the acute stage or by a delay in treatment. Just as in the treatment of acute otitis media, too much faith has been put in one-shot or 24-hour treatment of acute sinusitis. If antibiotics are indicated, they should be continued until the infection has subsided.

Signs of complications. Certain signs occurring with, or shortly after, apparent subsidence of acute sinusitis are danger signals. The following symptoms should alert the physician to the possibility that infection may have spread from the involved sinus and is threatening important structures:

1. Generalized persistent headache
2. Vomiting
3. Convulsions
4. Chills or high fever
5. Edema or increasing swelling of the forehead or eyelids
6. Blurring of vision, diplopia, or persistent retro-ocular pain
7. Signs of increased intracranial pressure
8. Personality changes or dulling of the sensorium
9. Any combination of signs and symptoms in which the patient appears to be more ill than he should be with uncomplicated sinusitis (includes any sudden increase in white blood cells above 20,000)

When any of these symptoms or signs are present, complications must be suspected and every effort made to find the probable site of origin. Thus, in addition to the careful evaluation of the condition of the sinusitis, a general survey must be made to rule out other acute infections that may be the cause of the generalized symptoms, such as pneumonia.

Orbital cellulitis. When infection spreads from the ethmoid sinuses through the lateral ethmoid wall, it may cause a diffuse cellulitis of the periorbital tissues. A chill may accompany the initial invasion. The temperature rises, and there is dull pain deep in the involved eye. Edema and sometimes mild inflammation of the eyelids and the region of the inner canthus occur early. As the process develops, the eyeball begins to protrude, usually in a straightforward direction. Eye movements become painful, but the eyeball can be moved until the inflammation is far advanced and the proptosis pronounced. Later the conjunctiva becomes red, edematous, and thickened (chemosis). The patient is acutely ill. Still later the eyeball may become completely

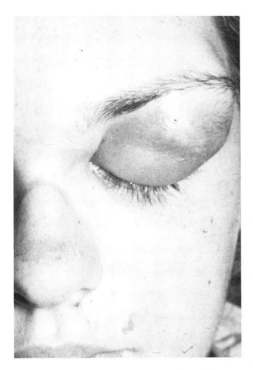

FIG. 17-1. Acute frontal sinusitis with a subperiosteal abscess extending into the upper lid.

fixed, the lids swollen and red, and the conjunctiva so edematous that the lids do not close over it.

Antibiotics must be given in large doses. A combination of two or more antibiotics may be necessary to effect a resolution of the infection. Early recognition and prompt, adequate treatment will prevent serious late sequelae.

Periorbital abscess. When infection extends through the lateral ethmoid plate but does not penetrate the periorbita, pus collects between the bone and the periorbita, producing a periorbital abscess. The general symptoms are not as severe as those caused by orbital cellulitis. There is an increase in fever, some pain during motion of the eye, and edema in the region of the inner canthus. The eye may slowly be forced slightly outward and downward. There is little or no chemosis of the eyeball. Pressure over the inner canthus will cause pain. If unrecognized or neglected, the abscess may later break into the cone of the eye muscles and produce orbital cellulitis.

Such periorbital abscesses must be drained to prevent spread to the eye or the dura. An incision (Fig. 16-13) around the inner canthus of the eye and subperiosteal separation of the periorbita from the ethmoid wall will allow drainage. After drainage and the use of adequate chemotherapy, recovery is almost always certain.

Cavernous sinus thrombosis. Cavernous sinus thrombosis occurs when there is extension of infection through the venous pathways (usually the angular vein) to the cavernous sinus (Fig. 17-2). A septic thrombus forms. The symptoms occur abruptly and are severe. Chills and a rise in temperature as high as 106° F. are the rule. Pain deep in the eyes is present. The patient is in an extremely toxic condition, sometimes semicomatose. The third, fourth, and sixth cranial nerves are closely associated with the cavernous sinus. Initially, there is selective ocular palsy, which helps to differentiate the condition from orbital cellulitis, in which complete ophthalmoplegia is the rule. Eventually the infection affects both eyes, and complete fixation, lid edema, and chemosis develop. If cavernous sinus thrombosis is unrecognized or inadequately treated, death may occur in 48 to 72 hours.

Treatment consists of large doses of antibiotics, usually given intravenously and continuously. Also, the administration of heparin, in doses to keep the clotting time prolonged, has increased the number of cures. In spite of adequate management, more than 50% of patients with cavernous sinus thrombosis die.

Meningitis. Infection from the frontal, ethmoid, or sphenoid sinuses may spread through the inner table of bone to the meninges or to the frontal lobe of the brain. Extension of infection occurs most often as a result of septic thrombophlebitis. Veins within the submucosa of the sinuses pierce the skull and join with dural veins. *Sterile* thrombosis of these veins is the normal protective mechanism by which the body prevents such extension. However, in some abrupt infections, particularly those that occur as a result of the patient's swimming and diving, bacterial invasion may be so rapid that sterile thrombi may not have time to form. A chill usually marks this invasive stage, but several days may elapse after the chill before the symptoms of intracranial disease occur. Purulent invasion may also occur as a result of long-standing and neglected chronic sinusitis in which erosion of the bone of the inner table has occurred. Then, during an acute episode, extension may occur because the normal barrier of the skull is absent.

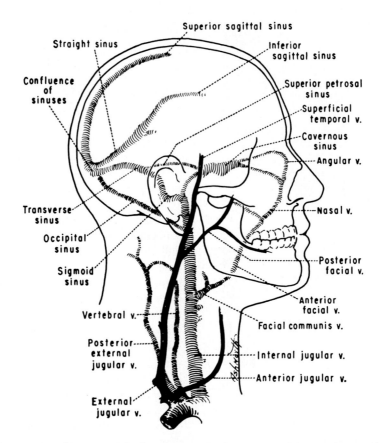

FIG. 17-2. Venous drainage of the brain. Note the continuity of the nasal vein, the angular vein, and the cavernous sinus. Note also the transverse sinus, the sigmoid sinus, and the internal jugular veins.

The symptoms of meningitis following sinusitis are the same as those of meningitis from any cause—stiff neck, chills, semicoma or coma, localized convulsions, headache, and vomiting. Spinal fluid examination and culture must be performed early to find the causative organism. General supportive measures, fluids given intravenously, and massive doses of antibiotics are required. The prognosis is good if treatment is started promptly and continued long enough.

Epidural abscess. An epidural abscess is more difficult to diagnose than meningitis. After an initial invasive stage (usually a chill), symptoms and signs are minimal. The white blood cell count may be only slightly elevated. There is often a predominance of lymphocytes in the differential blood cell count. Dull, persistent headache is common. There may be tenderness to percussion of the skull over the involved dura.

Late in the course of disease there may be erosion of the inner table of the skull over the abscess. When headache persists and the patient's general condition does not suggest a subsiding sinusitis, daily evaluation of his condition, including consultation with a neurosurgeon, is necessary. Otherwise, an epidural abscess cannot be recognized before it spreads to the brain or ruptures into the subarachnoid space to produce meningitis.

Treatment consists of providing drainage by removing the full thickness of the skull over the abscess. Recovery is then the rule.

Subdural abscess. Occasionally, a subdural abscess occurs. Even more rarely, epidural hemorrhage takes place. Both require daily evaluation of symptoms and signs by the otolaryngologist and the neurosurgeon.

Brain abscess. Abscesses of the frontal lobe of the brain are often difficult to recognize. The

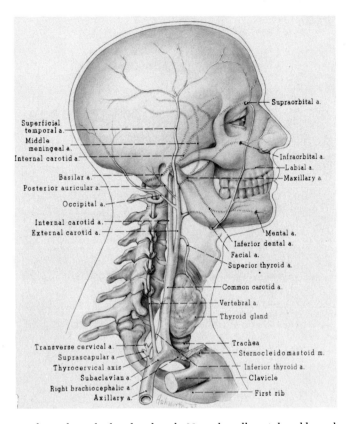

FIG. 17-3. Arterial supply to the head and neck. Note that all peripheral branches are from the external carotid system. The internal carotid artery does not give off branches until it reaches the cranial cavity. (From Jacob, S.W., and Francone, C.A.: Structure and function in man, ed. 2, Philadelphia, 1970, W.B. Saunders Co.)

frontal lobe is frequently called a "silent" area of the brain because disease here must be extensive to produce any obvious neurologic signs. A brain abscess must be suspected when a patient with sinusitis appears to be responding well to treatment and yet continues to have signs of retained pus. Slight personality and mood changes may occur. There may be slight weakness of the facial muscles on the side opposite the involved lobe. Signs of increased intracranial pressure occur late in the disease process. Careful daily observation of the ocular fundi may reveal an early papilledema, which does not occur in epidural abscess. Ultimately the diagnosis is made when confirmatory signs appear. Encephalograms, ventriculograms, and trephination may be required before the diagnosis is established. Cooperation with the neurosurgeon is important.

• • •

In general these complications must be recognized and managed before any operative approach to the sinus infection is attempted. If any infection remains in the sinuses after the complication is under control or drainage has been established, definitive surgery on the sinuses should be performed to prevent future recurrence of the intracranial infection.

Osteomyelitis of the skull. Since antibiotics and chemotherapeutic drugs have been available, the incidence of osteomyelitis of the skull has diminished steadily. It still occurs in undertreated or neglected patients. The primary signs of this complication are (1) continuation of low-grade fever, (2) dull headache, and (3) slow development of a doughy, tender thickening of the periosteum over the infected bone (Fig. 17-4). Edema of the upper lids is common. The patient does not have overwhelming symptoms. Rather, he appears chronically ill. Roentgeno-

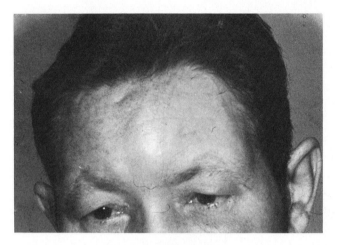

FIG. 17-4. Doughy swelling over the left frontal sinus, typical of osteomyelitis—often called Pott's puffy tumor.

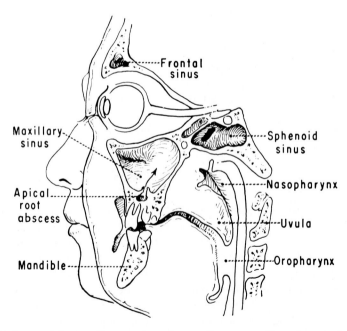

FIG. 17-5. Relation of the maxillary teeth to the maxillary sinus. Note the apical root abscess, a cause of sinusitis of dental origin and of oroantral fistula.

grams of the skull may show localized decalcification or destruction of bone. Treatment is best delayed until definite roentgenologic evidence of bone change is present.

Treatment demands excision of the full thickness of the involved portion of the skull to a point somewhat beyond gross evidence of infected bone and to the extent that normal dura is visible in all areas around the involved one. If bone removal is extensive, a plastic or metal plate can be placed at a later date to protect the underlying brain from external injury.

Osteomyelitis of the superior maxilla. Osteomyelitis of the superior maxilla is rare. It may occur spontaneously in infants and young children as a result of sinusitis or serious dental infection. In adults it is *almost always caused by unnecessary intranasal procedures performed while a patient is suffering from acute maxillary sinusitis.* Removal of polyps, fracture of turbinates, and puncture of the antrum should *always* be avoided during the acute stage of maxillary sinusitis.

When osteomyelitis occurs, the soft tissue over the maxillary sinus becomes red, swollen, and tender. There are signs of spreading infection with sepsis. Pus pours into the nose. If treatment is neglected, osteomyelitis rapidly spreads to involve the entire maxilla, the orbit, and the lateral wall of the nose. Subperiosteal abscesses, slough of necrotic bone, and spreading cellulitis of the face may occur. Septicemia or further extension to the cavernous sinus may complicate the condition in the untreated patient. Treatment may be prolonged unless it is instituted early. It may involve excision of sequestra or, occasionally, of the entire maxilla.

Oroantral fistula. An oroantral fistula connects the maxillary sinus with the oral cavity. In the mouth the fistula usually opens in the space left by an extracted molar. Roots of the molars extend almost to the floor of the maxillary sinus. Sometimes when a tooth is extracted, a root may be forced into the sinus or the thin bony plate may be fractured. If so, a fistula may develop (Fig. 17-5). When it does, a purulent discharge drains from the maxillary sinus into the oral cavity. The pus is usually foul and green. Large oroantral fistulas will not respond to nonoperative treatment.

Carcinoma of the maxillary sinus is a second cause of oroantral fistulas. As the cancer grows, it destroys the bony floor of the sinus. Eventually the tumor erodes into the oral cavity. Then granular, fungating tissue appears on the gingiva, and a probe will pass upward into the maxillary sinus. A biopsy establishes the diagnosis.

When the fistula results from dental infection after extraction of a tooth, conservative treatment should be attempted first. Most newly created fistulas can be closed by suturing the gingival tissues. If infection develops, appropriate antibiotics should be given and the sinus should be irrigated. If the condition has been present for several months, with or without treatment, a Caldwell-Luc operation is performed and the fistula is closed. Mere curettement of the tract and closure of a flap over the fistula will not suffice—the maxillary sinus must be thoroughly cleaned. When a large fistula is present, plastic flaps from the palatal or buccal mucosa may be necessary to close the opening. When the fistula is the result of malignancy, more radical surgical (maxillectomy) or irradiation therapy is indicated.

Mucocele and pyocele. When there is complete blockage of the nasofrontal duct or of the ducts of one or more of the ethmoid sinuses, no mucus can drain from the sinus into the nose (Fig. 17-6). Since the mucosal lining of the sinus continues to produce mucus, the result is slow development of swelling above and medial to the eyeball. This is caused by erosion of the floor of the frontal sinus or of the lateral wall of the ethmoid labyrinth as a result of pressure from

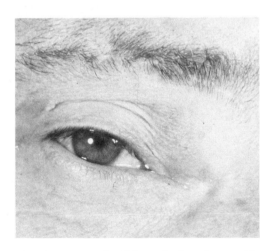

FIG. 17-6. Mucocele of the right frontal sinus. Note that the eye is displaced downward and outward.

the retained mucus. Such swelling occurs slowly, and it may take years to become evident. The eye is slowly pushed downward and outward, eventually giving rise to diplopia. There is no redness, inflammation, or pain. Except for diplopia, there are no visual changes.

Examination of the nose usually shows no abnormality. Sometimes evidence of a past intranasal operation can be seen. The cardinal sign is a rubbery mass under the inner third of the supraorbital ridge. The mass is smooth and partially compressible. Often a firm edge can be felt where the mucocele joins the remaining uneroded bone. The eye can be moved in all directions, but there is restriction of motion upward and inward. When the swelling is great, the eyeball is forced partially out of the orbit, giving a downward and outward proptosis.

Roentgenograms show a loss of continuity of the bony supraorbital ridge or displacement of the bony floor of the frontal sinus (Fig. 17-7).

Chronic dacryocystitis may cause swelling at the inner canthus of the eye (Figs. 17-8 and 17-9), but such swelling is usually *below* the medial canthal ligament. The swelling of a mucocele is above *and* medial to the eyeball.

If a mucocele becomes infected, it is called a pyocele. Treatment is directed toward the infection and must include surgical management of the mucocele.

In most instances a carefully taken history reveals that some intranasal manipulation or surgery was performed many years previously. Attempted cannulization of the nasofrontal duct or removal of turbinates may have caused scar tissue formation that blocks the normal ostia. Sometimes a facial injury or fracture may have caused the block. In any event, the block occurs years before visible signs of the mucocele appear.

Treatment is operative. The area is opened in the same manner as for a radical frontoethmoid operation. The usual finding is a large cavity filled with thick, tenacious mucus. It is lined with a thin, secreting membrane. The entire membrane is removed along with any remaining ethmoid air cells. A new opening is made into the nose and is kept open during the postoper-

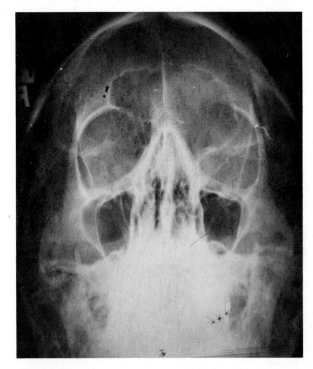

FIG. 17-7. Roentgenogram (Waters view) of a mucocele in the left frontal sinus. Note that the floor of the sinus is depressed into the orbit to cause proptosis.

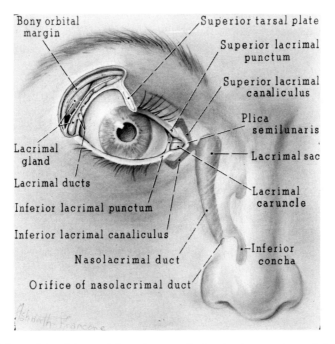

FIG. 17-8. Relationship of the eyelids and eye to the lacrimal apparatus and the nose. (From Jacob, S.W., and Francone, C.A.: Structure and function in man, ed. 2, Philadelphia, 1970, W.B. Saunders Co.)

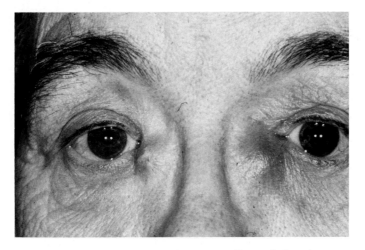

FIG. 17-9. Chronic dacryocystitis. Note that the swelling is *below* the inner canthus.

ative period by means of a mucosal flap or plastic tube. Total cure is the rule. The eye assumes its normal position as soon as the postoperative tissue reaction has subsided.

Malignant exophthalmos. Malignant exophthalmos is not a complication of sinusitis. Nevertheless, it produces signs and symptoms similar to some of the complications of sinusitis. Since treatment involves the sinuses, the condition is discussed with sinusitis.

Malignant exophathalmos is the result of an endocrine disturbance of the pituitary-thyroid relationship. The exact mechanism is unknown. It most often occurs in a person who has had hyperthyroidism and who a short time before the exophthalmos had a thyroidectomy. The endocrine upset produces an increase in the amount of orbital fat. The fat increase may occur slowly or rapidly. If enough fat is produced, the eyes are forced out by the pressure of the fat in the muscle conus behind the eyeball. There may be enough pressure behind the eyes to cause protrusion of the eyeball to a point where the lids cannot close over the globe. Edema, chemosis, and inflammation of the conjunctiva occur, and the cornea is in constant danger of injury from drying (drying often produces corneal ulcers). In addition, the optic nerve is stretched and vision is threatened. In the advanced stage, malignant exophthalmos is an ophthalmologic emergency.

In the early stage of the disease, treatment of the endocrine disturbance may arrest the fat increase before serious damage to the eyes occurs. If proptosis is increasing and vision is decreasing despite medical management, surgery must be performed. There are several procedures. All are designed to create a space into which the orbital fat can expand. This removes the threat to vision and allows the globe to return to an early normal position in the orbit.

The most successful operation is one in which the space of the ethmoid and frontal sinuses is used. A routine exenteration of all the ethmoid air cells is performed through an incision around the inner canthus of both eyes. The floor of the frontal sinus is removed, as is all of the lining mucosa of the frontal sinus, and the periorbita is incised. The fat, usually under considerable pressure, then moves out from the conus of the eye and occupies the space that was previously the air space of the sinuses (Fig. 17-10). This al-

lows the eyeball to return to its usual place in the orbit, relieves the tension on the optic nerve, stops the conjunctival edema, and once more allows the lids to protect the cornea. If treatment is neglected or if the condition is unaffected by medical treatment, the increased fat production will lead to total blindness unless surgery is performed.

A similar release of the orbital fat can be accomplished by removing the lateral wall of the orbit or by removing the floor of the orbit and using the space of the maxillary sinus. However, neither of these procedures is as satisfactory as the frontoethmoid decompression. Removal of the roof of the orbit has been recommended. This method is effective, but it places the fat and periorbita in direct contact with the inferior dura under the frontal lboe. As a consequence, the eye pulsates with each pulsation of the cerebrospinal fluid. This procedure also is not as satisfactory as the frontoethmoid approach.

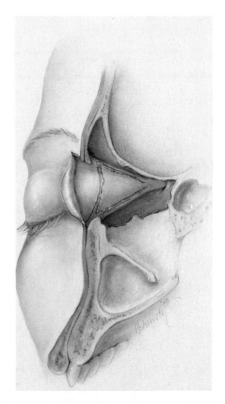

FIG. 17-10. Orbital conus after removal of the ethmoid cells, the medial wall of the orbit, and the floor of the frontal sinus for malignant exophthalmos. Note incisions in the periorbita for release of orbital fat.

TUMORS OF THE NOSE AND SINUSES

Tumors of the external nose. Both squamous cell carcinoma and basal cell carcinoma attack the external nose. The squamous cell lesions usually grow faster and may metastasize to the neck at any stage. Basal cell lesions often remain very small for a long period and then gradually spread locally. They do not metastasize. In advanced stages, the basal cell carcinoma may erode the entire nose and adjacent cheek and cause the patient's death (Fig. 17-11). Treatment of either type of carcinoma in the early stages should be very successful. Wide local excision is necessary. Other malignant tumors of the external nose are unusual.

Rhinophyma is a benign tumor caused by an overgrowth of sebaceous glands of the tip of the nose (Fig. 17-12). Sometimes the condition is marked and produces lobulated tumors, so that the patient is said to have a "potato nose." Treatment is simple and effective. The excess tissue is shaved off until the nose has a normal configuration. The area is allowed to epithelize, or a skin graft is applied.

Tumors of the internal nose. *Squamous papillomas* occur in the nasal vestibule. They cause lcoal irritation and are easily removed by excision or diathermy. Nasal polyps, the most common tumors of the nose, arise from the sinuses or their ostia and then hang into the nose.

Nasal polyps are discussed in Chapter 15 (pp. 217 to 218).

Inverted nasal papilloma. An inverted papilloma of the nose and sinuses is a rather unusual tumor that, although histologically benign, is clinically malignant, since it may by continuity involve adjacent structures beyond the interior of the nose. Furthermore, there is a strong ten-

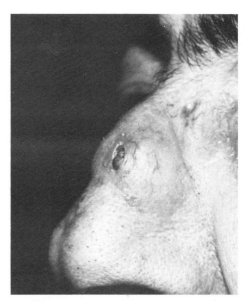

FIG. 17-11. Basal cell carcinoma. Note how the tumor undermines the skin.

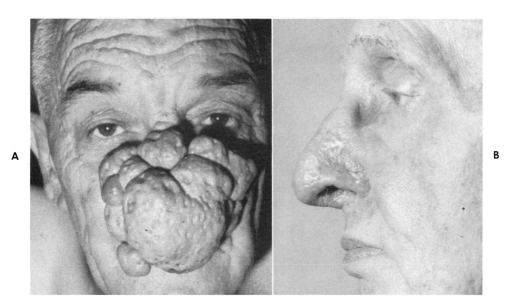

FIG. 17-12. A, Large rhinophyma. **B,** Appearance of the nose in another patient after removal of a rhinophyma without a graft. (**A,** Courtesy Dr. James A. Harrill, Winston-Salem, N.C.)

dency toward recurrence if the lesion is not completely excised. The usual symptom is nasal obstruction. Visual examination of the nose reveals a fleshy papillary exophytic growth filling one or both nasal passages. Irradiation is contraindicated, but adequate surgery will usually cure the patient.

Tumors of the sinuses. Carcinoma of the *maxillary sinus* causes no early symptoms. When the tumor is large enough, it may erode into the nose and cause nasal obstruction or bloody discharge. If it erodes the periosteum of the posterior or lateral wall of the antrum, there is persistent pain in the face. The pain may follow the distribution of the second division of the fifth cranial nerve. If there is erosion of the superior wall of the antrum, the orbital contents may be displaced upward and produce proptosis and double vision (Fig. 17-13). If the superior alveolar ridge is invaded, the maxillary teeth may become loose.

The diagnosis is usually confirmed by biopsy. In some instances a specimen for biopsy can be obtained from the nose. When the tumor has not invaded the nose, it may be necessary to open the antrum through a Caldwell-Luc incision to obtain a specimen (Fig. 16-12).

Successful treatment demands complete surgical excision of the maxilla. The surgery is performed through an incision that begins along the lateral border of the nose, is extended through the upper lip in the midline, and is continued laterally along the upper alveolus (Weber-Ferguson incision) (Figs. 17-14 and 17-15). All the soft tissue of the maxillary region of the face is reflected laterally. The entire maxilla is then resected. In addition, it may also be necessary to resect the contents of the orbit if the superior wall of the maxilla, which is the same as the floor of the orbit, has been invaded. The resulting defect is grafted with a split-thickness skin graft. After healing occurs, a dental prosthesis is made that replaces the resected hard palate and floor of the nose. This allows nearly normal speech and swallowing.

Irradiation alone for carcinoma of the antrum is usually palliative. A combination of irradiation and maxillectomy may be more effective than either procedure alone. There remains controversy regarding the time of the irradiation. Some physicians prefer to use a tumor dose of supravoltage roentgenotherapy 8 to 10 weeks before the maxillectomy is performed. Others favor similar irradiation after the maxillectomy. The relative value of these two approaches has not yet been determined.

Just as with any other malignant condition, early diagnosis here greatly improves the surgical result. To that end, use of a *diagnostic antrotomy* through a Caldwell-Luc incision (Fig. 16-12), a relatively benign procedure, is advocated by many when there seems to be a possibility of antral carcinoma or when the course of a unilateral sinusitis is prolonged and different from what was expected. Also, a screening roentgenogram (Waters view) is incorporated by some clinics in multiphasic screening programs for patients above 40 years of age.

Malignancy in the *frontal sinus* is more unusual than in the maxillary sinus. It is likely that there will be no early symptoms. Nasal bleeding, pain, or even proptosis may be the first symptom. Treatment is usually a combination of surgery and irradiation. The prognosis is poor.

Carcinomas are more common in the *ethmoid sinus* than in the frontal sinus. The nose fills with tumor (Fig. 17-16), the eye is pushed outward, and shortly thereafter the skin near the inner canthus breaks down. Cure is occasionally brought about by external ethmoidectomy and later irradiation therapy.

Malignancy of the *sphenoid sinus* is rare.

Benign tumors of the sinuses include chiefly osteoma (Fig. 17-17) and chondroma. These tumors enlarge very slowly. Symptoms are due to pressure on, or obstruction of, drainage channels. Osteoma and chondroma are easily removed through external operations on the sinus. Small *exostoses*, found in the frontal sinus, are different from osteomas in that they do not enlarge. *Mucoceles*, which the examiner may easily confuse with neoplasms, are discussed on pp. 243 to 244. *Mixed salivary gland* tumors are found occasionally in the maxillary sinus. *Polyps* in the sinuses, particularly in the maxillary sinus, are often reported by the radiologist as tumors. Of course, a polyp is a tumor, but it is entirely benign and usually causes no symptoms. Such a polyp is seen on the x-ray film as a smooth, rounded mass. Treatment is unnecessary. *Fibrous dysplasia* (of bone), a benign growth in which bone is softened and replaced by relatively avascular, abnormal fibrous tissue, occurs in the maxillary, ethmoid, and frontal

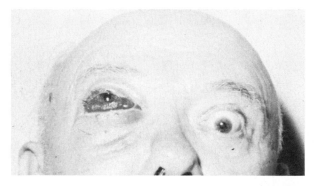

FIG. 17-13. Carcinoma of the maxillary sinus. Note the conjunctival edema and proptosis.

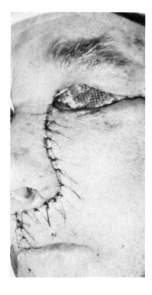

FIG. 17-14. Weber-Ferguson incision after suture. Note that it was necessary to remove the eye. The entire maxilla is easily removed through such an incision. When healed, the scar is almost invisible.

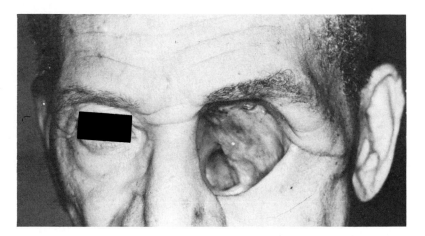

FIG. 17-15. Postoperative defect after maxillectomy and exenteration of the orbit. If the orbit is not removed, there is no severe external deformity.

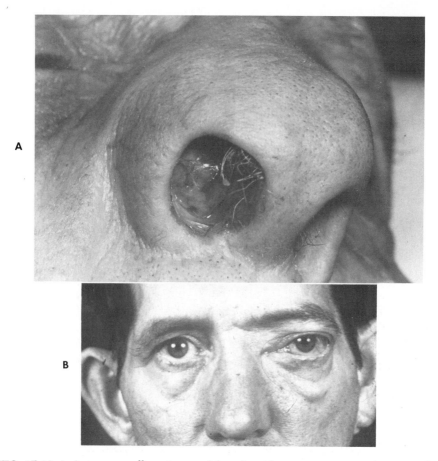

FIG. 17-16. **A,** Squamous cell carcinoma of the ethmoid sinus appearing at the external nares. **B,** Carcinoma of the ethmoid sinus. Note lateral displacement of the eye.

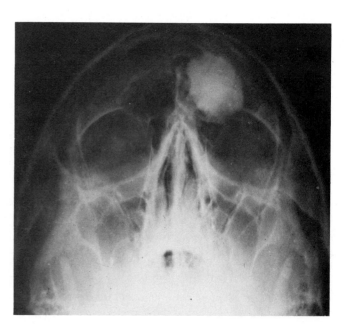

FIG. 17-17. Osteoma of the frontal sinus.

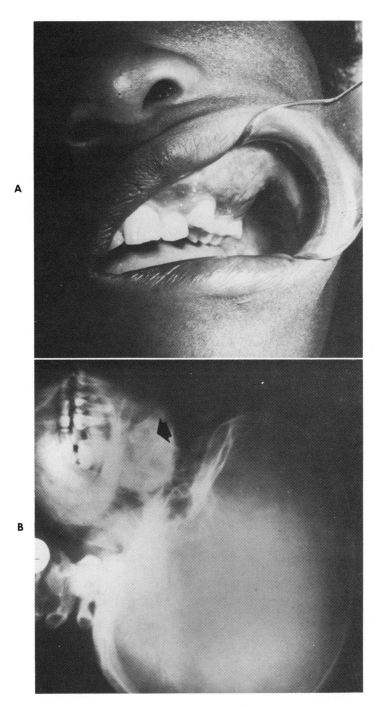

FIG. 17-18. A, Fibrous dysplasia of the maxilla. **B,** Lateral roentgenogram of skull showing fibrous dysplasia of maxilla.

sinuses. It is a rare condition that causes deformity and obstruction of the sinus ostia, displacement of the eye, nasal obstruction, and erosion of the full thickness of the skull. The treamtent is surgical removal of the tumor with preservation of all other bony and soft tissue structures (Fig. 17-18).

SELECTED READINGS

Arlen, M., and others: Chondrosarcoma of the head and neck, Am. J. Surg. **120:**456, 1970.

Blaugrund, S., and Parisier, S.C.: Benign tumors of the nasal sinuses, Otolaryngol. Clin. North Am. **4:**143, 1971.

Bortnick, E.: Neoplasms of the nasal cavity, Otolaryngol. Clin. North Am. **6:**801, 1973.

Boysen, M.: Osteomas of the paranasal sinuses, J. Otolaryngol. **7:**366, 1978.

Bridger, M.W.M., Beale, F.A., and Bryce, D.P.: Carcinoma of the paranasal sinuses: review of 158 cases, J. Otolaryngol. **7:**379, 1978.

Cheng, V.S.T., and Wang, C.C.: Carcinomas of the paranasal sinuses: study of 66 cases, Cancer **40:**3038, 1977.

Dupin, C.L., and LeJeune, F.E.: Nasal masses in infants and children, South. Med. J. **71:**124, 1978.

Fauci, A.S., and Wolff, S.M.: Wegener's granulomatosis, Medicine **52:**535, 1973.

Fechner, R.E., and Lamppin, D.W.: Midline malignant reticulosis; a clinicopathologic entity, Arch. Otolaryngol. **95:**467, 1972.

Gallagher, T.M., and Boles, R.: Symposium; treatment of malignancies of paranasal sinuses. I, II, and III, Laryngoscope **80:**924, 1970.

Harrison, D.F.N.: Lateral rhinotomy: a neglected operation, Ann. Otol. Rhinol. Laryngol. **86:**756, 1977.

Hawkins, D.B., and Clark, R.W.: Orbital involvement in acute sinusitis, Clin. Pediatr. **16:**464, 1977.

Kolmer, J.W., Wallenborn, P.A., Jr., and Crowgey, J.E.: Cavernous sinus thrombosis complicating sinusitis and orbital cellulitis, Va. Med. Mon. **93:**134, 1966.

Kotner, I.M., and Wang, C.C.: Plasmacytoma of the upper air and food passages, Cancer **30:**414, 1972.

Kurchara, S.S., and others: Role of radiation therapy and of surgery in the management of localized epidermoid carcinoma of the maxillary sinus, Am. J. Roentgenol. Radium Ther. Nucl. Med. **114:**35, 1972.

Larsson, L.G., and Martensson, G.: Maxillary antral cancers, J.A.M.A. **219:**342, 1972.

Montgomery, W.W.: Surgery of the frontal sinuses. In Bernstein, L., editor: Symposium on surgery of the nasal sinuses, Otolaryngol. Clin. North Am. **4:**97, 1971.

Ogura, J.H.: Surgical results of orbital decompression for malignant exophthalmos, J. Laryngol. Otol. **92:**181, 1978.

Pound, E., and others: Fibrous dysplasia (ossifying fibroma) of maxilla; analysis of 14 cases, Ann. Surg. **161:**406, 1965.

Rao, A., and others: Maxillary sinusitis and cancer: the role of polytomography, Am. J. Radiol. **131:**321, 1978.

Rubin, P.: Cancer of the head and neck; nose, paranasal sinuses, J.A.M.A. **219:**336, 1972.

Schenck, N.L., and Ogura, J.H.: Esthesioneuroblastoma; an enigma in diagnosis, a dilemma in treatment, Arch. Otolaryngol. **96:**322, 1972.

Schramm, V.L., Myers, E.M., and Kennerdell, J.S.: Orbital complications of acute sinusitis: evaluation, management, and outcome, Otolaryngology **86:**221, 1978.

Sheffield, R.W., Cassisi, N.J., and Karlan, M.S.: Complications of sinusitis: what to watch for, Postgrad. Med. **63:**93, 1978.

Suh, K.W., and others: Inverting papilloma of nose and paranasal sinuses, Laryngoscope **87:**35, 1977.

Want, C.C.: Radiotherapeutic management of transitional cell carcinoma of the nasopharynx, Cancer **28:**566, 1971.

18 ANATOMY OF THE EAR

External ear. The external ear consists of the auricle and the external auditory canal.

AURICLE. *Cartilage* (elastic type) and *skin* make up the entire auricle except for the dependent lobule, which contains no cartilage. The skin is closely attached in front but is looser behind. This explains why hematomas are more common anteriorly than posteriorly. The skin is also easily separated posteriorly and is thinner than most of the skin elsewhere in the body. Without a protective layer of fat and with essentially only one layer of blood vessels, the auricular skin is more subject to frostbite than any other part of the body.

The *muscles* that attach the auricle to the head (temporal bone) are innervated by the facial nerve. Lower animals have great control of their auricular muscles and may even use them to increase their hearing acuity. In humans, however, the muscles are small and serve no practical function. There are three—the anterior, superior, and posterior auricularis muscles.

The *lymphatics* drain anteriorly, inferiorly, and posteriorly. Lymphadenopathy behind the ear in patients with external otitis (or with an infection in the adjacent scalp) may confuse the examiner. The ear is pushed forward and the patient looks as though he has acute mastoiditis. Also, in external otitis a node just anterior to the tragus is commonly palpable.

The *sensory nerve supply* of the auricle has several sources. The great auricular nerve, the lesser occipital nerve, the auricular branch of the vagus nerve (Arnold's nerve), and the auriculotemporal nerve (from the mandibular) all contribute. Note that the fifth, seventh, and tenth cranial nerves, in addition to cervical nerves, are involved. Any one or more of these pathways may allow disease in other areas of the mouth, nose, throat, or neck to produce pain in the ear *(referred otalgia)*. The various parts of the auricle are shown in Fig. 18-1.

EXTERNAL AUDITORY CANAL. The external auditory canal (Fig. 18-2) ends blindly at the tympanic membrane. It is oblique, so that its superior wall is about 5 mm. shorter than its anteroinferior wall; this accounts for the oblique positions of the tympanic membrane. Furthermore, the canal bends, and it is necessary to straighten it by upward traction on the auricle before the eardrum can be examined easily. The outer half of the ear canal is cartilaginous, and the inner half is bony—except in the infant, in whom ossification has not yet occurred. The skin lining the cartilaginous canal is thick and contains fine hairs, sebaceous glands, and special glands that produce cerumen. The cartilage of the ear canal is continuous with that of the auricle. It should be noted that the cartilaginous portion is oval on section and forms an incomplete circle, since the roof is usually made of fibrous tissue. Other deficiencies, known as the *fissures of Santorini*, may also occur in the cartilage, and it is said that these minute openings provide potential pathways for infection or tumor to spread between the parotid gland and the mastoid.

In the adult the external auditory canal is approximately 24 mm. long, the bony canal being somewhat longer than the cartilaginous one. About 7 mm. from the tympanic membrane it forms a constriction known as the *isthmus*. Inferiorly and anteriorly, beyond the isthmus and just external to the lower part of the eardrum, is the *tympanic sulcus*. Debris often collects here, especially in patients with external otitis. It is a difficult area to clean. Another problem is caused by the anterior part of the bony canal, which often is so prominent that one cannot see all of the drumhead. This is a complicating fac-

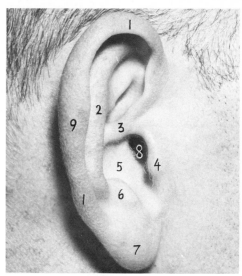

FIG. 18-1. Auricle. *1*, Helix. *2*, Antihelix. *3*, Crus of helix. *4*, Tragus. *5*, Concha. *6*, Antitragus. *7*, Lobule. *8*, External auditory meatus. *9*, Darwin's tubercle.

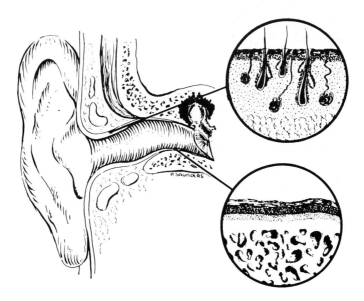

FIG. 18-2. External auditory canal. *Upper inset*, Cartilaginous ear canal shows hair follicles, sebaceous glands, and ceruminous glands. *Lower inset*, Thin epithelium attached to the bone.

tor at the time of tympanoplasty, when all of the drumhead must be seen. Drilling away of the overhang of bone may be necessary.

Anterior to the ear canal is the temporomandibular joint. Otalgia is sometimes produced when disease of the joint causes referred pain to the ear. A test of this possibility is to press the index finger into each temporomandibular joint while the patient's mouth is open and ask him to bite down. As he does so, he may wince with pain because of tenderness in one or both tem-

poromandibular joints. Superiorly and posteriorly the osseous canal is very thin and is directly under the mastoid antrum. Acute mastoiditis may cause periostitis and sagging of this portion of the ear canal. In chronic mastoiditis a cholesteatoma may erode this thin bony plate (sometimes called the scutum—"shield") and appear in the ear canal external to the annulus. Epithelium lining the bony half of the ear canal is very thin and contains no hair or glands. The epithelium is also very delicate, and often the

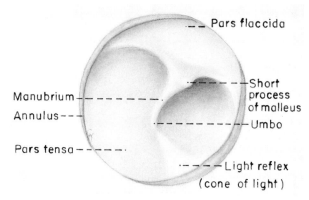

Pars flaccida

Short process of malleus

Manubrium

Umbo

Annulus

Pars tensa

Light reflex (cone of light)

FIG. 18-3. Landmarks of the right tympanic membrane. The size of the pars flaccida is exaggerated in this drawing.

slightest trauma produces a hematoma. The anatomy of the *tympanic membrane* (Fig. 18-3) is discussed in Chapter 23.

Middle ear. The middle ear, or tympanic cavity, has been likened to a drum, covered as it is by the tightly stretched tympanic membrane. The word "eardrum" therefore refers properly to the tympanic cavity, whereas the drumhead is the tympanic membrane. In popular usage, however, the word "eardrum" is used synonymously with the terms "tympanic membrane" and "drumhead."

The middle ear, or tympanic cavity, is a roughly oblong space lined with mucous membrane. The portion directly behind the tympanic membrane is sometimes spoken of as the mesotympanum, but there is an almost equally large area directly above known as the epitympanum, or attic, and it is here that the bodies of the incus and malleus are located (Fig. 18-4). A smaller part of the middle ear, known as the hypotympanum, lies below the level of the promontory and round window. Sometimes, if the bony floor of the hypotympanum is dehiscent, the dome of the jugular bulb may protrude upward into the middle ear space and be seen through the tympanic membrane, inferiorly, as a bluish bulge.

All the walls of the middle ear, except the lateral wall, are bony. The part of the lateral wall covering the mesotympanum is the tympanic membrane. Anteriorly the eustachian tube (Fig. 18-4) leads downward and medially to the nasopharynx. Medially, directly opposite the tympanic membrane, is a domelike prominence called the promontory. This is the basal turn of the cochlea. Posteriorly and superiorly

the stapes fits into the oval window. Posteriorly and inferiorly is the round window niche. The seventh cranial nerve, in the fallopian canal, crosses the medial wall of the middle ear. It passes just above the oval window. The middle ear opens posteriorly into the mastoid antrum. The connecting passage is called the aditus ad antrum (Fig. 18-9).

OSSICLES. In the middle ear are the three auditory *ossicles*—malleus, incus, and stapes. These tiny bones, each modeled with great delicacy, are entirely covered with middle ear mucosa. They serve to connect the tympanic membrane with the oval window and represent the normal pathway of sound transmission across the middle ear space. The malleus has a head, neck, handle (manubrium), and short process. The handle and short process are embedded in the layers of the eardrum. The head and neck extend above the upper margin of the tympanic membrane into the epitympanum (attic) (Fig. 18-5). The head of the malleus articulates with the body of the incus. With a capsule and supporting ligaments, the articulation is a true joint. The incus has two crura, one long and one short. The short crus is directed backward, rests on the posterior bony wall, and acts as a fulcrum on which the incus rotates. At the end of the long crus is a short articular facet called the lenticular process, which connects to the head, neck, anterior and posterior crura, and footplate (Fig. 18-6). The footplate closes the oval window. An annular ligament connects the oval window and the footplate. Additional anatomic description of the ossicles and tympanic membrane may be found in Chapter 23.

Two *muscles* attach to the ossicular chain.

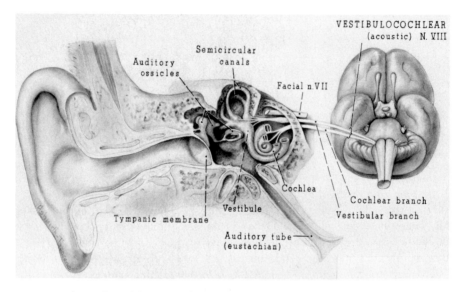

FIG. 18-4. Relationship of the external ear, middle ear, and inner ear. Note the ossicles of the middle ear, the relationship of the cochlea and semicircular canals, and the location of the eustachian tube. Note that the head of the malleus and the body of the incus are *superior* to the eardrum. (From Jacobs, S.W., and Francone, C.A.: Structure and function in man, ed. 2, Philadelphia, 1970, W.B. Saunders Co.)

FIG. 18-5. Lateral view of the right middle ear after the drumhead has been removed. The chorda tympani nerve passes behind the malleus but in front of the long crus of the incus. The stapedial tendon joins the neck of the stapes.

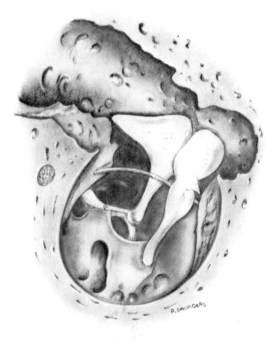

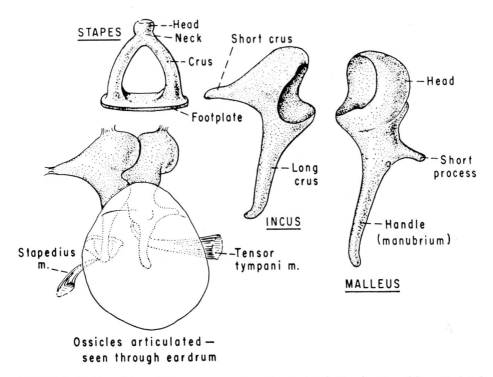

FIG. 18-6. Ossicles of the middle ear—separate and articulated. The drawing of the articulated ossicles is of a right ear.

The tensor tympani muscle originates from a bony semicanal above the eustachian tube. It emerges as a tendon near the neck of the malleus. The tendon turns sharply around the processus cochleariformis and attaches to the neck of the malleus. The tensor tympani muscle is supplied by a branch of the fifth nerve. Its action is to tense the tympanic membrane by pulling the handle of the malleus inward. The stapedius muscle is the smallest muscle in the body. It arises from a bony pyramid in the posterior wall of the middle ear and attaches to the neck of the stapes. It is supplied by a branch of the seventh nerve. Its action is to tilt the stapes posteriorly and to fix it in the oval window. It is believed to help protect the internal ear from sudden loud sounds by preventing abnormal excursion of the footplate.

Eustachian tube. The pharyngotympanic tube of Eustachius connects the middle ear and the nasopharynx. Opening into the lateral wall of the nasopharynx just above the plane of the floor of the nose, it is lined with respiratory mucous membrane. The cartilaginous, or medial, portion of the eustachian tube (nearest the nasopharynx) is about 24 mm. long, and the osseous portion (nearest the middle ear) is approximately 12 mm. long. The diameter is greatest at the pharyngeal end, narrowing to an isthmus at the junction of the cartilaginous and bony portions.

The function of the eustachian tube is to provide an air passage from the nasopharynx to the ear to equalize the pressure on both sides of the eardrum. If pressure in the external auditory canal is greater than that in the middle ear, the eardrum is retracted. If pressure in the middle ear is greater than that in the external canal, the eardrum will bulge outward.

The eustachian tube, which is normally passively closed, has the least resistance to opening when the head is erect; tipping the head forward or backward increases the resistance. The tube is opened by the action of the tensor and levator muscles of the palate. It opens briefly, for $1/10$ to $1/5$ second, during swallowing, but not necessarily with every swallow. In otitis media, when pus is present in the middle ear, the pus does not ordinarily drain through the eustachian tube since the tube has been closed by edema. Pus under pressure in the middle ear tends to rupture through the drumhead rather than drain into the nasopharynx.

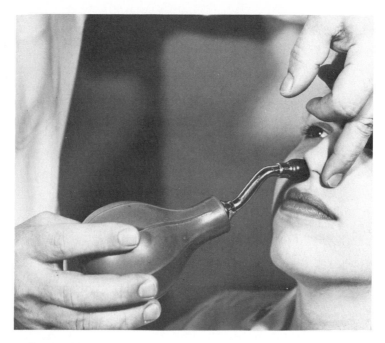

FIG. 18-7. Inflation of the eustachian tube by increasing pressure in the nasopharynx with a Politzer bag during the act of swallowing.

The eustachian tube can be opened, and air can be forced into the middle ear by increasing the air pressure in the nasopharynx. One way to increase air pressure is to attempt to blow air against the resistance of the closed mouth and nose. Many persons are unable to do so. Another method is to close one side of the nose and force air into the other nostril as the patient swallows (Fig. 18-7). Swallowing closes the nasopharynx. Still another method is to place a curved metal catheter against the nasopharyngeal opening of the eustachian tube. The catheter is passed along the floor of the nose and turned into the tube, and air is blown gently through the catheter (Fig. 18-8).

Temporal bone. The temporal bone is formed by the fusion of four distinct portions—the squamous, petromastoid, and tympanic portions and the styloid process. Usually the petromastoid portion is separated into the petrous and mastoid portions. The squamous (scalelike) portion shows on its inner aspect the vertical groove for the middle meningeal artery and irregular depressions for the convolutions of the temporal lobe of the brain. The root of the zygoma extends anteriorly from the squamous portion and forms the articular process of the temporomandibular joint. Abnormalities of this joint may produce pain, frequently *referred to the ear*.

Mastoid. The mastoid (breastlike) process of the temporal bone provides externally an attachment for the sternocleidomastoid and digastric muscles. The cortex of the bone covers a honeycomb of air cells, each of which interconnects, and the thin mucous membrane of each cell is continuous with that of the middle ear. The mastoid air cells are separated from the dura of the temporal lobe and from the cerebellum by thin cortical bone (the inner table) (Fig. 18-9).

At birth the mastoid process is present, but it is small. It is filled with diploic bone. During the first 2 to 6 years of life the diploic bone is gradually replaced by air cells that bud off from the mastoid antrum. The mastoid antrum is the first and largest air cell and connects directly to the middle ear through the aditus. In a well-pneumatized temporal bone, tracts of air cells extend deep behind the internal ear, under the middle ear, and into the petrous portion of the temporal bone, which houses the internal ear. Cells often extend into the root of the zygoma, superior and anterior to the middle ear.

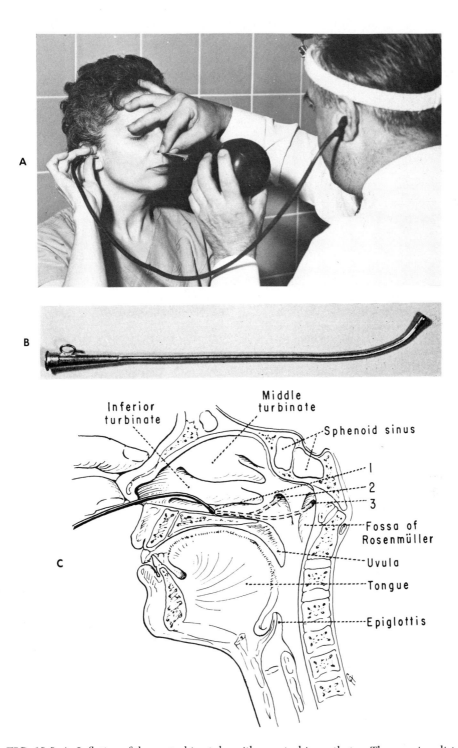

FIG. 18-8. A, Inflation of the eustachian tube with a eustachian catheter. The examiner listens through the auscultation tube to be sure air enters the middle ear. **B,** Eustachian catheter. **C,** Insertion of the eustachian catheter. *1,* Insertion of the catheter along the floor of the nose. *2,* Sliding the catheter forward into the mouth of the tube. *3,* Turning the catheter tip into the fossa of Rosenmüller.

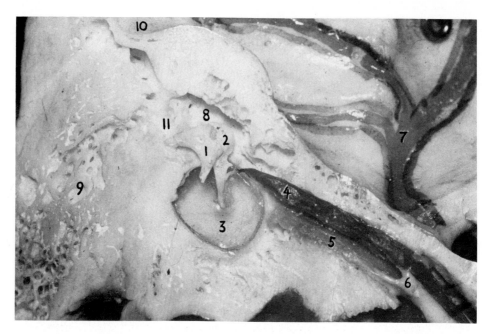

FIG. 18-9. Left ear seen from the medial aspect with the petrous apex, cochlea, and labyrinth removed. *1*, Incus. *2*, Malleus. *3*, Tympanic membrane. *4*, Tensor tympani muscle. *5*, Eustachian tube (osseous portion). *6*, Eustachian tube (cartilaginous portion). *7*, Middle meningeal artery. *8*, Epitympanum. *9*, Mastoid air cells. *10*, Middle cranial fossa. *11*, Aditus ad antrum.

The mastoid is close to the following important intracranial structures:

1. Superiorly, the dura of the temporal lobe
2. Posteriorly, the cerebellar dura
3. Posteriorly, the sigmoid sinus. The sigmoid sinus continues forward and downward until it reaches the anterior limits of the mastoid; then it turns sharply upward to form the jugular bulb; the jugular bulb lies under the floor of the middle ear (Figs. 18-10 and 18-11).
4. Anteriorly, the internal carotid artery, which passes upward into the cranial cavity

The *blood supply* of the middle ear and mastoid is from branches of the internal maxillary artery, a branch of the external carotid system. The *nerve supply* of the middle ear and mastoid is from branches of the fifth, seventh, ninth, and tenth cranial nerves. Branches of these nerves form the tympanic plexus on the promontory. The small fibers lie in grooves in the bone of the promontory just beneath the mucosa of the middle ear (Fig. 18-12). Disturbances of other parts supplied by these nerves, such as the *teeth, tongue, tonsils, and larynx, may cause referred pain to the ear.*

The *petrous* (rocklike) portion of the temporal bone fits into the base of the skull between the sphenoid and occipital bones and separates the middle cranial fossa from the posterior cranial fossa. As its name implies, it is a hard bone. It houses the end organs of the auditory and vestibular systems. On its posterior surface is found the internal auditory meatus, which transmits the seventh and eighth cranial nerves.

Inner ear. The inner ear is that portion of the ear composed of the end organ receptors for hearing (the cochlea) and equilibrium (the labyrinth). Both are contained in the petrous portion of the temporal bone. The bony capsule that surrounds these organs is the most compact bone in the body. These structures are protected from mechanical damage to a greater degree than almost any other body structure. In addition to the hard bone that surrounds the cochlea and labyrinth (called the otic capsule), the membranous end organs are surrounded by fluid (perilymph) and filled with fluid (endolymph). This fluid is important in the protection

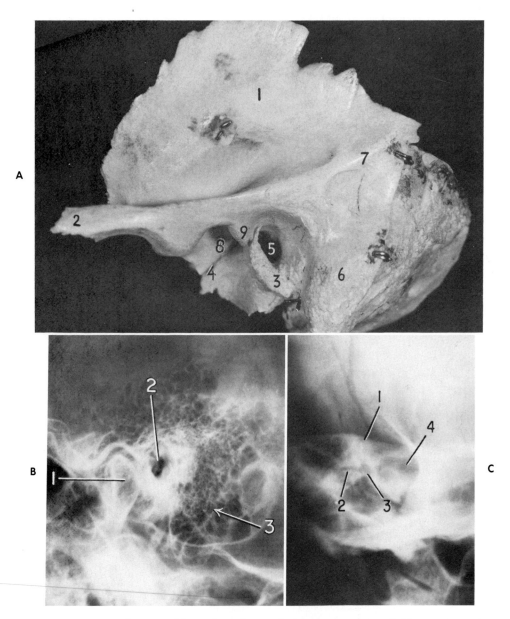

FIG. 18-10. A, Left temporal bone, lateral view. *1,* Squamous portion. *2,* Zygomatic portion.
3, Tympanic portion. *4,* Petrotympanic fissure. *5,* External auditory meatus. *6,* Mastoid portion. *7,* Linea temporalis. *8,* Temporomandibular joint. *9,* Articular tubercle. **B,** Roentgenogram of the left temporal bone, Law position. *1,* Mandibular condyle. *2,* External auditory
canal. *3,* Mastoid cells in the body and tip. **C,** Roentgenogram of the right temporal bone,
Stenver's position. *1,* Superior semicircular canal. *2,* Horizontal semicircular canal. *3,* Vestibule. *4,* Internal auditory meatus.

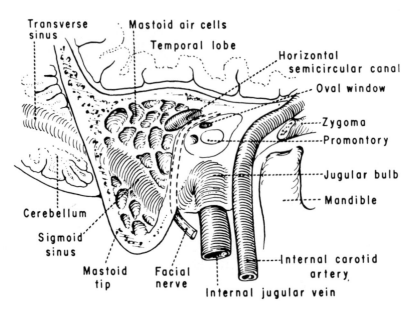

FIG. 18-11. Composite drawing of the right ear, showing the relationship between the middle ear, the mastoid, and surrounding structures.

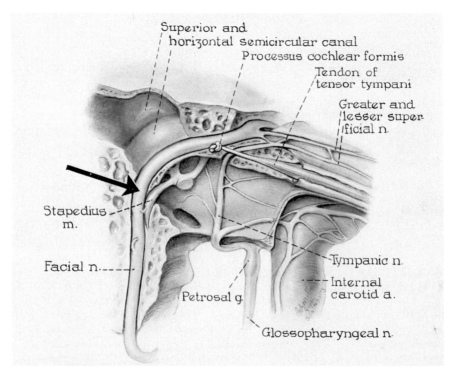

FIG. 18-12. Medial wall of the middle ear. Note the tympanic plexus of nerves over the promontory. The arrow indicates the beginning of the vertical course of the facial nerve.

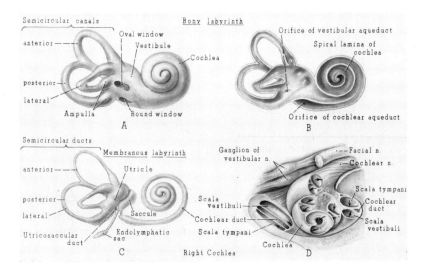

FIG. 18-13. **A** and **B,** Bony labyrinth. **C,** Membranous labyrinth. **D,** Cochlea opened up, with its relationship to the seventh and eighth cranial nerves shown. (From Jacob, S.W., and Francone, C.A.: Structure and function in man, ed. 2, Philadelphia, 1970, W.B. Saunders Co.)

of the end organ. It acts as a cushion against abrupt movements of the head. The membranous cochlea and labyrinth literally "float" in fluid.

The endolymph in the cochlea and labyrinth is a continuous closed system with no ducts (Fig. 18-13). Fluid changes within the endolymphatic system occur as a result of osmotic transfers across the permeable membrane between the endolymph and perilymph. The perilymphatic fluid surrounding the membranous inner ear is continuous with the subarachnoid space through the aqueduct of the cochlea, a small canal through bone, which provides direct exchange of fluid with the spinal fluid. Because of the lack of barriers between the cochlea and the labyrinth, injury or disease frequently affects both hearing and equilibrium.

COCHLEA. The cochlea is coiled upon itself like a snail shell and makes two and one-half turns. It lies in a horizontal plane. The basal end (the largest in diameter) is the medial wall of the middle ear, that is, the promontory (Figs. 18-4 and 18-11). There are three compartments within the cochlea. Two of these, the scala vestibuli (associated with the oval window) and the scala tympani (associated with the round window), contain perilymph. The third, the cochlear duct, contains endolymph. The membranous wall on which rests the delicate end organ of hearing is called the basilar membrane (Figs. 18-14 to 18-16). The membranous cochlear duct connects with the saccule located in the vestibule of the labyrinth. The exact function of the saccule is unknown.

The neural end organ for hearing is the organ of Corti. It rests on the basilar membrane. The organ of Corti extends along the entire length of the cochlea except at the helicotrema, where the scala tympani and the scala vestibuli join. Approximately 24,000 hair cells project from the neuroepithelium. When these hairs are bent or distorted, sound, which has been a mechanical force, is converted into an electrochemical impulse. Later, in the temporal cortex, it is interpreted as understandable sound.

By selective destruction of various areas of the cochlea in experimental animals, the cochlea has been "mapped." Thus it is known that high-pitched sounds stimulate the basal portion of the cochlea and low-pitched sounds stimulate the apical end. The area of the cochlea closest to the middle ear (represented by the promontory) is stimulated by sound in the frequency range between 3000 and 5000 cycles per second (Fig. 18-17).

The cochlea receives its blood supply from a branch of the basilar artery. The cochlear ar-

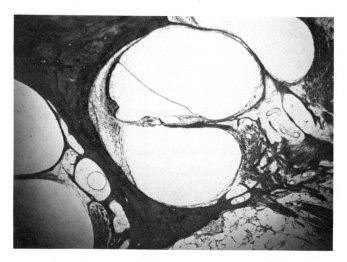

FIG. 18-14. Cross section of the cochlea (monkey). (Courtesy Dr. Merle Lawrence, Ann Arbor, Mich.)

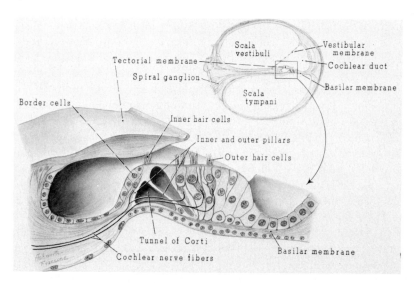

FIG. 18-15. Cross section of the cochlea. The organ of Corti is shown in detail. (Compare with Figs. 18-14 and 18-16.)

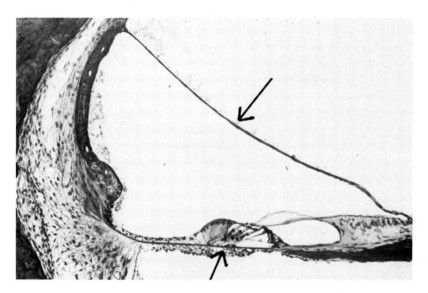

FIG. 18-16. High-power view of a cross section of the cochlea (monkey). The upper arrow indicates the membrane between the cochlear duct and the scala vestibuli (Reissner's membrane). The lower arrow indicates the organ of Corti, resting on the basilar membrane. (Courtesy Dr. Merle Lawrence, Ann Arbor, Mich.)

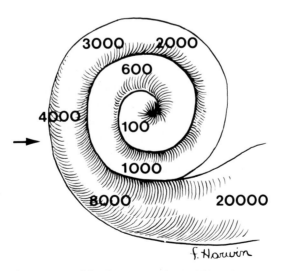

FIG. 18-17. Schema showing sound localization in the cochlea. The arrow points to the region of the promontory.

tery is one of the terminal branches of the internal auditory artery. It is an end artery, and there is no collateral circulation to the cochlea.

Sound impulses received by the cochlear hair cells travel from the cochlea through ganglion cells, axons of which form the cochlear portion of the eighth cranial nerve. The eighth nerve leaves the posterior surface of the petrous portion of the temporal bone through the internal auditory meatus and almost immediately enters the pons. The auditory cortex is located in the superior and transverse gyrus of the temporal lobe.

VESTIBULE. The vestibular portion of the inner ear is composed of the utricle and three semicircular canals (Fig. 18-13). Both ends of each semicircular canal open into the utricle. The semicircular canals are known as the lateral (horizontal), the superior (anterior vertical), and the posterior (posterior vertical) canals. They are situated so that the two horizontal canals are in the same plane, whereas the superior canal of one side is in the same plane as the posterior canal of the opposite side (Fig. 18-18). In other words, the three canals have the same relationship to one another as two walls and the floor at the corner of a room. The floor represents the plane of the horizontal canal. When the head is held erect, the horizontal canal is not quite horizontal. Instead, the head must be inclined 30 degrees forward to bring the horizontal canal parallel to the floor (Fig. 18-19).

The relationship of the canals to one another and to the head can be demonstrated with the hands and arms. If the left elbow is held against the left side and the forearm and hand are placed in front of the body with the palm up, the palm will approximate the plane of the horizontal semicircular canal. If the right hand is then bent at a right angle at the carpophalangeal joint and placed on the palm of the left hand (Fig. 18-20), the fingers of the right hand will indicate the plane of the superior canal and the palm of the right hand will indicate the plane of the posterior canal of the *left* labyrinth. The planes and relationships of the right labyrinth can be demonstrated by reversing the hands.

The membranous semicircular canals are much smaller than the bony canals and are supported in the perilymph by minute fibrous strands (Fig. 18-21). Near the utricle each canal

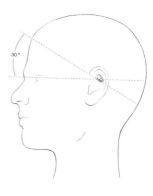

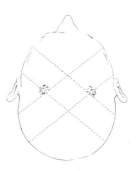

FIG. 18-18. Relationship of the semicircular canals to the plane of the erect head and to each other.

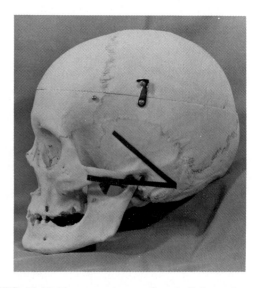

FIG. 18-19. Tape superimposed on skull shows the 30-degree angle between the normal erect position and the anatomic plane of the horizontal semicircular canal. The head is tipped 30 degrees down to bring the horizontal canal into a truly horizontal position.

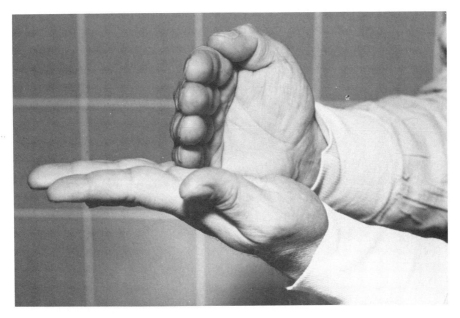

FIG. 18-20. Hands representing the semicircular canals of the left labyrinth. The palm of the left hand represents the horizontal canal; the palm of the right hand, the posterior canal; and the fingers of the right hand, the superior canal.

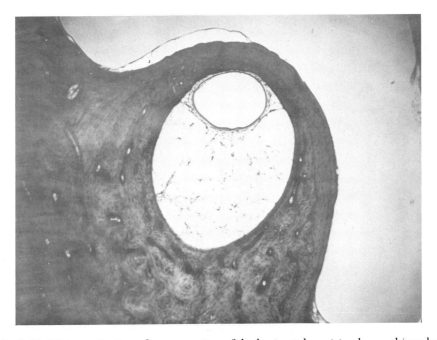

FIG. 18-21. Microscopic view of a cross section of the horizontal semicircular canal (monkey). Note the size of the clear endolymphatic (membranous) canal and the fine supporting stroma in the perilymphatic space. (Courtesy Dr. Merle Lawrence, Ann Arbor, Mich.)

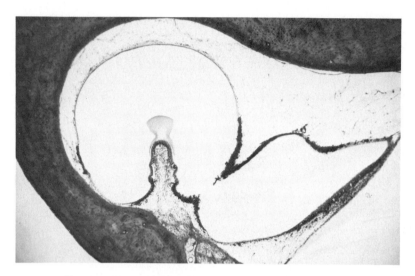

FIG. 18-22. Ampullated end of a semicircular canal, where it joins the utricle (guinea pig). The brushlike structure projecting into the ampulla is the crista. (Courtesy Dr. Merle Lawrence, Ann Arbor, Mich.)

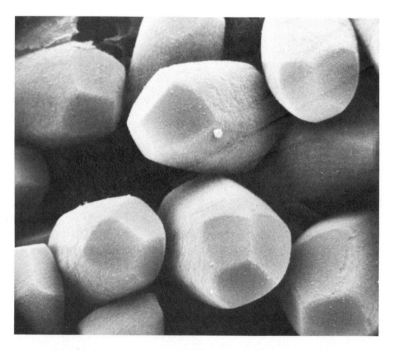

FIG. 18-23. Scanning electron microscope photograph shows otoconia (squirrel monkey) magnified 5,000 times. Crystals are calcium carbonate in calcite form. (Courtesy Dr. David Lim, Columbus, Ohio.)

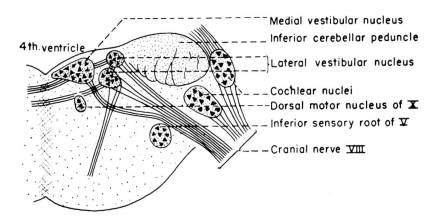

FIG. 18-24. Vestibular and cochlear nuclei in the brain stem. (From DeWeese, D.D.: Dizziness; an evaluation and classification, Springfield, Ill., 1954, Charles C Thomas, Publisher.)

is enlarged. This enlargement is known as the ampulla, or ampullated end of the canal. In each ampulla is found the specialized neuroepithelium, which is the end organ for equilibrium. This end organ is known as the crista of the semicircular canal (Fig. 18-22). Additional specialized epithelium is present in the utricle.

The utricle is concerned with static equilibrium. It regulates the sense of position in space and is stimulated by gravity, centrifugal force, and linear movements. Small (microscopic) granules of calcium carbonate known as *otoconia* are believed to initiate static responses owing to the effect of gravity on them (Fig. 18-23). Stimulation of the utricle produces compensatory eye positions, the head-righting reflex, and alterations in muscle tone. The semicircular canals are stimulated by rotation or acceleration in any direction. Inertia is the primary stimulus. The right and left canals always function together (except during artificial stimulation) (see the section on tests for labyrinthine reactions, p. 300).

The axons from the utricle and semicircular canals join to form the vestibular portion of the eighth cranial nerve. On reaching the brain stem, the cochlear and vestibular portions of the eighth nerve divide and terminate in their respective nuclei (Fig. 18-24). The vestibular nuclei lie on the floor of the fourth ventricle and are separated from the cochlear nuclei by the inferior cerebellar peduncle. The vestibular nuclei have connections with the nuclei of the third, fourth, and sixth cranial nerves through

the medial longitudinal bundle and with the ventral motor gray cells of the spinal cord through the vestibulospinal tract. Fibers also connect to the cerebellar cortex through the inferior cerebellar peduncle. The dorsal motor nucleus of the tenth nerve lies in close approximation to the vestibular nuclei in the brain stem (Fig. 18-24). It undoubtedly accounts for the vagal symptoms of nausea, vomiting, and pallor that accompany severe vertiginous attacks.

The saccule, utricle, and semicircular canals receive their blood supply from the vestibular artery, which is a terminal branch of the basilar artery. It is formed from the confluence of the two vertebral arteries arising from the subclavian artery.

SELECTED READINGS

Bast, T.H., and Anson, B.J.: The temporal bone and the ear, Springfield, Ill., 1949, Charles C Thomas, Publisher.

DeWeese, D.D.: Dizziness; an evaluation and classification, Springfield, Ill., 1954, Charles C Thomas, Publisher.

Farrior, J.B.: Radiographic anatomy of the temporal bone, Rochester, Minn., Am. Acad. Ophthalmol. Otolaryngol. (manual)—reprinted from Med. Radiogr. Photogr. **26**:90, 1950.

Lim, D.J.: Human tympanic membrane, Acta Otolaryngol. **70**:176, 1970.

McNally, W.J., and others: A symposium on the utricle, Trans. Am. Otol. Sci., p. 12, 1956.

Pulec, J.L.: Abnormally patent eustachian tubes; treatment with injection of poly-tetrafluoroethylene (Teflon) paste, Laryngoscope **77**:1543, 1967.

Pruzansky, S.: The temporomandibular joint, Otolaryngol. Clin. North Am. **6**(2):523, 1973.

Saunders, W.H., and Paparella, M.M.: Atlas of ear surgery, ed. 3, St. Louis, 1980, The C.V. Mosby Co.

19 PHYSIOLOGY OF HEARING

Decibel system. Before hearing is discussed, it is necessary to explain the decibel, the measurement commonly used in dealing with hearing loss. The decibel system is a logarithmic method of dealing conveniently with large numbers. The range of the human ear is so great that it requires such a method. An infinitesimal movement of hair cells is enough to cause faint hearing, and yet a *trillion-fold increase* in energy produces a sound pressure that is still tolerable to the ear. Such an enormous increase in sound pressure is expressed as 120 decibels. For practical purposes, the decibel system as it is used is shown in Table 1. The intensity of sounds produced in various situations is shown in Table 2.

It is important to understand that the decibel is a ratio—*not an absolute value*. The decibel compares the relationship between two sound intensities. Thus if we say that one sound is of so many decibels, we mean that it is more intense than a reference level by that much. When hearing is tested with the audiometer and the setting is changed from a reading of 0 decibels to a reading of 60 decibels, there is an energy increase of 1 million times. Even so, the sound increment of 60 decibels above threshold is not excessively loud. Roughly, it represents the sound pressure exerted by a moderately loud voice several feet from the ear.

A percentage description of hearing loss is unsatisfactory, because the pure tone signals used in audiometric tests are not all of equal importance in speech or in other common environmental sounds. The results obtained by taking the numerical values of hearing loss for each frequency and then using these values to compute a one-figure percentage are misleading. Instead, hearing loss is better expressed by recording auditory acuity for each frequency (in

TABLE 1. Relation of decibels to energy

10 decibels	10× increase in power
20 decibels	100× increase in power
30 decibels	1,000× increase in power
60 decibels	1,000,000× increase in power
120 decibels	1 trillion× increase in power

decibels). The readings may then be plotted on a chart to make an audiogram.

External ear and hearing. The external ear consists of the auricle and the external auditory canal. In humans the auricle does little to increase the sensitivity of hearing. Its occasional absence in congenital or traumatic conditions is not associated with an appreciable loss of hearing. On the other hand, occlusion of the external auditory meatus affects hearing seriously.

Actually, provided that the good ear is turned toward the sound source, monaural hearing is only slightly less acute than binaural hearing. But if the head is turned, hearing may be reduced as much as 20 decibels in some frequencies. A more serious handicap of unilateral deafness is the patient's inability to localize a sound source. We are able to determine the direction of a sound because sound waves reach the two ears at slightly different times and intensities.

If the auditory canal of a person with normal hearing is occluded tightly by the examiner's finger, the resultant hearing loss is generally no greater than 40 decibels. This loss still permits the patient to hear a low or moderately loud voice. A common mistake in testing hearing is to assume that one ear is adequately masked by the finger when actually it is not. The patient then receives credit for better hearing than he has.

Earplugs and other safety devices to protect the ear from excessive noise are worthwhile,

TABLE 2. Intensity of sound in different situations (approximate)

Decibels	Situation
140	Air raid siren
	Jet engine (pain felt in ear)
130	Tickle (sensation)
	Aircraft engine (close)
120	Loud shot (1 foot)
	Thunder
110	
	Aircraft engine
100	Boiler shop
	Discomfort for pure tones
	Riveting machine
90	
	Train
	Air hammer (pneumatic)
80	
	Heavy traffic
70	
	Truck (outside)
60	Average street traffic
50	Ordinary spoken voice
	Vacuum cleaner
	Automobile
40	
	Average office
30	Quiet room
	Usual home
20	Soft whisper
	Rural area
10	
0	Threshold of hearing

although they are often not very popular. However, it must be remembered that the attenuation of sound provided by these devices is only partial and that uncomfortable and even harmful noise can still affect the ear in some industrial and military situations.

Tympanic membrane and hearing. The tympanic membrane separates the external auditory meatus from the middle ear. Sound waves that strike the drumhead are partially reflected back into the ear canal and partially transmitted across the drumhead. Of the transmitted waves, some cross the tympanic cavity and enter the round window (Fig. 19-1). Other sound enters the oval window via the chain of ossicles (Fig. 19-2). In the patient with normal hearing, as explained later, sound waves entering the oval window contribute a great deal more to hearing than that sound reaching the cochlea by aerial transmission across the tympanic cavity to the round window. In animal experiments interruption of the ossicular chain, for example, dislocation of the incus from the stapes (Fig. 19-3), reduces hearing about 60 decibels. Then, additional removal of the drumhead, malleus, and incus improves hearing about 15 decibels because these structures, when not connected to the stapes, impede sound waves.

Perforations of the tympanic membrane exert a variable effect on hearing, depending on their size and location and whether there are associated changes in the middle ear. Without audiometric studies, the examiner may be unable to detect hearing loss resulting from small tympanic perforations. In general, uncomplicated tympanic perforations reduce hearing from as few as 5 to as many as 20 decibels. The loss extends throughout the entire frequency range, although it may be greater in some frequencies than in others. Perforations near the attachment of the malleus are especially serious because they contribute to loss of effective action of the ossicular chain. Some patients with almost complete loss of the tympanic membrane can still understand a loud whisper at a distance of 2 feet. *The condition of the ossicles, particularly freedom of motion of the stapes in the oval window, is more important to hearing than is an intact tympanic membrane.* Of course, many patients with tympanic perforations have a loss of hearing greater than 20 decibels, but in them the greater loss generally is due to additional disturbances in the conduction mechanism of the middle ear (for example, ossicular destruction or dislocation, stapedial fixation, or middle ear adhesions).

Middle ear and hearing. The transfer of sound pressure from a gaseous medium (air) to a liquid

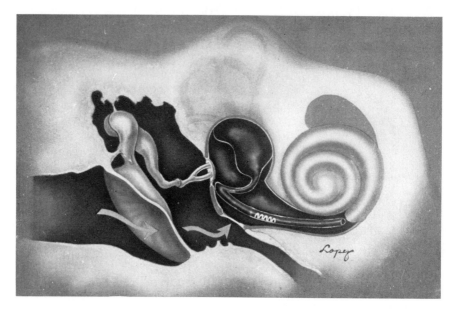

FIG. 19-1. Round window (aerotympanic) route. By aerial transmission across the middle ear, some sound waves enter the round window, but they are relatively ineffective. (Courtesy Dr. Merle Lawrence, Ann Arbor, Mich.)

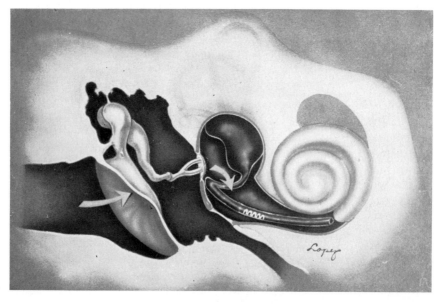

FIG. 19-2. Oval window (ossicular) route in the normal patient. The effective sound waves are those that cross the chain of ossicles to enter the oval window. (Courtesy Dr. Merle Lawrence, Ann Arbor, Mich.)

FIG. 19-3. Dislocation of the incus from the stapes. A 60-decibel (million-fold) hearing loss results because (1) sound waves are largely reflected and absorbed by the eardrum and ossicles and (2) sound waves that do cross the middle ear enter both windows almost simultaneously. There is a cancellation effect.

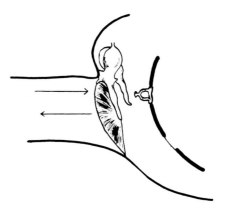

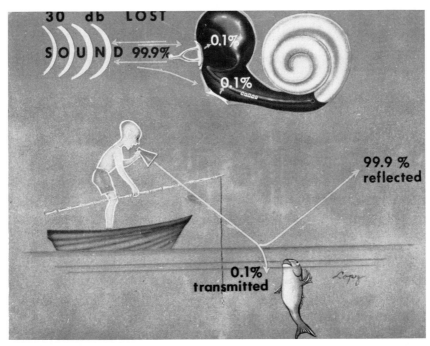

FIG. 19-4. Sound transfer from air to water. At any air-water interface there is a 30-decibel loss of sound energy. This is just as true in the ear as in the sea. (Courtesy Dr. Merle Lawrence, Ann Arbor, Mich.)

medium (endolymph) results in a tremendous loss of energy. In an analogy, Wever and Lawrence point out that fishermen may talk in their boats without much likelihood of disturbing the fish. The reason is that 99.9% of the sound energy of their voices is reflected from the surface of the lake back into the air. Only 0.1% enters the water (Fig. 19-4). On the other hand, the fishermen should be very careful not to stamp on the floor of the boat or splash into the water with their hands. The example illustrates clearly a task of the ear. It must transfer energy from a gaseous to a liquid medium without in-

curring a serious loss en route. The loss of 99.9% of energy is expressed as 30 decibels, about the level at which a person begins to complain that he has a hearing problem.

TRANSFORMER ACTION (Fig. 19-5). To help overcome this great loss of energy, the middle ear acts as a mechanical transformer. There are two mechanical devices built into the middle ear that help to restore most, but not all, of the sound pressure lost in the transfer.

LEVER SYSTEM. Because the handle of the malleus is somewhat longer than the long crus of the incus, the ear gains a small mechanical

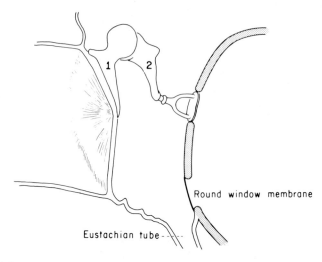

FIG. 19-5. Middle ear transformer system. Note that the handle of the malleus (*1*) compared to the long crus of the incus (*2*) adds an advantage of 1.3 to 1, allowing a gain in sound energy of only 2.5 decibels. However, the areal ratio of the tympanic membrane–footplate is much greater. The effective ratio is 14:1 and corresponds to a 23-decibel gain.

advantage. Actually, the gain is minimal and restores only 2 or 3 decibels of the 30-decibel loss caused when sound pressure in air is transferred to a liquid medium. In certain otologic operations the drumhead is repositioned and placed directly on the stapes (after removal of the incus). A birdlike ear with a single columella results; yet there may be nearly normal hearing.

TYMPANIC MEMBRANE–FOOTPLATE RATIO (AREAL RATIO, OR HYDRAULIC RATIO). Far more important than the lever action is the ratio between the area of the large tympanic membrane and the tiny footplate of the stapes. This ratio is given somewhat different values by various observers. Wever and Lawrence assign an actual ratio of 21:1 but an effective ratio of 14:1. The difference between the two values is due to the fact that not all parts of the tympanic membrane are equally effective in transmission of sound. The 14:1 ratio corresponds to 23 decibels.

Thus *the transformer action of the middle ear* recovers about 25 to 27 of the 30 decibels lost when sound waves pass from air to liquid. The remaining 3 to 5 decibels are forever lost.

MIDDLE EAR MUSCLES. The stapedius muscle (supplied by the seventh nerve) and the tensor tympani muscle (supplied by the fifth nerve) have nothing to do with the acuity of hearing. Instead, they are protective mechanisms. They react reflexly when there is a loud sound. The stapedius inhibits action of the stapedial footplate, and the tensor tympani diminishes excursions of the manubrium. Actually, a sudden sharp sound, too fast for the latent period of either muscle, enters the cochlea unchanged. More prolonged sounds may be diminished 10 decibels—enough attenuation to help protect the inner ear against very intense sounds (such as those over 100 decibels).

PHASE RELATIONSHIPS. In the person with normal hearing, the intact drumhead not only contributes to the very important areal ratio (tympanic membrane–footplate ratio) but also *shields sound from the round window.* In doing so, it changes the phase relationship between the oval and round windows so that there is less likelihood that a wave will cancel itself by entering both windows simultaneously.

To further clarify phase relationships and the way in which sound waves travel in the cochlea, let us consider the patient with chronic otitis media who has lost most of the eardrum and two auditory ossicles (Fig. 19-6). In this patient, simultaneously and with equal intensity, sound waves may strike the stapedial footplate and the membrane closing the round window. Because the oval window opens into the scala vestibuli and the round window opens into the scala tympani, and because these channels are on the opposite sides of the basilar membrane (which supports the organ of Corti), the effect could be

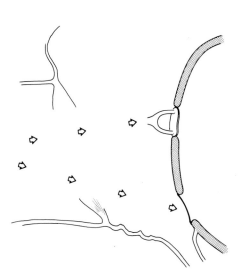

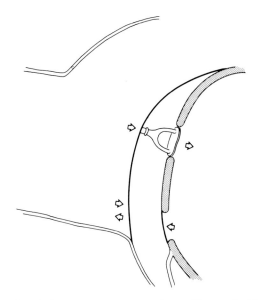

FIG. 19-6. Here the malleus, incus, and tympanic membrane are destroyed—the middle ear has lost its transformer action. Additional hearing loss is caused by exposure of both windows to approximately equal sound pressures. Total loss is 45 to 55 decibels.

FIG. 19-7. Type III tympanoplasty. The negligible lever action is lost, but the important areal ratio is restored, and there is sound protection for the round window. There is a free tissue graft on the stapes.

the same as that produced by placing equal pressure on the two ends of an open U tube filled with water. There would be no displacement of fluid because of a cancellation effect. Similarly, a microphone placed equidistant between two identical sources of sound may pick up very little sound. It is in a zone of silence caused by a cancellation effect.

In practice, when sound waves can enter both windows, total deafness never results but the hearing loss may be worsened. Conversely, it is sometimes possible to improve hearing in a patient without an eardrum by occluding the round window with some substance that will partially reflect sound waves. Alternatively, in the operation known as *tympanoplasty*, if a tissue graft can be laid across the middle ear so as to touch the stapes but leave an air pocket about the round window, hearing is improved (Fig. 19-7). The reason is that sound waves are transmitted through the graft directly to the stapes and the oval window (columella effect, as in the bird), whereas sound waves striking the part of the graft covering (but not touching) the round window are mostly reflected back. There is no cancellation effect because more sound energy enters one window than the other and also because the waves are thrown out of phase. This

sound protection for the round window is one of the two basic principles applied in restoring hearing through tympanoplasty.

Sound in the cochlea. Under normal conditions the most effective sound waves are those transmitted across the drumhead and the chain of ossicles to the oval window. The footplate of the stapes, closing the oval window, is held in position by an annular ligament, which allows the stapes to vibrate according to the frequency and intensity of a sound wave. Thus a weak signal causes minimal displacement of the footplate, whereas exceptionally intense sound waves actually produce discomfort by causing the ossicles to rattle.

As the footplate of the stapes rocks in the oval window, sound pressure is transmitted directly to the perilymph of the inner ear. The perilymph does not circulate but acts as a protective cushion for a fragile membranous tube, the cochlear duct. In the cochlear duct there is endolymph. As sound pressure displaces the perilymph, the endolymph is likewise displaced, and the final receptors of hearing, the hair cells, are distorted. At this point, sound, which was a mechanical force, is transformed into an electrical response.

In order for a pressure wave to pass through

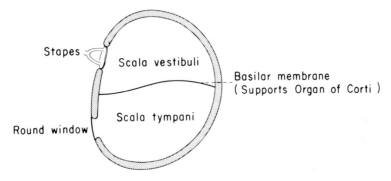

FIG. 19-8. Basic diagram for Figs. 19-9 to 19-11. (Adapted from Wever, G., and Lawrence, M.: Physiological acoustics, Princeton, N.J., 1954, Princeton University Press.)

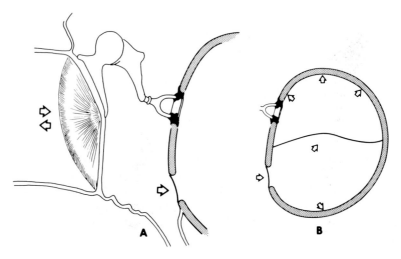

FIG. 19-9. Footplate otosclerosis. **A,** Very little sound can enter the cochlea. **B,** With only one window open, any sound energy from the round window spreads throughout the cochlea uniformly, so that the basilar membrane is not appreciably displaced.

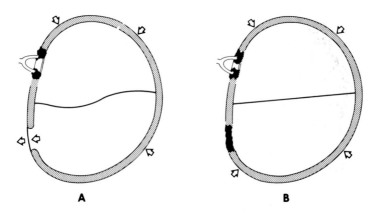

FIG. 19-10. Bone conduction in otosclerosis. **A,** Otosclerosis (with an open round window) does not diminish the compressional type of bone conduction. **B,** Rarely, otosclerosis closes both windows. All sound reflects, and the patient has minimal hearing. The opening of either window would reestablish the compressional type of bone conduction. The opening of both windows would reestablish air conduction.

liquid (an almost noncompressible substance) housed by an unyielding chamber (the cochlea), there must be openings at either end of the channel. In the cochlea, one opening is the oval window and the other is the round window. Again, a hollow glass U tube filled with water may be used as an analogy. Both ends must be "open" in order that finger pressure on a rubber diaphragm (over one end) can effectively transmit pressure waves to the opposite end. Older investigators misunderstood the function of the round window in the normal ear. Some thought that the sound waves that were most effective in producing hearing entered the cochlea via the round window. They ignored the transformer action of the middle ear. Now it is agreed that the great mechanical advantage offered when sound energy is directed across the auditory ossicles explains the true pathway. The round window in the person with normal hearing serves chiefly as a relief hole in the bony cochlear capsule.

Organ of Corti. In order for hearing to occur, it is necessary that sound waves move or distort the hair cells, the final receptors of hearing. Any condition that prevents sound from distorting the hair cells reduces hearing accordingly. For example, in *otosclerosis* (Figs. 19-9 and 19-10), a formation of abnormal bone locks the footplate of the stapes in the oval window. Hearing is reduced even though the round window remains open. Sound waves that do reach the cochlea, rather than passing directly from one window to the other across the basilar membrane and distorting hair cells en route, are reflected back because the ankylosed stapedial footplate obstructs the oval window. Since there is ineffective displacement of the hair cells, hearing by air conduction is reduced. However, in otosclerosis, hearing by bone conduction remains normal. As long as one window remains open (closure of both windows by otosclerosis is rare), sound waves may cause displacement of the endolymph, as demonstrated in Fig. 19-10.

In an ingenious procedure (the fenestration operation) (Figs. 19-11 and 25-13) used to relieve deafness resulting from otosclerosis, a new window is created in the horizontal semicircular canal. The perilymph in this channel connects with the same channel (scala vestibuli) as does the oval window. Thus the new window is on the opposite side of the basilar membrane from the round window (scala tympani). This new arrangement again permits sound pressure to escape in a manner that displaces the hair cells, and hearing is restored.

The hair cells of the organ of Corti are susceptible to injury by oxygen deprivation, drug toxicity, mechanical injury (usually in the form of noise), and other forms of trauma. Until recently many authorities thought that nutrients for the organ of Corti and the hair cells came

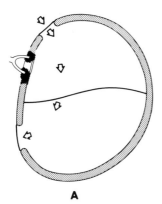
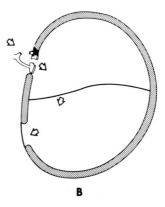

A   **B**

FIG. 19-11. Effect of operations for otosclerosis. **A,** Fenestration operation. The new window on the *vestibular* side of the cochlea reestablishes a normal sound pathway (another opening into the scala tympani obviously would not permit effective displacement of cochlear fluids). Even so, loss of middle ear transformer action leaves the patient with an average hearing loss of 27 decibels. **B,** Stapes mobilization operation—anterior crurotomy technique. Theoretically, normal hearing can be restored.

from the endolymph in which they are bathed. Lawrence has demonstrated that modiolar vessels leading to the capillary loops beneath the basilar membrane are a true source of nutrients for the organ of Corti.

• • •

In summary, if we are to hear, hair cells must be stimulated by physical distortion or displacement. Such stimulation is normally produced when sound, amplified by the transformer action of the middle ear, enters the scala vestibuli via the oval window, deflects hair cells as it crosses the basilar membrane, and then escapes through the round window.

The discussion in Chapter 25 on tympanoplasty (p. 367) and Fig. 25-21 should be helpful in relating the physiology of hearing to disease conditions.

SELECTED READINGS

Allan, G.W., and Habib, M.: The effects of increasing the cerebrospinal fluid pressure upon the cochlear microphonics, Laryngoscope 72:423, 1962.

Davis, H., and Walsh, T.E.: The limits of improvement of hearing following the fenestration operation, Laryngoscope 60:273, 1950.

On the function of middle ear and eustachian tube, Acta Otolaryngol. (supp. 182), 1963.

Guild, S.R.: Hearing by bone conduction, Ann. Otol. Rhinol. Laryngol. 52:246, 1944.

Lawrence, M.: Recent investigations of sound conduction; the normal ear, Ann. Otol. Rhinol. Laryngol. 59:1020, 1950.

Lawrence, M.: Some physiological factors in inner ear deafness, Ann. Otol. Rhinol. Laryngol. 69:480, 1960.

Lawrence, M.: Effects of interference with terminal blood supply on organ of Corti, Laryngoscope 76:1318, 1966.

Lawrence, M., Wolsk, D., and Litton, W.B.: Circulation of the inner ear fluids, Ann. Otol. Rhinol. Laryngol. 70:753, 1961.

Lempert, J.: Fenestra nov-ovalis; a new oval window for the improvement of hearing in cases of otosclerosis, Arch. Otolaryngol. 34:880, 1941.

Rauch, S., and others: Arguments for the permeability of Reissner's membrane, Laryngoscope 73:135, 1963.

Shambaugh, G.E.: Surgery of the ear, Philadelphia, 1959, W.B. Saunders Co.

Simkins, C.S.: Functional anatomy of the eustachian tube, Arch. Otolaryngol. 38:476, 1943.

Simmons, F.B.: Individual sound damage susceptibility; role of middle ear muscles, Ann. Otol. Rhinol. Laryngol. 72:528, 1963.

Wever, E.G.: The mechanics of hair-cell stimulation, Ann. Otol. Rhinol. Laryngol. 80:786, 1971.

Wever, E.G., and Lawrence, M.: The functions of the round window, Ann. Otol. Rhinol. Laryngol. 57:579, 1948.

Wever, E.G., and Lawrence, M.: Physiological acoustics, Princeton, N.J., 1954, Princeton University Press.

Wever, E.G., Lawrence, M., and Smith, K.R.: The middle ear in sound conduction, Arch. Otolaryngol. 48:69, 1948.

Wullstein, H.: The restoration of the function of the middle ear in chronic otitis media, Ann. Otol. Rhinol. Laryngol. 65:1020, 1956.

Zollner, F.: The prognosis of the operative improvement of hearing in chronic middle ear infections, Ann. Otol. Rhinol. Laryngol. 66:907, 1957.

20 EVALUATION OF HEARING

HEARING LOSS

Loss of hearing can be either partial or total. It can be present in low, middle, or high frequencies and in any combination. Only when it is total or nearly total (more than 85 to 90 decibels below normal) do we speak of deafness. To say that a person with a 60-decibel loss of hearing is deaf leads to the erroneous assumption that nothing can be done to improve his hearing. Hearing loss implies a partial loss of function; only the profoundly damaged ear is unable to respond to amplified sound. For practical purposes, a person begins to be socially incapacitated when his hearing loss in *both* ears reaches or exceeds 40 decibels in the speech frequencies (300 to 3000 cycles). A bilateral hearing loss of more than 40 decibels in these frequencies, if not medically or surgically correctable, indicates the need for a hearing aid.

Sensorineural hearing loss. Also referred to as a perceptive or nerve type of hearing loss, sensorineural hearing loss is due to disease within the cochlea, in the cochlear nerve, or in the brain. The causes may be infection, trauma, toxic substance, degenerative disease, or congenital abnormality. For example, purulent labyrinthitis may destroy the inner ear; mumps is a common cause of severe unilateral deafness; a skull fracture may sever the eighth nerve or injure the organ of Corti; intense noise may destroy cochlear hair cells; kanamycin and other drugs sometimes cause deafness; the deafness of old age (presbycusis) is due to senile degenerative changes; congenital nerve deafness may be due to hereditary factors or intrauterine disease (for example, rubella in a pregnant woman).

Injury to the organ of Corti produces a special type of sensorineural hearing loss that differs from both conductive hearing loss caused by middle ear disease and hearing loss caused by nerve fiber or brain disease. In the inner ear sound is transformed from mechanical into electrical energy; any physiologic disturbance at this site is apt to result in a serious and complicated hearing loss.

To distinguish between hearing loss resulting from end organ disease (cochlear deafness) and hearing loss resulting from nerve fiber or central disease, certain special examinations are used. These are described later (pp. 287-290, p. 293).

Conductive hearing loss. Conductive hearing loss contrasts sharply with sensorineural loss. It occurs in patients with external or middle ear disorders such as otitis media, otosclerosis, and perforated eardrum. Patients with only conductive loss have a normal inner ear. They are hard of hearing because there is a defect in the mechanism by which sound is conducted to the inner ear. Such persons hear perfectly if only the sound is amplified sufficiently. Thus they can use hearing aids very satisfactorily. Patients with sensorineural hearing loss, and especially those with cochlear disease, often use hearing aids less satisfactorily.

In contrasting sensorineural loss with conductive loss, it is worthwhile to note that disorders producing sensorineural hearing loss do not cause changes in the appearance of the tympanic membrane. On the other hand, *disorders producing conductive loss (except otosclerosis) nearly always cause alterations in the normal appearance of the drumhead.*

• • •

Congenital deafness is the term used to indicate a hearing loss presumably present since birth or occurring so early in infancy that the time of onset cannot be determined.

Mixed hearing loss means that both the conducting mechanism and neural components are involved.

Simulated hearing loss indicates that an apparent loss of hearing is not due to organic disease. It may result from a functional (involuntary) disorder, or it may represent malingering.

HEARING TESTS

Hearing tests commonly employed include those using the whispered and spoken voice, the watch tick, tuning forks, and similar devices that are readily available. The tests yield much knowledge if they are employed intelligently. However, the results obtained are likely to be more qualitative than quantitative, particularly when evaluated by inexperienced examiners. Better quantitative determinations are made with the electrically calibrated audiometer. Such an instrument produces sound of known intensity—either pure tone signals (at various frequencies) or actual speech (recorded or "live").

Whispered and spoken voice tests. The examiner who uses his voice to test a patient's hearing must have had experience enough to know how well his own voice is heard at different distances and how to vary the intensity of his voice so that each patient is tested under similar conditions. One method is to begin testing with a very low whisper, the lips about 2 feet from the patient's ear and directed toward the ear. The examiner exhales as strongly as possible and then whispers. In a quiet room a patient with normal hearing can repeat what is said to him. If he cannot understand a low whisper, the examiner uses a medium whisper and finally a loud whisper. The spoken voice is then used in the same manner as the whisper. The examiner gradually increases the intensity of his voice until the patient responds correctly.

Another technique is for the examiner to maintain a constant intensity for his whispered or spoken voice but to vary the distance. Thus, his report might read:

Whispered voice	Left ear, 1 foot
Spoken voice	Left ear, 6 feet

Obviously this technique leaves much to be desired with regard to masking, since it depends on the patient to occlude one ear effectively while his other ear is being tested.

Although a rapidly moving fingertip in the opposite ear canal will mask a whisper, a more intense sound is necessary to mask anything louder than a low voice. Usually the Bárány noisebox is used (Figs. 20-3 and 20-7, *B*).

Care must be taken in the choice of word material used to test hearing. Questions that can be answered by yes or no should be avoided. It is better to have the patient repeat familiar bisyllabic words (known as spondee words), such as *snowball, cowboy,* and *mousetrap,* or to ask a question such as, "Do guns shoot bullets or flowers?" Also, it is very important to be certain that the patient cannot read the examiner's lips (Fig. 20-1). On the other hand, after hearing has been checked, a test for lipreading ability should be given to obtain information regarding the patient's adjustment to his hearing loss. To do so, the examiner whispers or speaks below the level at which the patient can hear while the patient observes the lips closely.

Patients with sensorineural hearing loss often hear a spoken voice much better than a whisper, even a loud one. The reason is that they tend to have a greater loss in high than in low frequen-

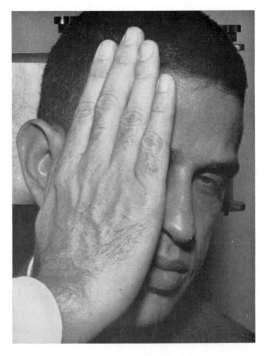

FIG. 20-1. Voice test. Examiner's hand shields the eyes of the person being tested to make certain he does not lipread.

cies, and the whisper contains more high frequencies than does the spoken voice.

The watch tick. Many patients first discover their hearing loss when they find themselves unable to hear a watch ticking.

The watch tick is a high-pitched sound, and it is used in testing patients with high-frequency deafness. It is a poor method to use exclusively (as is any one test) because it tests only a portion of the hearing range. Since watch ticks vary greatly in intensity, information cannot easily be compared when examiners use different watches.

Tuning fork tests. Tuning fork tests for hearing acuity remain an important part of the otologic functional examination. A common error is to use the wrong fork. *The 128-cycle tuning fork commonly used to test vibratory sense should not be used.* When such a low frequency is used, the patient has difficulty differentiating between feeling the vibrations and hearing them. Inaccurate results are therefore obtained. The most useful tuning forks for testing hearing are those with vibrating frequencies of 256, 512, and 1024 cycles per second. For some testing, a fork that vibrates at 2048 cycles per second may be used.

A tuning fork should be stroked between the thumb and index finger, gently tapped on the knuckle (Fig. 20-2), or carefully activated with a rubber reflex hammer. Most *beginners strike the fork too hard* or strike it on a hard surface and thus produce overtones as well as too intense a sound. *Hearing tests are performed near threshold.* A patient becomes fatigued if he must wait too long or answer too often while a strongly activated fork dies down. When tuning forks are used for testing, masking may be necessary (Fig. 20-3). Tuning forks, as employed in the Weber, Rinne, and Schwabach tests, are useful within certain limits in the differentiation between conductive and sensorineural hearing losses (Table 3).

NORMAL RESPONSES (**NO HEARING LOSS**). When a vibrating tuning fork is placed on the maxillary incisors or in any midline position of the skull, sound waves travel through the skull, activate the cochlear fluids, and cause hearing. When both ears are normal, the sound is heard at equal loudness in both ears. When the vibrating fork is placed on one mastoid process, it is heard in that ear a certain length of time before it gradually dies away. Then, if without reactivation the fork is replaced opposite the external auditory meatus, the sound will again be heard and again slowly die down. Normally, a tuning fork is heard twice as long by air conduction as by bone conduction. In other words, stimula-

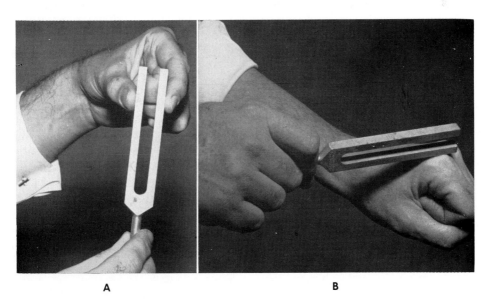

A   **B**

FIG. 20-2. Activating the tuning fork. Hearing is tested at *near-threshold* levels; therefore the fork should be made to ring softly. **A,** Stroking the fork. **B,** Tapping the fork gently on the knuckle.

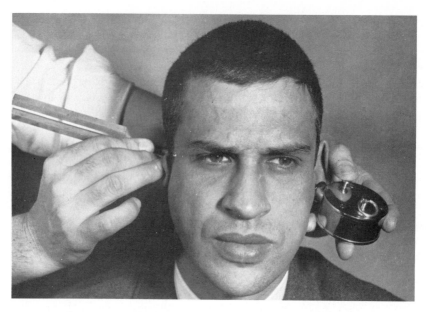

FIG. 20-3. Use of a noisebox to mask the ear not being tested. Unless the opposite ear is excluded from the test, the examiner may never know for certain which ear hears the fork.

TABLE 3. Tuning fork tests for normal hearing, conductive hearing loss, and sensorineural hearing loss

	Weber (bone only)	Rinne (air-bone)	Schwabach (bone only)
Normal	Not lateralized	Positive AC > BC	Equal
Conductive loss	Lateralized to poorer ear	Negative BC > or = AC	Patient hears longer than examiner
Perceptive loss	Lateralized to better ear	Positive AC > BC	Examiner hears longer than patient

tion of the hair cells causes hearing regardless of how the vibrations reach the cochlea. Because the middle ear route is more efficient, however, the normal ear *hears sound conducted by air longer than sound conducted by bone.*

WEBER TEST (Fig. 20-4). In the Weber test a tuning fork is placed on the maxillary incisors or anywhere in the midline of the skull. A patient with *conductive* hearing loss hears the sound in the poor ear provided that he has normal hearing in the opposite ear. The reason is that ordinary room noise always present in the usual testing situation tends to mask the normal ear but the poor ear with conductive loss, not hearing such noise, has a better chance to hear bone-conducted sound.

If there is *sensorineural* loss in one ear and the opposite ear is normal, the same fork is heard louder in the good ear.

Strike a tuning fork and place it on your skull in the midline. You will hear it in both ears. Now occlude one ear tightly with your finger. You will immediately hear the sound of the fork in the plugged ear, and it will be louder. You have not increased your hearing acuity, but you have eliminated some of the ever-present environmental sound (ambient noise) from one ear. There is a temporary conductive hearing loss in one ear.

RINNE TEST (Fig. 20-5). The Rinne test is performed by *alternately* placing a ringing tuning fork opposite one external auditory meatus and on the adjacent mastoid bone. The normal ear hears a tuning fork about twice as long by air conduction as by bone conduction. In well-developed conductive loss, the normal ratio is reversed. In lesser conductive losses, the air-bone relationship may not be completely re-

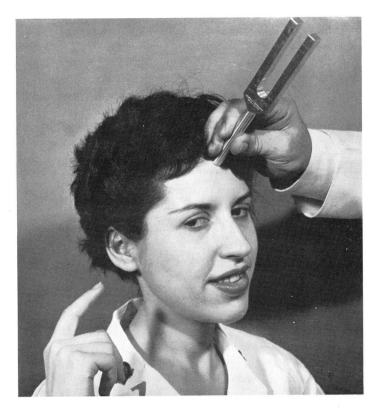

FIG. 20-4. Weber test. Patient indicates that the sound is heard louder in the right ear. This may mean either a conductive loss in the right ear or a sensorineural loss in the left ear. Another good place to hold the fork is on the maxillary teeth.

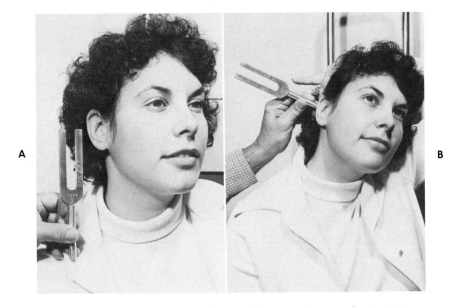

FIG. 20-5. Rinne test: air conduction (**A**) versus bone conduction (**B**).

versed but the ratio is altered so that sound by bone conduction is heard relatively longer (a 1:1 ratio). The patient hears just as long, or even longer, by bone conduction. Patients with sensorineural loss, on the other hand, hear better by air conduction than by bone conduction. They maintain the normal ratio, although hearing is reduced by both air and bone conduction.

Arbitrarily, a patient's Rinne test is said to be positive when he hears longer by air than by bone conduction and negative when the reverse is true.

SCHWABACH TEST (Fig. 20-6). The Schwabach test permits the examiner to compare his own normal hearing by bone conduction with the patient's hearing by bone conduction. The test is performed by *alternately* placing a vibrating tuning fork on the patient's mastoid process and on the examiner's mastoid process. When either the patient or examiner stops hearing the tone, the number of seconds that the other continues to hear is recorded. If the examiner's hearing is normal, he will hear the tone several seconds longer than will a patient with sensorineural hearing loss. However, if the patient with a hearing loss continues to hear the tone after the examiner can no longer hear it, it follows that the patient has a normal sensorineural pathway

(at least for that tone) and a conductive hearing loss. He hears the tone longer in the involved ear because this ear, when the conductive mechanism is damaged, need compete no longer with the masking effect of the room noise to which the examiner's ear is subjected.

POINTS TO REMEMBER. The following points should be remembered in performing tuning fork tests:

1. The correct forks must be used (preferably those with frequencies of 256, 512, 1024, and 2048 cycles per second).
2. The forks must be applied to the proper region of the mastoid because not all parts of the mastoid are equally satisfactory for testing. Trial and error is often necessary in determining the best place to apply the fork.
3. Intermittent rather than continuous application of the forks to the bone is important.
4. The tines of the forks should be directed at the ear—not held obliquely (where theoretically there should be no sound at all). Hold a tuning fork to your own ear and rotate it slowly. You will note that the tone increases and diminishes in intensity, depending on the position of the tines with respect to the external auditory meatus.

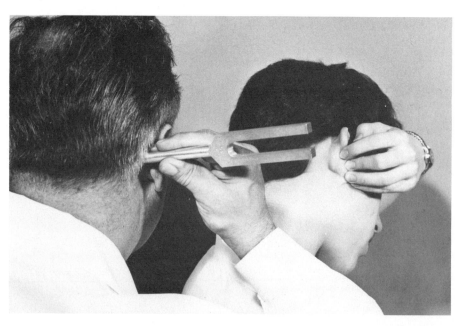

FIG. 20-6. Schwabach test. Examiner's and patient's hearing are compared by *bone conduction*.

5. Most beginners ring the fork too loudly. The fork should be made to ring softly rather than loudly because the purpose of the test is not to determine how intense a sound the patient can tolerate but rather the point at which he can just hear. Ring the fork by stroking it between the index finger and the thumb.

6. Doubtful or conflicting results must be rechecked several times.

7. A sound-treated room is not required, but a quiet room is necessary.

Pure tone audiometry. Most quantitative measurements of hearing are made by using the pure tone audiometer. This electrical device produces pure tones that can be varied according to frequency and intensity. Plotting the intensity against the frequency provides a chart such as that shown in Fig. 25-3, *A*. In the chart it can be seen that there is a drop in the hearing in higher frequencies and that normal hearing is preserved in lower frequencies. The same approximate information is obtainable by using tuning forks, but less easily and less accurately.

Seven frequencies from 125 cycles per second to 8000 cycles per second are tested by first presenting the tone loud enough for the patient to hear distinctly and then seeking the threshold level for the frequency. The patient signals by raising a finger, pressing a button, or simply saying, "I hear it."

Both air conduction and bone conduction measurements are made at threshold levels. In special situations, above-threshold measurements are also made.

The pure tone electric audiometer is the basic instrument used in modern audiometry. It is a moderately complicated device, and it holds many opportunities for error. Results should be checked by tuning forks and the ordinary whispered and spoken voice tests.

The zero (0) reference level of a clinical audiometer refers to a level obtained by testing normal human ears. It is therefore an *average* of the sound intensity that can just be detected by the *average* normal ear. It is spoken of as the threshold of normal hearing for pure tones. Most audiometers show decibels in minus as well as plus values. When a person can hear a given frequency at −10 decibels, it merely means that he can hear that frequency better than the person with *average* hearing. Similarly,

when the threshold of an ear is no more than 25 decibels above zero, the hearing is considered to be normal, although not quite as good as average.

The most important range of hearing for speech is between the frequencies of 300 and 3000 cycles per second. Testing is performed above and below these frequencies to more thoroughly map the ability of the ear to receive sound and to indicate minimal losses (particularly in the high tones) of which the person is unaware. The human ear can detect sounds from 20 cycles per second to 20,000 cycles per second. Audiometers could be constructed to test all these frequencies, but from a practical point of view little additional diagnostic information would be obtained.

Recent experiments with higher frequency testing (12,000 to 15,000 cycles per second) may prove to be of value in early detection of cochlear damage resulting from drug toxicity. If reliable, such tests could dictate cessation of a toxic drug before significant cochlear damage occurs. Such high-frequency tests might also provide an earlier warning of eighth nerve damage from a progressive lesion such as acoustic neuroma.

Actually, hearing in the human ear is most acute at about 1000 cycles. In the audiometer other frequencies at which the ear is less sensitive are automatically brought up to equal loudness with the 1000-cycle tone when those frequencies are dialed.

For many years the need for an international standard reference zero for pure tone audiometers has been recognized. The American standard reference levels, published in 1951, differed significantly from those of the British standard, used in most European countries. The International Organization for Standards took this matter under advisement in 1955. The British standard had been established 15 years after the American standard and had the advantage of better equipment, acoustic conditions, and techniques. The British standard turned out to be about 10 decibels less than the American standard. After several years of discussion and verification, all studies were combined to form a new international standard, which was published in 1964. The new standard has been approved by the American Academy of Otolaryngology and by the American Speech-Lan-

TABLE 4. Conversion table to change
ASA 1951 to ISO 1964

Frequency (cycles per second)	Decibels (+ or −)
125	9
250	15
500	14
1000	10
1500	10
2000	8.5
3000	8.5
4000	6
6000	9.5
8000	11.5

guage Hearing Association on the basis that the levels are (1) more accurate in depicting normal thresholds, (2) reproducible from country to country, and (3) more likely to reduce confusion and ambiguity in the future. The new standard has been officially accepted by the American National Standards Institute (ANSI). Audiometers in use before the acceptance of the new standard can be recalibrated with minimal expense. At the present time the American standard (ASA 1951) can be corrected to the international standard (ISO 1964) by adding the corrections listed in Table 4. To change the ISO 1964 to ASA 1951, the same corrections are subtracted from the audiometric readings in the various frequencies.

When an audiogram is being charted, the proper standard, according to the calibration of the audiometer used, should be clearly indicated, that is, ASA 1951 or ISO 1964.

Importance of masking. While one ear is being tested, the opposite ear must be excluded from the test. Failure to mask the good ear is a very common error and one that leads the examiner to think the patient is hearing the signal in the poor ear (which is being tested). When testing is done by air conduction, it is important to mask the good ear if the difference in the hearing level of the two ears is more than 30 decibels. Masking is especially important in testing by bone conduction and has to be used with both tuning fork and audiometer examinations. *The greater the discrepancy in hearing between the ears, the greater will be the need for masking the better ear.*

A finger tightly fitted into the meatus will mask the sound of a low or medium whisper, but it may not obscure the sound of a loud whisper or low voice (Fig. 20-7, *A*). Moving the fingertip briskly in the ear canal will provide a better masking level. This method of masking is used when the examiner's voice is louder than the low or medium whisper. Still louder sounds that must be blocked out—for example, the medium voice or loud voice—require a more effective mask than a mere finger in the ear canal. A device such as the Bárány noisebox, placed in one ear to produce a loud noise, will effectively mask even a loud voice (Fig. 20-7, *B*). Some physicians use a stream of air from a compressed air pump. Audiometers are equipped with a masking sound that can be varied in intensity.

Most important of all is simply remembering to mask. Masking seems obvious when vision is being tested (one eye is always shielded), but it is very commonly disregarded when hearing is being tested.

Speech audiometry. A speech audiometer is essentially the same instrument as the pure tone audiometer, but it reproduces the spoken voice rather than pure tones. The spoken voice may be the so-called live voice of the examiner, or it may be a recorded voice.

In addition to testing the patient with sound transmitted through earphones, "free field" testing also is used. Here the patient sits before a loudspeaker and listens to speech or word material. The difficulty of the listening task is increased by simultaneously adding background noise from another speaker. Such noice approximates normal listening conditions.

SPONDEE WORDS. Spondee words are easily understood, bisyllabic, equally stressed words, such as *birthday, hothouse, toothbrush, horseshoe, airplane, northwest, whitewash, hot dog, hardware,* and *woodwork.*

The level at which the listener correctly repeats half the words (and misses the other half) is called his speech reception threshold (SRT). In most persons this measurement correlates closely with the measurement found by pure tone audiometry.

PHONETICALLY BALANCED WORDS. Phonetically balanced (P-B) words are one-syllable words such as *an, yard, carve, us, day, toe, felt, stone, hunt,* and *ran.*

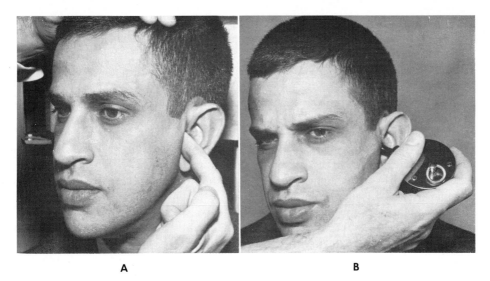

FIG. 20-7. Masking the ear not being tested. **A,** A moving finger will mask the examiner's whispered or low voice but not a loud voice. **B,** Bárány noisebox being used to mask more intense sound. A loud noise in the left ear usually has little effect on the right ear.

All of them are familiar. They have been selected so as to approximate the distribution of speech sounds in ordinary conversation. P-B words are presented (through earphones) at an intensity approximately 30 decibels above the speech reception threshold as measured by spondee words. In other words, P-B words are given at an *optimal intensity*.

The person with normal hearing will hear and correctly repeat 95% to 100% of these words. The patient with inner ear hearing loss will fail to achieve a satisfactory score. He may score 80%, or he may miss every word. No matter how loudly P-B words are presented, the patient with severe inner ear hearing loss fails to make an adequate score. In fact, if the intensity is increased beyond the range of his most comfortable loudness, his score may even become worse. Such a patient is said to have a poor *discrimination ability*.

In contrast to the patient with cochlear disease, patients with a conductive loss score high on this test. All that is required for them to hear well is *amplification*. Thus they can use hearing aids very satisfactorily.

The patient with poor discrimination ability hears sound and realizes that someone is speaking but cannot satisfactorily distinguish between similar words. Patients often remark, "I can hear you, but I can't understand you." Such patients have difficulty in group conversation or when listening against a background of noise. A poor discrimination score is one evidence that a deaf person may not be able to use a hearing aid satisfactorily. The hearing aid makes sound louder, but it often fails to make sound more intelligible; only normally functioning hair cells can do that.

Special auditory phenomena. Certain auditory phenomena known to be associated with inner ear hearing loss help to pinpoint the lesion. A description of these auditory phenomena will also enable the reader to understand better the hearing problems of the patient with cochlear hearing loss.

RECRUITMENT. Recruitment is defined as an abnormally rapid increase in loudness. (Loudness is the subjective awareness of sound as contrasted to sound intensity. Thus, even if a sound is made 20 decibels more intense, it may be no louder if the patient still cannot hear it.)

A person with normal hearing (listening through earphones) interprets any two sounds having the same intensity as being equally loud. As long as the sound pressure remains the same in both ears, regardless of whether the intensity is increased or decreased, he continues to interpret the sounds as being equally loud. If one sound is initially less intense than the other, the normal listener hears it as less loud than the other. He continues to do so as long as both sounds are made equally louder or softer.

When cochlear disease is unilateral, as for example, in Meniere's disease, one ear may exhibit recruitment and the other ear may not. Sounds of equal intensity, presented at threshold levels, will be heard by the good ear but not by the recruiting ear because it is partially deafened and cannot hear faint sounds at all. The phenomenon of recruitment is apparent when the sound intensity is raised sufficiently for the recruiting ear to hear. A relatively small increase beyond the level at which the ear first hears brings the loudness up to equal loudness with the normal ear. In other words, there is an *abnormally rapid increase in loudness in the recruiting ear.*

Some patients show hyperrecruitment—the loudness in the recruiting ear becomes even greater than that in the normal ear, although the sound intensities are the same. Other patients exhibit incomplete recruitment.

A simple test for recruitment may be performed with only a tuning fork of fairly high pitch (1024 cycles per second). If only one ear inhibits recruitment, then when the fork is struck *lightly* and presented alternately to each ear, the patient will report that it sounds louder in the good ear than in the deaf ear. If the fork is then struck very *strongly* and is presented to the good ear, the patient will remark that it is very loud. When the fork is transferred imme-

diately to the deafened ear in which recruitment is present, the patient may wince or even jerk away. He will say that the fork now sounds equally loud in both ears (recruitment) or even louder in the recruiting ear (hyperrecruitment), whereas originally sound from the lightly struck fork was barely perceptible in the poor ear.

Another illustration of recruitment is provided by testing the patient with a two-channel audiometer. At 20 decibels the poor ear hears nothing (Fig. 20-8, *A*). In fact, the first sound that the patient hears in his poorer ear may be at 50 decibels. At 50 decibels the sound is heard very faintly in the recruiting ear but seems reasonably loud when transferred to the opposite, normal ear. Increasing the sound intensity only 20 decibels (to 70 decibels) makes the sound suddenly just as loud in the poor ear as in the normal ear at 70 decibels; *in the recruiting ear there is suddenly a loud sound where just previously there was none* (Fig. 20-8, *B*).

The phenomenon of recruitment is not definitely explained. According to one authority, it represents degeneration of a number of hair cells or cochlear fibers. Such degeneration makes it impossible for the patient to hear weak signals; however, when a strong stimulus is presented, the cochlear nuclei suddenly are completely saturated by way of the remaining healthy fibers. However, this explanation still fails to explain hyperrecruitment.

The phenomenon of recruitment accounts for the irritable remark of the person who seemingly cannot hear and yet says, when the speak-

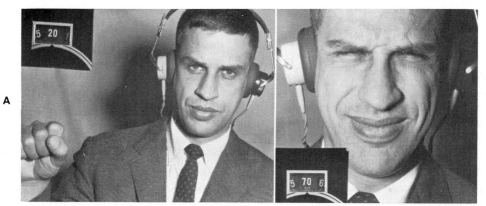

FIG. 20-8. Demonstrating recruitment. **A,** Patient fails to hear a low-level (20-decibel) sound. **B,** At 70 decibels (ordinarily not unpleasant), sound has suddenly become very intense in the recruiting ear and the patient winces.

er raises his voice sharply, "You don't have to shout at me, you know." At first he hears nothing or hears indistinctly, but when the sound level becomes great enough to cause recruitment, he hears the speaker's voice at its actual loudness or more loudly. Because the loudness increases rapidly, he finds it unpleasant.

Recruitment is one reason that patients with inner ear hearing loss are sometimes poor candidates for hearing aids. They have a very narrow range of tolerance between the intensity at which they are just able to hear and the intensity at which sound suddenly becomes painfully loud.

When recruitment is suspected, the patient should be asked if sudden loud noises are painful to his ears or if he notices that loud sounds are more unpleasant in his poor ear than in his good one. If he has recruitment (and particularly if he has hyperrecruitment), he will answer yes.

DIPLACUSIS. Diplacusis is a second phenomenon manifested by patients with cochlear disease. Like recruitment, it is produced by disease in the organ of Corti and not by disease involving the nerve fiber. Diplacusis has nothing to do with conductive or middle ear hearing loss.

Patients with diplacusis may dislike music because sounds are discordant or instruments seem out of tune. When the same sound is heard at a different pitch in each ear, the hearing becomes confused and ability to discriminate speech is decreased.

A simple test for diplacusis is performed by presenting the same tuning fork to each ear alternately and asking the patient if he hears the same pitch in each ear. Many patients confuse loudness with pitch; therefore this point must be made clear. It may be necessary to repeat the test with forks of various frequencies (512, 1024, and 2048 cycles per second) because diplacusis is not necessarily present in all frequencies.

LOSS OF AURAL DISCRIMINATION. A person is said to have good aural discrimination if he can properly distinguish between speech sounds that he hears. This permits him to interpret the sounds correctly as intelligible words.

Discrimination ability is a measure not of how keenly we hear but of how accurately or meaningfully we hear. In cochlear hearing loss, the patient's discrimination ability may be markedly reduced, but patients with conductive hearing loss have no difficulty in word discrimination.

Aural discrimination is tested with the speech audiometer, using P-B words, or with a simple discrimination test made by saying to the patient very clearly and at optimal loudness, "Repeat these words: *sin, thin, fin.*" The normal patient or the patient with conductive deafness will repeat the words correctly. Patients with sensorineural hearing loss often have great difficulty in distinguishing among the high-pitched consonant sounds: *s*, *th*, and *f*. They usually repeat one of the words three times because they hear only the sound "in" and then guess at one of the consonants. Of course, care must be taken to prevent the patient from reading the examiner's lips.

Specialized audiologic tests. Specialized audiologic tests are useful in helping to pinpoint the site of hearing loss—for example, middle ear, cochlea, cochlear nerve, or central. They also help to differentiate patients with functional hearing loss from those with organic loss.

BÉKÉSY AUDIOMETER TEST. The Békésy audiometer presents automatically either an interrupted or a continuous pure tone at continuously variable frequencies. By pressing and releasing a lever, the subject causes the testing signal to become more intense and less intense while the frequency varies continuously. In this way he conducts his own audiogram. A needle traces the audiogram on paper.

The critical factors are the difference between the thresholds for the interrupted and continuous tones and the number of responses per unit of time. These findings give information of value in differentiating between cochlear and eighth nerve sites of hearing loss. They also help distinguish middle ear from inner ear hearing loss.

Békésy tracings are reported as types I, II, III, IV, and V. This typing has some diagnostic value by itself but *must not* be used as a single criterion. The results should be correlated with other pure tone, speech, or special tests. The different Békésy types are usually interpreted as follows:

Type I. There is interweaving of the pulsed and continuous tones throughout the *entire* frequency range. This type is characteristic of normal hearing or conductive hearing loss.

Type II. There is interweaving of the two tones in the low tones through 1000 cycles with separation of the tones above 1000 cycles. The separation is about 20 decibels, with the continuous tone paralleling the pulsed tone in the higher frequencies. This pattern is characteristic of cochlear pathology.

Type III. The pulsed tone agrees with conventional pure tone audiometer results, but the continuous tone shows a rapid decline from the beginning frequency and drops quickly to the limits. This pattern correlates highly with retrocochlear (eighth nerve or central) pathology.

Type IV. There is a separation of the two tones below 500 cycles, and the separation continues throughout all the frequencies. This type correlates also well with retrocochlear pathology.

Type V. The pulsed tone drops below the continuous tone in certain frequencies. This is seen most often in functional hearing loss (psychogenic hearing loss or malingering).

SHORT INCREMENT SENSITIVITY INDEX TEST. The short increment sensitivity index (SISI) test presents a constant pure tone to the patient. Superimposed on this continuous tone are short pips of 1-decibel increments. Individuals with normal hearing have difficulty detecting these pips, whereas persons with cochlear involvement hear most of them. Thus the SISI test distinguishes sharply between patients with cochlear involvement and those with other kinds of loss.

THRESHOLD TONE DECAY TEST. In the threshold tone decay test the subject is presented with a sustained pure tone at his threshold level. He signals with a raised finger as long as he hears the tone. If the tone becomes inaudible (decays) before 1 minute, the intensity is increased. This procedure is continued until the tone is heard for 1 entire minute. Various frequencies are used in the test.

A person with normal hearing usually continues to hear the tone a full 60 seconds at levels 5 to 10 decibels above his threshold. Significant tone decay requiring an increase of 20 decibels, or even 50 to 60 decibels, before the tone is heard a full minute is seen in Meniere's disease and in cochlear nerve involvement. This phenomenon usually occurs in high tones only. Eighth nerve tumors often show marked tone decay in all frequencies.

Tests for nonorganic hearing loss. The following tests are used to differentiate between a functional (nonorganic) hearing loss and an organic one or varying degrees of each. A functional hearing loss is one that is either psychogenic, caused by malingering, or overlaid on an organic loss. Functional hearing losses are always sensorineural, not conductive, but often there is an overlay of functional loss on a pre-existing conductive loss.

DELAYED FEEDBACK TEST. In the delayed feedback test the person whose hearing is being tested is asked to read simple printed material. After his normal reading time is recorded, he is asked to read the same passage again, but this time a microphone is switched on and his voice is recorded on a tape. After a slight time lapse, usually ⅕ second, the recorder plays the person's voice back to him through earphones (in one or both ears).

In effect, the person finds himself reading one or two words ahead of what he must listen to. This delayed feedback is so confusing that some people cannot read at all, whereas others stumble over a phrase or in some audible way show that they are having trouble. Most important, the reading time is prolonged. This test is useful in demonstrating that a person does hear in one or both ears. If he could not hear, his reading would be unaffected.

SHADOW CURVE. A "shadow curve" is produced normally when a patient is presented with intense sound to a unilateral dead ear through earphones. Because the sound travels across his head to his normal ear, he should report hearing it. Some patients with nonorganic hearing loss say that they hear no sound at all, whereas, of course, they should report some hearing because of the "shadow curve" effect.

PSYCHOGALVANIC SKIN RESISTANCE AUDIOMETRY (Fig. 20-9). In the psychogalvanic skin resistance (PGSR) test the person being tested is conditioned reflexly much like Pavlov's dog. Two finger electrodes are placed. An audiometer makes a sound in the person's ear. One second later he receives a light electric shock on the finger. The shock produces sweating, and

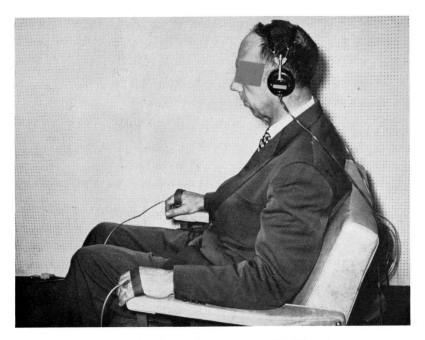

FIG. 20-9. Psychogalvanic skin resistance (PGSR) audiometry.

the moisture reduces skin resistance between two electrodes. After a series of tones and shocks, most patients are conditioned; 15% to 20% of patients cannot be satisfactorily conditioned. In a conditioned patient sound alone (without the shock) causes sweating and consequently a lowering of skin resistance. A change in the galvanometer reading every time a sound is presented to the patient is evidence that he hears.

This test is also useful in young children, who cannot be tested with conventional methods.

DOERFLER-STEWART TEST. The basis of the Doerfler-Stewart test is that the introduction of noise during testing confuses the patient. If he is malingering, for example, he cannot remember well his previous thresholds. Aslo, the *Lombard effect* may be noticed; as the noise in the patient's ear increases, his voice becomes louder if he talks or reads aloud.

LOMBARD TEST. The basis for the Lombard test is the normal monitoring of intensity of one's own voice that occurs during speaking. While the subject is reading aloud from printed material, a masking signal is delivered into one ear (if a unilateral loss is claimed) or both ears (if a bilateral loss is claimed). If he starts to read

louder, it is an indication that he hears the masking noise and therefore that there is a functional loss.

STENGER TEST. The basis for the Stenger test is that normally there is a psychophysiologic reaction that causes a shifting of the position of sound to the ear receiving the greater stimulus. If a tone of the same frequency is presented to both ears, but with the intensity greater in one ear than in the other, the tone is heard *only* in the ear receiving the more intense sound (assuming normal hearing or an equal organic loss in each ear).

The test is particularly useful in a person who claims a greater loss in one ear than in the other. A tone is presented to the poorer ear and then to the good ear. Both intensities should be above the previously determined threshold for the better ear. If the patient has a functional loss, he will claim one of two things: (1) that he doesn't hear the tone at all, and then he can be shown that the better ear had an above-threshold tone in it all the time (which he couldn't hear because of the louder tone in the "poorer" ear); or (2) that he hears the tone only in the good ear, and then the intensity is turned down in the good ear until there is no sound at all. The earphone is removed from the "poorer" ear to demonstrate that the sound he claimed to hear in the good ear came from the earphone on the "poorer" ear.

In practice, unmasking the patient in this way is not always recommended because of the psychologic disturbance that may result.

SWINGING VOICE TEST. In the swinging voice test the tester reads a story to the subject, who wears earphones. The tester switches dials constantly so that the story reaches first one ear, then the other, then both, and so on. The story is so composed that it makes sense to a person with a true organic loss and to a patient with functional loss—but the stories as related by the subjects come out differently. If the person relates any of the words of the story presented to his supposed bad ear (the one he claims a loss in), he does have useful hearing in that ear.

A typical test is shown below.

Impedance audiometry. Impedance audiometry makes use of an entirely different approach to testing hearing than does traditional audiometry. Normally, sound travels through the external auditory canal and impinges on the tympanic membrane and vibrates it, and in turn these vibrations are transmitted across the chain of auditory ossicles to the fluids of the inner ear. Some of the sound energy, however, on striking the drumhead is not transmitted but is reflected back into the auditory canal. It is this reflected energy that is measured by impedance audiometry. Measurement of impedance provides an indication of the flow of sound energy through the structures of the auditory periphery, particularly the middle ear. Changes in impedance reflect the presence and type of middle ear pathology.

Impedance audiometry measures the compliance (or its reciprocal, impedance) of the auditory system. The more compliant the system, the more sound energy it will absorb; the

stiffer the system, the more energy it turns back into the external canal.

One method using the impedance principle to provide evaluation of the status of the middle ear function is called tympanometry. Typically, tympanometry makes use of a specially constructed earpiece with three separate openings. One opening is connected to a sound source (oscillator, potentiometer, and loudspeaker). Through this opening a probe tone is delivered into the sealed external auditory canal. A second opening connects to a microphone and balance meter. It measures the sound pressure in the ear canal, including the sound generated by the sound source and the sound reflected at the eardrum. The device does not measure directly the sound transmitted across the middle ear. The third opening connects to an air pressure pump and manometer. Through this port one is able to alter air pressure within the external auditory canal and thus set up various conditions affecting sound transmission, which then can be compared with that of the normal ear.

Maximum sound energy is transmitted when the air pressure in the middle ear is approximately that of the surrounding air. If air pressure is increased in the canal until the tympanic membrane and ossicular chain are effectively immobilized or locked in place, no sound (or minimal sound) is absorbed through the middle ear. Similarly, a negative pressure may be produced in the external canal and the same locking effect produced. By plotting the ear's compliance on one axis and air pressure on the other, we obtain a tympanogram. Some ears with disease will show more compliance (less impedance) than normal, whereas in others the reverse is true. Consider the condition otosclerosis, in which the footplate of the stapes is firmly locked in place. The tympanogram should show greater impedance to sound transmission

Good ear	Bad ear	Both ears
Two little boys,	their baby sister,	and their mother and father
spent their vacation,	fishing and swimming,	at the ocean.
The boy's father,	whose name was Bill,	built the children
a large castle of sand,	and driftwood.	When the tide
came rushing in,	that evening at suppertime,	all of his hard work,
was washed out,	into the bay,	and destroyed by a huge wave.

than in a normal ear. Some have referred to this as a "stiff ear," and we can measure the amount of stiffness by tympanometry. A more flaccid system than normal would result if, for example, the incus had been dislocated.

Impedance audiometry is of particular value in young children because a voluntary response is not required. If normal tympanometric patterns are obtained, conductive hearing loss can be ruled out and the need for bone conduction audiometry is eliminated. At this stage of its development impedance measurement will not serve as well as conventional pure tone audiometry to give accurate measurements of hearing acuity.

Impedance audiometry also is used to measure the acoustic reflex. This reflex is normal and occurs when sound stimulation produces a contraction of the stapedius muscle. There is a change in compliance as the muscle contracts and pulls on the stapes. With the acoustic probe sealed in the nontest ear, a sound is delivered to the ear being tested. Bilateral contractions of the stapedius muscle should occur if the sound is loud enough—usually 70 to 80 decibels above threshold—and the resulting change in compliance is demonstrated on the tympanogram. There are several important conditions that may affect the stapedial reflex response and thus give an abnormal measurement. To consider one example, refer to the discussion of recruitment, a common finding in Meniere's disease, on p. 287. In patients with recruitment, sound stimulation of the impaired ear at no more than 40 decibels above threshold may result in a reflex response in the opposite (probe) ear instead of the expected 70- to 80-decibel level. On the other hand, in retrocochlear lesions such as acoustic neuroma, there may be no reflex at all or the "tone decay" phenomenon may be evident (see p. 290).

Using impedance audiometry for assessing the acoustic reflex could be informative in the case of a malingerer who claims severe deafness in one ear. If a tone presented in that ear causes a stapedial reflex in the other ear, he obviously is not totally deaf in the test ear.

Impedance audiometry does not replace pure tone or speech testing but may, in some instances, be a valuable adjunct to conventional testing.

Audiologic methods for infants and children.

Infants and young children cannot be tested by conventional methods and require special testing. In infants under 6 months of age the startle reflex, or its absence, can be a clue to whether the infant hears. Later in the first year, the infant will attempt to localize sound. As the child becomes older, the play element is used in testing. The psychogalvanic skin test can also be used.

Brain stem evoked response, a measure of electrical activity in the auditory pathway similar to electroencephalography, is a relatively new measure of auditory function. It is used together with the sensorineural test battery to localize lesions in the auditory pathway and to determine hearing levels in otherwise untestable patients (infants, mentally retarded patients, patients with functional hearing loss).

Brain stem evoked response is a completely objective test that requires only that the patient remain quiet during the examination. Sedation can be used. Electrodes are attached to the earlobes and forehead, and auditory stimuli are presented to either ear to evoke a response. A series of rapid click sounds (25 per second) provides the stimulus. A computer averages the resulting waveforms from samples of thousands of results and prints them.

The measurement of the latency from the stimulus to the appearance of waveforms and the appearance of characteristic waveform patterns are compared to norms. The appearance of recognizable waveforms for different frequencies establishes thresholds, and the latencies of waves one to five are then measured. The results may indicate the location of a lesion in the auditory pathway. Wave one represents activity in the cochlear nerve, wave two in the cochlear nucleus, wave three in neurons of the superior olivary complex, wave four in the lateral lemniscus, wave five in the inferior colliculus, and wave six in the medial geniculate body (Fig. 20-10).

Brain stem evoked response is used successfully in young children, including newborns. At the present time it is probably the most reliable test for the very young child. In addition, the test can be reliably used to detect suspected posterior fossa lesions affecting hearing, such as acoustic neuroma.

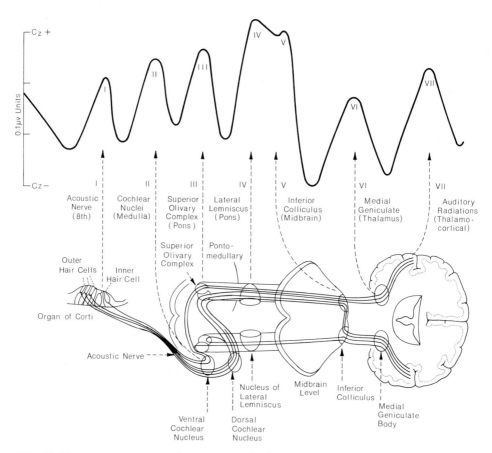

FIG. 20-10. Schematic tracing of brain stem evoked audiometry (BSEA), indicating the levels of the central nervous system responsible for the various wave patterns.

With these and other methods, it is possible to determine hearing levels in infants and young children.

The importance of determining, if possible, the presence of a significant hearing loss in an infant or a child under 2 years of age cannot be overemphasized. In order to learn speech, a child must hear. If enough residual hearing is present (if the child is hard of hearing), amplification of sound with a hearing aid is necessary early in life. Hearing aids have been successfully used by infants under 6 months of age. If the hearing loss is profound (if the child is deaf), it is necessary to begin sense training very early in life so that the child will be able to learn lip-reading (speech-reading) as well as the early simple vocal sounds. Most specialized schools for the hard-of-hearing or the deaf accept children for training before the age of 3 years to provide the extra training necessary to compensate for the loss of hearing. There is always educational delay, even with normal or superior intelligence.

The physician should never adopt the attitude, "Let's see him again in a year—he will probably outgrow it." When parents, or more frequently grandparents who have raised a child with normal hearing, are concerned enough to seek medical advice for a suspected hearing problem in an infant or a child under 2 years of age, every effort should be made to determine, if possible, whether the hearing is normal or defective. If there is any suspicion of significant hearing loss, special tests, which may need to be repeated, should always be performed.

SELECTED READINGS

Beery, Q.C., and others: Tympanometric pattern classification in relation to middle ear effusion, Ann. Otol. Rhinol. Laryngol. **84**:56, 1975.

Bess, F.H., and others: Use of acoustic impedance measurement in screening for middle ear disease in children, Ann. Otol. Rhinol. Laryngol. **87**:288, 1978.

Carhart, R., and Jerger, J.F.: Preferred method for clinical determination of puretone thresholds, J. Speech Hear. Disord. **24**:330, 1959.

Egan, J.J.: Békésy audiometry, Ear Nose Throat J. **59**:3, 1980.

Davis, H., and Hirsh, S.K.: Brain stem electric response audiometry (BSERA), Acta Otolaryngol. **83**:136, 1977.

Goodhill, V., Rehman, I., and Brochman, S.: Objective skin resistance audiometry, Ann. Otol. Rhinol. Laryngol. **63**:22, 1954.

Goodman, W.S., and others: Audiometry in newborn children by electroencephalography, Laryngoscope **74**:1316, 1964.

Guide for evaluation of hearing handicap, J.A.M.A. **241**:2055, 1979.

Hoople, G.D., and others: Clinical study of bone conduction audiometry, Ann. Otol. Rhinol. Laryngol. **63**:785, 1954.

House, J.W.: Brainstem audiometry in neurotologic diagnosis, Arch. Otolaryngol. **105**:305, 1979.

Jerger, J., and others: The acoustic reflex in eighth nerve disorders, Arch. Otolaryngol. **99**:409, 1974.

Johnson, E.W.: Auditory findings in 200 cases of acoustic neuromas, Arch. Otolaryngol. **88**:598, 1968.

Liden, G., Harford, E., and Hallin, O.: Automatic tympanometry in clinical practice, Audiology **13**:126, 1974.

McCandless, G.A., and Thomas, G.K.: Impedance audiometry as a screening procedure for middle ear disease, Trans. Am. Acad. Ophthalmol. Otolaryngol. **78**:98, 1974.

Mokotoff, B., Schulman-Galambos, C., and Galambos, R.: Brain stem evoked responses in children, Arch. Otolaryngol. **103**:38, 1977.

Olsen, W.O., Noffsinger, D., and Sabina, K.: Acoustic reflex and reflex decay, Arch. Otolaryngol. **101**:622, 1975.

Sanders, J.W., Josey, A.F., and Glasscock, M.E.: Audiologic evaluation in cochlear and eighth nerve disorders, Arch. Otolaryngol. **100**:283, 1974.

Stockard, J.: Detection and localization of occult lesions with brain stem audiometry responses, Mayo Clin. Proc. **52**:761, 1977.

21 THE LABYRINTH

PHYSIOLOGY

When the utricle or semicircular canals are stimulated, definite reactions are expected. The greater the stimulation, the more violent the reactions will be. The important reactions are nystagmus, past pointing, and falling. Vertigo, nausea, vomiting, and sweating accompany the severe reactions because the dorsal motor nucleus of the tenth nerve is located near the vestibular nuclei in the brain stem (Fig. 18-24).

Motion of the endolymph inside the membranous semicircular canals stimulates the hair cells of the cristae located in the ampullae of the semicircular canals (Fig. 21-1). Distortion of the hair cells sets up a chain of reflexes that produces contractions in the eye muscles, in the neck muscles, and in the muscles of the trunk and extremities. In normal persons these reactions restore the body position when any force throws it out of balance. The contractions of the muscles after artificial stimulation of the labyrinth throw the body out of balance. Unsteadiness, accompanied by a feeling of dizziness, is then produced.

If a patient complains of dizziness or vertigo, it is helpful to know whether the labyrinth is functioning normally. This information can be obtained by means of artificial stimulation of the semicircular canals. The reactions produced are then compared with the known normal reactions.

Nystagmus. Disturbances of the labyrinth and some disturbances of the central nervous system produce a type of nystagmus known as labyrinthine or central nystagmus. A slow movement of the eye in one direction is followed by a rapid compensatory movement in the opposite direction. In other words, the motion is *rhythmic.*

Another type of nystagmus is produced by ocular abnormalities and is called optic or optokinetic nystagmus. Such nystagmus differs from labyrinthine or central nystagmus in that both excursions of the eye are of equal amplitude. Also, the amplitude is greater and the motion tends to be wandering or pendulous rather than rhythmic.

The varieties of nystagmus are referred to by many terms. The following are the most commonly used:

Horizontal nystagmus—occurring in the horizontal plane

Rotary nystagmus—occurring in the frontal plane

Vertical nystagmus—occurring in the sagittal plane

Perverted nystagmus—any deviation from that expected

Variable nystagmus—a different direction in each eye

Positional nystagmus—seen in a change of head position

Spontaneous nystagmus—occuring spontaneously

Induced nystagmus—produced by artificial stimulation

First-degree nystagmus—noted only when the eyes look in the direction of the rapid component

Second-degree nystagmus—noted when the eyes look straight ahead

Third-degree nystagmus—noted when the eyes look in the direction of the slow component

Spontaneous nystagmus indicates a disease process except when it occurs during extreme lateral gaze. Vertical nystagmus usually indicates central nervous system disease. Some-

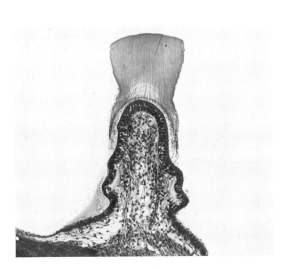

FIG. 21-1. High-power photomicrograph of the crista of a semicircular canal (guinea pig). This is the sensory end organ for kinetic equilibrium. (Courtesy Dr. Merle Lawrence, Ann Arbor, Mich.)

times it indicates *bilateral* ear disease. Perversion of the expected response from artificial stimulation indicates central nervous system disease.

Induced nystagmus (see Bárány test and Caloric tests, p. 300) is horizontal when the head is tipped 60 degrees backward and rotary when the head is tipped 30 degrees forward. First-degree and second-degree nystagmus are considered normal after artificial stimulation. Third-degree nystagmus is abnormal unless the stimulus is excessive.

Nystagmus can be observed more easily when +20-diopter lenses (Fresnel glasses) are placed over the eyes. They not only magnify the eyeball but also prevent the patient from fixing his eyes on an object. Fixation can overcome fine nystagmoid movements and lead the examiner to think that no nystagmus is present. Observation of the ocular fundus through an ophthalmoscope will sometimes demonstrate fine nystagmus that cannot otherwise be seen.

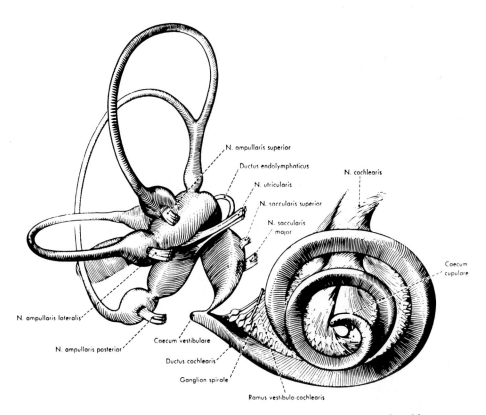

FIG. 21-2. Drawing of the labyrinth and cochlea showing the vestibular and cochlear nerves. (Courtesy Abbott Laboratories, Chicago, Ill.)

TESTS FOR POSITIONAL NYSTAGMUS. Nystagmus may be induced by changes in the position of the head. The tests are not difficult and are performed as follows:

The patient is seated on an examining table in the erect position and then is assisted in assuming the supine position. The eyes are observed for nystagmus. After 30 or 40 seconds the patient is helped in turning his head and body to the right while remaining in a horizontal position. After another interval of 30 to 40 seconds he is returned to the supine position, and after another, similar delay of 30 to 40 seconds he is turned to the left while supine. During each of these maneuvers the examiner should assist the patient and be certain that the head and body turn together as one unit. If the head is turned independently of body motion, reflexes from the neck muscles may be initiated, which may alter the reactions. After each assumption of a new position, the eyes are carefully observed for nystagmus. The patient is then returned to the supine position. After another delay, the head is dropped backward over the end of the table and again any evidence of nystagmus is noted. The patient is then returned to the supine position and, finally, helped to sit erect again. After each new position the eyes are carefully observed by having the patient look straight ahead and then to the right and left in extreme lateral gaze.

The normal person will exhibit no nystagmus during these maneuvers. If nystagmus is induced in any position, it is recorded, including the direction of the nystagmus and its duration. It is often helpful to wait 30 to 40 minutes and repeat the test or to have the patient return at another time to repeat it. Consistently reproducible results may add to other findings and aid in diagnosis of a specific disease or assist in localizing pathology.

Past pointing and falling. Stimulation of the labyrinth produces past pointing and falling as well as nystagmus. Past pointing and falling always occur in the direction of flow of the endolymphatic fluid.

In the test for past pointing, the patient sits facing the examiner. The patient then closes his eyes and keeps them closed during the test. He is asked to put his arms in front of him and point both index fingers toward the examiner. The examiner then places his two index fingers under the fingers of the patient (Fig. 21-3, *A*). The opposing fingers of the patient and examiner should touch to give the patient a point of reference. The patient is told to raise both arms and hands (Fig. 21-3, *B*) and then to lower them, attempting to return to the examiner's fingers. This task is easy for the normal person to accomplish. When the labyrinth has been stimulated or there is a lack of normal sense of position, the patient will be unable to bring his fingers back to the examiner's fingers. The patient's fingers will deviate to the right or left (Fig. 21-3, *C*).

The patient should be tested, with eyes closed, before the ear is stimulated with warm or cold water. This preliminary test indicates to the examiner whether the patient has *spontaneous* past pointing and reassures the patient that the test is not complicated.

After labyrinthine stimulation, falling reactions are demonstrated by having the patient stand with the eyes closed and the feet together. A tendency to fall toward the right or left ear is noted. We say toward the right or left ear rather than toward the right or left side, because if the patient turns his head to one side, he falls toward the stimulated ear, that is, to the front or back rather than to the side. This is the basis for the Romberg test.

• • •

There is an apparent discrepancy in the fact that all three labyrinthine reactions do not occur in the same direction. The reason is that the direction of nystagmus was originally named by the direction of the rapid component. In other words, a nystagmus in which the slow component is to the left and the rapid component is to the right is called nystagmus to the right. Actually, the *slow component of nystagmus is the labyrinthine component.* Therefore past pointing, falling, and the slow component of nystagmus do occur in the same direction and in the direction of the flow of the endolymph.

Labyrinthine reactions

Falling ———————————→

Past pointing ———————————→

Slow nystagmus ———————————→

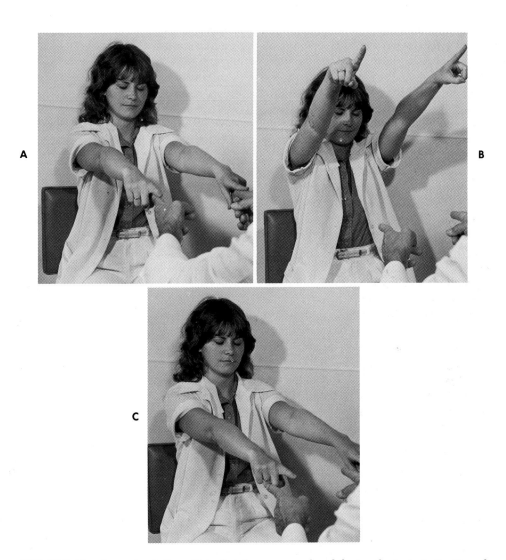

FIG. 21-3. Test for past pointing. Note that the eyes are closed during the test. **A,** Position of hands and arms immediately after caloric stimulation. **B,** Patient is raising arms vertically with elbows straight. **C,** Patient has lowered arms and is past pointing to the left.

TESTS FOR LABYRINTHINE REACTIONS

Bárány test. A chair designed to turn in a complete circle can be used to test labyrinthine reactions. The construction of the chair also allows the patient's head to be held in different positions. For the test the chair is turned at a specified rate of speed (usually 10 turns in 20 seconds) and stopped suddenly. Although the patient's body stops moving, his endolymph continues to move because of its momentum. The endolymph bends the sensory hairs in the ampullae of the semicircular canals, which produces falling, past pointing, nystagmus, and subjective vertigo.

The Bárány turning test was formerly widely used, but now it is employed only in special circumstances. Because the Bárány test stimulates both labyrinths simultaneously, it is less useful in most clinical situations than is caloric testing. More information can be obtained when each labyrinth is tested separately. The Bárány test is useful in working with laboratory animals.

Caloric tests. The semicircular canals can be stimulated by introducing either water or air (above or below body temperature) into the external auditory canal. Water below body temperature, when directed against the tympanic membrane, causes endolymphatic fluid to flow in a downward direction. Water above body temperature sets up convection currents in the opposite direction, causing the fluid in one or more canals to rise. Motion of the endolymphatic fluid distorts the hair cells and produces the labyrinthine reactions.

If the head is inclined 30 degrees forward, the lateral semicircular canal assumes a horizontal plane (Fig. 18-19) and the vertical canals are perpendicular. Cold or warm caloric stimulation then sets up convection currents in the vertical canals. When the head is tipped 60 degrees backward, the lateral semicircular canal is vertical and therefore can be stimulated by convection currents. Although all three canals are stimulated simultaneously to some extent, careful testing may indicate more damage to one part of the labyrinth than to another.

The results of the tests are interpreted as normal, hyperactive, hypoactive, or absent. When no reaction can be obtained from the semicircular canals, the labyrinth is said to be dead. Before and after stimulation the patient is examined for nystagmus, past pointing, and falling.

Cold caloric testing can be done by several methods. One is to douche the ear with cold water at 20° C. until nystagmus begins (Fig. 21-4). A 1-quart canister is filled with water. The head is tipped 30 degrees forward, and the water is allowed to run through a rubber tube into the ear canal. When nystagmus begins, the irrigation is stopped. This method of caloric testing causes maximal stimulation of the semicircular canals.

A second method is to direct ice water against the eardrum through an ear speculum (Fig. 21-5). The patient either is seated with the head tipped 30 degrees forward or is placed in a supine position with the head tipped 60 degrees backward. Twenty-diopter glasses are placed over the eyes to abolish accommodation. Ice water is directed against the eardrum from a Luer-Lok syringe through a 22-gauge needle for a specific number of seconds. After a short latent period labyrinthine reactions begin. The eyes are observed for nystagmus, testing for past pointing is performed, and falling reactions are noted.

If no reaction is stimulated by the original test, the duration of stimulation is increased, usually doubled. In the average normal individual 10 to 12 seconds of ice water stimulation will induce mild vertigo, definite nystagmus, and a tendency to lean or fall in one direction. When no reaction occurs with 10 to 12 seconds of stimulation, the test is repeated with 20 to 30 seconds of stimulation. If there is still no reaction, the stimulus is increased until reaction or no reaction occurs.

This test is known as the Kobrak caloric test and is convenient for office use. It affords minimal (that is, threshold) stimulation and can be made quantitative by varying the duration of the stimulation against the eardrum.

When properly used, the Kobrak caloric test can assist the physician by indicating whether the labyrinth is reacting normally and is hypoactive or hyperactive, or whether no labyrinthine response is present (that is, the labyrinth is "dead").

Regardless of which method is used, 10 to 15 minutes of rest is allowed between the tests on the two ears. If the second ear is tested too soon after the first ear and before the stimulation of

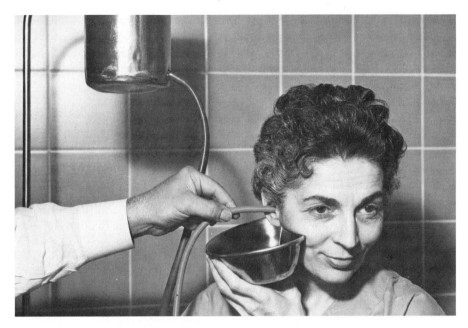

FIG. 21-4. Caloric testing by douche (maximal stimulation).

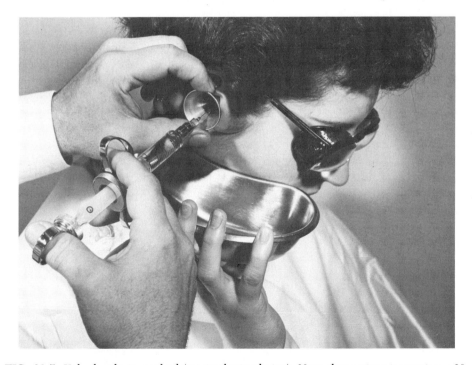

FIG. 21-5. Kobrak caloric method (minimal stimulation). Note that patient is wearing +20-diopter lenses and that the head is tipped 30 degrees forward.

the first ear has completely disappeared, a false reaction of hypoactivity may be found on the second ear. This is true because stimulation of opposite ears gives opposite directions to the labyrinthine reactions.

With either method the expected reactions are nystagmus in the opposite direction from the ear stimulated and past pointing and falling toward the ear stimulated. Warm caloric tests give reactions opposite those obtained by cold caloric tests.

Directional preponderance. Still another method of testing labyrinthine responses is that of alternate cold and warm caloric stimulation, which combines the information obtained from both. Each ear is douched for 40 seconds with water that is 7° C. above and below body temperature (30° and 44° C.). An appropriate rest period is allowed between tests. After each stimulation (warm or cold) the duration of the resulting nystagmus is measured in seconds. Abnormal function of the labyrinth or of its higher central nervous system connections is indicated when there is an increase in nystagmus in one direction and a decrease in the other direction. This is known as directional preponderance. The test must be performed under controlled conditions. With proper control it can occasionally provide information helpful in localizing unilateral lesions of the labyrinth, the eighth nerve, the vestibular nuclei, and the temporal lobe.

Galvanic tests. In galvanic tests electrodes are attached to the body, one being placed near the labyrinth. Galvanic current is then used to stimulate the semicircular canals, and the resultant reactions are observed. This method is, however, seldom used.

Electronystagmography. Electronystagmography (ENG) is a test that records the position and movement of the eyeball by recording the changes in the electrical field around the eye when there is a change in position of the eye. Since the cornea of the eye carries a positive electrical charge and the retina a negative charge, it is possible to place electrodes near the eye and to record eye motion through an amplifier and on a recorder. Thus a permanent record is made on prepared graph paper, allowing later study and actual mathematical calculations of amplitude, direction, and speed of nystagmus. Obviously, this can be used to record either spontaneous nystagmus or induced nystagmus. In the usual test a recording is made of the resting state of eye motion (there is always some motion), and the direction, speed, and ampli-

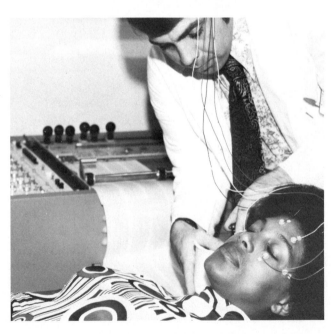

FIG. 21-6. Electronystagmography. Patient undergoing caloric stimulations as nystagmus is recorded on a graph.

tude of nystagmus are measured after stimulation of the labyrinth by both warm and cold water or warm and cold air. The temperature of the stimulating fluid is carefully controlled, adequate periods of rest between different stimulation times are allowed, and all eye motions are recorded. The test is performed in a dark room or with the eyes closed to eliminate, as far as possible, the accommodative and fixative functions of the eye, which may suppress eye movements caused by the stimulus (Fig. 21-6).

This test supplies a permanent record that can be compared with known abnormal patterns or used to compare changes in the reactions in a given individual at different times. Although valuable in carefully selected cases, the test is time consuming, requires a trained technician, and makes careful calibration of the instrument a necessity.

As in all functional tests of hearing or labyrinthine reaction, ENG must be used as an aid in diagnosis only and integrated with other available information, including the medical history and other physical findings. The test is rarely diagnostic by itself.

Drugs affecting vestibular testing. The following drugs exert an effect in nystagmus, and if a history that includes the use of these drugs is not taken, erroneous testing results will be obtained during vestibular tests and electronystagmographic tracings.

1. *Alcohol* causes positional alcohol nystagmus (PAN) when the patient is in the right-ear-down or left-ear-down position. During drunkenness the nystagmus beats toward the floor, and during "hangover" it beats toward the ceiling. It is stronger with the eyes closed than with the eyes open. The cause is unknown.

2. *CNS depressants* cause suppression of all types of vestibular nystagmus. This effect is believed to be caused by the sedative effects of these drugs. It is well known that drowsiness, whether drug induced or not, suppresses nystagmus.

3. *Barbiturates* cause vestibular nystagmus to be stronger with eyes open than with eyes closed. This effect, known as "failure of visual suppression of nystagmus," is important in the interpretation of the caloric test, where it would be otherwise regarded as a sign of a posterior fossa lesion. This effect is believed to be caused by selective blocking of multisynaptic vestibulo-oculomotor pathways through the reticular formation.

4. *Alcohol, barbiturates, phenytoin (Dilantin), or other CNS depressants* all can cause degeneration of smooth pursuit movements. Higher levels cause horizontal gaze nystagmus, and still higher levels can cause upbeating nystagmus during upward gaze.

Comment. Clinically it is important to remember to use the same technique on all patients. Comparison between different patients and also between the right and left ears of the same patient is then possible. Regardless of what technique is used, and assuming it is the same from patient to patient, *the mechanics are of secondary importance. Interpretation is of primary importance.* The ability to interpret results is acquired only by repeated personal experience with a given technique.

SELECTED READINGS

Barber, H.O.: Positional vertigo and nystagmus, Otolaryngol. Clin. North Am. **6**:169, 1973.

Barber, H.O.: Diagnostic techniques of vertigo, J. Vertigo **1**:1, 1974.

Barber, H.O., and Stockwell, C.W.: Manual of electronystagmography, ed. 2, St. Louis, 1980, The C.V. Mosby Co.

Benitez, J.T., Bouchard, K.R., and Choe, Y.K.: Air calorics: techniques and results, Ann. Otol. Rhinol. Laryngol. **87**:216, 1978.

Daroff, R.B., and Hoyt, W.F.: Supranuclear disorders of ocular control systems in man. In Bach-y-rita, P., Collins, C., and Hyde, J., editors: The control of eye movements, New York, 1971, Academic Press, Inc.

Gay, A.J., and others: Eye movement disorders, 1974, St. Louis, The C.V. Mosby Co.

Lim, D.J.: Vestibular sensory organs, Arch. Otolaryngol. **94**:69, 1971.

Naunton, R.F., editor: The vestibular system, New York, 1975, Academic Press, Inc.

(See also selected readings at the end of Chapter 29, pp. 408 to 409.)

22 DISEASES AND ABNORMALITIES OF THE EXTERNAL EAR

DISEASES AND ABNORMALITIES OF THE AURICLE

Congenital malformations. The auricle may be deformed because it is too small *(microtia)*, too large *(macrotia)*, or improperly shaped. Rarely, it is altogether absent. Absence of the auricle is often associated with atresia of the external auditory canal.

Atresia of the ear canal causes a conductive type of hearing loss; if only the auricle is missing, there is no appreciable hearing loss, because in humans the auricle contributes very little to hearing (Fig. 25-9).

"Lop" ear, or outstanding auricle, is fairly common and can be readily corrected by plastic surgery (Fig. 22-1, *A*). It is necessary to cut and re-form the conchal cartilage. Mere excision of the skin from behind the ear does not hold the auricle back permanently.

Sometimes an *accessory auricle* appears as a tag of skin, or skin and cartilage, in front of the tragus. Remnants of the first branchial apparatus may persist and produce a sinus tract or a dimple just anterior to and above the tragus (Fig. 22-1, *B*).

Neoplasms. Carcinoma of the auricle is not uncommon. The cancer may be either basal cell or squamous cell carcinoma (Figs. 22-2 and 22-3). When the lesion is advanced, the diagnosis is obvious, but small growths are often overlooked. Any ulcerated, crusted, or indurated lesion that fails to heal should be excised and ex-

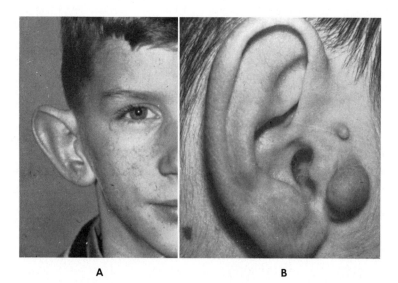

A   **B**

FIG. 22-1. **A,** Outstanding auricle, or lop ear. Note absence of an anthelix. **B,** Two accessory auricles in another patient. This pretragal position is common.

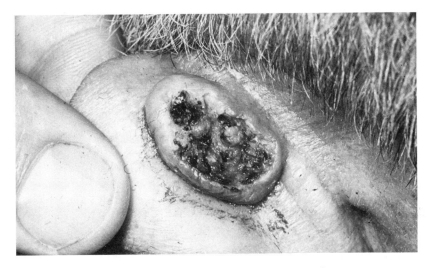

FIG. 22-2. Basal cell carcinoma on the posterior surface of the auricle. Treatment consisted of excision of the auricle. These lesions burrow under the skin (rodent ulcer).

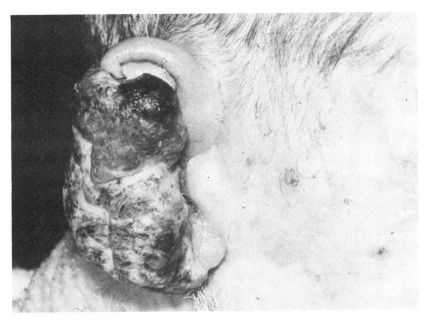

FIG. 22-3. Squamous cell carcinoma of the ear. Treatment included wide local excision and a skin graft.

amined. Approximately 80% to 85% occur on the external ear; 10% to 15% are seen in the external canal.

Treatment of carcinoma of the auricle (either basal cell or squamous cell) is usually successful if the lesion is *excised widely enough.* Such lesions tend to burrow subcutaneously beyond the visible limits of the tumor. Inadequate excision leaves cancer behind. *The first consideration in the treatment of malignant neoplasms is adequate removal.* The cosmetic result is secondary. Sometimes the entire auricle must be excised and bare bone of the skull exposed. A skin graft can be placed either at the time of excision or after granulation tissue has developed. Irradiation therapy is also effective but generally is used less often than surgery.

When carcinoma of the external ear invades the bony ear canal or the mastoid, the prognosis is much worse than when the cancer is limited to soft tissues. Such cases may require excision not only of the entire ear but also of the temporal bone to control the cancer.

Trauma. The ear may be cut or torn from the head during fights, in automobile accidents, or on the playing field. Because the blood supply is good, such wounds heal very well. The physi-cian should be careful not to discard tissue unnecessarily. Often auricular tissue that looks nonvital recovers, and even if torn completely from the head, an ear can be reattached successfully at times. The ear is kept cool in a physiologic solution, and anticoagulates may be given. Strict aseptic technique is important in handling and cleaning the tissues. The use of fine sutures and careful closure of skin, subcutaneous tissue, and perichondrium in layers gives the best result. Gauze or cotton should be placed behind the ear before ear dressings are applied, so that the ear is not crushed painfully against the skull. A pressure dressing may increase the chance of perichondritis.

Frostbite of the auricle is difficult to treat. Some authorities still advise gentle warming of the frostbitten ear with snow; others believe that the final result is determined at the time of the injury and that any type of treatment is of little use.

Cauliflower ear is the result of an injury (often repeated injuries) to the ear. There is bleeding between the cartilage and perichondrium (hematoma) (Fig. 22-4, *A*). When the blood organizes, scarring occurs, and the auricle is deformed (Fig. 22-4, *B*). If there is infection, the

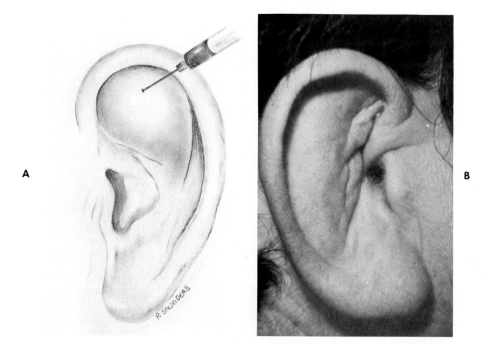

FIG. 22-4. A, Aspiration of a hematoma. **B,** Perichondritis deforming the auricle.

final result is worse. When a hematoma is seen soon after an injury, the blood should be aspirated with sterile technique and a pressure dressing that molds itself to the curves of the ear should be carefully applied. However, the hematoma often re-forms, and aspiration may have to be repeated several times.

One should differentiate between *perichondritis* and *chondritis* of the auricular cartilage. Perichondritis implies an early state of inflammation. In chondritis, there are infection and breakdown of the cartilage itself, so that in addition to antibiotic therapy, surgical intervention, including excision of the infected cartilage and thorough drainage, is usually required.

Perichondritis and chondritis must be treated early and aggressively for the optimal result. Parenteral antibiotics appropriate for the causative organism are indicated, sometimes for several weeks. Since *Pseudomonas* and *Staphylococcus* are the most common causative bacteria, antibiotics to which they are usually sensitive should be used when culture results are not yet known. Any collection of purulent material should be incised and drained. All necrotic cartilage must be removed. If any cartilage is questionable, it should be removed to obtain the best final result. Irrigation three or four times daily by way of a small polyethylene tube,

inserted beneath a *nonpressure* dressing, enhances the resolution of this serious infection. A saline solution containing polymyxin B, bacitracin, neomycin, or a combination of these is recommended. Previous sensitivity to neomycin should be taken into consideration.

Keloids. Keloids, massive overgrowths of reparative (scar) tissue, form predominantly in blacks but are also seen in whites (Fig. 22-5). About the ear they are most commonly attached to the lobule as the result of the ear's having been pierced for earrings, but they may occur after any type of trauma to the auricle (Fig. 22-6). The best treatment is excision followed by repeated injections of a long-acting steroid such as methylprednisolone acetate (Depo-Medrol) or triamcinolone acetonide (Kenalog) into the suture line area.

Painful nodule. Painful nodule of the helix (chondrodermatitis nodularis chronica helicis) is the name given to small indurated areas of chondritis along the superior rim of the auricle (Fig. 22-7). The condition is quite painful, and the cause is unknown. Treatment is injection of a long-lasting steroid or excision.

Sebaceous cysts. Sebaceous cysts often appear just behind the lobule of the ear or in the meatus of the canal (Fig. 22-8). The content of the cyst is sebum, a soft, cheeselike material. If

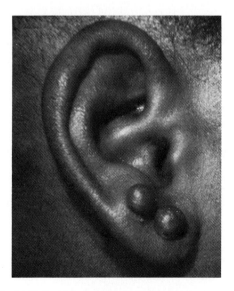

FIG. 22-5. Double keloid after two attempts to wear an earring requiring pierced lobules.

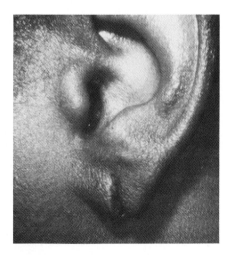

FIG. 22-6. Laceration of earlobe from torn-off earring.

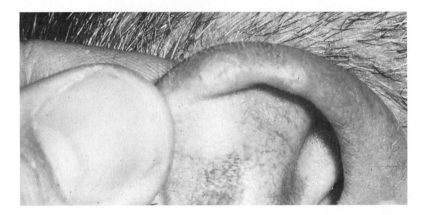

FIG. 22-7. Painful nodules of the auricle.

FIG. 22-8. Large sebaceous cyst in a characteristic location.

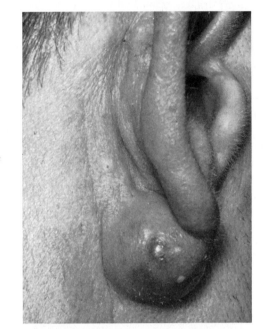

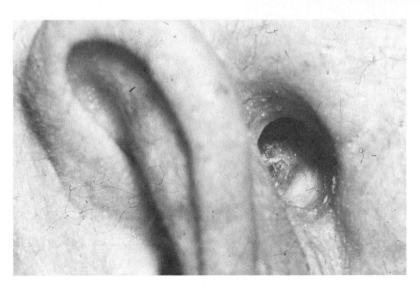

FIG. 22-9. Postauricular fistula leading into the mastoid antrum.

the cyst becomes infected, it enlarges rapidly and is painful. Treatment in the acute stage is incision and drainage and the use of hot compresses. If the cyst recurs, all of its lining should be excised.

Postauricular fistulas (Fig. 22-9). In the past, mastoidectomy was complicated occasionally by postauricular fistulas, but now, with improved techniques, they are rare. Except for their appearance, they are usually asymptomatic. Closure of such fistulas is readily possible.

DISEASES AND ABNORMALITIES OF THE EXTERNAL AUDITORY CANAL

Cerumen. Cerumen, or earwax, is formed by special glands in the cartilaginous ear canal. Its purposes are to lubricate the skin of the ear and to entrap foreign material entering the canal. Normally, cerumen, which is produced only in small amounts, dries in the ear canal and is forced out bit by bit during mastication and talking.

EXCESSIVE CERUMEN AND IMPACTED CERUMEN. Some patients have overactive glands that produce excessive accumulations of wax in the ear canal. Other patients have impacted cerumen because their ear canals are tortuous and small, or abnormally narrow at one point. Still other patients have an abnormal type of cerumen (often associated with dermatosis) that does not dry and flake out but remains very soft. Eventually it fills the ear canal.

If occlusion of the canal is complete, the ear feels blocked or full and the patient is hard of hearing. Tinnitus may be present, and occasionally there is dizziness. Ordinarily there is no pain. Not infrequently a patient who gets water in his ear while swimming or taking a shower finds that he has suddenly lost his hearing in one ear. This may be due to increased bulk of the earwax as a result of water absorption or to the water's becoming trapped beyond the wax.

Inspection reveals a ball of wax completely occluding the canal. Sometimes the patient has pushed the cerumen inward toward the drumhead. Often an ear appears to be completely occluded, and yet the patient has no symptoms. In such an instance there is a tiny slit where the meatus is clear, which suffices to transmit sound pressure and maintain normal hearing.

Treatment consists of removing the wax by irrigation or with a cerumen spoon. In irrigating the canal, one need not worry that the force of the stream will injure the eardrum, provided that space is left around the syringe to allow water to escape. Ordinarily, tap water is used, but *it must be at body temperature*, or vertigo will develop from vestibular stimulation. After irrigation the canal should be dried by inserting a small length of cotton with bayonet forceps (Fig. 1-9). Removing the wax with a cerumen spoon requires skill. The epithelium that lines the osseous ear canal is exquisitely sensitive and may bleed when touched. The eardrum itself is less likely to be injured. The cerumen spoon should be smooth edged and must be used under direct vision through an ear speculum. When possible, it is better to insert the spoon and pull the wax outward en masse rather than pick it out in pieces. Usually there is a narrow slit superiorly where the cerumen spoon can be inserted (Fig. 1-8).

Occasionally cerumen may be impacted and so dry that it cannot be removed painlessly. In such an instance the patient is instructed to instill a few drops of hydrogen peroxide or mineral oil several times daily for 2 or 3 days to soften the wax. Then it can be removed easily be irrigation. Another preparation that may be used is

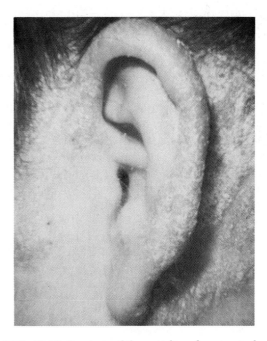

FIG. 22-10. Psoriasis of the auricle and postauricular skin.

Cerumenex, a proprietary drug that is said to produce occasionally an inflammatory reaction if used too often.

Occasionally, desquamated epithelium is attached to the surface of a large mass of cerumen and looks white, like dead skin. In elderly men, cerumen often is admixed with long hairs and the two form a matted obstruction.

INADEQUATE CERUMEN. Too little cerumen may be more annoying to the patient than too much, because the ear canal is dry. There may be scaling and itching. This condition is not readily cured, but it may be improved by the application of suitable ear ointments. Occasionally an inadequacy of cerumen or an abnormal type of cerumen seems to be associated with dermatologic disorders such as seborrheic dermatitis or psoriasis (Fig. 22-10).

Keratosis obturans. Keratosis obturans is an example of a cholesteatoma of the external auditory meatus. The cause is undetermined. This is a rather unusual condition in which the cholesteatomatous mass is found in the floor of the osseous portion of the ear canal. The symptoms are pain, usually mild, and sometimes aural discharge. Treatment consists of burring away the underlying bone, using a dental engine and drill, so that new epithelium can grow across the ear canal.

Exostoses and chondromas. Exostoses in the ear canal arise near the tympanic membrane, where they are attached to the osseous ear canal. They are small, broad-based, bony hard lumps covered with normal epithelium. Often they are multiple, and usually they are bilateral (Fig. 22-11). Some authorities believe that exostoses form because of periosteal irritation resulting from swimming in cold water. Others believe that they result from embryologic maldevelopment. Exostoses are usually not large enough to hide all of the eardrum from view. Usually they are asymptomatic. Rarely, they cause obstruction. Treatment is usually unnecessary. If removal is indicated because of size, the operation may be performed directly through the meatus or through an endaural incision such as that used for mastoidectomy. Exostoses usually arise from the posterior wall of the ear canal, where their bases are in close relationship to the facial nerve.

Chondromas arise at a location more external to the drumhead than do exostoses, since chon-

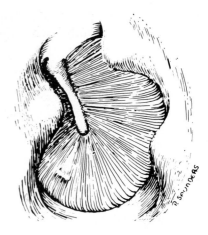

FIG. 22-11. Exostoses are often multiple and bilateral.

dromas spring from the cartilaginous ear canal. They are quite rare. Like the more common exostoses, they are asymptomatic unless very large.

Malignant tumors. Basal cell carcinomas, squamous cell carcinomas, and adenoid cystic carcinomas are found in the external auditory meatus. Basal cell carcinomas invade the meatus and the ear canal from the external ear. Squamous cell carcinomas may come from the skin of the auricle or from the parotid gland. They also may arise in the epithelium of the ear canal, middle ear, or mastoid.

The symptoms include drainage from the ear; deep, boring pain; hearing loss; and, in later stages, a peripheral type of facial paralysis. After pus is cleared from the ear canal, examination reveals a granular, readily bleeding tumor (Fig. 22-12). A biopsy establishes the diagnosis and differentiates the condition from an aural polyp (chronic otitis media). The diagnosis is usually not difficult when the lesion is extensive, but it may be overlooked if the tumor is visible only in the depth of the canal.

The prognosis of carcinoma of the ear canal is reasonably hopeful as long as the tumor is confined to the cartilaginous canal. Wide local incision and skin grafting may result in cure. However, if the osseous canal is invaded, treatment is compromised and the cure rate is greatly reduced. Radical mastoidectomy, followed by deep roentgenotherapy, is required to control cancer involving bone. In advanced cases, when clinical judgment indicates poor prognosis even with the combination of radical mastoidectomy

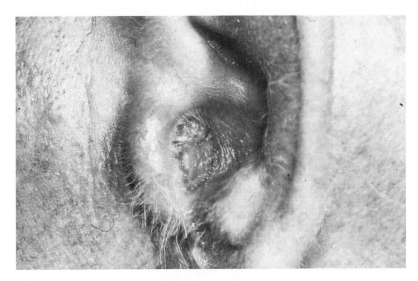

FIG. 22-12. Carcinoma of the external auditory meatus (and mastoid). This growth was bathed in pus and bled readily when touched.

and roentgen therapy, the entire temporal bone can be removed surgically. This operation, usually performed by the neurosurgeon and the otolaryngologist working as a team, is a last-resort, lifesaving procedure that carries a high operative mortality (30% to 50%) and, even when successfully accomplished, does not result in cure in all cases.

Adenoid cystic carcinoma (cylindroma) is a particularly vicious tumor; short-term survival rates are good, but long-term rates are very poor. Extremely wide surgical excision is needed for a good result.

Aural polyps. Aural polyps appear in the depth of the ear canal and are almost always covered with purulent discharge. They bleed easily. Larger polyps may appear at the external auditory meatus (Figs. 22-13 and 22-14).

The polyp may arise from within the external ear canal or from the middle ear. It may consist of granulation tissue, or it may be edematous mucosa of the middle ear. Polyps composed of granulation tissue may be partially covered by squamous epithelium, but they still look much redder and bleed more easily than do mucosal polyps. In either case polyp formation indicates chronicity.

The symptoms are a foul, purulent discharge (particularly from the polyp composed of granulation tissue) and partial deafness if the polyp

arises in the middle ear or obstructs the ear canal. Sometimes bleeding occurs.

The examiner must determine whether the polyp arises from epithelium of the ear canal or protrudes into the canal through a perforation of the tympanic membrane. The ear canal should be carefully cleansed by wiping, gentle suction, or irrigation. When the polyp can be seen more clearly, it may be moved gently with a probe to determine its relationship to the eardrum. Often a polyp fills a perforation so completely that the opening cannot be readily demonstrated.

The polyp is cut off near its base with small-cup forceps or a wire snare. This maneuver invariably causes annoying bleeding, which is best controlled by applying aqueous epinephrine, 1:1000, on a cotton pledget. It is best not to avulse a polyp, particularly if it comes from a perforation in the posterosuperior quadrant, because there is danger of disturbing the stapes or the facial nerve. After excision, the base of the polyp may be trimmed again, if necessary. Antibiotic ear drops are useful to reduce the associated infection.

Polyps arising from the external canal (external otitis) heal rapidly after treatment because there is no underlying bone disease. Polyps arising in the middle ear are often secondary to chronic mastoiditis or chronic otitis media,

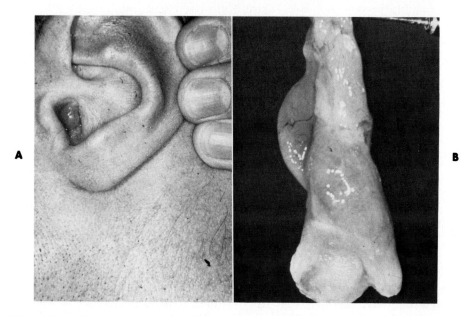

FIG. 22-13. A, An aural polyp attached to the promontory of the middle ear. There was a tympanic perforation through which the polyp hung. The polyp was bathed in foul pus. Chronic mastoiditis was also present. **B,** Same polyp as shown in **A.**

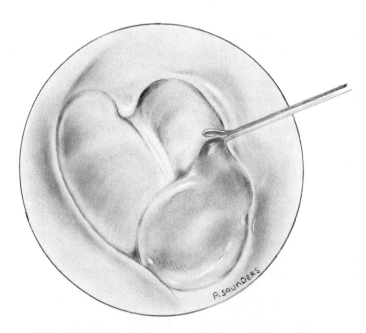

FIG. 22-14. Polyp being grasped with a middle ear forceps.

and their definitive treatment depends on successful management of the associated infection.

Foreign bodies. Obstruction of the ear canal is commonly caused by inanimate and vegetable foreign bodies placed in the ear by young children. Cotton is the most common foreign body in the ear canal in adults. Small stones, pieces of wood, peas, beans, paper, and the like are fairly commonly found in the ear canals of children. Sometimes there are no symptoms. The doctor often finds the foreign body during a routine examination. At other times there may be pain, or pus may drain from the ear. Occasionally an insect will fly or crawl into the ear canal and cause great distress by beating its wings and crawling about (Fig. 22-15).

Treatment usually consists of removal of the foreign body with delicate forceps or a cerumen spoon or by irrigation. When an insect is in the canal, an oily substance, such as mineral oil or olive oil, should first be dropped into the ear to immobilize and smother the insect. It can then be removed by gentle irrigation.

The external auditory canal is very sensitive to touch and, as previously mentioned, the skin over the bony canal is thin, bleeds easily, and forms subepithelial hematomas from minor trauma. Therefore the removal of a solid foreign body (a bead, BB shot, or piece of wood) carries

a definite risk of additional trauma to the ear if the patient is not completely cooperative or the removal is difficult. *Whenever the removal is painful enough to make the patient unable to remain quiet* (which is often true of children), *further attempts without anesthesia should not be made.* The patient should be hospitalized and the foreign body removed with the patient under light general anesthesia. If a difficult removal is attempted without anesthesia, the foreign body may be forced through the eardrum into the middle ear, resulting in subsequent hearing loss or chronic infection. Trauma to the canal of the ear, if significant, also causes stenosis of the external canal, which may require operative correction and grafting to again obtain a patent external auditory canal.

Hematoma. A hematoma of the epithelium lining the osseous part of the external ear canal is easy to produce inadvertently by wiping too hard with a cotton applicator or other instrument. This epithelium is so delicate that sometimes only the slightest trauma produces a hematoma. On the other hand, the epithelium lining the cartilaginous, or external, half of the ear canal is thick and not as sensitive.

Effects of mastoid disease. In acute mastoiditis, the posterosuperior part of the osseous ear canal may sag downward and look red. The sag-

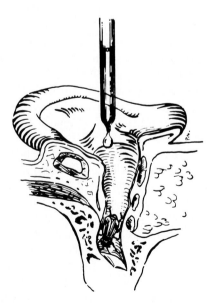

FIG. 22-15. An insect in the ear canal. The dropper contains oil.

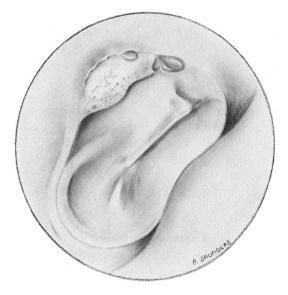

FIG. 22-16. Cholesteatoma in the epitympanum that has eroded the bone of the ear canal adjacent to the annulus. Chronic mastoiditis with a discharge of foul pus was present.

ging is due to periostitis. This sign is important in differential diagnosis of acute mastoiditis and other diseases causing aural pain and discharge.

In *chronic mastoiditis*, the superior part of the ear canal is occasionally eroded by a cholesteatoma (a mass of desquamated squamous epithelium) in the epitympanum and mastoid antrum so that there is a perforation into the ear canal adjacent to the eardrum (Fig. 22-16). If a cholesteatoma is present, it looks like white, cheesy material (Fig. 24-11) and usually is bathed in a foul discharge. If the cholesteatoma has dropped out or has been removed by treatment, only a dark hole remains and the ear may be dry.

Temporomandibular joint dysfunction. Temporomandibular joint infection is mentioned here to call attention to the fact that disorder of the temporomandibular joint, generally unilateral, is not uncommon and is a frequent cause of pain referred to the ear. The patient, who complains chiefly of earache, is surprised to learn that the cause of his pain is in the jaw joint, a point readily demonstrated to him by having him open his mouth widely and pressing an index finger in each joint. As he closes sharply, he winces. Radiation of temporomandibular joint pain to the temporal area and the entire side of the head is common. If dental occlusion is faulty, correction of the bite may be necessary. In most cases, however, simple measures are enough to give relief. Appliction of heat and analgesics, and sometimes the injection of 1% lidocaine (Xylocaine), into sensitive points adjacent to the joint, and especially into the masseter muscle, may help.

Referred otalgia. Referred otalgia is common as a cause of ear pain. When no obvious aural condition causes the patient's pain, the physician must search carefully in all areas of the head and neck for signs of an inflammation or neoplasm that could produce the pain.

EXTERNAL OTITIS

External otitis is a general term used for inflammatory diseases of the auricle and the external auditory canal.

External otitis may be caused by either infections or a dermatosis or both. Either bacteria or fungi may produce the infectious type. Fungi cause a larger proportion of infections in tropical climates, whereas bacteria cause most external

otitis in temperate zones. As might be expected, external otitis is much more common in the summer than in the winter.

External otitis may be associated with an infection of the face or scalp such as infectious eczematoid dermatitis; however, it more commonly occurs as a primary infection and is limited to the ear canal or the auricle, or both. The normal ear canal harbors *Staphylococcus albus* and diphtheroids but no pathogenic organism. The bacteria most commonly cultured from patients with external otitis are *Pseudomonas aeruginosa* (pyocyaneus), *Proteus vulgaris*, staphylococci, and streptococci. The pyocyaneus organism is especially common. "Swimmer's ear" is a special type of external otitis that occurs in patients who get contaminated water in the ear. These patients often have wax in the ear that absorbs water, macerates the skin of the canal, and affords a basis for infection.

Pathogenic yeast forms include *Aspergillus niger*, which produces a black growth, *Candida* organisms, *Penicillium* organisms, and others.

Acute external otitis. In the *mild stage* of acute external otitis, there is mild to moderate pain that is aggravated by movement of the auricle or tragus. There may be low-grade fever or discharge (often sticky and yellow) from the ear canal. If the ear canal is swollen shut or obstructed by debris, there may be partial loss of hearing and the feeling of a blocked ear.

In the *severe stage*, there is often intense pain. The entire side of the head aches and throbs. Some patient will not permit aural examination because of pain. There is usually a discharge from the ear. The hearing may be diminished, and the ear feels blocked. Examination reveals the external auditory canal to be swollen or entirely closed. Often the tragus and external meatus are also swollen. A sticky yellow or purulent discharge may ooze or pulsate from the ear canal. The temperature may be as high as 104° F. Movement of the tragus or traction on the auricle aggravates the pain because such movements are transmitted to the swollen ear canal (Fig. 22-17). Some patients refuse to permit such manipulation. The increase in pain caused by movement of the external ear is an important consideration in differential diagnosis between acute external otitis and otitis media (since both of these conditions may produce ear pain and aural discharge).

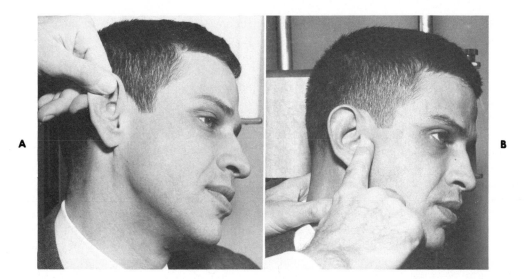

FIG. 22-17. A, Traction on the auricle is painful in acute external otitis. **B,** Pressure on the tragus is also painful.

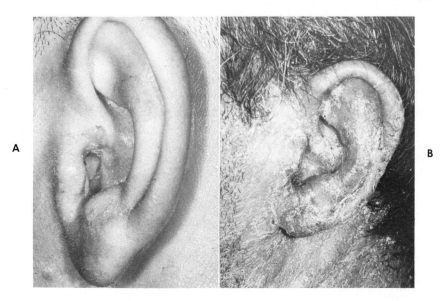

FIG. 22-18. A, Acute external otitis. Note swelling of the ear canal and lymphadenopathy in front of the tragus. **B,** Chronic scaling in external otitis associated with seborrheic dermatitis.

If an ear speculum can be inserted, the canal is seen to be swollen and the epithelium soggy and pale. Often there is desquamated epithelium and wax in the canal. Sometimes, however, the canal may be red instead of pale, or the epithelium may be dry instead of wet. Lymphadenopathy is common; tender nodes may be felt anterior to the tragus, behind the ear, or in the upper neck. Sometimes postauricular adenopathy or cellulitis is so great as to

push the auricle forward. In such an instance the condition must be differentiated from the subperiosteal abscess of acute mastoiditis.

When the auricle is infected, the skin oozes and crusts (Fig. 22-18, *B*). Pustules may be present, and the ear is swollen and tender. The infection may spread to the face or into the scalp, or it may have originated there. Usually infections of the ear canal cause much greater pain than do infections of the auricle alone because the epithelium of the ear canal cannot stretch much without producing pain.

In acute external otitis, the eardrum often cannot be seen well because of the swelling of the ear canal. When it is possible to see the eardrum, its color may be normal or it may be red like the ear canal.

Chronic external otitis. In chronic external otitis, itching, rather than pain, is the chief complaint. Excoriation of the ear canal frequently occurs as a result of scratching. The manipulations used in cleaning the ears, which patients usually find a little unpleasant or even painful under normal conditions, are welcomed by most patients with chronic external otitis. Aural discharge is present in some patients with chronic external otitis, but not in all. Hearing is unaffected unless debris accumulates and fills the ear canal. If an acute infection develops in the patient with chronic external otitis or if the epithelium is broken as a result of scratching, pain may become a major symptom.

The epithelium of the ear canal or auricle, or both, is thickened and red (Fig. 22-18, A). Both the ear canal and the surface of the drumhead are remarkably insensitive to the usual cleaning with cotton applicators. Aural discharge is frequently present. When it is, the odor may be moderately foul but not as foul or penetrating as in patients with certain types of middle ear disease. In contrast to acute external otitis, in the chronic form there is usually no pain when the auricle or tragus is manipulated.

Differential diagnosis. Principally, external otitis must be differentiated from otitis media. The list of symptoms may be very nearly the same. In *severe stages*, both groups of patients have pain and fever and sometimes aural discharge. The data in Table 5 should serve as a guide in differentiating between the two conditions.

Treatment of acute and chronic forms. In the *mild stage* of acute external otitis, the patient does not require narcotics—aspirin or similar analgesics suffice. Heat relieves discomfort and may be provided by a heat lamp, hot wet compresses, or a heating pad. A medicated wick of cotton or narrow gauze may be inserted gently into the ear canal when the canal is occluded as a result of swollen epithelium. Such a wick may be wet with any of a number of medications. A very effective one is Burow's solution (5% aluminum acetate). Either the 5% solution or a solution reduced in strength with an equal amount of water may be used. Antibiotic ear drops, with or without hydrocortisone, are widely available and are very useful (although more expensive). Drops containing polymyxin B (Aerosporin), neomycin, and bacitracin are effective against the usual bacteria that infect the ear. Also, these drugs do not sensitize the patient to the more common antibiotics, which might be used orally later. Neomycin may, if used over a period of time, sensitize the skin, causing atopic (allergic) dermatitis when used again.

In the *severe stage* of acute external otitis, when the patient's ear canal is swollen and fever and pain are present, additional treatment with a systemic antibiotic such as erythromycin or penicillin is advisable. These medications should be used in full dosage for several days. *Cultures are important as a guide to treatment.* When pain is severe, aspirin alone is not sufficient; codeine, 32 mg. or more every 2 or 3 hours, is required.

TABLE 5. Differential diagnosis of acute external otitis and acute otitis media

	Acute external otitis	Acute otitis media
Season	Summer	Winter
Movement of tragus painful	Yes	No
Ear canal	Swollen	Normal
Eardrum	Normal (or red)	Perforated or bulging
Discharge	Yes	Yes—but through a perforation
Nodes	Frequent	Less frequent
Fever	Yes	Yes
Hearing	Normal or decreased	Always decreased

Local treatment begins with careful cleansing of the ear canal. In general, only bland, soothing liquid preparations, with or without antibiotics and hydrocortisone, should be used for the patient with acute external otitis. Ointments often make the acute form worse; they are better reserved for patients with chronic external otitis. When the auricle is infected, the use of cotton or gauze compresses soaked with Burow's solution U.S.P., half strength, or with a saturated boric acid solution is good local treatment. In addition, systemic antibiotic medication may be required.

Rarely, a fulminant bone-destroying infection (so-called malignant external otitis) caused by the *Pseudomonas* organism is seen. When it does occur, the patient is almost always diabetic. In diabetics, as in other patients with severe *Pseudomonas* infection, hospitalization and parenteral treatment with potent antibiotics such as gentamicin or carbenicillin are required.

Often, *chronic* external otitis is due to a dermatosis such as seborrhea or psoriasis. More frequently a bacterial or fungal infection produces the condition. Occasionally an allergic reaction may cause or complicate chronic external otitis (Fig. 22-19). Allergic reactions from preparations such as nail polish, hair dye, hair spray, and permanent wave lotions are common enough to deserve special mention. Dermatitis from these substances may be baffling until

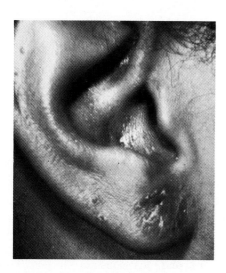

FIG. 22-19. Atopic dermatitis resulting from sensitivity to the metal in an earring.

one thinks to inquire about their use. The condition clears rapidly when the offending agent is discontinued.

Careful cleansing of the ear canal is absolutely essential as the first step in treatment. It is usually done by repeatedly wiping the canal with cotton applicators. Special care should be given to the inferior tympanic sulcus just external to the annulus because debris that collects here may delay healing (Figs. 22-20 and 22-21). When the chronic form of external otitis is due to infection, antibiotic ointments containing neomycin, bacitracin, and polymyxin (with or without hydrocortisone) may be used locally, two or three times daily, for a week or longer. Often, cortisone preparations seem to help chronic external otitis for a time and then their effectiveness diminishes or is lost. Other ointments that do not contain antibiotics are also effective, particularly when the external otitis is due to a dermatosis rather than to an infection. A good prescription is given below:

℞	Phenol	0.9 gm.
	Salicylic acid	0.9 gm.
	Precipitated sulfur	0.9 gm.
	Petrolatum q.s. ad.	30.0 gm.

Sig. Apply to ear canals once or twice daily.

This ointment, a mild exfoliating agent and antipruritic, may be used for an indefinite period or until the condition clears. Sometimes, however, it is impossible to cure chronic external otitis. The condition improves or is apparently cured but later recurs. Patients should be taught how to apply ear ointments. *Commercially prepared applicators are too thick.* The physician should demonstrate how to wind cotton on a toothpick so that a small tuft is left on one end (Fig. 1-6).

The most important single treatment in chronic external otitis is meticulous removal of all debris from the ear canal and the surface of the tympanic membrane. In all forms of external otitis, exclusion of water from the ear canal is all important.

Fungal infections. Fungal infections of the ear canal, common in the tropics, also occur occasionally in temperate climates. Fungal infections of the external ear canal are usualy easy to diagnose even without culture technique, since mycelia and hyphae of the fungi growth can be readily seen with the operating microscope un-

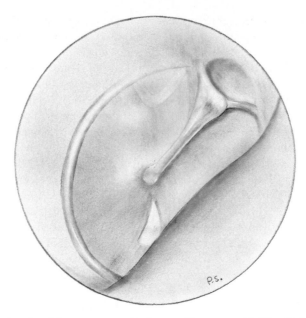

FIG. 22-20. Landmarks of the tympanic membrane. (Compare with Fig. 18-3.) The prominent ear canal partly hides the drumhead anteriorly.

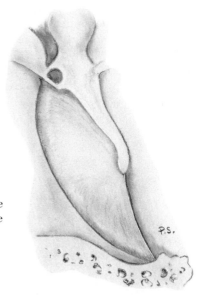

FIG. 22-21. Manubrium and short process of the malleus embedded in the tympanic membrane. Note the inferior sulcus just external to the eardrum.

der 6× or 10× magnification. The most common fungi affecting the ear are *A. niger, C. albicans* (monilia), and yeastlike fungi. *A. niger* forms a black or grayish blotting paper–like mass in the ear canal, and when this is removed, the underlying epithelium appears hyperemic and edematous and is often denuded of epithelium. Not all fungal infections of the ear canal produce symptoms, since many times the growth is saprophytic and simply is a formation found on wax and other debris in the ear and is not invading the tissue. If there is a lack of response to what would ordinarily be adequate treatment, one must consider the possibility of diabetes.

Very careful cleansing of the ear canal and

the application of an exfoliating ointment, such as that described for chronic external otitis, or 2% salicyclic acid in alcohol is usually effective. Ointments and creams containing nystatin, such as Mycolog (with neomycin, gramicidin, and a corticosteroid) and Mycostatin ointment or cream, are available as treatment for *Candida* organisms; nystatin, however, is not effective against other organisms. Amphotericin B (Fungizone) is effective and is available as a cream, lotion, or ointment. For infection with *Aspergillus* not responding to nystatin, a 1% solution of thymol in ethyl alcohol can be effective. It is usually applied on a cotton wick, which is left in place in the ear canal for several hours and then replaced. Gentian violet (2%) in 95% alcohol has been used successfully. It does stain the tissues, which makes evaluation of the progress toward cure difficult. One of the most effective treatments is the use of 25% M-cresyl acetate (Cresylate) drops in the ear three times daily, after careful preliminary cleaning of the external auditory canal.

Irradiation therapy for external otitis is contraindicated because the effects of repeated exposures are undesirable.

Furunculosis. Furunculosis is a type of localized external otitis in the outer half of the ear canal, where there are glands and hair follicles that may become infected. Aural discharge from chronic otitis media predisposes the patient to furunculosis. Unless there is an associated otitis media, the eardrum is normal. Even a small furuncle causes *severe pain* until it breaks spontaneously or is incised. The symptoms and findings are similar to those of an acute external otitis except that the furuncle is more localized. Osteomas of the ear canal are sometimes mistaken for furuncles, but osteomas are not tender or red. Also, they occur in the osseous, rather than in the cartilaginous, ear canal.

If the furuncle is ready to be opened, the apex is incised. General anesthesia may be required. In earlier stages, an ear wick wet with half-strength Burow's solution may be inserted to relieve pain. Local heat also affords relief. Codeine may be required. Antibiotics are given systemically, especially if there is fever or cellulitis of adjacent tissues.

Surgical treatment is rarely indicated but can be very effective in selected cases. When the patient has had external otitis for years and the ear canal is virtually closed by swollen, tough epithelium, and after various medical treatments have been given a fair trial and have failed, excision of the epithelium and the application of a thin split-thickness graft skin are indicated. Often the surgeon enlarges the cartilaginous and bony meatus at the same time. He may or may not remove the outer squamous layer of the tympanic membrane, depending on whether it, too, is severely affected.

Relapsing polychondritis. Although all cartilage is vulnerable, cartilage of the ear is most commonly involved in this inflammatory connective tissue disease. Destruction of the nasal septal cartilage and peripheral arthropathy are also frequently seen. Fever, the most common clinical sign, is too nonspecific to aid in diagnosis. Abnormalities of the special sense organs, including episcleritis and inner ear dysfunction, are almost always present. Laboratory findings are varied and nonspecific but often include anemia, elevated erythrocyte sedimentation rate, albuminuria, and abnormal serum protein electrophoresis. Microscopic findings are not pathognomonic, but a biopsy of affected cartilage should be performed. Inflammatory changes, loss of basophilic staining of cartilage, chrondrolysis, and invasion by fibrous connective tissue suggest this disorder.

The cause of relapsing polychondritis remains obscure. An autoimmune mechanism triggering enzymatic breakdown of the chondroitin matrix may be responsible. An acute attack is usually controlled by 30 to 60 mg. prednisone or its equivalent, daily in divided doses. This dosage may be reduced, but a suppressive dosage of 5 to 10 mg. prednisone should be continued. Flare-ups may occur even then, and more aggressive medical therapy must be reinstituted. Rest, sedation, and general supportive measures should be maintained if necessary, particularly for patients whose course is complicated by generalized arthropathy. Elective surgical procedures should be performed only during remission and, even then, only with corticosteroid coverage.

Granular external otitis. In granular external otitis, the external auditory canal contains granulation tissue, usually with a sessile base in the inner aspect of the canal. The symptoms are drainage and sometimes pain. During treatment the granulations are gently removed with small-cup forceps; the ear canal then may be packed with Gelfoam and the Gelfoam soaked with an antibiotic-hydrocortisone solution. In the case of a severe and unrelenting granular external otitis, one must consider the possibility of so-called malignant external otitis, particularly if the patient is diabetic (see p. 317).

Herpes zoster. A viral infection of the geniculate ganglion may produce vesicles that break after a short time and then leave a crust either in the posterior aspect of the ear canal or on the posterior aspect of the drumhead. If the auriculotemporal branch of the trigeminal nerve is affected, there will also be lesions on the auricle. There probably is no effective treatment for this painful condition.

SELECTED READINGS

Becker, W., and others: Atlas of otorhinolaryngology and bronchoesophagology, Philadelphia, 1969, W.B. Saunders Co.

Chandler, J.R.: Malignant external otitis: further considerations, Ann. Otol. Rhinol. Laryngol. 86:417, 1977.

Chen, K., and Dehner, L.: Primary tumors of the external and middle ear, Arch. Otolaryngol. 104:247, 1978.

Clairmont, A.A., and Conley, J.J.: Uses and limitations of auricular composite grafts, J. Otolaryngol. 7:249, 1978.

Clemons, J.E., and Connelly, M.J.: Reattachment of a totally amputated auricle, Arch. Otolaryngol. 97:269, 1973.

Conley, J., and Schuller, D.: Malignancies of the ear, Laryngoscope 86:1147, 1976.

Davenport, G., and Bernard, F.D.: Experience with mattress suture technic in correction of prominent ears, Plast. Reconstr. Surg. 36:91, 1965.

Gross, C.W.: Soft tissue injuries of the lips, nose, ears, and preauricular area, Otolaryngol. Clin. North Am., June 1969.

Guralnick, W., Kaban, L.B., and Merrill, R.G.: Temporomandibular joint afflictions, N.Engl. J. Med. 299:123, 1978.

Herzon, F.S.: The prophylactic use of antibiotics in head and neck surgery, Otolaryngol. Clin. North Am. 9:781, 1976.

Holmes, E.M.: Otoplasty, Arch. Otolaryngol. 83:156, 1966.

Lawrence, R.A., Schechter, G.L., and Carson, D.L.: Reconstruction of the burned ear, Otolaryngol. Clin. North Am. 5:667, 1972.

Martin, R., Yonkers, A.J., and Yarington, C.T.: Perichondritis of the ear, Laryngoscope 86:664, 1976.

McCaffrey, T.V., McDonald, T.J., and McCaffrey, L.A.: Head and neck manifestations of relapsing polychondritis: review of 29 cases, Otolaryngology 86:473, 1978.

Mohs, F.: Chemosurgery: microscopically controlled surgery for skin cancer, Springfield, Ill., 1978, Charles C Thomas, Publisher, Ch. 1, 2, 5.

Mustarde, J.O.: The correction of prominent ears using simple mattress sutures, Br. J. Plast. Surg. 16:170, 1963.

Senturia, B.H.: Diseases of the external ear, Springfield, Ill., 1957, Charles C Thomas, Publisher.

Senturia, B.H.: External otitis, acute diffuse; evaluation of therapy, Ann. Otol. Rhinol. Laryngol. 82:1, 1973.

Smathers, G.R.: Chemical treatment of external otitis, South. Med. J. 70:543, 1977.

Stroud, M.H.: Treatment of suppurative perichondritis, Laryngoscope 88:176, 1978.

Tanzer, R.C.: Microtia: long-term follow-up of 44 reconstructed auricles, Plast. Reconstr. Surg. 61:161, 1978.

23 THE TYMPANIC MEMBRANE

Layers. The tympanic membrane (drumhead) is made up of two layers of epithelium—the outer layer is squamous and the inner layer is cuboidal—and a middle layer of fibrous tissue. The fibrous layer is incomplete at the small portion of the eardrum that is enclosed between the anterior and posterior malleolar ligaments or folds. The part of the drumhead with a fibrous layer is known as the *pars tensa;* the tiny remaining portion (Shrapnell's membrane) is called the *pars flaccida* (Fig. 18-3). The latter is attached loosely to the squamous portion of the temporal bone, and this region of attachment is known as the tympanic *incisura Rivini* or the incisura tympanica.

Normal position. The tympanic membrane is slightly cone shaped, like the diaphragm of a loudspeaker. It is also slightly inclined, so that the upper part is more external, or closer to the examiner's eye, than the lower part. Both the concavity of the drumhead and its position relative to the ear canal normally vary somewhat and may be greatly altered in disease.

Annulus. The fibers of the tympanic membrane condense peripherally into a fibrocartilaginous ring called the annulus, which fits into the tympanic sulcus. The annulus is not a complete ring: there is a break in it superiorly between the anterior and posterior malleolar ligaments, and this deficiency of the ring is known as the notch of Rivinus (incisura tympanica). The portion of the tympanic membrane closing this area is the pars flaccida, so called because it lacks a fibrous layer.

Normal variations in color. The color of the normal tympanic membrane is usually described as pearl gray. However, there is a slight variation in color in many apparently normal membranes. Particularly, there is a difference in the vascularization seen along the annulus and around the manubrium and malleolar folds. Also, as a result of minimal tympanosclerosis (see p. 327), there may be a fine, white mottling, making the drumhead look more dense or thicker than normal.

Landmarks. The primary landmark in otologic examination is the *malleus*. The *long process* and the *short process* of the malleus are embedded in the tympanic membrane (Figs. 23-1 to 23-3). The short process stands out like a tiny knob at the upper end of the manubrium (long process or handle). The *anterior* and *posterior malleolar folds* are directed upward and outward from the short process. The *umbo* is at the lower end of the malleus, and from here the *light reflex* is directed anteriorly and inferiorly. The head and neck of the malleus are in the epitympanum (or attic) and cannot be seen during otologic examination (Fig. 18-6).

In some normal ears the *long process of the incus* may be seen behind the malleus in the posterosuperior quadrant of the drumhead. The incus is at a deeper level than the malleus and is not attached to the tympanic membrane. Therefore the incus is seen only when the tympanic membrane is not thickened or is more translucent than usual. The *chorda tympani nerve* arches high across the back side of the drumhead and is visible in the posterosuperior quadrant in an occasional normal ear (Fig. 23-3).

Significance in diagnosis. The tympanic membrane may be regarded as a translucent window through which the middle ear can be viewed. With the exception of fixation of the stapedial footplate in the oval window (otosclerosis) and rare disarticulations of the middle ear ossicles, *virtually all diseases of the middle ear reflect their presence by alterations in the position, color, or integrity of the tympanic membrane.* Inflammatory change within the layers of the

FIG. 23-1. Right tympanic membrane. Note that the curved line passing behind the handle of the malleus is the usual position of the chorda tympani. The dotted right angle in the posterosuperior area is the normal position of the incudostapedial joint. Sometimes these two structures can be faintly seen through an intact tympanic membrane. (See also Figs. 1-14 and 18-3.)

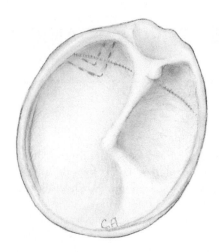

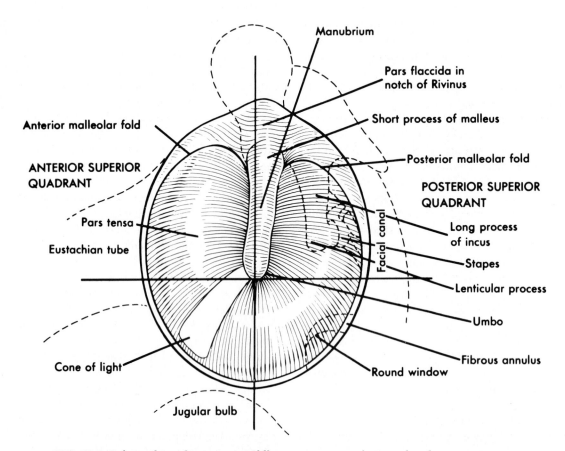

FIG. 23-2. Relationships of important middle ear structures to be considered in myringotomy. Often the incudostapedial joint can be seen dimly through the intact tympanic membrane. (From Saunders, W.H., and Paparella, M.M.: Atlas of ear surgery, ed. 2, St. Louis, 1971, The C.V. Mosby Co.)

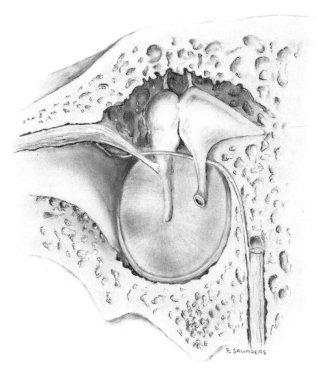

FIG. 23-3. Tympanic membrane and ossicles seen from the middle ear side. The chorda tympani nerve leaves the facial nerve and crosses just behind the drumhead (between the malleus and the incus).

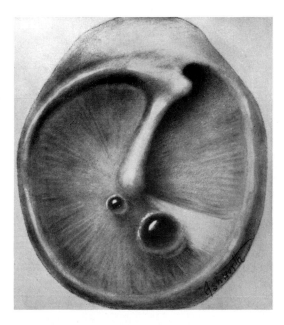

FIG. 23-4. Myringitis bullosa. These small vesicles are seen in viral infection at times and may also be present in herpes zoster oticus.

tympanic membrane may cause vesicles to form (Fig. 23-4). Even in otosclerosis there is sometimes a faint pink blush on the promontory that shines through the membrane (Schwartze's sign). In serous otitis media, for example, the drumhead is almost always retracted and is often amber. Sometimes an air-fluid level can be seen (Fig. 23-5), or there may be bubbles of air scattered about in amber liquid (Fig. 23-6). In purulent otitis media, pus under pressure pushes the drumhead outward (bulging drumhead) (Fig. 23-7). The usual landmarks either become faint or cannot be seen at all. Middle ear adhesions cause an irregular retraction, or the drumhead may be plastered to the promontory. A cholesteatoma in the mastoid or epitympanum is usually associated with a tympanic perforation and a foul discharge. Rarely, a cholesteatoma is seen through an intact drumhead. In that case the tympanic membrane looks white and full but has a more localized bulging than it would were the bulging caused by otitis media. Also, palpation of the drumhead elicits a

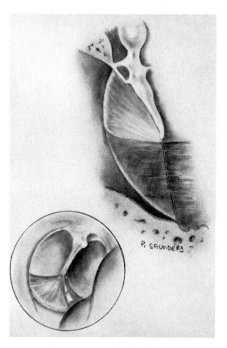

FIG. 23-5. Air-fluid level behind the tympanic membrane. *Inset,* Typical appearance of a retracted drumhead and meniscus.

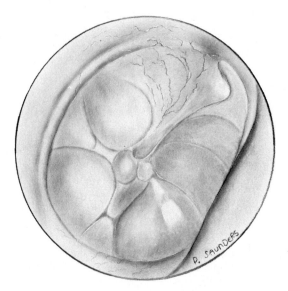

FIG. 23-6. Bubbles of air in serous otitis media. The bubbles move about when the examiner tilts the patient's head or exerts pressure against the drumhead with a pneumatic otoscope.

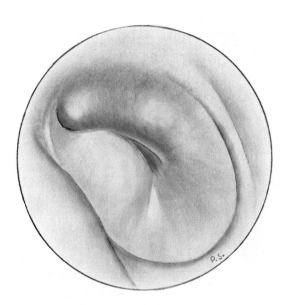

FIG. 23-7. Bulging tympanic membrane.

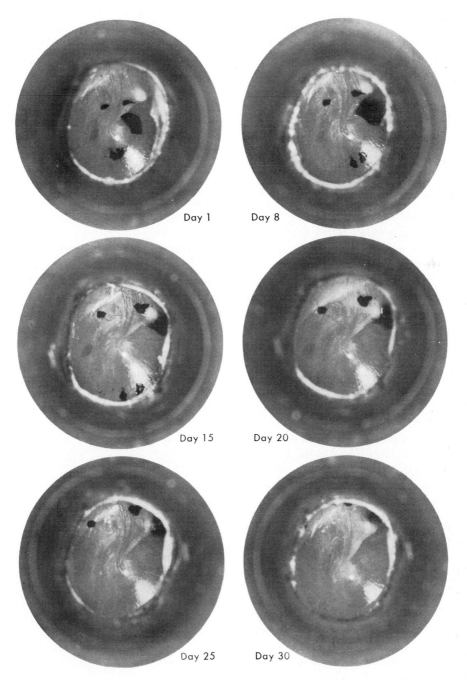

Day 1   Day 8

Day 15   Day 20

Day 25   Day 30

FIG. 23-8. Photographs taken at intervals over a month to show migration of various colored ink dots over the tympanic membrane. The dots continued to migrate over the canal after passing over the annulus. (Courtesy Dr. W.B. Litton, Iowa City, Iowa.)

sensation of probing a doughy mass, as if a solid rather than a liquid were filling the middle ear.

Proper diagnosis of middle ear and mastoid disease depends on a good look at the tympanic membrane. To that end, every effort should be made to clean the ear canal and the surface of the drumhead.

Epithelial migration. It is known that there is a peculiar movement of epithelial cells across the surface of the tympanic membrane. This movement is called epithelial migration and can be demonstrated by placing a tiny dot of ink or other marking substance on the eardrum. After several weeks the dot has moved. It continues to do so until it is no longer on the tympanic membrane but is actually in the ear canal (Fig. 23-8). In this way the squamous debris that otherwise would accumulate at the deeper end of the auditory canal is cleaned out, and the canal is kept open. Epithelial migration also accounts for the eventual extrusion of the small plastic tubes that are placed through the tympanic membrane in patients with serous otitis media. These tubes are slowly moved toward the periphery of the drumhead and extruded.

Anesthesia. Because the outer layer of squamous epithelium is derived from skin and is not mucous membrane, customary methods of obtaining topical anesthesia for mucous membrane surfaces are useless. Solutions of cocaine or tetracaine (Pontocaine), which afford excellent anesthesia for mucous membranes or denuded skin, are completely ineffective when applied to the intact eardrum. The application of a saturated solution of liquid phenol, however, will produce anesthesia immediately. A tiny, tightly wound metal applicator is touched to this liquid, and the end of the applicator is applied to a small area of the tympanic membrane. The membrane instantly turns a dead white, and there is absolute anesthesia at this site, so that a myringotomy may be made painlessly. Another preparation, Bonain's solution, provides anesthesia because it contains phenol. Bonain's solution is made by mixing together three crystals that shortly become liquid: 2 gm. phenol, 2 gm. cocaine alkaloid, and 2 gm. menthol.

Anesthesia of the ear canal and tympanic membrane may also be produced by injecting a small quantity of local anesthetic such as lidocaine (Xylocaine) or procaine hydrochloride (Novocain) into the skin of the cartilaginous external canal at several points. A fine-gauge needle with a short bevel is necessary.

Myringotomy. Incision of the tympanic membrane is called myringotomy. Draining fluid from the middle ear, whether by incision or by needle aspiration, is called *paracentesis*. The only instruments needed for myringotomy are a very sharp knife and an aural speculum. When a very sharp blade is used, the normal drumhead (such as is found in patients with serous otitis media) may be opened with only little pain. Also, incision of the bulging drumhead (forced outward by pus and gas in the middle ear) produces relatively little pain when a sharp blade is used. On the other hand, incision of the acutely inflamed drumhead causes severe pain.

Myringotomy is best performed posteriorly and inferiorly (Fig. 23-9), where the drumhead can readily be seen and where there are no ossicles to be injured. The membrane should not be incised above a line connecting the 9 and 3 o'clock positions. If the incision is too deep, the mucous covering the promontory may be cut. Although pain and bleeding ensue, the mistake is not serious.

Before the advent of the sulfonamides and antibiotics it was common practice to open the

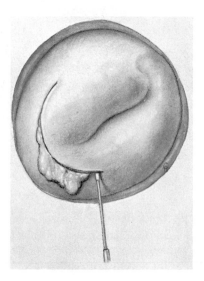

FIG. 23-9. Technique of myringotomy, right ear.

drumhead as wide as possible (often sweeping through a wide arc from back to front) because fibrin and inflammatory products would quickly seal a smaller incision. Today, in most patients with suppurative otitis media, such a generous incision may be unnecessary because the antibiotics that are usually given concomitantly greatly reduce the amount and duration of purulent drainage. Nevertheless, in patients with purulent otitis an incision larger than a mere nick or needle puncture should be made. A smaller opening is sufficient when serum or mucous is aspirated from the middle ear in patients with serous otitis media.

Needle paracentesis, performed with a short-bevel 20-gauge needle and a 2-ml. syringe, is another effective way of removing serous fluid.

COMMON MISTAKES. As mentioned previously, one mistake is to cut the mucous membrane covering the promontory. Another mistake, easiest to make in the infant, is to incise the ear canal instead of the drumhead.

MYRINGOTOMY AND HEARING. A common *misconception* is that myringotomy results in hearing loss. The following common circumstance may give rise to such a misconception: A child has otitis media, and the middle ear fills with pus, which causes the drumhead to bulge. A myringotomy is not immediately performed,

and the pus in the middle ear has an opportunity to cause ossicular destruction or to form fibrous adhesions. Finally a myringotomy is performed. When the purulent process subsides, any partial deafness that has resulted is erroneously ascribed to the myringotomy, *whereas it actually resulted from not performing the myringotomy promptly.* Even when repeated myringotomies are necessary, the tympanic membrane will usually heal perfectly and the hearing will remain normal.

Tympanosclerosis. Tympanosclerosis is a disorder of the middle ear and tympanic membrane that results as the aftermath of inflammatory disease. Long after a purulent otitis media has cleared and the tympanic perforation through which pus drained has healed, deposits of a hyaline material may be seen in the tympanic membrane, where they appear dead white or ashen gray and vary from a few distinct flecks to large, irregular, dense plaques (Fig. 23-10). Unless they are large and therefore affect the mobility of the drumhead, they have no appreciable effect on hearing. In the middle ear, however, the same deposits may seriously affect hearing, since they are prone to form around the footplate of the stapes, locking it in place. In the epitympanum, tympanosclerosis may form about the heads of the incus and malleus, fixing them. In either case the mobility of the ossicular chain is impaired and hearing is reduced accordingly. When one is considering the tympanoplasty operation to repair a defect in the drumhead and sees a heavy, white deposit of tissue in the remaining parts of the drumhead, one should suspect that the ossicles may be affected similarly.

Healed perforations. A perforated eardrum usually heals. Generally, healing takes place by regrowth of the inner and outer epithelial layers. Often the fibrous layer fails to proliferate. Then the healed area is thinner, more transparent, and also more flaccid than the rest of the eardrum. The healed portion moves in and out more readily than usual when alternating positive and negative pressures are produced in the ear canal with a pneumatic otoscope. In effect, the patient acquires a secondary flaccid membrane (Fig. 23-11).

When a perforation does not heal spontaneously, it may well be because the squamous

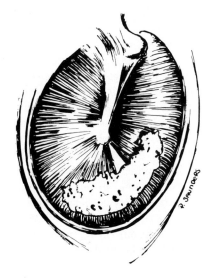

FIG. 23-10. Tympanosclerosis in the fibrous layer of the tympanic membrane.

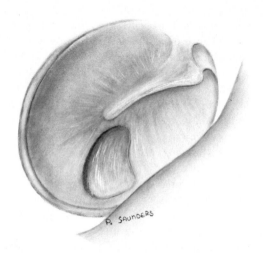

FIG. 23-11. Healed perforation. The healed area is often thinner, more flaccid, and more transparent than the rest of the eardrum.

epithelium has grown around the margins of the perforation, preventing primary closure. Cholesteatoma (Figs. 22-16 and 24-11) begins in this way, particularly when the perforation is marginal rather than central. Epithelium growing around the edges of the perforation continues to grow into the middle ear and mastoid (and especially into the epitympanum), where it desquamates and forms a cholesteatoma.

External otitis and the tympanic membrane. Localized infections in the ear canal such as furuncles do not affect the drumhead, but a generalized external otitis, either acute or chronic, may change the appearance of it. The outer layer of the eardrum is a continuation of the squamous epithelium lining the external auditory canal. Therefore it is subject to the same diseases. In patients with chronic external otitis the eardrum may look dull red or even thickened and leathery. Also, it is less sensitive than normal. Patients with *chronic* external otitis actually enjoy having the ear canal and drumhead cleaned, whereas normal patients or patients with acute external otitis find this procedure unpleasant or painful.

Granulation tissue on the tympanic membrane. Granulation tissue present in the general region of the eardrum usually is an indication that the drumhead has been perforated and that granulation tissue arising in the middle ear has protruded through the remaining membrane. Sometimes granulations are actually due to an inflammation of the squamous epithelium of the drumhead itself. Careful examination often discloses a pinhole perforation. Treatment of granulation tissue on the drumhead, if it is not associated with a middle ear infection, is most successful. The granulations are removed with small forceps, the base is cauterized with a silver nitrate bead, and antibiotic ear drops are instilled. Hydrocortisone, combined with an antibiotic such as neomycin, is also effective. To help maintain the eardrops in the canal, a piece of Gelfoam may be placed in the canal against the tympanic membrane. The Gelfoam (or a cotton wick) soaks up the drops and prevents their loss.

Trauma to the tympanic membrane. Trauma to the tympanic membrane may result from many causes.

PICKING THE EAR. The tympanic membrane is not as delicate as is usually thought. The warning "never clean the ear with anything smaller than the elbow" may be good advice, but actually the eardrum is less likely to be injured than is the very delicate epithelium covering the osseous ear canal. The fibrous layer between the two epithelial layers makes the eardrum a substantial structure. Many patients who pick their ears to remove wax or to relieve itching cause bleeding or pain. However, examination almost invariably reveals that the injury was to the ear canal near the drumhead rather than to the drumhead itself.

CONCUSSION. An explosion or a hard slap on the ear may easily tear the tympanic membrane, often resulting in severe pain and partial deafness. Tinnitus or vertigo may also be present. The middle ear may become infected. Occasionally there is dislocation of the ossicles. Treatment of the ruptured tympanic membrane consists of keeping a sterile cotton ball in the meatus and changing cotton as necessary. No irrigation, insufflation, or manipulative treatment is advisable. Some authorities recommend prophylactic treatment with antibiotics. Most traumatic perforations heal spontaneously in several days or weeks. If the eardrum does not heal, a myringoplasty may be performed.

BAROTRAUMA. Barotrauma, which may be caused by a too-rapid descent during air travel, for example, is a common cause of injury to the tympanic membrane. Ordinarily the eardrum is not perforated, but sometimes there is ecchymosis of the tympanic membrane. Bleeding into the tympanic cavity, another rather common result of barotrauma, produces a blue drumhead.

SKULL FRACTURE. Fractures through the base of the skull may tear the tympanic membrane. If the fracture line passes through the tympanic sulcus, there may be a steplike effect to the annulus when healing occurs.

HOT SLAG. Welders sometimes have a red-hot piece of slag fly into the ear. There is pain, and almost invariably an infection ensues that is difficult to clear. The patient is left with a perforation of the tympanic membrane caused when the hot metal burned its way through the drumhead. Frequently tympanoplasty, or even mastoidectomy and tympanoplasty, may be required to clear the infection and repair the defect in the tympanic membrane.

24 DISEASES OF THE MIDDLE EAR AND MASTOID

The most important diseases of the middle ear and mastoid are inflammations of various kinds and hearing losses. Tumors of the middle ear are rare. They are discussed in this chapter as well as in the chapters on the facial nerve (Chapter 30) and hearing losses (Chapter 25).

ACUTE INFLAMMATIONS OF THE MIDDLE EAR

Inflammation and infections of the middle ear are caused by extension of infection from the nose and nasopharynx. In rare instances traumatic perforation of the drumhead causes infection of the middle ear. In the presence of a long-standing perforation of the tympanic membrane, infection sometimes enters the middle ear through the external auditory canal.

Eustachian tube blockage. When the pharyngeal end of the eustachian tube is swollen and edematous, air cannot enter the tube. If the tube is blocked for any length of time, part of the air in the middle ear is absorbed into the capillaries. The eardrum becomes retracted as the negative pressure increases. A similar condition, often called aerotitis, occurs in flying, when in some persons the eustachian tube fails to open during the descent of an airplane (barotrauma).

Symptoms of eustachian tube blockage are mild, intermittent pain, mild hearing loss, and a feeling of fullness in the ear. Examination of the ear reveals a retracted eardrum. Its color is normal. Treatment is directed toward the nose and nasopharynx until all infection is cleared. As swelling of the tube subsides, air can again enter the middle ear and the condition clears up. If the blockage persists, inflation of the eustachian tube may help. The tube should not be inflated

while the nasopharynx is infected because suppurative otitis media might develop.

Acute catarrhal otitis media. Inflammation throughout the length of the eustachian tube and into the middle ear may occur without a actual bacterial invasion of the middle ear.

Symptoms are intermittent or continuous pain in the ear (which is usually mild), a feeling of fullness in the ear, and slight hearing loss. There may also be a subjective feeling of bubbling or crackling in the ear.

Examination shows that the eardrum has a dull appearance and that the capillaries around the periphery or along the handle of the malleus are dilated. Sometimes the entire eardrum is mildly inflamed. The drumhead does not bulge. Tests for hearing are grossly normal. Treatment is the same as that for a blocked eustachian tube. Aspirin or occasionally codeine may be needed for pain. Antibiotics are unnecessary.

Acute suppurative otitis media. When virulent bacteria invade the middle ear, an acute suppuration occurs. Fluid and white blood cells enter the middle ear, and pus is formed. Otitis media is one of the most common infections of childhood. It may accompany any upper respiratory tract infection. Frequently it is a complication of the common cold, measles, scarlet fever, or influenza.

Severe, deep throbbing pain in the ear is the cardinal symptom. It is accompanied by an elevation in temperature as high as 104° to 105° F. in infants or children and 101° to 102° F. in adults. *There is definite hearing loss.* Slight dizziness, nausea, or vomiting may occur. The pain increases steadily for several hours or several days. If the pressure in the middle ear becomes great enough, the eardrum ruptures. A mixture of blood and pus is then discharged from the ear, and the pain is relieved.

Examination shows pus in the canal if the eardrum has ruptured. After the ear has been cleaned, a pulsating discharge may be seen coming through the perforation. The eardrum is thick, red, and dull. If rupture has not occurred, the eardrum appears fiery red and dull. It bulges, and its normal landmarks are not visible. Hearing is reduced for both the whispered and the spoken voice. There is usually pain during pressure over the mastoid antrum.

Antibiotics should be given in full dosage. Penicillin is the drug of choice for empirical selection, except when the patient is sensitive to this drug; in any case, antibiotic sensitivity studies are important. When sensitivity to penicillin is known to exist, sulfonamides, erythromycin, tetracyclines, or broad-spectrum antibiotics may be used. Clean cotton should be kept in the outer ear to prevent the purulent discharge from infecting the lobule or skin of the face and neck. After rupture or myringotomy, medication for pain is rarely necessary.

Antibiotics should be continued in full dosage until the *ear is dry, the eardrum looks normal, and the hearing is normal.*

Myringotomy (incision of the drumhead) is indicated when there is bulging of the drumhead. Myringotomy is usually performed to drain pus from the ear in patients with acute suppurative otitis media or to release serum from the middle ear in patients with serous otitis. The instruments required are an ear speculum and a myringotomy knife (which has a small blade and a long handle; the blade may be sharpened on one or both edges). A good source of light is necessary. The head mirror provides the best lighting (Fig. 24-1). (See also Fig. 1-2.)

Myringotomy may be performed under general anesthesia, local anesthesia, or no anesthesia at all. A thin, normal eardrum may be opened without anesthesia and almost with no pain, *but a sharp knife must be used.* A slightly inflamed eardrum is usually more painful and requires local anesthesia. The most satisfactory method of obtaining partial or complete local anesthesia is to place a small piece of cotton moistened with Bonain's solution against the

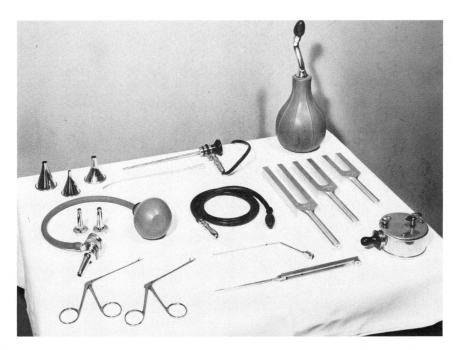

FIG. 24-1. Instruments necessary for complete examination of the ear. *Top row,* Ear speculums, eustachian catheter, nasopharyngoscope, Politzer bag. *Middle row,* Pneumatic otoscope, auscultation tube, tuning forks. *Bottom row,* Middle ear forceps, small suction tip, myringotomy knife, noisemaker for masking.

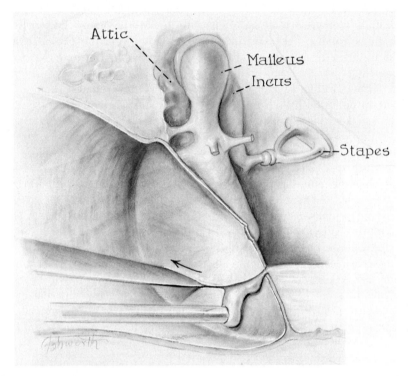

FIG. 24-2. Type of myringotomy used for acute suppurative otitis media. (See also Fig. 23-9.)

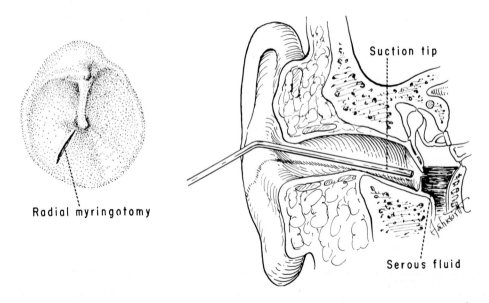

FIG. 24-3. Radial myringotomy and suction of fluid from the middle ear in serous otitis media.

eardrum and leave it in place approximately 5 minutes. Equivalent anesthesia can be attained by touching the eardrum for a few seconds with a tiny applicator moistened with a saturated solution of phenol. *Bonain's solution* consists of equal parts of cocaine alkoloid, phenol, and menthol. Because of the phenol in this solution, it should not be left against the eardrum for a long time and *should not be used if the canal or eardrum is wet.*

Iontophoresis, using lidocaine and epinephrine, has been used to produce anesthesia of the eardrum. It is effective in producing anesthesia of the intact, noninflamed tympanic membrane, such as is seen in serous otitis media. It is not as effective in an inflamed, thickened, and bulging tympanic membrane.

General anesthesia is used in almost every adult patient with acute suppurative otitis media and in older children who require myringotomy. The acutely inflamed eardrum is thick, and pain is severe when the eardrum is touched. General anesthesia need last only a few minutes. Usually no anesthetic is given when the eardrum of an infant is incised.

There are two types of myringotomy—circumferential and radial. Circumferential myringotomy (Fig. 24-2) allows wide drainage and is used to remove fluid or pus under pressure. The incision is begun by placing the knife against the eardrum in its posterosuperior portion, below the malleolar folds. It should be made carefully to avoid injury to the medial wall of the middle ear. It is carried down and forward, with the knife blade kept 2 to 3 mm. away from the drum margin. It ends in the anteroinferior quadrant of the eardrum. A cotton pledget, placed in the canal, will absorb the blood and fluid that are released. Radial myringotomy (Fig. 24-3) is sufficient to release serum from the middle ear. The incision extends from near the umbo to a point 1 to 2 mm. from the drum margin. The same precautions regarding depth of the incision in circumferential myringotomy also apply to radial myringotomy.

Acute serous otitis media (otitis media with effusion). The cause of serous otitis media is not always known. It may accompany or follow viral diseases or episodes of allergy, it may occur spontaneously without signs of other disease, or it may occur following an airplane flight, most often in the person who travels by air while he has an upper respiratory infection. Symptoms are a feeling of fullness in the ear and hearing loss. There may be a vague feeling of top-heaviness.

Examination may reveal one of several changes in the eardrum. The drum is usually slightly retracted but occasionally is in normal position. The entire drum may be amber colored, or the lower half may be amber colored and the upper half normal in appearance. The amber coloration is due to the presence of a transudate in the middle ear. Often a fine black line will be seen running across the eardrum. This line, looking like a horsehair, is the meniscus of a fluid level. If blood is present in the middle ear, the eardrum appears blue or black. Sometimes air bubbles can be seen through the drum, giving it a ground-glass appearance. Any of these findings indicate the presence of fluid in the middle ear (Figs. 23-5 and 23-6).

Careful statistical studies have shown that 60% to 70% of children have had at least one episode of otitis media before their third birthday. Approximately one third of all children in the United States have had three or more such infections by the age of 3. The frequency of such infection is higher in children with cleft palates.

It is becoming increasingly evident that otitis media in early childhood contributes to early (and often unsuspected) hearing loss. The loss is often mild enough to go undetected until routine testing is done when the child enters school at the age of 5 or 6. It is most often due to residual (usually sterile) fluid in the middle ear. Careful follow-up study has shown that 70% of children retain middle ear effusion (fluid) for 2 weeks after the acute infection has subsided, 40% for 1 month, and 20% for 2 months or longer. Some children retain antibiotic-resistant bacteria in the middle ear after the subsidence of the acute disease.

Many patients with serous otitis media recover spontaneously or after inflation of the eustachian tube. Fluid may persist until a myringotomy is performed and the fluid is aspirated from the middle ear or blown into the external canal by inflation of the eustachian tube. Myringotomy for removal of serous fluid may be adequate when it is smaller than that required for treatment of acute suppurative otitis media.

Eustachian tube blockage, catarrhal otitis media, and serous otitis media are rarely accom-

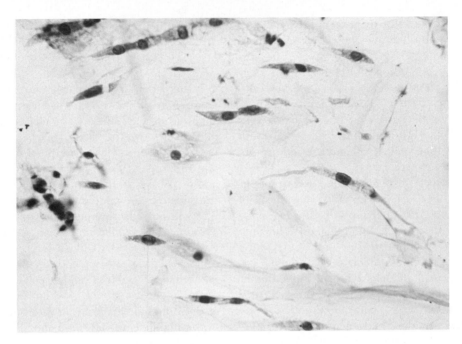

FIG. 24-4. High-power microphotograph of thick mucoid secretion removed from a patient with neglected serous otitis media. Note the fusiform fibroblasts, which, if not removed, might form adhesions and produce permanent hearing loss.

panied by complications. Hearing loss may persist if these conditions are neglected and fluid remains in the middle ear for weeks or months. In some cases serous fluid, if it is unrecognized and therefore allowed to persist, may thicken (Fig. 24-4) and organize to cause permanent hearing loss.

Acute mastoiditis. Acute mastoiditis was a common complication of acute otitis media before the advent of sulfonamides and antibiotics. It is still seen rarely in patients in whom otitis media has not been treated or has been inadequately treated. It occurs when pus has been left in the middle ear and a myringotomy has not been performed or when an infection has not been treated with the correct antibiotic.

Symptoms are a slowly increasing, thick, purulent discharge from the ear, dull aching behind the ear, and a low-grade fever (temperature of 99° to 100° F.). When acute mastoiditis is not accompanied by complications, examination usually demonstrates a copious, thick purulent discharge filling the external auditory canal. After the canal has been cleaned, the eardrum appears dull, edematous, and thick. Sometimes the eardrum is still intact if inadequate doses of antibiotics have been used. Pressure over the

mastoid process produces deep bone tenderness. Firm pressure is necessary to demonstrate tenderness in contradistinction to the light pressure required to elicit the tenderness of acute external otitis. There may be sagging of the soft tissue lateral to the eardrum. X-ray examination of the temporal bone may be necessary to confirm the diagnosis. Characteristic findings are clouding of the mastoid air cells and decalcification of the bony walls between the cells (Fig. 24-5).

Before the use of sulfonamides and antibiotics, *treatment* almost always required an operation. Today, if only clouding of the mastoid air cells and early decalcification of bone are visible, massive doses of antibiotics plus wide myringotomy usually cure the disease. If destruction of bone has occurred, an operation may still be necessary. The operation for acute mastoiditis is *simple mastoidectomy.* It can be performed through a postaural incision or an endaural incision. Both incisions give the same exposure (Fig. 24-6, *A*). All mastoid cells are removed. The inner table of bone over the dura is left intact, and the middle ear is not disturbed. A myringotomy is performed to drain the middle ear. Antibiotics are continued post-

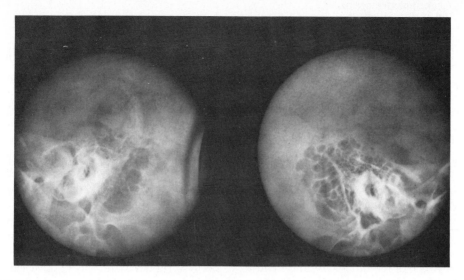

FIG. 24-5. Comparative study of the right and left mastoids. The roentgenogram on the right shows normal cells. In the roentgenogram on the left the cells are indistinct and clouded, and some intercellular walls have disappeared. This is typical of acute mastoiditis.

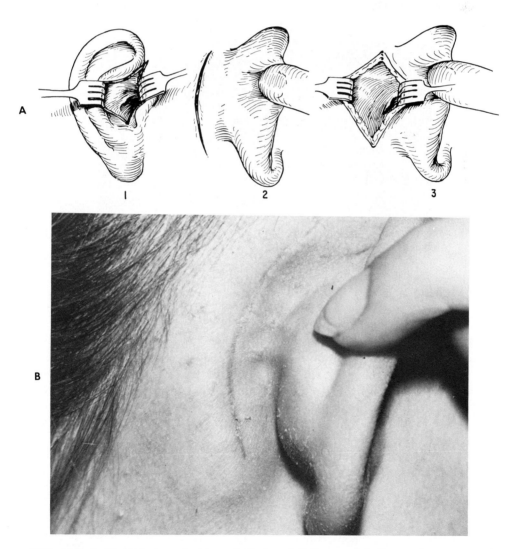

FIG. 24-6. A, Mastoidectomy incisions. *1,* Endaural. *2,* Postaural. *3,* Postaural incision open. **B,** Postaural incision 10 days after the operation.

operatively. Complete healing (Fig. 24-6, *B*) usually occurs in 7 to 10 days. Hearing is unaffected.

Complications of acute mastoiditis are caused by extension of infection from the mastoid to contiguous structures. The complications take different forms, as follows.

There may be erosion of the bone protecting the facial nerve. Inflammation of the nerve then produces *paralysis of the facial muscles*. Differential diagnosis and management of facial paralysis are discussed in Chapter 30.

Extension of infection through the inner table may cause *meningitis*. The symptoms and treatment of this type of meningitis are the same as for meningitis from any other cause. When meningitis orginates in the mastoid, the causative bacteria will be a gram-positive coccus 90% of the time.

Extension of infection through the inner table

may also cause an epidural or *brain abscess* of the temporal lobe or of the cerebellum. The diagnosis of an epidural abscess is more difficult to establish than the diagnosis of meningitis. Dull, persistent headache, recurring mild fever, and minor changes in the sensorium are the usual symptoms. An abscess of the temporal lobe of the brain causes slowly increasing signs of an expanding intracranial lesion. Papilledema is usually slight, and gross neurologic signs are infrequent, since the temporal lobe is a relatively silent neurologic area of the brain. An abscess of the cerebellum may produce ataxia. Papilledema is often severe, and a coma may occur abruptly. When any of these symptoms or signs are associated with otitis media or mastoiditis, neurologic and neurosurgical consultation is imperative.

Thrombosis of the sigmoid sinus occurs when infection spreads through the dura over the pos-

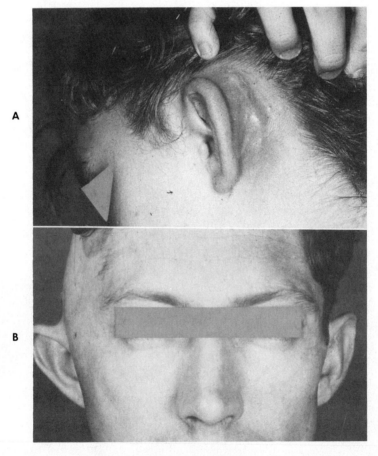

FIG. 24-7. A, Postauricular subperiosteal mastoid abscess. **B,** Subperiosteal abscess in the zygomatic cells on the right. The ear is displaced laterally by the abscess.

terior fossa. An infected thrombus forms inside the sigmoid sinus. The thrombus may extend backward through the transverse sinus or downward to the jugular bulb. Such a thrombus is always accompanied by septicemia. A septic fever, with temperature spikes to 104° or 105° F., is characteristic. There may be tenderness over the jugular vein in the neck on the involved side. Treatment demands administration of antibiotics in maximal dosage, followed by a mastoidectomy and removal of the infected thrombus from the sigmoid sinus. This is accomplished by removal of the inner table of the mastoid, incision of the outer dural layer of the sinus, and removal of the thrombus until free venous bleeding is obtained from both the superior and inferior limbs of the sinus. If the thrombus has extended to the jugular bulb, it is necessary to ligate the jugular vein in the neck.

Invasion of the internal ear by infection produces *suppurative labyrinthitis*, which is manifested by whirling vertigo with nystagmus, nausea, vomiting, tinnitus, and sensorineural hearing loss. If neglected, the infection may extend through the labyrinth and cause meningitis. Treatment, again, consists of administration of antibiotics in maximal dosage and sometimes drainage of the labyrinth through the mastoid. Following suppurative labyrinthitis, there is usually total hearing loss and a dead labyrinth.

When infection in a mastoid causes erosion through the outer cortex, a *subperiosteal abscess* is produced. This is manifested by temperature elevation and deep fluctuation of soft tissue. A subperiosteal abscess may form over the mastoid process. In this instance the fluctuation is behind the ear (Fig. 24-7, *A*). If the erosion comes from the zygomatic mastoid cells, the swelling and fluctuation are superior and anterior to the ear (Fig. 24-7, *B*). Rarely, erosion will occur through the medial aspect of the mastoid tip, causing abscess formation deep to the attachment of the sternocleidomastoid and digastric muscles and producing pain, swelling, and tenderness under the mastoid or between the mastoid tip and the mandible. This type of subperiosteal abscess is known as a *Bezold's abscess.*

CHRONIC INFLAMMATIONS

Chronic suppurative otitis media. Neglected or recurrent infection of the middle ear may eventually produce a chronic change in the mucosa of the ear or destruction of the periosteum covering the ossicles. The infection then tends to become chronic.

Chronic infection of the middle ear is much more common in persons who had ear disease in early childhood. Disease of the ear in infancy and early childhood may arrest the normal pneumatization of the mastoid (Fig. 24-8). It is possible that the same process alters the mucosa of the middle ear, so that it is more susceptible to recurrent infection than is the normal ear. Most patients with chronic suppurative otitis media have a small, undeveloped, and acellular mastoid, which can be demonstrated with roentgenograms (Fig. 24-9).

Any otitis media that is virulent enough to destroy parts of the eardrum or the ossicles damages the middle ear to such an extent that chronic disease may ensue. Scarlet fever and measles were the common offenders before the use of antibiotics. Today this result is much less common. Hypertrophied adenoid tissue, which

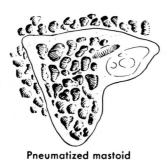

Pneumatized mastoid

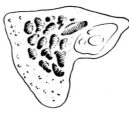

Partially pneumatized mastoid

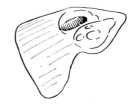

Contracted (infantile or sclerotic) mastoid

FIG. 24-8. Types of mastoid pneumatization. Otitis media in infancy or early childhood can arrest normal pneumatization at any stage.

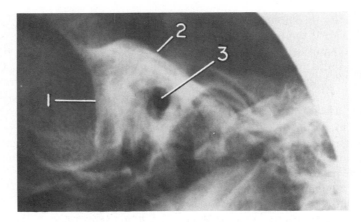

FIG. 24-9. Roentgenogram of an infantile type of temporal bone with no pneumatized cells. *1*, Anterior wall of the sigmoid sinus. *2*, Tegmen between the mastoid and the middle fossa. *3*, External auditory canal. (Compare with Fig. 24-5.)

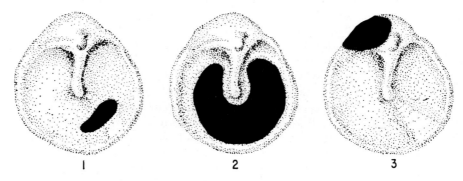

FIG. 24-10. Three common tympanic perforations. *1*, Small central perforation (hearing is usually good). *2*, Large central perforation around the handle of the malleus (hearing is usually poor). *3*, Marginal perforation of Shrapnell's membrane (hearing is usually good). Cholesteatomas commonly occur in patients with a marginal perforation.

causes chronic eustachian tube obstruction, tends to produce recurrent and chronic middle ear infection. Neglected acute otitis media may initiate chronic changes at the time of the original infection.

The term "chronic suppurative otitis media" implies *permanent perforation* of the eardrum. Recurrent episodes of acute otitis media, even though frequent and occurring off and on for years, are not considered to be chronic suppurative otitis media unless there is a permanent perforation of the eardrum. In chronic otitis media, there are many different types of perfor-

ation. Some have considerable diagnostic and prognostic value. When perforation does not involve the margin of the eardrum, it is considered to be a *central* perforation (Fig. 24-10, *1* and *2*). The term "central" means that some eardrum remains at all points around the circumference of the perforation. When the annulus or the margin of the drum is destroyed, the perforation is called *marginal* (Fig. 24-10, *3*). The distinction between central and marginal perforation in prognosis cannot be overemphasized. Central perforation indicates a more benign disease process than does marginal perforation. A

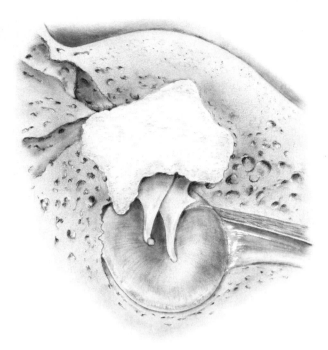

FIG. 24-11. Cholesteatoma viewed from the medial side of the left eardrum. Usually the surrounding bone is less pneumatized. (Compare with Fig. 22-16.)

cholesteatoma is less likely to occur when there is only a central perforation. Surgery for chronic suppurative disease of the middle ear is most often necessary when the perforation is marginal. Multiple perforations of the eardrum should arouse suspicion of tuberculosis.

A special type of chronic condition of the middle ear is known as a *cholesteatoma* (Figs. 24-11 and 22-16). It occurs most often when there is a marginal perforation of the eardrum that allows squamous epithelium from the external auditory canal to grow into the middle ear. The epitympanum (attic) of the middle ear may then become lined by squamous epithelium. As squamous epithelium grows, it desquamates, and keratin and cellular debris collect inside the middle ear. Slow enlargement of the cholesteatoma leads to expansion into the mastoid antrum. After 5 to 20 years bony destruction may cause erosion of important adjacent structures. Pathologically, cholesteatomas are identical to epidermoid inclusion cysts. They occur in other parts of the skull when an ectodermal inclusion has been left beneath the bony surface. They are more common in the ear, however, and are

more dangerous because of the contiguous structures they may damage.

The constant *symptom* of *chronic suppurative otitis media is a painless discharge* from the ear, which may be foul smelling or nearly odorless. There may be periods of days or weeks with no discharge, but the discharge always recurs. It is frequently made worse by an upper respiratory tract infection. When discharge from an ear begins during an upper respiratory disease and is unaccompanied by pain in the ear, it can be assumed that there is a permanent perforation of the drum. Occasionally there is slight discomfort in the ear. Pain in the ear in patients with chronic suppurative disease is a danger sign indicating possible complication.

Hearing loss is always present. It may vary from minimal loss, when the perforation is small, to as much as 50 to 60 decibels when the ossicles are destroyed or fixed by tympanosclerosis. The loss is usually of the conductive type, but in some patients one must expect a cochlear or sensorineural component producing a mixed type of loss. The cochlear involvement probably is the result of the toxic effect of pus in the middle ear on the permeable round window, causing chemical lymph change and finally endorgan disease. It is somewhat surprising that not all patients with chronic (or even acute) suppurative otitis media suffer cochlear damage.

Pain or vertigo is *not* expected to be present in *uncomplicated* chronic suppurative otitis media. *The presence of either symptom may indicate an impending complication.* Deep, persistent pain may indicate the presence of pus under pressure. It may also indicate irritation of the dura or a brain abscess. Vertigo indicates irritation of the labyrinth or erosion of the bone of the labyrinth. Either symptom may be an indication for an early operation.

A particular type of vertigo is seen in some patients with a cholesteatoma. They become dizzy when the ear is cleaned, and the physician can produce dizziness by increasing the pressure in the external auditory canal. Most often the vertigo in these patients is momentary, but it may be so violent that the patient falls. Nausea and vomiting do not occur. Such a patient probably has a fistula in the horizontal semicircular canal. A fistula can be present through the bony labyrinth (exposing the membranous labyrinth), but the patient does not have continuous vertigo.

To demonstrate a fistula, the air in the external auditory canal is compressed, usually by inserting the tip of a Politzer bag into the external meatus and compressing the rubber bulb (Fig. 24-12). Alternatively, a pneumatic otoscope may be used or thumb pressure may be exerted on the external canal. When a fistula is present, compression of the air causes an immediate conjugate deviation of the eyes toward the opposite side, a sudden feeling of whirling or propulsion, and a tendency to fall. This is called the *fistula test.* While performing the test, the physician should guard the patient lest the patient fall out of his chair. A positive fistula test is an indication for an early operation.

In chronic suppurative disease of the middle ear, many pathologic changes can occur. Perforations vary from small, clean holes to complete destruction of the eardrum. Sometimes the handle of the malleus remains, but the rest of the eardrum is destroyed. Granulation tissue or polyps may be present in the middle ear. A polyp may obscure the eardrum when it ex-

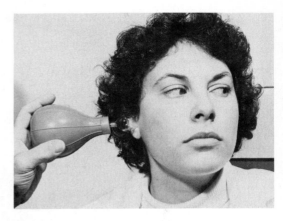

FIG. 24-12. Fistula test done with a Politzer bag. Note conjugate deviation of the eyes to the left (with positive pressure), indicating a labyrinthine fistula. Negative pressure should cause conjugate deviation of the eyes to the right.

trudes into the external auditory canal through a perforation. A cholesteatoma is seen as a shiny white or opalescent mass. The drum and its perforations may be obscured by pus or crusted discharge. All pus and foreign matter must be carefully removed by wiping or suction before the ear can be examined.

Lillie has contributed a useful classification of chronic suppurative disease of the middle ear. His classification gives four groupings.

Type I. The first type is characterized by a thin, usually odorless discharge coming from a perforation of the anteroinferior quadrant of the eardrum. The discharge is more mucoid than purulent, it comes primarily from the eustachian tube, and it is often increased during upper respiratory tract infections. There is no evidence of destruction of the middle ear contents.

Type II. There is a larger perforation of the eardrum, and it may be associated with polyps, granulation tissue, and some destruction of the ossicles. The discharge is thick and purulent and has a fetid odor. There is no evidence of attic disease. The perforation of the eardrum does not involve the margin of the drum in any area.

Type III. There is a perforation that is marginal in at least some areas. There is evi-

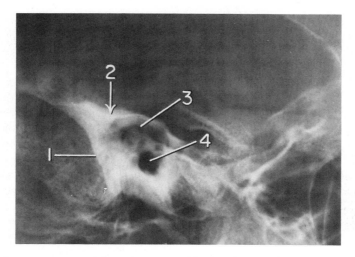

FIG. 24-13. Roentgenogram of the right temporal bone. The rounded radiolucency above and behind the external canal is destruction due to a cholesteatoma. *1,* Anterior margin of the sigmoid sinus. *2,* Floor of the middle fossa. *3,* Destruction by cholesteatoma. *4,* External auditory canal. The lumen of the superior semicircular canal can also be seen.

dence of attic disease. The discharge is scanty. A cholesteatoma is often present. Type II changes may also be present.

Type IV. All examples of chronic suppurative otitis media accompanied by a complication such as meningitis, brain abscess, or facial paralysis are included in this group. A cholesteatoma is present in almost all patients with Type IV disease.

Roentgen examination of the temporal bone of patients with chronic suppurative otitis media usually shows the mastoid to be small and without air cells. Sclerosis of bone, evidenced by increased calcification, is almost always present. Any areas of bone destruction indicate that the pathologic process has extended beyond the middle ear. Such areas of destruction may be varied in size and extent. Their presence suggests that an operation should be performed. If a cholesteatoma has extended into the mastoid, the roentgenogram often shows a sharply defined, rounded area of radiolucency surrounded by sclerotic bone (Fig. 24-13).

Polytomography is now widely used in most clinics in addition to standard roentgenographic techniques because this technique better defines the middle and inner ear structures.

Medical treatment of chronic suppurative otitis media consists of the use of local medications in the ear and eradication of any contributing factors. Careful removal of granulation tissue, polyps, and visible cholesteatomas will allow local medication to reach the areas of infection more adequately. Aural irrigation using several ounces of normal saline solution at *body temperature* often will do much to clean up disease in the middle ear and epitympanum. Saline irrigations may be carried out twice daily, the ear dried as carefully as possible, and then antibiotic drops instilled. Various powders may be beneficial. They are usually blown into the middle ear by the physician. Ear drops containing antibiotics or other drugs known to inhibit bacteria are commonly used. The patient instills the drops three or four times daily. Examples of types of powders and drops often used are as follows:

Ear drops

℞   Boric acid powder   1.2 gm.
    Bichloride of mercury   0.012 gm.
    Alcohol, 70%, q.s.   30.0 ml.
Sig. 4-8 drops in ear 3 or 4 times daily.

℞   Acetic acid, 2%   30.0 ml.
Sig. 4-8 drops in ear 3 or 4 times daily.

(NOTE: This is used specifically for infections caused by *Bacillus pyocyaneus*)

Many antibiotics are effective when dissolved in suitable vehicles. Those most commonly used are chloramphenicol (Chloromycetin), bacitracin, polymyxin B, neomycin, and hydrocortisone. They can be used singly but are more generally used in combination. The drugs are available in standard mixtures under trade names. Rarely can the druggist make them up from a written prescription. The drops are used several times daily.

Streptomycin in saline solution can be used. It is ordinarily given after other drops have not been effective. It should not be used over a prolonged period because bacteria quickly become resistant to it.

Powders

℞ Sulfanilamide powder ⎫
   Sulfathiazole powder ⎬ Equal parts
   Zinc peroxide powder ⎭

Sig. Blow in ear with powder blower 3 times daily.

℞ Iodine   0.3 gm.
   Solvent ether   4.0 ml.
   Boric acid powder   30.0 gm.
   (Dissolve iodine in ether. Mix with boric acid powder until dry.)

Sig. Blow in ear with powder blower 3 or 4 times daily.

Individual powders that are effective against specific bacteria determined by culture can be blown into the ear by the physician, or the patient can be instructed in the use of a powder blower to instill the powder. Commonly used powders are sulfanilamide, sulfathiazole, urea, and boric acid.

Systemic antibiotics have not proved helpful in chronic suppurative otitis media except when there is a superimposed acute process. When there is an acute exacerbation in a chronically infected ear, systemic antibiotics are essential. Often, unsuspected destruction of bone has occurred from the chronic disease, allowing an acute process to invade important deep structures and produce complications. In the absence of pain or signs of complication, local treatment may be necessary for months or years.

Many different bacteria may be associated with chronic suppurative otitis media. Some are virulent, and others are common saprophytes. The appearance and odor of the discharge may be helpful in identifying certain bacteria. *Pseudomonas aeruginosa* is a common invader and causes a green discharge. *Escherichia coli* may be introduced by finger contamination and has the characteristic odor of coliform bacilli. *Proteus* bacilli cause a foul or fetid odor. Culture of the discharge is important. Staphylococci, streptococci, gram-negative bacilli, and pneumococci, as well as diphtheroids, are commonly present. Most often a culture grows several different bacteria. *Sensitivity studies should be performed.* However, antibiotics that are effective in vitro are not always effective in vivo. Repeated cultures may be necessary when the response to treatment is inadequate.

Surgical treatment of chronic suppurative otitis media requires radical mastoidectomy or a modification of radical mastoidectomy. A *radical mastoidectomy* can be performed through an endaural or postaural incision. All mastoid air cells, granulations, and pus are removed. Next, the posterior wall of the external auditory canal is removed. Then the remnants of the eardrum, the ossicles (except the stapes), and all mucosa of the middle ear are removed. Finally the tensor tympani muscle is removed. The middle ear orifice of the eustachian tube is cleaned of infected mucosa. The resulting cavity heals by the ingrowth of epithelium from the skin of the external canal. The cavity can be grafted, but the former method is preferable. In some instances the cavity formed by removal of the mastoid cells can be filled with muscle. A flap is fashioned from the temporalis muscle, leaving a pedicle for the blood supply, and is turned down into the mastoid cavity. The cavity thus created is smaller than usual and requires a minimum of postoperative care. Such a flap should not be used unless *all* infected tissue has been removed.

When a perforation of the eardrum is small and high in the posterior margin of the drum, and when the disease involves the epitympanum but not the middle ear, hearing is often nearly normal. The middle ear may be normal except for the changes in the attic, a common situation when a cholesteatoma is present. Then a *modified radical mastoidectomy* is performed. This operation differs from the radical mastoidectomy in that the middle ear structures and the eardrum are preserved. The eardrum is left attached to the skin of the external auditory canal (posteriorly), and both are used to seal the middle ear from the mastoid cavity. After modified radical mastoidectomy the hearing should be

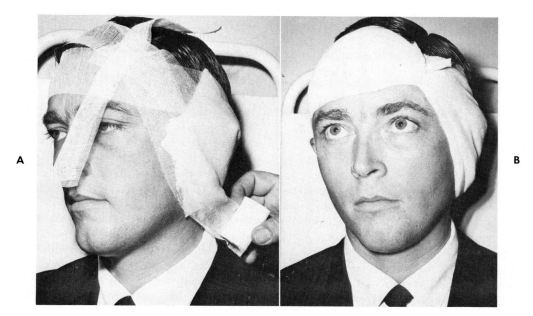

FIG. 24-14. A, Good mastoid dressing requires enough gauze around the ear to form a mound. Note the figure eight method of bandaging—high on the head opposite the ear and low on the ear. Note also the gauze tie placed *under* the bandage before starting. **B,** Completed dressing. Note that the gauze tie has been used to lock the head bandage at the point where the figure eight is narrowest.

serviceable and better than after radical mastoidectomy. After either radical mastoidectomy or modified radical mastoidectomy, the epithelium-lined cavity is open to the outside through a slightly enlarged external meatus. It can thus be cleaned from time to time. Both procedures are designed to cure infection and provide the patient with a safe ear.

Sometimes an ear that has been chronically infected can be made dry and safe by medical treatment rather than by an operation. Occasionally spontaneous cessation of a chronic discharge will occur. There may still be an open perforation of the eardrum, a partially eroded ossicle, or adhesive bands that impede the normal mobility of the eardrum and the ossicles. In the absence of a cholesteatoma the ear is considered to be safe, but hearing is diminished. The hearing loss is conductive in type (see Chapter 25). Often it is possible and desirable to consider reconstruction of the sound-conducting mechanism in an effort to restore part or all of the hearing loss.

Such reconstructive procedures are known as *myringoplasty*, when only a perforation is re-

paired, or *tympanoplasty*, when the middle ear structures are rebuilt or replaced by prostheses (see pp. 367-373). Reconstructive techniques require magnification and the use of fascial grafts, cartilage, bone, perichondrium, silicones, Teflon, and stainless steel wire. Each case must be considered individually, and a decision as to the exact method of reconstruction must often be made in the operating room after the middle ear has been exposed and the extent of the mechanical derangement observed. The necessary tissues are obtained from the ear itself or from nearby tissues such as the fascia of the temporalis muscle or the perichondrium of the tragus. In properly selected patients, who have normal or nearly normal cochlear function, good results can be obtained more than 50% of the time.

Complications of chronic suppurative otitis media are the same as those occurring in acute mastoiditis, that is, meningitis, epidural abscess, brain abscess (temporal lobe or cerebellar), thrombosis of the sigmoid sinus or jugular vein, septicemia, suppurative labyrinthitis, facial paralysis, and subperiosteal abscess.

Chronic (or recurrent) serous otitis media. Recurrent accumulation of fluid in the middle ear presents a serious threat to hearing. Although chronic serous otitis media has been recognized for many years, the incidence has increased only since the early 1940s.

Chronic serous effusion of the middle ear may be caused by overgrowth of lymphoid tissue in the nasopharynx, chronic sinus infection, or allergy of the nose and nasopharynx. Hypometabolism may be the underlying cause for recurrence of middle ear effusion. A lowered resistance to infection, usually evidenced by low gamma globulin in the blood plasma (hypogammaglobulinemia or agammaglobulinemia), may contribute to recurrent effusion.

Inadequate treatment of acute suppurative otitis media may lead to recurrent serous otitis. The common practice of treating acute otitis media with antibiotics for 24 to 48 hours without myringotomy often leaves a low-grade, smoldering infection that recurs repeatedly until a thick mucoid effusion remains in the middle ear for weeks or months. Even though this fluid is sterile, the middle ear does not absorb it. *Inadequate treatment of acute or subacute suppurative otitis media is believed to be the largest single factor responsible for the increased incidence of chronic serous otitis media.*

Finally, the physician must remember that chronic serous otitis media in an adult may be caused by carcinoma of the nasopharynx. When *unilateral* effusion occurs in an adult, nasopharyngeal carcinoma should always be suspected and every possible diagnostic measure should be used to prove or disprove its presence.

Symptoms of chronic serous otitis media are minimal. Hearing loss characterized by fluctuation is the most common symptom. An annoying feeling of heaviness of the head on one side may also occur. Sometimes certain sounds are distorted. There is no pain or fever. There is no discharge from the ear.

Examination of the ear is often deceiving. Minimal changes occur in the tympanic membrane. Sometimes a fluid level is visible, but more often there is only dulling of the normal shiny appearance of the eardrum or minimal retraction. An audiogram shows a conductive hearing loss. Sometimes a diagnostic myringot-

omy must be performed to differentiate chronic serous otitis media from unilateral or bilateral otosclerosis. In otosclerosis, the middle ear is dry and normal in appearance when the eardrum is opened.

A history of fluctuating hearing loss in a child, usually suspected by the parents or a teacher, should immediately make the physician think of a middle ear effusion and calls for an audiogram even though the eardrum appears to be normal.

Surgical treatment of serous otitis media is discussed in Chapter 25 under "Conductive Hearing Loss" (p. 361). Prevention of recurrence or ultimate cure may require an investigation of the metabolism, blood count, allergies, or level of gamma globulin in the blood plasma. In addition to removal of fluid from the middle ear, treatment must be directed toward control of any possible systemic cause. Even then, treatment may fail.

Abnormal patency of the eustachian tube occurs when there is loss of tissue about the eustachian tube orifice. One cause is recent severe loss of weight. The symptoms are autophony and fullness in the ear, which are relieved when the patient becomes recumbent. Patients can even hear themselves breathe, and the too-free exchange of air along the tube is annoying. Insufflation of a 4:1 mixture of boric and salicylic acid powder into the tubal orifice is a useful diagnostic test as well as a temporary treatment.

A method that produces more lasting relief is the injection of polytetrafluoroethylene paste into the anterior wall of the eustachian tube orifice. This method seems to be useful in the treatment of an abnormally patent eustachian tube. Although not always successful, this method of treatment works well enough to be used for the occasional patient with persistent marked symptoms.

TUMORS OF THE MIDDLE EAR

Tumors of the middle ear are rare. The three most common types are neurofibroma of the facial nerve (discussed in Chapter 30), squamous cell carcinoma, and glomus jugulare tumor.

Squamous cell carcinoma. Squamous cell carcinoma of the middle ear may occur after long-standing chronic suppurative otitis media. It also occurs spontaneously. A discharge from the ear, often blood tinged, is the only early symptom. Eventually there is hearing loss on the affected side. In the advanced stage, pain and facial paralysis are common. Diagnosis is made by a biopsy of tissue removed from an ulcerating, fungating mass seen through the ear speculum.

Treatment must be radical. Irradiation alone has been unsuccessful in effecting a cure. Rarely, a thorough radical mastoidectomy preceded or followed by irradiation may eradicate all tumor cells. However, a complete resection of the temporal bone is usually necessary to prevent recurrence. The prognosis, therefore, in squamous cell carcinomas of the middle ear is poor regardless of the treatment.

Glomus jugulare tumor. A glomus jugulare tumor arises from the glomus bodies located in the adventia of the dome of the jugular bulb. Identical tumor tissue may be found on the medial wall of the middle ear attached to a tiny arteriole. In this case the tumor is referred to as *glomus tympanicum*. Such tumors ordinarily are small and are of much less serious import than glomus jugulare tumors. The carotid body tumor looks the same microscopically as the glomus tumor, and similar tumors have been found in numerous other parts of the head and neck, where they are sometimes called chemodectoma or nonchromaffin paraganglioma. These tumors grow slowly and may remain unnoticed for years. In reported cases, the average length of time from the original symptoms to the diagnosis is 7 to 8 years.

Early symptoms may be tinnitus, slight hearing loss, or a throbbing pulsating discomfort. Later, pain, dizziness, total unilateral deafness, and multiple cranial nerve paralyses are seen. The striking feature of this tumor is its tendency to bleed profusely when manipulated. Spontaneous hemorrhage is rare but does occur. Any episode of profuse bleeding following manipulation of a mass in the external canal or in the middle ear should make the physician suspect that a glomus jugulare tumor is present. Clinically the erroneous diagnosis of granulation tissue polyp is often made.

Only a biopsy will establish the correct diagnosis. When neglected, a glomus jugulare tumor expands slowly and causes extensive destruction of the mastoid and the internal ear. It may also extend intracranially. A carotid angio-gram, as well as a retrograde dye study of the internal jugular vein, is considered essential in diagnosis. Aneurysm of the internal carotid artery may mimic a glomus tumor in symptoms and appearance, and an angiogram will distinguish between the two. Even more important, an angiogram will demonstrate the size and position of the tumor.

Treatment may be either surgical or by irradiation therapy. In the case of *glomus tympanicum*, often all that needs to be done is to reflect the drumhead, as would be done for stapedectomy, and to excise the small red tumor on the promontory. In the case of *glomus jugulare*, surgery may be formidable and complete surgical removel is not always possible. Irradiation therapy, although it does not destroy the tumor, causes it to shrink and prevents progression of symptoms.

SELECTED READINGS

Bast, T.H., and Anson, B.J.: The temporal bone and the ear, Springfield, Ill., 1949, Charles C Thomas, Publisher.

Becker, W., and others: Atlas of otorhinolaryngology and bronchoesophagology, Philadelphia, 1969, W.B. Saunders Co.

Davison, F.W.: Prevention of recurrent otitis media in children, Ann. Otol. Rhinol. Laryngol. **75:**735, 1966.

Farrior, J.B.: The radical mastoidectomy; anatomical considerations in surgical technique, Surg. Gynecol. Obstet. **89:**328, 1949.

Frenkiel, S., and Alberti, P.W.: Traumatic thermal injuries of the middle ear, J. Otolaryngol. **6:**17, 1977.

Gardner, G., and others: Combined-approach surgery for removal of glomus jugulare tumors, Laryngoscope **87:** 665, 1977.

Hough, J.V.D.: Congenital malformation of the middle ear, Arch. Otolaryngol. **78:**335, 1963.

Howie, V.M., Ploussard, J.H., and Lester, R.L., Jr.: Otitis media, a clinical and bacteriological correlation, Pediatrics **45:**29, 1970.

Juhn, S.K., and others: Pathogenesis of otitis media, Ann. Otol. Rhinol. Laryngol. **86:**481, 1977.

Lack, E.E., and others: Paragangliomas of the head and neck region: clinical study of 69 patients, Cancer **39:**397, 1977.

Lewis, J.S.: Carcinoma of the ear, Arch. Otolaryngol. **97:** 41, 1973.

Lim, D.J., and Birck, H.G.: Ultrastructural pathology of the middle ear mucosa in serous otitis media. Ann. Otol. Rhinol. Laryngol. **80:**838, 1971.

Lim, D.J., and Shimada, T.: Secretory activity of normal middle ear mucosa, Ann. Otol. Rhinol. Laryngol. **80:**319, 1971.

Love, J.T., and Caruso, V.G.: Civilian air travel and the otolaryngologist, Laryngoscope **88:**1732, 1978.

Meltzer, P.E.: Treatment of thrombosis of the lateral sinus, Arch. Otolaryngol. **22:**131, 1935.

Ogura, J.H., Spector, G.J., and Gado, M.: Glomus jugulare and vagale, Ann. Otol. Rhinol. Laryngol. **87:**622, 1978.

Olson, A.L., and others: Prevention and therapy of serous otitis media by oral decongestants: double-blind study in pediatric practice, Pediatrics **61:**679, 1978.

Paparella, M.M., Brady, D.R., and Hoel, R.: Sensorineural hearing loss in chronic otitis media and mastoiditis, Trans. Am. Acad. Ophthalmol. Otolaryngol. **74:**108, 1970.

Paparella, M.M., and Kim, C.S.: Mastoidectomy update, Laryngoscope **87:**1977, 1977.

Paparella, M.M., and others: Pathology of sensorineural hearing loss in otitis media, Ann. Otol. Rhinol. Laryngol. **81:**632, 1972.

Proctor, C.A.: Intracranial complications of otitic origin, Laryngoscope **76:**288, 1966.

Rosenwasser, H.: Glomus jugulare tumors, Arch. Otolaryngol. **88:**29, 1968.

Schuknecht, H.F.: Pathology of the ear, Cambridge, Mass., 1974, Harvard University Press, pp. 241-247.

Shambaugh, G.E., Jr.: Surgery of the ear, Philadelphia, 1959, W.B. Saunders Co.

Sinha, P.P., and Aziz, H.I.: Treatment of carcinoma of the middle ear, Radiology **126:**485, 1978.

Veltri, R.W., and Sprinkle, P.M.: Serous otitis media, Ann. Otol. Rhinol. Laryngol. **82:**297, 1973.

25 HEARING LOSSES

Communicative disorders constitute the greatest number of handicapping disabilities in the United States. Studies by the National Center for Health Statistics and the Centers for Disease Control indicate that more people suffer from hearing, speech, and language impairment than from heart disease, venereal disease, paralysis, epilepsy, blindness, tuberculosis, cerebral palsy, muscular dystrophy, and multiple sclerosis combined. Direct federal expenditures for services and programs for the communicatively handicapped are estimated to be at least $500 million per year. This includes the costs of special education, vocational rehabilitation, hearing aids, and training professional personnel. According to the Department of Health and Human Services, the yearly loss of earnings caused by communicative disorders is a staggering $1.75 billion.

Hearing loss affects 16.2 million Americans. Of these, 3 million are school-age children. However, hearing loss is most common among the elderly. Almost half of those needing help are over 65 years of age; reliable statistics indicate that over 6 million persons in this age group have a hearing disorder. More than 11.5 million Americans suffer from *uncorrected* hearing handicaps.

Studies by family practice physicians indicate that inflammation of the middle ear in children is the second most prevalent disorder seen by the family physician, the first being the common cold. The incidence of hearing loss in children is between 2% and 4%. In almost one third of hard-of-hearing children, the problem can be traced to something that happened before or during birth. These causes include German measles (rubella) contracted by the mother in the first trimester of pregnancy, influenza, shingles, other viral diseases, and certain drugs.

Hearing loss has *major* socioeconomic implications. In 1979, according to the Department of Health and Human Services, such disorders had a direct cost of approximately $410,445,000 for the education, management, and compensation of those with hearing problems.

Hearing losses fall into two broad categories—conductive and sensorineural. Each has a variety of causes.

SENSORINEURAL HEARING LOSS

Sensorineural hearing loss (Fig. 25-1) occurs when the cochlea or the eighth nerve is damaged. This damage may take place before birth, during delivery, or later in life.

Hereditary deafness. Hereditary deafness may be the result of a defect in the genes of the parents that prevents normal development of the cochlea. When this is the cause, there is often more than one deaf child in the family. However, sometimes the siblings of a deaf child have normal hearing and there is no familial history of deafness. Intermarriage of persons with hereditary deafness should be discouraged, since their likelihood of having deaf offspring is greater than that of other people.

There are many types of hereditary deafness recognized, and the easiest grouping to remember seems to be one based on associated abnormalities. Types *not* associated with other abnormalities include dominant types of congenital severe deafness, progressive nerve deafness, unilateral deafness, low-frequency hearing loss, and mid-frequency hearing loss. Recessive forms also occur in all these types.

Types of hereditary deafness with associated integumentary anomalies include Waardenburg's syndrome, albinism with congenital deafness, piebaldness with congenital deafness, and others.

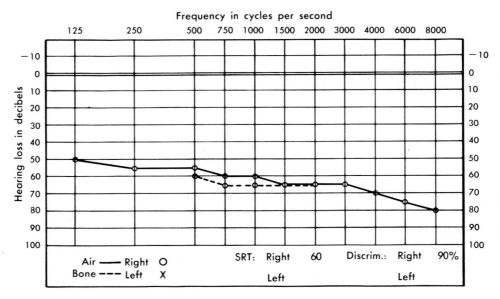

FIG. 25-1. Audiogram of profound sensorineural hearing loss in the right ear. Both bone conduction and air conduction are far below the usable range. The normal discrimination score (90%) suggests that good hearing should be obtained with proper amplification.

Eye conditions and disorders of the nervous system may be associated with hearing loss.

Skeletal disorders associated with deafness include Crouzon's disease (craniofacial dysostosis), Treacher-Collins syndrome (mandibulofacial dysostosis), van der Hoeve's syndrome (osteogenesis imperfecta), Paget's disease, craniometaphyseal disease, and others.

In Alport's disease hereditary deafness is associated with nephritis, and in Pendred's disease deafness is associated with goiter. There are many other types of hearing loss that have been described—not always, however, of the sensorineural type. Otosclerosis, for example, a common cause of conductive hearing loss, is transmitted in an autosomal dominant manner. Otosclerosis is not clinically manifested at birth but affects hearing first, and then progressively, in the second and third decades of life. Ossicular deformities of the middle ear, such as an absent incus or stapes or a fused incus and malleus, are commonly associated with congenital atresia of the external auditory canal.

Congenital deafness. Congenital deafness may be caused by toxicity or by trauma. When a pregnant woman contracts German measles (rubella) during the first trimester of pregnancy, her child may be deaf. Pregnant women who have not had German measles and who have been exposed to the disease should be given immune globulin or vaccine to present them from contracting it. If a pregnant woman is treated with drugs that may damage the inner ear, such as quinine or streptomycin, the cochlea of the fetus may be damaged. Prolonged anoxia in a newborn infant may damage the cochlea and produce hearing loss. It may also cause cerebral palsy. Trauma during delivery may sometimes cause intracranial hemorrhage and damage to the cochlea or to the eighth nerve. Erythroblastosis fetalis often damages the cochlea.

Congenital syphilis must always be considered as a cause of otherwise unexplained sensorineural hearing loss. The onset of deafness may be in adolescence or adult life, and one or both ears may be affected. The cause of the deafness is often rather bizarre; there are remissions and exacerbations. Often vertigo is present, and then the symptoms may be virtually indistinguishable from those of Meniere's disease. The patient may or may not have been treated for syphilis; in either case the serology test is not always positive. The presence of other signs of congenital syphilis helps in establishing the diagnosis. Treatment is with modern antisyphilitic drugs. Steroids sometimes help.

Waardenburg's syndrome. Waardenburg's syndrome was described in 1951. If all features are present, the patient may have a white forelock, eyes of different colors (heterochromia), an epicanthal fold, and deafness. The eyes may appear widely spaced, and some patients show hypertrichosis of the eyebrows. Frequently, one or more of these findings, but no deafness, may appear in a family and be repeated for several generations until a deaf child is born. The deaf child may have none of the other characteristic features and may be fitted into the Waardenburg classification only because of the other features that have occurred in members of the family. As is the case with other types of hereditary sensorineural deafness, there is no effective medical or surgical therapy.

Traumatic hearing loss. Traumatic hearing loss is usually due to direct injury to the internal ear or to the eighth nerve. Skull fractures, hemorrhage (or thrombosis), and explosive blasts are the usual causes. Occasionally the internal ear is damaged during operations on the temporal bone or during intracranial operations. Meningitis often causes damage to the eighth nerve, in which event the infection may extend to the cochlea. Infection of the inner ear may be associated with otitis media or with mastoiditis. Scarlet fever can cause cochlear damage out of proportion to the damage it produces in the middle ear. Particularly in infants and children, cochlear damage sometimes occurs during or after a high temperature. Mumps shows a specific affinity for the inner ear. *It is the most common cause of profound sensorineural unilateral deafness in childhood.*

Deafness resulting from drug toxicity. Drug toxicity is an increasingly important cause of sensorineural hearing loss. This is emphasized in the following summary by Robert E. Brummett, whose research in this field is widely recognized.

Organ specific toxicity of drugs is now recognized to be a serious problem. This type of toxicity is known to affect the eye, liver, kidney, heart, blood, and bone marrow, as well as the ear. Organ specific toxicity to the ear is usually referred to as ototoxicity. There are many different classes of drugs reported to produce ototoxicity, and the effect ranges from production of permanent deafness to temporary tinnitis. The drugs that are most well known in this regard are the aminoglycoside antibiotics, the salicylate analgesics and quinine and related antimalarials.

Ototoxicity resulting from all of the aminoglycoside drugs is qualitatively similar. However, there are quantitative differences. Aminoglycoside-induced ototoxicity is often complicated by factors related to their absorption and elimination. Because this class of drugs is poorly absorbed from the gastrointestinal tract it is sometimes mistakenly assumed that they are without danger from this route of administration. In fact, the 3% of the large doses administered orally that is absorbed represents about one-third of the dose that might be administered parenterally. This route of administration *can* result in ototoxicity, especially in patients with renal disease. Another related problem occurs when these drugs are used to irrigate wounds. It is assumed that, because the drugs are poorly absorbed from intact skin, they are also poorly absorbed when used topically on wounds. In fact, aminoglycoside antibiotics are rapidly absorbed from wounds, and blood levels that are ototoxic can easily be achieved. The sole mechanism for the elimination of the aminoglycoside antibiotics is by renal excretion. Their renal clearance is the same as the renal clearance of creatinine, and thus any impairment of renal excretion of creatinine will be reflected in impaired excretion of the aminoglycoside antibiotic, necessitating appropriate dosage adjustment. Aminoglycoside antibiotic ototoxicity results from rather selective destruction of the sensory hair cells of the organ of Corti. The most sensitive cells are those in the basal turn of the cochlea because high frequency sounds are processed in this region. The initial hearing loss involves high frequency sound. The hair cells are incapable of regeneration so that the ototoxicity is permanent. In general the magnitude of the ototoxicity is related to both the daily dosage and the duration of therapy. A unique feature of the ototoxicity is that is might not be detected during the period of drug administration, but can occur days to weeks after therapy has terminated. Another unique feature of aminoglycoside ototoxicity is that it can be unilateral. Ototoxicity is known to occur *in utero* when women are given aminoglycoside antibiotics while they are pregnant. Ototoxicity is also reported to occur in experimental animals after the drugs are placed in the middle ear space.

Aminoglycoside antibiotics have been shown to interact with loop-inhibiting diuretics such as ethacrynic acid. This interaction is reported to occur in both man and experimental animals, and can occur with all of the aminoglycoside antibiotics and all of the loop-inhibiting diuretics. (Although such as interaction appears to occur only with loop-inhibiting diuretics, a similar interaction can occur with non-aminoglycoside antibiotics such as viomycin, capreomycin, polymyxin B and even cis-platinum.) This interaction results in the destruction of cochlea hair cells. It appears that there is no such effect on the vestibular portion of the inner ear.

In laboratory animals it has been clearly demonstrated that excessively loud noise, and concurrent administration of aminoglycoside antibiotics, results in augmented ototoxicity. The relationship of these findings to the clinical use of the drugs is not known at this time, but it would seem prudent to keep the noise exposure of patients receiving these drugs to a minimum.

Non-steroidal anti-inflammatory drugs such as aspirin are reported to produce a temporary hearing loss and tinnitis in patients receiving large doses. In most cases both the hearing loss and the tinnitis disappear when drug therapy has been terminated. There are a few cases of permanent ototoxicity reported, but the data are not very convincing. There are no well controlled animal studies that demonstrate permanent cochlea lesions following the administration of these drugs.

Many other types of drugs are reported to be ototoxic. Of these the most serious toxicity appears to be produced by drugs such as quinidine and other antimalarial drugs, and cisplatinum. Other drugs such as nitrogen mustard, 6-aminonicotinamide, viomycin and vancomycin have been reported to produce permanent ototoxicity. Erythromycin, in very large doses, has been reported to produce a temporary hearing loss, and minocycline has been reported to produce temporary unsteadiness.

The iatrogenic nature of drug-induced ototoxicity should be borne in mind by physicians prescribing drugs with such a propensity.*

Drugs that may cause hearing damage are listed in Table 6.

Presbycusis. Presbycusis is the term given to hearing loss associated with the aging process. It is probably the result of atrophy of the ganglion cells in the cochlea. The degenerative changes producing this type of hearing loss parallel those that occur in other tissues of the body as senility approaches. Presbycusis is characterized by bilateral gradual loss of hearing. Beginning with a loss of the high tones, it slowly progresses to involve the middle and lower tones (Fig. 25-2).

*From Brummett, R.E.: Drug-induced ototoxicity, Drugs **19:**412-428, 1980.

TABLE 6. Drugs known to produce cochlear and vestibular toxicity or to produce symptoms (hearing loss, dizziness, tinnitus) related to the inner ear

Toxic to cochlea and/or labyrinth
Amikacin
Chloramphenicol (topically)
Chloroquine
Cis-platinum
Dibekacin
Dihydrostreptomycin
Ethacrynic acid
Furosemide (Lasix)
Gentamicin
Kanamycin
Neomycin
Netilmycin
Nitrogen mustard
Quinidine
Quinine
Salicylates
Sisomycin
Streptomycin
Tobramycin
Vancomycin
Viomycin
Causing the symptom dizziness
Antihypertensives
Barbiturates
CNS depressants
Estrogens
Phenothiazines
Phenylbutazone
Oral contraceptives

Hypothyroidism. Whether congenital or acquired, hypothyroidism causes recognizable changes in the ear. Deafness is the principal symptom. In cretins the hearing loss is often severe and is sensorineural in type. It is not correctable. Acquired hypothyroidism is also sensorineural but is less severe and is reversible. The actual pathologic change that produces the hearing loss is unknown, but proper replacement of circulating thyroxine with oral medication, as for any hypothyroid state, will usually correct the hearing loss.

Occupational hearing loss. Occupational hearing loss may be caused by injuries such as explosive blasts, accidents that involve the head, or intense heat. The results of such injuries vary widely. The canal may be fractured, the ear-

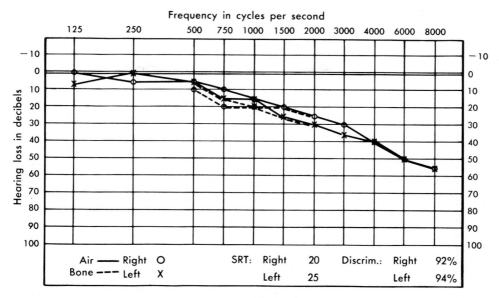

FIG. 25-2. Audiogram of moderate-degree presbycusis. Note that both ears are equally involved.

drum may be destroyed, the ossicles may be disrupted, or the internal ear may be damaged or destroyed. These conditions are due to concussion, hemorrhage, or tearing of the soft tissue of the cochlea or vestibule. They may occur singly or in combination. Each presents a different problem and must be handled according to the symptoms present.

When the middle or the internal ear has been accidentally opened by trauma, strict asepsis should be observed even during routine examination of the ear. If infection is introduced by the instruments used in examination, suppurative labyrinthitis and occasionally meningitis may occur.

NOISE-INDUCED HEARING LOSS. Hearing loss caused by loud noise is the most common and most important type of occupational hearing loss. Exposure to industrial noise levels greater than 85 to 90 decibels for months or years causes cochlear damage. In the early stage there is a loss of hearing at or near the frequency of 4000 cycles per second (Fig. 25-3). Later the damage extends to both the higher and lower tones. The lowest tones are affected least. Considerable damage can take place before a worker is aware of hearing loss because speech reception is not altered seriously until the hearing loss is greater than 40 decibels (ISO, 1964) in the speech fre-

quencies (500, 1000, and 2000 cycles per second).

Noise-induced hearing loss has two phases. The first is known as *temporary threshold shift* (TTS). The term means that the human ear, when exposed to sound loud enough to affect it, will show a loss of sensitivity to sound, that is, a raise in threshold for sound. If the hearing returns to its previous level after the noise has been removed, the shift has been temporary and no permanent damage has occurred. On the other hand, if the hearing does not return to its previous level, permanent damage has ensued. This second phase of damage is the *permanent threshold shift* (PTS). A temporary threshold shift can be superimposed on permanent damage. The ears of some people are more easily damaged by noise than are those of others.

Hearing loss caused by noise has become a serious economic problem. Individual workers and unions have filed suits totaling millions of dollars against industries, insurance carriers, and state industrial accident commissions. Compensation and liability laws are being studied and changed. New laws in some states now make the last employer responsible for all previous noise-induced hearing loss. For this reason and because conservation of hearing is so important, many industries require pre-em-

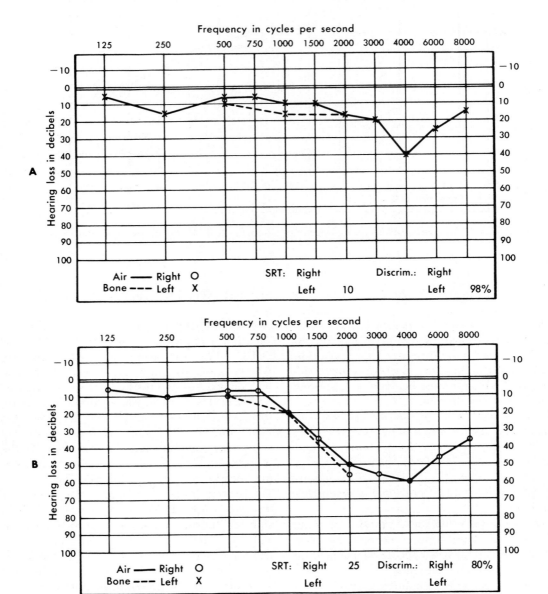

FIG. 25-3. Noise-induced hearing loss. **A,** Early damage—worst at 4000 cycles per second. **B,** More serious loss—damage has spread to middle tones. Damage is still greater at 4000 cycles per second. Note loss of discrimination due to high-tone loss.

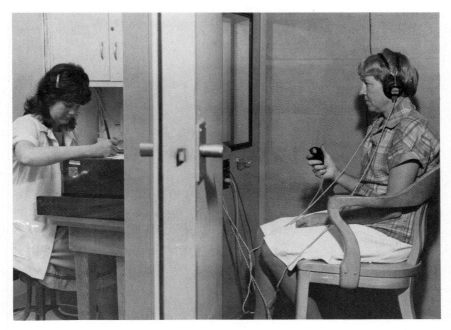

FIG. 25-4. Industrial hearing screening (audiometry) on the job in a sound-treated booth. The door is closed during the test.

ployment audiometric examinations (Fig. 25-4). Persons who work where noise is above the 85- to 90-decibel level are required to have periodic hearing tests so that cochlear impairment can be detected. When hearing loss is found, the worker may be transferred to a less noisy area.

If it is necessary for a person to continue working in the area of high noise level, he can use ear protectors, or plugs, as they are often called. These plugs are inserted into the external auditory canal, and in some persons they reduce the noise reaching the middle ear by 10 to 30 decibels. Earplugs are usually made of rubber or malleable plastic and come in several sizes to fit different auditory canals. Some protectors are custom made; they are molded to the individual ear canal by impression techniques. They offer a better seal but are more expensive. In most industries the standard plugs are used.

In industries with extremely high noise levels, such as jet engine factories, simple earplugs do not afford enough protection. In such factories, where the sound level may reach 140 decibels, workmen wear earplugs, muffs over the ears, and, finally, a large shield over the entire head (Fig. 25-5).

When the hearing has been damaged by noise, it is important that the worker remain away from noise for several weeks before a final hearing evaluation is made to avoid complicating any compensation award for permanent loss when part or all of the loss may be temporary.

Hearing loss associated with firearms such as the M-16 rifle, and also with guns used in sports, can readily occur. The loss tends to be substantially greater in the left than in the right ear for a right-handed person shooting from the shoulder. With revolvers, the hearing loss is equal in both ears. Patients should be warned that if firing guns causes tinnitus, a sensation of fullness in the ears, or temporary hearing loss, they probably should not fire guns or else should wear suitable ear protectors.

Also of interest is the observation that high-intensity music, such as rock-and-roll, is quite capable of producing hearing loss. Typical readings of 110-decibel sound-pressure levels at 30 feet from the loudspeaker will produce a severe temporary threshold shift in about 16% of listeners.

In 1970 the Congress of the United States passed the Occupational Safety and Health Act (Williams-Steiger Act), which was signed into

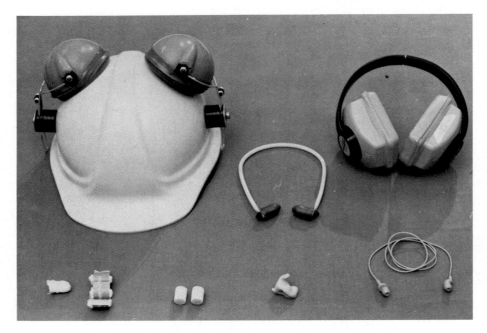

FIG. 25-5. Typical industrial ear defenders. *Above, left and right,* Earmuffs. *Below and center,* Earplugs.

law by the president. This law supplements and supersedes, in some instances, the provisions of the Walsh-Healey Public Contracts Act, passed in 1969. Although the act covers many aspects of occupational safety, it has specific provisions regarding occupational hearing losses. It makes mandatory certain industrial conservation-of-hearing actions that shall be taken by industry. The law has the following provisions:

1. Sets maximal permissible noise levels and exposures
2. Demands protection against the effects of noise when certain specified noise levels are exceeded
3. Differentiates intermittent and continuous noise, the latter being defined as noise with intervals between maximal peaks of 1 second or less
4. Requires industry to use *feasible* administrative and/or engineering controls to protect against excessive noise exposure
5. Demands the provision of personal protective equipment if other controls (as noted in provision 4, above) are ineffective
6. Requires a "continuing, effective hearing conservation program" to be administered in all cases in which sound levels exceed the values stated in the act

Thus industry, with the necessary help and advice of the medical and audiologic professions, will be required to perform extensive hearing testing and to provide sound-treated construction, sound-protected equipment, sound-treated booths for workmen in certain areas, and many other changes, such as those in work schedules and in the distance of workers from machinery.

Monetary compensation for hearing loss caused by industrial noise exposure is unique because the compensation is often awarded even though the injury (hearing loss) has not required time off the job or loss of wages. The actual dollar amount of compensation varies from state to state. Attempts are being made to standardize such awards on a national level. Therefore, before the physician calculates a percentage of loss caused by occupational noise, he must be aware of the legal method of calculating such loss in his own state.

Hearing loss resulting from endolymphatic hydrops (Meniere's syndrome). Endolymphatic hydrops causes a fluctuating type of sensorineural hearing loss of low tones (Fig. 25-6). As the disease progresses, the loss becomes greater, involves all tones, and may even become total. Usually it is unilateral. Recruitment of loudness

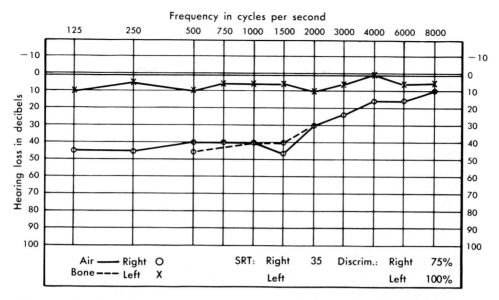

FIG. 25-6. Audiogram of typical hearing loss seen in patients with endolymphatic hydrops (Meniere's syndrome). Note the sensorineural loss of low tones. Note also that the loss of discrimination is more serious than one would expect with fairly good high-tone hearing.

and diplacusis are often demonstrated in labyrinthine hydrops (see Chapter 20).

Other causes of sensorineural hearing loss are tumors of the posterior fossa, particularly in the cerebellopontine angle; multiple sclerosis; cochlear invasion by otosclerosis; and idiopathic losses, the origins of which may never be determined.

Acoustic neuroma. Acoustic neuroma as a cause of hearing loss is rather rare, but it deserves special attention because of its great importance. Usually the first symptom is tinnitus; the onset of hearing loss may be delayed months or years. In *late* stages there will be vertigo of a constant, usually mild type, and finally facial paralysis as the seventh and eighth cranial nerves are compressed in the internal auditory canal. Tumors that grow large enough to expand into the cerebellopontile angle produce the symptoms of an intracranial space-occupying lesion.

Early diagnosis of acoustic neuroma is made on the basis of a suspicion of unilateral sensorineural hearing loss or tinnitus. Special hearing tests may pinpoint the site of the lesion and thus differentiate between a cochlear and a neural hearing loss. One common finding is that the patient's *discrimination score is unduly poor in comparison with his ability to hear pure tones.* Roentgenograms of the internal auditory meatus (especially in the Stenver's projection), made with a planigraphic or polytomographic technique, may show a widening of the internal auditory meatus. If widening has taken place, or even if it has not but acoustic neuroma is still suspected, a pantopaque study of the acoustic meatus (using only 1 ml. of dye) may show a characteristic filling defect. A computed tomographic (CAT) scan may be even more specific (Figs. 25-7 and 25-8).

Treatment is by surgical removal. Small and medium-size tumors can be resected through a middle cranial fossa or translabyrinthine approach, whereas large tumors are probably best approached through the posterior cranial fossa by neurosurgical techniques.

Sudden deafness. Sudden deafness, unilateral and sensorineural, and usually profound, may appear instantaneously in a person who just previously had no apparent hearing loss. Some patients say they hear a "click" in one ear and then realize they are deaf in that ear. Others go to bed hearing normally but wake up deaf in one ear and thus are uncertain must when their deafness commenced. Subsequently, over a period of days or weeks, this profound loss may

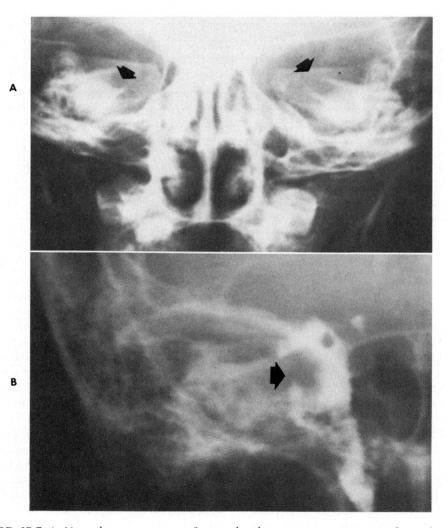

FIG. 25-7. A, Normal roentgenogram of internal auditory meatuses. Arrows indicate the right and left meatuses. **B,** Pantopaque dye study showing acoustic tumor in the internal auditory meatus.

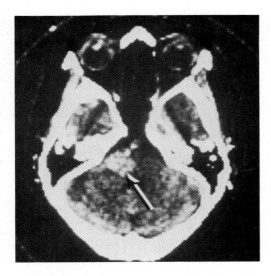

FIG. 25-8. CAT scan. Arrow points to acoustic tumor.

lessen, at least a little, and in some cases there is complete recovery.

Vertigo as an associated symptom is inconstant. Some patients become sick and vomit and are incapacitated for several days. Others have only a transient and mild vertigo lasting for a few hours. Many have no vertigo. Caloric tests do not always correlate well with the degree of vertigo. Tinnitus, although common, is not always present.

The clinical entity of sudden, profound, sensorineural, unilateral hearing loss was long considered a vascular accident, but more recently, viral factors began to be recognized as causative. We have long known, for example, that mumps is the most common cause of profound unilateral hearing loss in children, but who would suspect that in a child or an adult *without* obvious parotitis, mumps viremia could be a cause? Yet this virus, along with other viral agents, is now clearly demonstrated as a cause of sudden deafness. It seems clear that sudden unilateral sensorineural hearing loss unrelated to otitis media or to trauma may be the result of any one of a number of etiologic agents.

Exploratory tympanotomy may demonstrate a leakage of perilymph fluid into the middle ear through a fistula in the round or oval window, or both. These leaks may occur spontaneously or be caused by sudden exertion or trauma.

Idiopathic sudden deafness has been treated with a great variety of drugs, including vasodila-tors and steroids, but it is not certain whether any of them have been helpful. The only alternative to treatment, however, is to do nothing, and most physicians prefer to hospitalize these patients and offer therapy with either steroids or vasodilators, or both. If a patient is seen soon after the loss occurs (1 to 3 days), strict bed rest for 3 to 4 days may be the most effective management.

Treatment. There is no known specific treatment for hearing loss caused by cochlear or eighth nerve damage, except in labyrinthine hydrops. In spite of many attempts to treat patients with such hearing loss with vitamins, vasodilators, antibiotics, steroids, and other means, the only improvement obtained comes from the ability of the body to repair injured tissue. The best procedure for reducing the incidence of perceptive hearing loss is prevention of the known causes. When perceptive hearing loss is greater than 40 decibels (ISO, 1964) in the speech frequencies, usable hearing can be attained with an electric hearing aid.

CONDUCTIVE HEARING LOSS

Conductive hearing loss occurs when sound cannot reach the cochlea. The blockage may be due to abnormality of the canal, eardrum, or ossicles, including the footplate of the stapes. Lesions central to the footplate produce sensorineural hearing loss.

Hearing loss owing to obstruction of the external auditory canal. The external auditory canal can be obstructed by impacted cerumen, foreign bodies in the canal, tumors, and swelling of the canal during infection of the external ear. The most common cause is impacted cerumen. Still another cause is atresia of the external auditory canal, a congenital condition in which the external auditory canal fails to develop normally. It is sometimes associated with a mandibular deformity or an underdeveloped pinna. There may be bony closure of the external canal with a normal pinna, or there may be complete absence of the canal and external ear.

A syndrome related to maldevelopment of the external ear is known as Treacher Collins syndrome or sometimes as mandibulofacial dysostosis (Fig. 25-9). In addition to abnormality of the external and middle ear, there are agenesis of the mandible, poorly developed eyelashes in the medial part of the lower lid, and hypoplasia

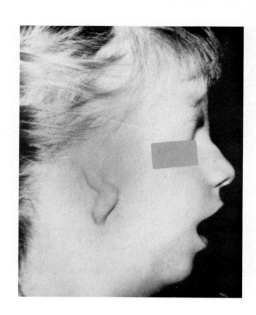

FIG. 25-9. Treacher Collins syndrome. Note the atretic ear canal, underdeveloped pinna, and recessed, underdeveloped mandible.

of the malar bones. There is a marked hereditary tendency in this condition. The hearing loss may be the result of both external and middle ear deformities. Treatment may be possible both for correction of certain cosmetic deformities and for improvement of the hearing loss.

The Pierre Robin syndrome is characterized by hypoplasia of the mandible, usually associated with a tendency of the tongue to fall posteriorly and block the pharynx. The same condition may be part of the Treacher Collins syndrome, but when it occurs independently, without other anomalies, it is known as Pierre Robin syndrome and is not associated with abnormalities of the ear.

Hearing loss owing to damage to the eardrum and middle ear. The eardrum may be affected as the result of thickening (as in tympanosclerosis), scarring, perforation, or retraction. Hearing loss in the middle ear may be caused by liquid (pus, serum, or blood), absent or decreased mobility of the ossicles (tympanosclerosis or otosclerosis), adhesions, tumors, or dislocated or absent ossicles (congenital or acquired).

Hearing loss resulting from otosclerosis. Otosclerosis is the most common cause of conductive hearing loss (Fig. 25-10) in people between the ages of 15 and 50 years. It is a hereditary defect of unknown cause. According to postmortem studies, 10% of the white population have otosclerosis. It is not common in blacks. Women are affected more often than men.

In otosclerosis, dystrophy occurs in the bony labyrinth (otic capsule). Normal bone is absorbed and replaced by otosclerotic bone, which is highly vascular and tends to overgrow the normal bony labyrinth. When the otosclerotic bone advances posteriorly from its usual site of origin (immediately anterior to the oval window), it causes progressive fixation of the footplate of the stapes, which is manifested by a slowly progressive conductive hearing loss. In women it may progress more rapidly during or immediately after pregnancy, but no definite causal relationship has been established. The eardrum usually appears normal. Occasionally a faint pink blush can be seen through the eardrum. This coloration is called Schwartze's sign and represents the vascularity in active otosclerotic bone.

Hearing loss is usually first noticed in the late teens or early twenties. Both ears are usually affected, but not always. Although otosclerosis characteristically produces more conductive hearing loss, it can involve neural elements and cause a mixed hearing loss or a sensorineural hearing loss. *If cochlear function is normal or near normal*, the hearing loss produced by otosclerosis can be improved by surgical means.

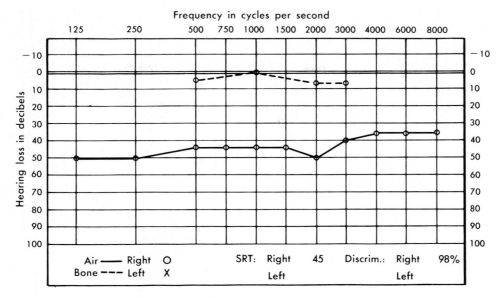

FIG. 25-10. Audiogram typical of otosclerosis (right ear). The normal bone conduction response indicates excellent cochlear function. This is reinforced by a normal discrimination score. Corrective surgery (stapedectomy) or a properly fitted hearing aid should provide excellent hearing.

Treatment. In most patients with conductive hearing loss the condition can be improved by treatment, and normal hearing can be restored in many. Treatment of hearing loss from occlusion of the external auditory canal is discussed in Chapter 22. Loss of hearing caused by disease of the middle ear is corrected partially or completely by treatment of the underlying disease, discussed in Chapter 24 as well as here.

The surgical treatment for conductive hearing loss resulting from various causes is described below.

HEARING LOSS RESULTING FROM CONGENITAL ATRESIA (Fig. 25-11). In almost all patients with atresia, the cochlea is functioning. Therefore a bone-conduction hearing aid can be worn to restore hearing loss. Restoration of useful hearing is also possible by means of an operation. The steps of the procedure recommended are as follows:

1. A simple mastoidectomy is performed through a postaural incision (Fig. 24-6).
2. The middle ear is located, and the bony plate that represents the tympanic membrane is removed. A new canal is fashioned from the bone.
3. If the malleus and incus are fused, they are removed. The stapes is left. If the malleus and incus are normal and mobile, they are left in place.
4. The entire cavity (mastoid and middle ear) is covered with a skin graft applied to the malleus or to the head of the stapes. The cavity is packed firmly.
5. An external opening is made in the soft tissue.
6. *Later*, if a satisfactory hearing improvement is not maintained, the skin graft can be lifted from the horizontal semicircular canal and a fenestration operation performed (see pp. 361 to 362).

The operation described is usually not recommended if the atresia is unilateral and the uninvolved ear has normal hearing.

HEARING LOSS RESULTING FROM OTHER CONGENITAL DEFECTS. Sometimes patients with conductive hearing loss (but not otosclerosis) have a normal or nearly normal tympanic membrane and a history of deafness since early life. The diagnosis is not readily apparent, and it may be necessary to explore the middle ear to ascertain the cause of hearing loss and to correct it

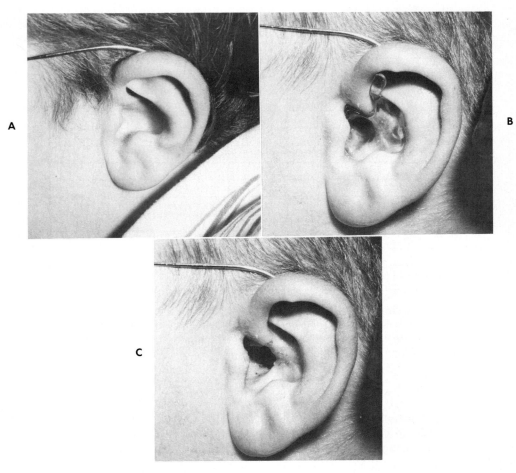

FIG. 25-11. A, Congenital atresia of the external auditory canal. The pinna is well formed in the patient shown. However, it may be small, distorted, or absent entirely. **B** and **C,** Surgical correction of atresia of the external auditory canal. **B,** Postoperative skin-lined cavity is kept open by an acrylic mold. **C,** Final result after healing; the mold is discarded. (From DeWeese, D.D.: Portland Clin. Bull. **8:**63, 1954.)

if possible during the same operative procedure. A transcanal approach is used, and a flap is turned similar to the one used for stapedectomy (Fig. 25-16).

Once the drumhead is reflected, the middle ear can be inspected. One may find, for example, a missing long crus of the incus or a missing lenticular process of the incus. In the former, the remaining part of the incus may be pulled down from the epitympanum and repositioned on the head of the stapes or between the stapes and malleus. If only the lenticular process is absent, a piece of cartilage from the tragus may be removed and wedged between the head of the stapes and the long crus of the incus.

Sometimes the bodies of the incus and malleus are fused by tympanosclerosis in the epitympanum and must be removed to free the ossicular chain. If the superstructure of the stapes is missing and the body of the incus still remains, it is possible to establish a connection between the malleus and the stapedial footplate by removing and modeling the incus and carefully interposing it, or a prosthetic incus may be used to connect the malleus and footplate.

Thus there are a great many variations in the middle ear anatomy that must be anticipated with congenital middle ear problems. Most of them are amenable to surgery, but usually exploratory tympanotomy is necessary before one

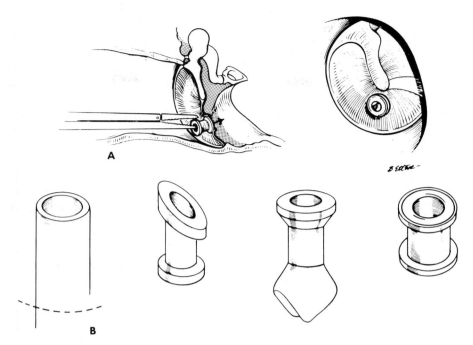

FIG. 25-12. A, Plastic tubular buttons in place through the tympanic membrane. **B,** Various types of plastic tubes and buttons used in serous otitis media.

can be certain as to just what technique will be required.

HEARING LOSS RESULTING FROM SEROUS OTITIS MEDIA. Removal of serum or thick mucoid secretion from the middle ear is necessary in some patients with serous otitis media. A myringotomy is performed. The incision of the tympanic membrane is made in a radial direction, and liquid is removed by suction. Tenacious fluid must be removed by using both suction and small middle ear forceps (Fig. 24-3). Both types of fluid may also be forced out of the middle ear by gentle inflation of the eustachian tube.

In adults myringotomy through the normal eardrum can be performed with little pain, even without anesthesia. In children a short period of anesthesia may be necessary. If there are no other contributing factors, the hearing often returns to normal immediately.

Patients with chronic (recurrent) serous otitis media may require myringotomy on many occasions. Sometimes it is beneficial to perform a myringotomy and to insert a polyethylene tube or a Teflon button (Fig. 25-12) through the eardrum and into the middle ear. The tube also allows aeration of the middle ear and appears to hasten recovery of eustachian tube obstruction, which has helped to create negative pressure in the middle ear. The myringotomy heals around the tube or button after a few hours. Often such tubes are left for several months or until they extrude spontaneously.

In children serous otitis media is often associated with large or recurrent adenoids. An adenoid hypertrophied enough to block the eustachian tube must often be removed to prevent further formation of serous fluid in the middle ear. If fluid has collected in the middle ear several times, adenoidectomy may be the only measure that will prevent further middle ear damage. In such patients it is important to remove adenoid tissue thoroughly. The lymphoid tissue behind the eustachian tube orifice (Rosenmüller's fossa) must be removed *under direct vision* for best results.

HEARING LOSS RESULTING FROM OTOSCLEROSIS

FENESTRATION. Creation of a surgical window into the labyrinth for improvement of hearing loss resulting from otosclerosis was first reported in 1914. The first successful one-stage operation that maintained an open surgical window was reported in 1938 by Dr. Julius Lempert. Although rarely used now, it remains a practical and safe surgical approach to otosclerosis.

The fenestration operation does not alter the disease process. It merely creates a new window into the labyrinth. This new window serves the function of the obstructed oval window. Even if the otosclerosis later involves the cochlea and produces cochlear damage, useful hearing has been created during a productive period of life.

The steps in the fenestration operation are as follows:

1. The mastoid is exposed through an endaural incision. A partial mastoidectomy is performed.
2. The bony wall between the external auditory canal and the mastoid cavity is removed. A flap is formed from the skin of the external auditory canal.
3. The incus and the head of the malleus are removed. The stapes is left in its fixed position. The eardrum is partially mobilized.
4. A small window is slowly ground through the horizontal semicircular canal directly adjacent to the oval window.
5. The perilymphatic space is exposed, with the membranous labyrinth left intact. The skin flap attached to the eardrum is used to cover the new window and to seal off the middle ear. The cavity is then tightly packed.

This operation creates a mobile window into the labyrinth through which sound waves reach the cochlea. Thus the fixed stapes and immobile oval window are bypassed (Figs. 25-13 and 25-15).

The fenestration procedure is of great historical interest but is rarely performed today, since it has been supplanted by the various stapes mobilization and stapedectomy procedures. Because of loss of the mechanical advantage of the middle ear (some 27 decibels), the fenestration operation, which circumvents the middle ear, can never approximate normal hearing.

STAPES MOBILIZATION. Since 1876 attempts have been made to mobilize a fixed stapes. The early efforts gave poor results and were aban-

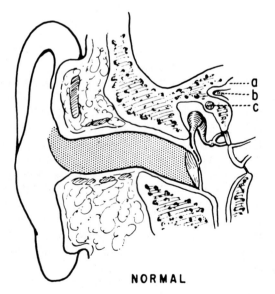 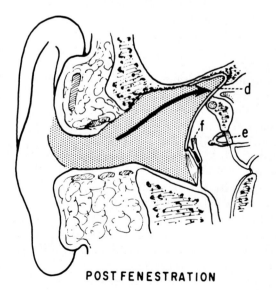

NORMAL   **POST FENESTRATION**

FIG. 25-13. Fenestration of the labyrinth for otosclerosis. *a*, Perilymphatic space of the horizontal semicircular canal. *b*, Membranous semicircular canal. *c*, Facial nerve. *d*, Skin of the ear canal attached to the eardrum and molded into the cavity to cover the fenestra made through the bony wall of the labyrinth. *e*, Stapes still fixed in the oval window. *f*, Neck of the malleus. The incus and the head of the malleus have been removed.

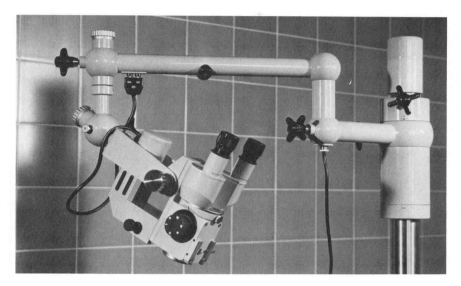

FIG. 25-14. Operating microscope used during stapes mobilization, stapedectomy, fenestration, and tympanoplasty. The parfocal lens system allows a change from 6- to 25-power magnification.

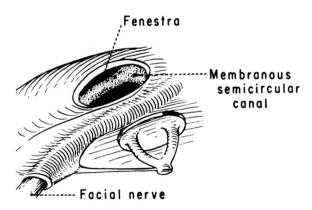

FIG. 25-15. Fenestra made in the horizontal semicircular canal for otosclerosis. The incus has been removed. The fenestra is ready to be covered by a flap fashioned from the eardrum and the skin of the external auditory canal.

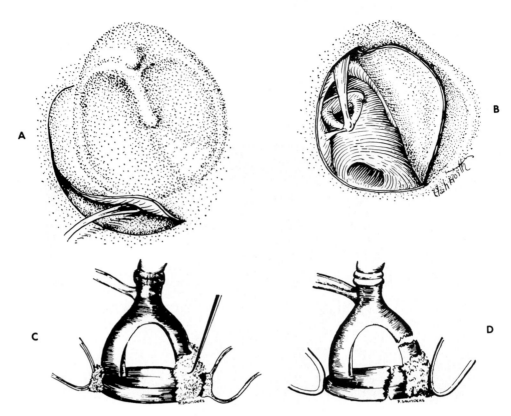

FIG. 25-16. Stapes mobilization. **A,** Incision in the posterior ear canal wall. **B,** Operative field seen through the ear speculum. **C,** Fracturing through the otosclerotic focus. **D,** Anterior crurotomy technique—the otosclerotic focus is bypassed.

doned about 1917. Subsequent improvements in lighting and in magnification (and the advent of antibiotics) enabled Dr. Samuel Rosen, in 1952, to carry out a successful mobilization operation.

The fenestration operation bypasses the fixed stapes and substitutes a new window for the immobile oval window. The stapes mobilization operation reestablishes the normal pathway of sound to the cochlea and improves hearing, often to normal. It is performed as follows:

1. With the patient under local anesthesia, two linear incisions are made in the posterior half of the external canal (Fig. 25-16, *A*). A third incision connects the first two incisions. The skin between the incisions is elevated.

2. Usually the incus and stapes are not immediately visible; bone of the ear canal is therefore removed for better exposure (Fig. 25-16, *B*).

3. Mobilization of the stapes is attempted under 10- to 25-power magnification by one of several methods: (1) application of pressure to the stapes through the crus of the incus, (2) application of pressure and manipulation directly to the head or neck of the stapes, (3) prying or chiseling of the otosclerotic bone around the footplate of the stapes, and (4) fracture of the anterior crus and cutting across the footplate to mobilize the posterior part of the footplate (Fig. 25-16, *C* and *D*).

4. The eardrum and the skin flap attached to it are replaced in normal position.

The advantages of stapes mobilization over fenestration are a shorter period of hospitalization, minimal postoperative care, and attainment of better hearing than can be produced by fenestration. When good mobilization is accomplished, the hearing improvement is immediate and dramatic. Such immediate improvement

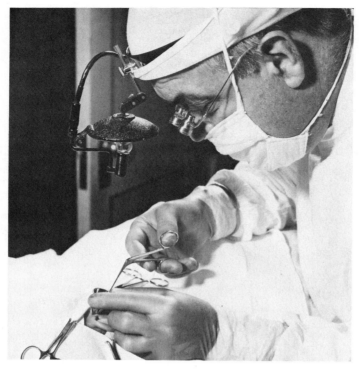

FIG. 25-17. Stapes mobilization and stapedectomy. Preliminary exposure of the middle ear is made through an ear speculum with a magnifying loupe. Note that the surgeon is wearing a head light. After exposure the operating microscope is used for greater magnification.

can be attained in 60% to 70% of properly selected patients. However, refixation of the stapes, either by new otosclerotic growth or by healing of the fractured footplate margin, occurs in approximately half of the successful cases.

The stapes mobilization procedure has been largely replaced by partial or total stapedectomy because of the high incidence of refixation of the stapes after mobilization. It is still indicated in carefully selected cases.

Both the fenestration and the stapes mobilization operations can impair hearing.

STAPEDECTOMY. When the initial good results of stapes mobilization began to fail, giving an overall, lasting result in less than 30% of patients, further procedures were devised. In 1957 Shea first reported success in removing the stapes with its footplate and replacing it with a prosthetic stapes made of polyethylene tubing. Since then, many modifications have been devised (Fig. 25-18).

Regardless of the method or material used to replace the stapes, the results of hearing improvement are statistically nearly identical. In properly selected patients who retain normal or nearly normal bone conduction, usable (and often normal) hearing can be restored 90% to 95% of the time.

Some patients do not improve in spite of careful stapedectomy and prosthetic replacement. The risk of damage to the cochlea and permanent (or total) hearing loss is reported to be from 2% to 6% of all ears operated on. This potential risk must always be considered before a decision is made to perform a stapedectomy. There are also patients who have initial good results but who later show slow cochlear damage.

In a few patients the overgrowth of otosclerotic bone is too dense to allow removal of the stapes. In some of these patients a hole can be drilled in the footplate and a Teflon piston attached to the incus can be inserted (Fig. 25-18,

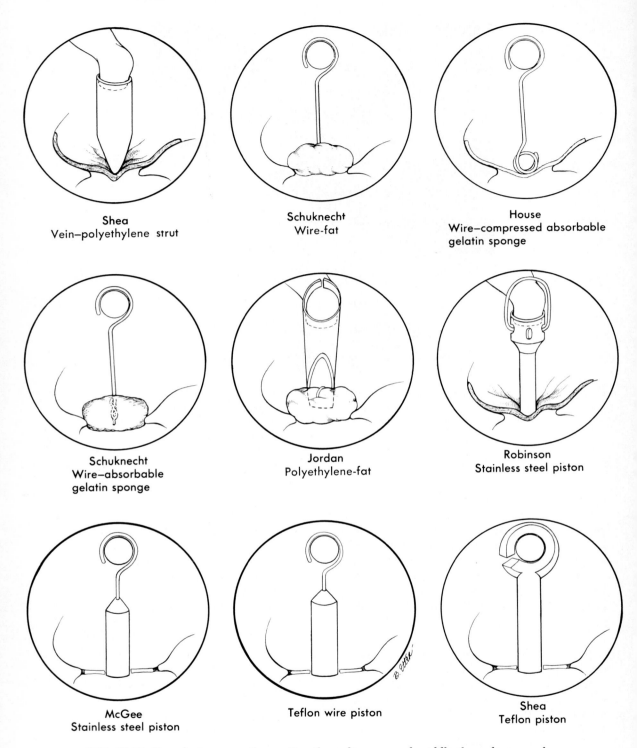

Shea
Vein—polyethylene strut

Schuknecht
Wire-fat

House
Wire—compressed absorbable
gelatin sponge

Schuknecht
Wire—absorbable
gelatin sponge

Jordan
Polyethylene-fat

Robinson
Stainless steel piston

McGee
Stainless steel piston

Teflon wire piston

Shea
Teflon piston

FIG. 25-18. Stapedectomy prostheses. Top three diagrams and middle three diagrams show various prostheses used after footplate has been removed. Bottom three diagrams indicate that the footplate has been "drilled" to precisely accept a prefabricated piston. (From Saunders, W.H., Paparella, M.M., and Miglets, A.W.: Atlas of ear surgery, ed. 3, St. Louis, 1980, The C.V. Mosby Co.)

5). In a few such patients fenestration is still the procedure of choice.

Good hearing may be maintained for many years. However, a high percentage of slowly progressive cochlear losses may occur. For this reason it may be best to delay performing a stapedectomy on the opposite ear of the same patient until 1 or 2 years after the first operation.

In some instances after a stapedectomy has been performed, there is incomplete closure of the oval window. Perilymph may then leak around the prosthesis and into the middle ear. If such a leak continues, the hearing level, which has been improved by the operation, may fluctuate widely or may suddenly diminish. Such changes may also be accompanied by tinnitus or by mild or very sudden intense vertigo. Whenever a patient who has undergone stapedectomy complains of fluctuating hearing, increasing tinnitus, or recurrent or abrupt vertigo, a perilymph leak should be suspected. Often the operation must be repeated and the leak repaired to preserve the hearing improvement and, in some cases, to prevent further serious and irreversible loss of hearing.

MEDICAL TREATMENT. In addition to the several surgical procedures devised for the correction of hearing loss caused by otosclerosis, a medical treatment has been suggested. Sodium fluoride is said to promote recalcification and inactivation of an actively expanding demineralized focus of otospongiosis, resulting in stabilization of a progressive sensorineural hearing loss. Thus the drug is used, not to correct the element of conductive hearing loss that has already taken place, but to prevent the superimposed sensorineural loss that sometimes occurs. Not all authorities are in agreement concerning the effectiveness of the treatment.

Various dosages are recommended. A common one is 40 to 60 mg. sodium fluoride daily for 6 months with 1,000 mg. calcium also taken daily at separate times from the fluoride.

HEARING LOSS RESULTING FROM CHRONIC SUPPURATIVE OTITIS MEDIA. The aim of most temporal bone surgery is eradication of infection. Radical or modified radical mastoidectomy requires removal of part or all of the eardrum, the mucosa of the middle ear, the malleus, and the incus. Such an operation is still necessary to control infection in some patients with extensive chronic suppurative otitis media. After the ears are free of infection, reconstruction by tympanoplasty may be possible. As a separate procedure, radical mastoidectomy is not performed nearly as often now as formerly.

TYMPANOPLASTY

Indications. Tympanoplasty is indicated in patients in whom chronic suppurative otitis media has produced a significant conductive hearing loss. The patient must have good nerve function (cochlear reserve) if hearing is to be improved. The greater the difference between the air and bone measurements, the greater are the chances for improvement. The operation is indicated especially in patients with bilateral ear disease. They suffer more from hearing loss than do patients in whom only one ear is affected.

It must be noted in passing that tympanoplasty may at times be performed for reasons other than improvement of hearing. For example, there are patients with a perforation of the tympanic membrane who have essentially normal hearing but who still need tympanoplasty to close the perforation. Others, who may have chronic suppurative otitis media but a sensorineural rather than a conductive hearing loss, still require tympanoplasty as part of an operative procedure to help clear infection, even though there is no likelihood of improving their hearing.

Tympanoplasty also may be used in patients with no perforation of the drumhead, such as those with traumatic defects (dislocation of the incus), those with congenital middle ear problems, and those in whom tympanosclerosis has fused the malleus to the incus. Here the problems are ossicular and may involve the use of metal or plastic prostheses, autogenous material (especially in incus transposition), or ossicles removed from cadavers. In these cases the results often are surprisingly good, since there is no concomitant infection.

Contraindications. Tympanoplasty is contraindicated in patients whose cochlear reserve is poor (as tested by bone conduction), in some patients whose conductive deafness is not due to chronic suppurative disease (for example, otosclerosis or serous otitis media), and in some patients with extensive mastoid disease that cannot be cleared effectively in a one-stage procedure that includes mastoidectomy and tympanoplasty. In such patients a two-stage procedure may be necessary—the first to clear infection and the second to reconstruct the hearing mechanism.

Principles. In Chapter 19 we learned that the normal ear provides a great mechanical advantage to sound pressure by means of a *transformer action.* This is made possible in small part by the lever action of the ossicles and in great part by the tympanic membrane–footplate ratio (areal ratio). This mechanical advantage afforded by the middle ear explains its chief purpose. It must regain as much as possible of the sound pressure that is lost when sound is transferred from air to a liquid medium. The transformer action of the middle ear is effective in recovering some 25 to 27 of the 30 decibels lost.

Also of importance in the normal schema of hearing is the sound protection afforded to the round window by the presence of an intact tympanic membrane. In the normal ear the round window acts as a relief hole for sound pressure driven into the cochlea across the ossicular chain. If it were not for this sound protection, sound waves could reach both windows simultaneously and cause a cancellation effect. If sound waves enter the round window in phase with those entering the oval window (as can occur where the eardrum is missing), there is a partial cancellation effect. But when the phase of the sound waves is shifted by the tympanic membrane, any sound waves entering the round window are thrown out of phase. The result may be a small summation effect that assists hearing. In chronic otitis media, in which the tympanic membrane (and often the malleus and incus) is partially or completely absent, sound waves can enter both windows with approximately equal intensity. Therefore there is a chance for partial cancellation. More important, with loss of the eardrum the areal ratio is lost or reduced. Then the transformer action of the middle ear becomes virtually nil.

Tympanoplasty improves hearing by reestablishing two important middle ear functions: (1) it restores the areal ratio (which is the chief component of the transformer action) and (2) it creates sound protection for the round window.

Originally five types of tympanoplasty were described, and for several years most surgeons used these groupings and patterned their surgery to fit. More recently, however, innovations have come about that do not conform to any of the original five types of tympanoplasty. These innovations are discussed below. In types I, II, and III tympanoplasty *both* the areal ratio *and* sound protection are restored (Table 7; Figs. 25-19 to 25-21). Autogenous tissue, usually fascia taken from the temporalis area but sometimes tissue from a vein or other tissue, is used to repair or replace the tympanic membrane and to seal a pocket of air (the new middle ear) in front of the round window. Types I, II, and III tympanoplasty are possible when enough of the ossicular chain remains (at least the entire stapes) to allow creation of a new areal ratio. Types IV and V, on the other hand, provide *only* sound protection for the round window; the areal ratio cannot be restored. In type IV

TABLE 7. Tympanoplastic procedures—as originally described

Type	Damage to middle ear	Methods of repair
I	Perforated tympanic membrane with normal ossicular chain	Closure of perforation; type I same as myringoplasty
II	Perforation of tympanic membrane with erosion of malleus	Closure with graft against incus or remains of malleus
III	Destruction of tympanic membrane and ossicular chain *but with* intact and mobile stapes	Graft contacts normal stapes; also give sound protection for round window
IV	Similar to type III but with head, neck, and crura of stapes missing; footplate mobile	Mobile footplate left exposed; air pocket between round window and graft provides sound protection for round window
V	Similar to type IV plus *fixed* footplate	Fenestra in horizontal semicircular canal; graft seals off middle ear to give sound protection for round window

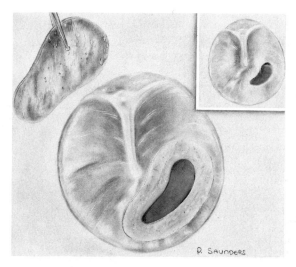

FIG. 25-19. Tympanoplasty—type I (also called myringoplasty). Usually, more of the squamous epithelium is removed from the tympanic membrane to give a broader base for the graft.

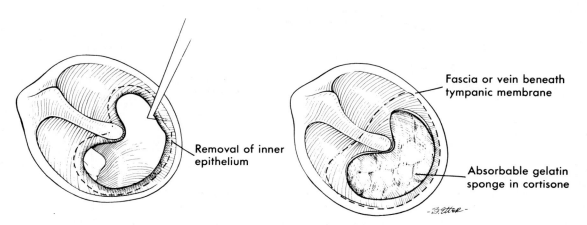

FIG. 25-20. Type I tympanoplasty (myringoplasty) performed by placing the graft against the medial surface of the drumhead. Epithelium is removed from the rim of the perforation, and the fascia or vein is placed beneath the tympanic membrane. Absorbable gelatin sponge must first be placed in the middle ear to support the graft against the undersurface of the drumhead. (From Saunders, W.H., and Paparella, M.M.: Atlas of ear surgery, ed. 2, St. Louis, 1971, The C.V. Mosby Co.)

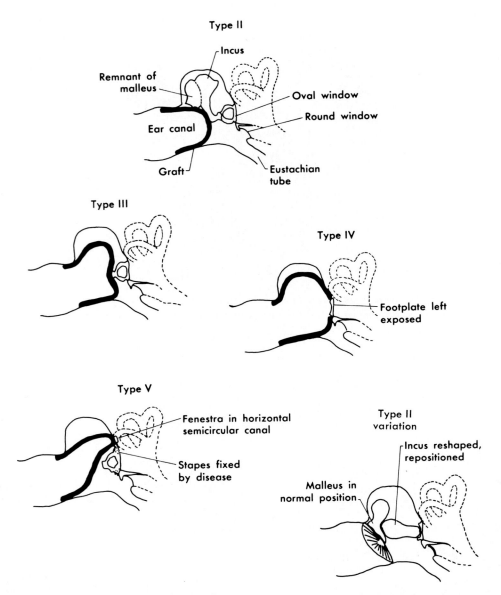

FIG. 25-21. Different types of tympanoplasty. In each diagram a graft (fascia, perichondrium) is indicated by the heavy line. The diagram of type V illustrates fenestration, and the diagram of the type II variation shows correction of an ossicular defect without a tympanic membrane perforation.

tympanoplasty only the footplate remains. In type V the footplate is fixed by disease, and a new opening into the inner ear must be made.

Thus, at least in theory, types I, II, and III tympanoplasty should result in normal hearing because they restore both the transformer action of the middle ear and sound protection for the round window. In types IV and V, however, even though good sound protection is established, the transformer action is lost. In these types the best hearing to be expected is that which would be present without the transformer action—a loss of about 25 to 27 decibels from normal.

INCUS INTERPOSITION. In incus interposition the incus is detached from the malleus (usually the long crus connecting the incus to the stapes has been destroyed when this procedure is needed). After the short crus and any remaining part of the long crus are cut off, the incus is drilled carefully to fit the head of the stapes and held in place by tiny pieces of Gelfoam. The incus may be notched at its other end to fit the malleus; it may contact only the head of the stapes and the covering graft of fascia when the malleus is missing. Sometimes this procedure is performed when there is no active suppurative disease—for example, in healed chronic otitis media in which the tympanic membrane is present, so that a fascial graft is not needed. In general, the use of either an autogenous or a homologous incus interposed between a mobile stapes and an intact tympanic membrane or fascia graft gives very good hearing, better than would ordinarily be achieved by type III or IV tympanoplasty. Even better results can be obtained if the interposed bone is drilled and shaped in such a fashion that there is *a secure fitting to the head of the stapes and at the handle of the malleus.* Thus a small facet will accommodate the head of the stapes, and a deep groove at the opposite end will fit the head or neck of the malleus. Good results demand a secure fit of all parts.

USE OF HOMOLOGOUS TYMPANIC MEMBRANE. Some surgeons now use a tympanic membrane, including the annulus and malleus, taken from a human cadaver. After the membrane is treated in a solution of alcohol, it is used as a graft, instead of fascia. Results are said to be good, but not enough evaluation has been done yet to be certain of the efficacy of this particular graft.

OTHER PROSTHESES. Sometimes, in place of an incus, a piece of cortical bone from the patient's mastoid is chiseled free and used to bridge the gap between a mobile stapedial footplate (when the head and crura are missing) and the tympanic membrane or fascia graft. Metal and plastic prostheses have also been used.

Modifications and innovations of plastic replacements for middle ear structures continue to be devised. An example is the partial ossicular replacement prosthesis (PORP) shown in Fig. 25-22. Similarly, the total ossicular replacement prosthesis (TORP) can substitute for the entire ossicular chain if the footplate of the stapes is intact. It is probable that in the future even more efficient and acceptable prostheses will be produced and used.

TECHNIQUES. Many different approaches and techniques are used. Some surgeons use a postauricular approach, whereas others use an endaural approach. The use of full-thickness or split-thickness skin grafts, the original grafting materials, has been abandoned. A sliding skin graft fashioned from the inner part of the canal of the ear can be used successfully. Most surgeons now use fascia as the grafting material of choice.

Tympanoplasty may be performed even in the presence of mastoid or middle ear disease such as infection or cholesteatoma. Some surgeons prefer, in extensively diseased ears, to perform the operation in stages. When a tympanoplasty is performed to correct defects caused by chronic suppurative otitis media, the results probably are better if the suppurative disease has been cleared first. Then all that remains to be accomplished is mechanical correction of the deficient sound-transmitting system. The operation can be combined, however, with mastoidectomy in patients with active suppurative disease. In fact, exploration of the mastoid is advised as a part of tympanoplasty whenever there appears to be any likelihood of such disease. Sometimes, good results are obtained when the posterior wall of the ear canal is left standing rather than being removed by radical or modified radical mastoidectomy, followed by a tympanoplasty.

The eustachian tube must be patent for the middle ear to be replenished with air. An air-filled middle ear is necessary if there is to be an air pocket between the graft and the round window.

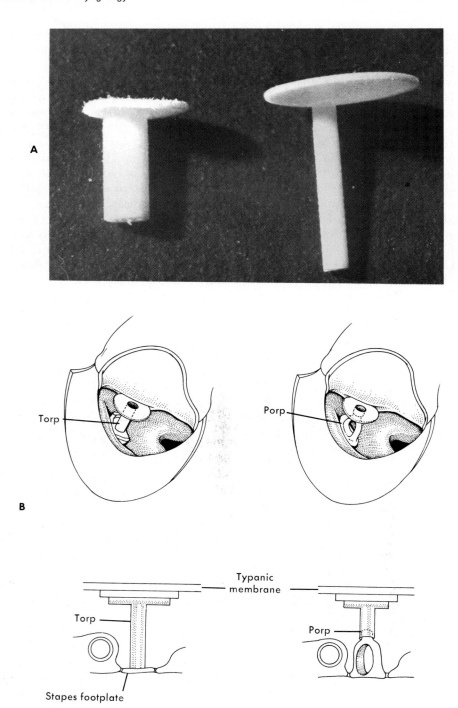

FIG. 25-22. A, *Left,* Partial ossicular replacement prosthesis (PORP). *Right,* Total ossicular replacement prosthesis (TORP). The PORP fits between the eardrum and the head of the stapes. The longer TORP fits between the eardrum and the footplate of the stapes. **B,** The left-hand figures (above and below) show total absence of the superstructure of the stapes. A TORP prosthesis is required. This may bridge from the footplate to the undersurface of a fascial graft, or it may bridge to the medial surface of the residual handle of the malleus. The right-hand figures (above and below) show the placement of the shorter PORP when most of the stapes still remains.

If the middle ear mucosa is in good condition, it is left undisturbed. However, if it has been replaced by squamous epithelium growing in from the ear canal through the perforated or absent drumhead, it must be removed. Then care is taken to interpose a nonadherent sheeting of Silastic between the denuded promontory and the new drumhead; otherwise, the fascia would adhere to the promontory and obliterate the middle ear space. In addition, Gelfoam often is placed in the middle ear space to support the new graft temporarily. As the Gelfoam is absorbed and the eustachian tube begins to ventilate the ear, an air channel is created from the tube to the round window. The fascial graft picks up a blood supply from the remains of the tympanic membrane or from the adjacent bony wall of the ear canal. As noted in Figs. 25-19 and 25-21, the fascia may be placed slightly external to the drumhead after its squamous epithelium is removed or internal to the drumhead, where it is invaginated through the perforation and supported by a bed of Gelfoam.

HEARING LOSS RESULTING FROM TRAUMA. Sensorineural hearing loss resulting from trauma was discussed previously. Trauma may cause hearing loss of the conductive type by lacerating the drumhead, dislocating or fracturing an ossicle, and so on. If such injuries do not repair themselves spontaneously, tympanoplasty or exploratory tympanotomy usually affords a good hearing result.

SELECTED READINGS

Bergsma, D.: Birth defects atlas and compendium, Baltimore, 1973, The Williams & Wilkins Co.

Black, F.O., and others: Congenital deafness, Boulder, Colo., 1971, Colorado Associated University Press.

Bohne, B.A., Ward, P.H., and Fernandez, C.: Rock music and inner ear damage, Am. Fam. Physician **15**:117, 1977.

Davis, K.R., and others: Computed tomography of acoustic neuroma, Radiology **124**:81, 1977.

Derkacki, E.L.: Office closure of central tympanic membrane perforation; a quarter century of experience, Trans. Am. Acad. Ophthalmol. Otolaryngol. **77**:53, 1973.

Eden, A.R., and Cummings, F.R.: Sudden bilateral hearing loss and meningitis in adults, J. Otolaryngol. **7**:304, 1978.

Farmer, J.C.: Diving injuries to the inner ear, Ann. Otol. Rhinol. Laryngol. **86**(suppl. 36), 1977.

Fox, M.S.: Industrial noise; its medical, economic, and social aspects, Am. J. Med. Sci. **223**:447, 1952.

Karmody, C.S., and Schuknecht, H.F.: Deafness in congenital syphilis, Arch. Otolaryngol. **83**:44, 1966.

Keim, R.J.: Sensorineural hearing loss associated with firearms, Arch. Otolaryngol. **90**:581, 1969.

Lempert, J.: Fenestra nov-ovalis; new oval window for improvement of hearing in cases of otosclerosis, Arch. Otolaryngol. **34**:880, 1941.

Lindsay, J.R., and Zajtchuk, J.: Concussion of inner ear; Edmund P. Fowler Memorial Lecture, N. Engl. J. Med. **282**:467, 1970.

Lowell, S.H., and Paparella, M.M.: Presbycusis: what is it? Laryngoscope **87**:1710, 1977.

Meyerhoff, W.L.: Medical management of hearing loss, Laryngoscope **88**:960, 1978.

Miller, R.R.: Deafness due to plain and long-acting aspirin tablets, J. Clin. Pharmacol. **18**:468, 1978.

Nadol, J.B.: Hearing loss as a sequela of meningitis, Laryngoscope **88**:739, 1978.

Paparella, M.M.: Differential diagnosis of hearing loss, Laryngoscope **88**:952, 1978.

Pulec, J.L., and others: A system of management of acoustic neuroma based on 364 cases, Trans. Am. Assoc. Ophthalmol. Otol. **75**:48, 1971.

Rosenhall, U., and others: Auditory function after *Hemophilus influenzae* meningitis, Acta Otolaryngol. **85**:243, 1978.

Saunders, W.H., Paparella, M.M., and Miglets, A.W.: Atlas of ear surgery, ed. 3, St. Louis, 1980, The C.V. Mosby Co.

Schuknecht, H.F., and others: Atrophy of the stria vascularis; a common cause for hearing loss, Laryngoscope **84**:1777, 1974.

Selters, W.A., and Brackmann, D.E.: Acoustic tumor detection with brain stem electric response audiometry, Arch. Otolaryngol. **103**:181, 1977.

Shambaugh, G.E., Jr.: Medical therapy of otospongiosis, O.R.L. Digest, March 1976, p. 9.

Shea, J.J., and Kitabchi, A.E.: Management of fluctuant hearing loss, Arch. Otolaryngol. **97**:118, 1973.

Valvassori, G.E., Naunton, R.F., and Lindsay, J.R.: Inner ear anomalies; clinical and histopathologic considerations, Ann. Otol. **78**:929, 1969.

Warkany, J.: Congenital malformations, Chicao, 1971, Year Book Medical Publishers, Inc.

Wolferman, A.: Twenty-five years of tympanoplasty: critical evaluation, Ann. Otol. Rhinol. Laryngol. **86**(suppl. 37, part 2), March-April 1977.

Wullstein, H.: Restoration of the function of the middle ear in chronic otitis media, Ann. Otol. Rhinol. Laryngol. **65**:1020, 1956.

26 TINNITUS

Tinnitus is defined as a noise or ringing in the ear. It is usually subjective and audible only to the patient. Occasionally it is objective and audible to the examining physician who employs certain techniques. When tinnitus is slight, it may be annoying only at night or when the usual environmental noise is low. During most of the day, and especially when busy at work, the patient does not notice the ringing. When tinnitus is continous and loud, it may actually interfere with hearing and be so annoying that a neurosis develops. In rare instances of extremely loud tinnitus a patient may consider suicide.

Tinnitus is often a sign of disease of the ear, and it may be the first or only sign of such disease. Thorough aural and general systemic examinations must be made. In many instances the cause cannot be determined. Sometimes, when there are no other signs or symptoms to aid in diagnosis, the cause can only be suspected.

Subjective tinnitus. Subjective tinnitus may arise from a disturbance of the external ear, tympanic membrane, ossicles, cochlea, eighth nerve, brain stem, or cortex. The character of the tinnitus does not aid in determining the site of the disturbance. However, certain conditions are known to give rise to one type of tinnitus more often than to another.

Cerumen in the external canal, perforation of the tympanic membrane, or fluid in the middle ear may cause subjective tinnitus. This type of tinnitus most often causes a muffling of other sounds and a change in the patient's voice. The patient may describe his voice as sounding hollow. The tinnitus is usually low pitched, and it may be intermittent.

Sometime in its course, otosclerosis is almost always accompanied by tinnitus, which may last for months or years and then disappear as the disease progresses. The tinnitus associated with otosclerosis is variable. There may be ringing, roaring, or whistling sounds. Several sounds may occur together. When present, the tinnitus is constant. It does not fluctuate widely.

Inflammation of the middle ear may be accompanied by tinnitus that is often pulsating in character. The tinnitus subsides with the inflammation. Chronic infection of the middle ear is rarely accompanied by tinnitus. This observation has given rise to speculation that tinnitus is caused by irritation of the tympanic plexus of the middle ear. When the plexus has been destroyed by chronic infection, tinnitus no longer occurs. Although this theory has not been proved, surgical excision of the tympanic plexus has been performed to relieve tinnitus. Although the original results seem to have been successful, the operation has been abandoned.

In presbycusis and after acoustic trauma, tinnitus is usually high pitched and ringing in character. In these conditions the pitch of the tinnitus is usually near the frequency at which the hearing loss is greatest.

When tinnitus follows exposure to accustomed acoustic trauma, such as that produced by the firing of a high-powered rifle, it frequently is associated with temporary hearing loss. *The patient should be told that tinnitus serves as a warning: if he continues to expose his ears to excessive noise, he may lose his hearing permanently.* Anyone with tinnitus after exposure to loud noise should be careful to protect his ears against the noise before repeating the experience.

Certain drugs cause tinnitus. The same drugs are known to damage the cochlea or the eighth nerve. Such tinnitus is usually high pitched and may continue after the drug has been stopped. Quinine and salicylates commonly produce tinnitus when used over a prolonged period of time. In some patients only a small, single dose causes the ears to ring. Streptomycin, dihydro-streptomycin, neomycin, kanamycin, and similar, chemically related drugs may cause both tinnitus and hearing loss. Heavy metals, such as arsenic used in the treatment of syphilis, may cause the same damage. Often the onset of tinnitus is a warning that the drug should be discontinued before irreversible hearing loss occurs.

Vascular changes in the central nervous system associated with arteriosclerosis or hypertension commonly cause a high-pitched tinnitus. In hypertension, the tinnitus will often fluctuate with the blood pressure.

Tumors of the posterior fossa, particularly in the cerebellopontile angle, produce tinnitus early in their course. Continuous high-pitched or low-pitched tinnitus *may be the first symptom* of an acoustic neuroma and may precede loss of hearing or disturbance of equilibrium by several years.

Unilateral tinnitus is one of the triad of symptoms characterizing labyrinthine hydrops (Meniere's disease). The characteristic sound is low pitched and, although continuous, fluctuates in intensity. It may become quite loud immediately preceding an acute attack of vertigo, and it may almost disappear after the attack. When the disease is under control, the tinnitus partially subsides but usually does not disappear. Distortion of sounds and diplacusis also accompany Meniere's disease and, along with the annoying tinnitus, make the patient's hearing even worse than it seems to be on the pure-tone audiogram.

Anemia and low blood pressure may produce a variable tinnitus of mild intensity. The tinnitus usually clears when the anemia is controlled or the blood pressure brought back to normal.

Syphilis of the central nervous system may produce tinnitus, usually high pitched and continuous. Attacks of epilepsy and migraine may be preceded by tinnitus.

Some patients hear certain vascular sounds that are interpreted as tinnitus. Perhaps head noise would be a better term for these sounds produced during venous congestion or when plaques are present in the walls of the carotid arteries (pulsating or "swishing" tinnitus synchronous with the heartbeat may be heard).

Pressure over the common carotid artery may abolish this tinnitus temporarily. Some loud cardiac murmurs are transmitted to the skull and are heard as a pulsating tinnitus. Vascular tinnitus is usually low pitched.

Finally, some types of tinnitus are neurogenic or functional in origin. They have no characteristic sound. Examination of the ear and central nervous system reveals no cause for the tinnitus. Often the tinnitus increases during emotional stress. This type of tinnitus is worse toward the end of the day than it is in the morning. Any type of tinnitus seems louder when the patient is fatigued.

Certain muscular sounds in the head and neck may be heard by the patient and disturb him. Chewing, stretching of the neck, tight closing of the eyes, or tight clenching of the jaws produces subjective sounds that any of us can hear. When a conductive hearing loss is present, all such sounds are accentuated because the masking effect of ambient noise is lost. Also, when a conductive hearing loss is present, motion of the eardrum and contraction of the muscles of the middle ear may become audible intermittently.

If a person hears organized sounds (such as voices or music) when no such sound is present, he is said to have auditory hallucinations. Central nervous system dysfunction is certain. Auditory hallucinations may occur in the psychotic person, but they may also be caused by localized or diffuse encephalitis of the temporal lobe of the brain.

Objective (audible) tinnitus. When a patient's tinnitus can also be heard by the physician, certain definite conditions are suggested. Audible tinnitus should be suspected when the tinnitus is blowing in character and coincides with respiration; when it is pulsating, biphasic, and rough in character; or when there is a rapid succession of clicking sounds. In order for audible tinnitus to be heard, the physician must place his ear against the patient's ear or use a stethoscope against the patient's external auditory canal.

A blowing tinnitus that coincides with inspiration, expiration, or both usually indicates an abnormally patent eustachian tube. This type of tinnitus is extremely distressing to the patient. It may appear after extreme weight loss in debilitated patients. Fortunately, most such instances of tinnitus are of short duration. Some relief can be obtained by repeating the Valsalva maneuver (swallowing with the mouth and nose obstructed to produce negative pressure in the nasopharynx).

Rarely, a patient will have tinnitus characterized by a series of sharp, regular clicks heard for several seconds or several minutes at a time. This type of tinnitus is almost always intermittent, although it may occur many times during the day. The cause is not definitely known, but the mechanism is understood. It is produced by tetanic contractions of the muscles of the soft palate, and the palate can be seen to contract spasmodically when the tinnitus is audible. The contractions are very small and rapid, approximately 175 to 200 a minute. Occasionally several injections of procaine hydrochloride (Novocain) or lidocaine (Xylocaine) into the palatal muscles on the involved side will break the reflex activity.

Audible tinnitus that is pulsating and synchronous with the heartbeat almost always indicates an arteriovenous aneurysm somewhere in the head or neck. Rarely, a carotid bruit is audible. The most common sites of arteriovenous aneurysms causing audible tinnitus are intracranial or are in the vessels immediately in front of the ear (anterior auricular artery). Arteriograms help locate the aneurysm. Resection of the aneurysm and ligation of the involved vessels are indicated.

Treatment. Tinnitus caused by changes in the external canal and middle ear can usually be relieved. The type accompanying acute or subacute middle ear disease disappears when the inflammation subsides. The tinnitus that accompanies otosclerosis cannot be treated except by surgical correction of the hearing loss. In most patients who have an operation for otosclerosis, the tinnitus disappears when the operation is successful but remains when the operation is unsuccessful (Fig. 26-1).

Tinnitus caused by disturbances in the cochlea, eighth nerve, and central nervous system cannot be treated specifically unless it is associated with a known disease and disappears with control of that disease. The majority of the patients cannot be treated successfully. In patients with a tinnitus of recent origin, vasodilation by the use of nicotinic acid may be of value. Mild sedation with phenobarbital may help. Occasionally potassium iodide in small doses over a long period may lessen the intensity of tinnitus. The true effect of these measures is hard to evaluate because there is *a tendency for all tinnitus to become less intense* or, at least, less annoying to the patient as time elapses.

Before 1978 specific medical treatment of tinnitus was of uncertain value. Since then, carefully controlled regimens including intravenous administration of lidocaine alone or in combination with carbamazepine (Tegretol) or phenytoin (Dilantin), or both, have shown some success in the management of some types of tinnitus. This method of treatment is still undergoing changes, and the site or sites of action of these drugs is tinnitus are unknown. Primidone (Mysoline) has also been used in combination with carbamazepine with some beneficial effect. None of these types of management is specific for tinnitus, but they offer future hope of tinnitus control in some patients. Since the causes of tinnitus are undoubtedly several rather than one, it is probable that control of tinnitus must wait for more precise localization of its origins.

When drug toxicity is the cause of tinnitus, withdrawal of the drug may stop the tinnitus. If cochlear damage has already occurred, the tinnitus may continue.

It is interesting to note that even sectioning of the eighth nerve, which has been performed many times for Meniere's syndrome and for acoustic neuroma, often fails to cause cessation of tinnitus. This raises the suspicion that central nervous system tinnitus is more common than is usually thought. It may also indicate that tinnitus represents autonomic dysfunction rather than a disturbance of the cochlea or eighth nerve.

Biofeedback, in conjunction with learned techniques of relaxation, has been used for control of tinnitus with variable success. These techniques are still in the early stage of study and are difficult to evaluate, but they may offer future help for the tinnitus sufferer.

When the loudness of a patient's tinnitus is matched by a similar sound from the audiometer presented to the unaffected ear, it is surprising how weak a signal is needed to match the tinnitus. The average is about a 10-decibel intensity, and often 5 decibels in the left ear, for example, will match with the tinnitus in the right ear. Twenty decibels matching is unusual.

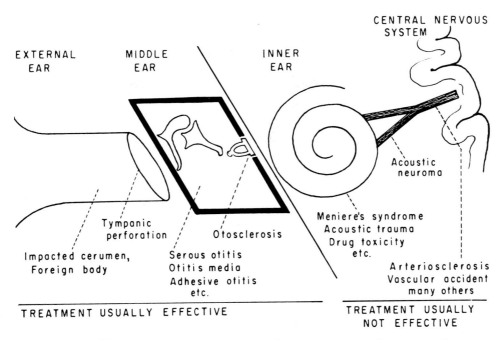

FIG. 26-1. Possible areas giving rise to tinnitus. The great majority of patients with tinnitus have the symptom from inner ear or central causes, not external or middle ear disorders.

It has been known for a long time that mild tinnitus is frequently masked by everyday sounds. Such tinnitus is unnoticed when the afflicted person is in ordinary room noise or outside in the traffic noise. Only in quiet surroundings, as at bedtime, is the tinnitus annoying. Even rather loud tinnitus is diminished by surrounding noise. Recent studies of this natural modifying of tinnitus have led to the development of electronic masking devices worn by the patient that in many cases can reduce the intensity of the tinnitus or mask it completely. Sometimes a hearing aid alone, since it amplifies external sound, not only improves hearing but also diminishes or stops the tinnitus while it is worn. A masking instrument can be used alone if tinnitus without hearing loss is the problem. The masking unit can also be incorporated with a hearing aid to relieve both hearing loss and tinnitus in some patients. This type of management is now widely used in the United States. Improvements in the instrument and further research will undoubtedly refine the technique in the future.

From the use of masking a phenomenon known as residual inhibition has been studied. Certain people have found that, if a masking device is used even for a short period of time, the tinnitus may be markedly diminished or absent for a period of time after the masking sound is removed. A few persons have been free of tinnitus for hours or longer after using a masking device for several hours. Residual inhibition is incompletely understood and will require further work to determine whether, or in what circumstances, it can be of practical value.

In the control of tinnitus the physician must remember that tinnitus is only a symptom and that a specific cause must be sought and eliminated if possible. Only when no treatable cause can be found should the symptom alone be treated. Tinnitus is sometimes a warning of other serious disease.

SELECTED READINGS

American Tinnitus Association Newsletter (various issues).

Berland, O.: No-mold fitting of hearing aids. In Dalsgaard, S.C., editor: Earmoulds and associated problems, Stockholm, 1975, Almqvist och Wiksell International, pp. 173-193.

Fowler, E.P.: Control of head noises; their illusion of loudness and of timbre, Arch. Otolaryngol. **37**:391, 1943.

Fowler, E.P., Sr.: Head noises in normal and disordered ears, Arch. Otolaryngol. **39**:498, 1944.

Hocks, R.: Earmold used in tinnitus maskers, useful in regular hearing aid fittings, Hear. Inst. **27**:11, 1976.

Pulec, J.L., and others: Tinnitus: diagnosis and treatment, Ann. Otol. Rhinol. Laryngol. **87**:821, 1978.

Quarry, J.G.: Unilateral objective tinnitus, Arch. Otolaryngol. **96**:252, 1972.

Reed, G.F.: An audiometric study of two hundred cases of subjective tinnitus, Arch. Otolaryngol. **71**:94, 1960.

Saltzman, M., and Ersner, M.S.: A hearing aid for the relief of tinnitus aurium, Laryngoscope **57**:358, 1947.

Shea, J.J., and Harell, M.: Management of tinnitus aurium with lidocaine and carbamazepine, Laryngoscope **88**:1477, 1978.

Somant, H.C., Gupta, S.K., and Gupta, O.P.: Palatal myoclonus, Ann. Otol. Rhinol. Laryngol. **79**:858, 1970.

Vernon, J.A.: The loudness (?) of tinnitus, Hear. Speech Act. **44**:17, 1976.

Vernon, J.A.: Attempts to relieve tinnitus, J. Am. Aud. Soc. **2**:124, 1977.

Vernon, J.A., and Schleuning, A.: Tinnitus: a new management, Laryngoscope **88**:413, 1978.

Vernon, J.A., A tinnitus clinic, Ear Nose Throat J. **56**:181, 1977.

27 SPEECH DISORDERS IN CHILDREN

David D. DeWeese, M.D.
Herold Lillywhite, Ph.D.

Because the otolaryngologist or the pediatrician is often the first person consulted when a child has a speech problem, it is important for the physician to understand the nature of speech deviations, what to do about them, and from whom to seek additional help.

Abnormal speech cannot be understood without a basic knowledge of normal speech development. When normal speech development is used as a standard, it is possible to evaluate the speech of a child at the age of 1 year. At any subsequent age, deviations that are severe enough to require therapy can be recognized.

During the first year of a child's life, attention should be focused on how he vocalizes, what sounds he makes, how he combines sounds, whether he is developing inflection, when he imitates, and how he responds to voice. Between the ages of 1 and 6 years the development and comprehension of speech should follow a general pattern. The normal pattern of language development from 1 month to 6 years of age is given in abbreviated form in Tables 8 to 10.

Critical periods in speech development. The first year of a child's life is extremely important in growth and development of language. Babbling, which begins at about 4 months of age, appears to be a rehearsal for the first words, which are spoken between 9 and 12 months of age. During this time a child learns to enjoy sounds and to make a variety of his own. This not only exercises the speech organs but also is the beginning of ear training.

Because the infant enjoys sounds, others around him repeat sounds to him. The mother often babbles with the child and thus teaches him that the sounds he makes have an effect on others. During this period, variations in pitch, inflection, and volume will begin. Some sound combinations that sound like words are produced. The word *mamma* is often the first combination. After the mother hears it and repeats it back to the child, it does not take long for him to learn that speaking the word *mamma* may satisfy many of his desires. Other words are learned by a similar repetition. This is the beginning of a vocabulary.

Normal development of language can be delayed by conditions that interfere with usual prelanguage activity. Congenital anomalies, birth trauma, delayed physical development, mental retardation, serious illness, or decreased hearing may prevent babbling as well as other prelanguage activities. Emotional trauma may have a similar effect. When language development is delayed, regardless of the cause, prelanguage actions seem to be essential. A 4-, 5-, or 6-year-old child who has never talked may begin by babbling. It is important that normal prelanguage activities are not hindered during the first year of life if later vocalization is to develop in the usual manner.

From the age of 12 to 18 months, slight language development occurs and speech may come to a virtual standstill. The child's time and attention during this period are directed toward exploration of his physical surroundings and learning to walk. Although this is the normal pattern, parents often become worried about lack of speech development during these

☐ Rewritten and partly quoted from Lillywhite, H.: Doctor's manual of speech disorders, J.A.M.A. **167:**850, 1958.

379

TABLE 8. Pattern of normal language development in vocalization
and response to vocal sound

Age (mo.)	Vocalization	Response to vocal sound
1	Cries, whimpers; produces some vowels and *k*, *g*, and *h*; makes explosive sounds	
2-3	Pitch higher; different cries for pain, hunger, and so on; some repetition, such as *gagaga*; added *m* and *ng*	May coo, sigh, gurgle, smile, or be soothed by pleasant adult voice; may cry in response to angry voice
4	Smiles, laughs, gurgles when comfortable; begins vocal play when alone; begins to use vowels and *m*, *k*, *g*, *b*, *p*, and *ng*	Imitation to other speech stops but reappears at 9 mo.; interruption of babbling causes to stop vocalizing
5	Increase of above; occasionally responds to parents' babbling	Responds to voices by turning eye or head; responds to friendly or angry tone; shows displeasure
6	Increase in rhythm and intensity; more noncrying sounds; nasal tones and tongue tip activity begin	Gestures begin in response to pleasant or angry tones
7	More variety; some sounds repeated several days; adds *d*, *t*, *n*, and *w*	Mostly rejects demands to imitate sounds; responds to gestures plus voice
8	Begins to imitate own vocal play of "mama," "dada," and so on, but not in response to adults; pitch and inflection change	Calls for attention; babbles with gestures; imitates hand clapping, and so on, accompanied by voice
9-10	More variety in crying and pitch, and more vocalizing than crying; makes effort to imitate others; can imitate; may use one word correctly	Retreats from strangers and others by crying; begins to comprehend "no no" and "dada"; may respond to "bye-bye" with gestures
11	Can imitate correct number of syllables and sounds heard; imitates some new sounds	Shows interest in words associated with objects or important activities
12	Accompanies vocalization with gestures; may acquire first true word or words; interested in isolated words connected with own needs and activities	May initiate animal sounds or adult exclamations; imitates the initial sound of adult words; often imitates 2- and 3-syllable words

months. After the age of 18 months language should develop rapidly. A vocabulary of 20 words at 18 months of age may increase to 250 words by the age of 2 years. At some time during this period a jargon stage occurs. The child's speech may sound like normal conversation except that most of it is unintelligible. This period of jargon may initiate parental concern.

The period from 2 to 4 years of age may be a critical one for normal language development. During this time the child attempts to use a rapidly increasing, and often inadequate, vocabulary to meet his expanding needs. He may often find himself without words to express his thoughts. He may then do as anyone might—hesitate, back up, repeat, or fill in the "ah, ah, ah" or "I, I, I, I." Sometimes he will block completely and give up attempts to finish his immediate flow of words. This may result in nonfluency and may be quite normal for many children at this age. It occurs more often and usually lasts longer in boys than in girls. Generally, if the nonfluency is not magnified by parental concern, the worst will disappear in about 6 months. Occasionally a child may remain in this stage of speech development for 1 or 2 years.

The period of nonfluency may become dangerous if parents and other children become disturbed and treat it as a problem. Adults may label this kind of speech stuttering or stammering. Constant corrections such as "Slow up," "Stop and start over again," "Don't talk so fast," or "Now, *think* what you are going to say" may create a problem where none should be.

TABLE 9. Pattern of normal language development in articulation and general intelligibility

Age (yr.)	Articulation	General intelligibility
1-2	Uses all vowels and consonants *m*, *b*, *p*, *k*, *g*, *w*, *h*, *n*, *t*, and *d*; omits most final consonants, some initial; substitutes consonants above for more difficult; much unintelligible jargon around 18 mo.; good inflection and rate	Words used may be no more than 25% intelligible to unfamiliar listener; jargon near 18 mo. almost 100% unintelligible; improvement noticeable between 21 and 24 mo.
2-3	Continues all sounds above with vowels but use is inconsistent; tries many new sounds, but poor mastery; much substitution; omission of final consonants; articulation lags behind vocabulary	Words about 65% intelligible by 2 yr.; 70% to 80% intelligible in context by 3 yr.; many individual sounds faulty but total context generally understood; some incomprehensibility because of faulty sentence structure
3-4	Masters *b*, *t*, *d*, *k*, and *g* and tries many others, including *f*, *v*, *th*, *s*, *z*, and consonant combinations *tr*, *bl*, *pr*, *gr*, and *dr*, but *r* and *l* may be faulty so substitutes *w* or omits; speech almost intelligible; uses *th* inconsistently	Speech usually 90% to 100% intelligible in context; individual sounds still faulty and some trouble with sentence structure
4-5	Master *f*, *v*, and many consonant combinations; should be little omission of initial and final consonants; fewer substitutes but may be some; may distort *r*, *l*, *s*, *z*, *sh*, *ch*, *j*, and *th*; no trouble with multisyllabic words	Speech is intelligible in context even though some sounds are still faulty
5-6	Masters *r*, *l*, *th*, and such blends as *tl*, *gr*, *bl*, *br*, and *pr*; may still have some trouble with glends such as *thr*, *sk*, *st*, and *shr*; may still distort *s*, *z*, *sh*, *ch*, and *j*; may not master these sounds until 7½ years	Good

It is often during this period that parents become worried and seek the advice of a physician. Usually the chief complaint is: "Johnny is stuttering (or stammering). What shall I do?" The usual advice to do nothing is good. It is necessary to explain to the parents that this stage or speech development is normal. They should understand that too much emphasis on speech at this stage may create a real speech problem. It would be far better if the parents and physicians would call this nonfluent speech "developmental nonfluency" rather than stuttering or stammering.

Between the ages of 3 and 6 years a problem may develop if parents or others expect too much articulation of sounds. Parents may become quite disturbed if the child does not use the *r*, *l*, *th*, *s*, *z*, *sh*, and *ch* sounds correctly. A study of Tables 8 to 10 will show that these sounds normally develop after 5 years of age and that the last four may not be used properly until 7 years of age. Problems such as reverting to baby speech, stuttering, or dyslalia may result from insisting that the child try to produce such sounds before he is ready to produce them.

Most children have adequate language for most situations when they are ready to start school. A few have not. These children suddenly find themselves confronted with a strange adult and a large group of unfamiliar children. Language that has previously met their needs in the family group may now be insufficient. Nonfluency may result. Many cases of stuttering apparently begin in kindergarten or in the first or second grade. Again, the proper handling of this nonfluency should be to accept it, provide security, and avoid stress until the child's language matures. Many children do not use their articulators well enough to pronounce sounds clearly when they begin school. Some do not reach this maturity until 7 or 8 years of age. Attempts to "help" the child, correct him, nag him, or emphasize his immature speech at this

TABLE 10. Pattern of normal language development in expressive speech and in comprehension of speech

Age (yr.)	Expressive speech	Comprehension of speech
1-2	Uses 1 to 3 words at 12 mo., 10 to 15 at 15 mo., 15 to 20 at 18 mo., about 100 to 200 by 2 yr.; knows names of most objects he uses; names few people, uses verbs but not correctly with subjects; jargon and echolalia; names 1 to 3 pictures	Begins to relate symbol and object meaning; adjusts to comments; inhibits on command; responds correctly to "give me that," "sit down," "stand up," with gestures; puts watch to ear on command; understands simple questions; recognizes 120 to 275 words
2-3	Vocabulary increases to 300 to 500 words; says "where kitty, " "ball all gone," "want cookie," "go bye-bye car"; jargon mostly gone; vocalizing increases, has fluency trouble; speech not adequate for communication needs	Rapid increase in comprehension vocabulary to 400 words at 2½ years, 800 words at 3 years; responds to commands using "on," "under," "up," "down," "over there," "by," "run," "walk," "jump up," "throw," "run fast," "be quiet," and commands containing 2 related actions
3-4	Uses 600 to 1,000 words, becomes conscious of speech; 3 to 4 words per speech response; personal pronouns, some adjectives, adverbs, and prepositions appear; mostly simple sentences, but some complex; speech more useful	Understands up to 1,500 words by 4 years; recognizes plurals, sex difference, pronouns, adjectives; comprehends complex and compound sentences; answers simple questions
4-5	Increase in vocabulary to 1,100 to 1,600 words; more 3- and 4-syllable words; more adjectives, articles appear; 4-, 5-, and 6-word sentences; syntax quite good; uses plurals; fluency improves; proper nouns decrease, pronouns increase	Comprehends from 1,500 to 2,000 words; carries out more complex commands with 2 to 3 actions; understands dependent clause, "if," "because," "when," "why"
5-6	Increase in vocabulary to 1,500 to 2,100 words; complete 5- and 6-word sentences, compound, complex, with some dependent clauses; syntax near normal; quite fluent; more multisyllabic words	Understands vocabulary of 2,500 to 2,800 words; responds correctly to more complicated sentences but is still confused at times by involved sentences

stage may again create a speech problem where none should have occurred.

Deviations from normal speech. Speech disorders generally fall into one or more of the following areas:

1. *Articulation* is the production of sound and sound combinations. Deviations in articulation account for 50% to 70% of all speech disorders.
2. *Stuttering* (or stammering) accounts for about 25% of all speech problems and usually is broken down into primary and secondary stages; the latter is the stage at which the individual himself considers his nonfluency to be a serious problem.
3. *Voice* refers to the processes of phonation and resonation. About 10% of all speech disorders include deviations of pitch, quality, or volume.
4. *Symbolization* refers to the association of meaning with language symbols in a normal manner. Inability to make this association is usually called aphasia or dysphasia. It is thought that 2% to 4% of speech problems may fall into this category.

The speech pathologist, in the diagnostic report, often uses other terms, such as *delay* (one or more aspects of language, such as articulation, vocabulary, or structure, have not developed according to chronologic age); *dyslalia* (articulation disorder caused by structural anomalies, impaired hearing, or functional causes); *dysarthria* (articulation disorder caused by central nervous system damage affecting speech or-

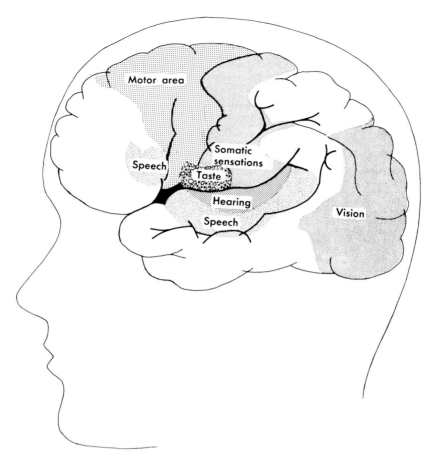

FIG. 27-1. Sensory and motor areas of the brain. Note the two areas for speech localization near the area for auditory reception.

gans); *dysphonia* (disorder of voice quality, pitch, or volume); *dysphasia* (defined above under area 4); *rhythm* (stuttering, stammering, or cluttering); *hypernasality* (too much nasal resonance); and *hyponasality* (too little nasal resonance).

Conditions that commonly cause speech disorders. The conditions generally responsible for speech disorders are discussed below.

LATE PHYSICAL DEVELOPMENT. Late physical development may retard coordination and cause dysfunction of speech organs, thus producing two types of faulty speech: delay in developing intelligible speech and articulatory distortion. In the latter problem, it is essential to evaluate the child's general developmental age. Speech therapy is usually most effective when the child

is reacting mentally and physically at approximately the 4-year-old level.

DENTAL MISALIGNMENT AND MALOCCLUSION. Dental misalignment and malocclusion most often cause articulation problems. The sibilant sounds, particularly *s* and *sh*, are often distorted. Orthodontic correction of the faulty structures is the most direct approach. Speech therapy is often necessary immediately after the correction has been made.

CLEFT LIP AND PALATE (Fig. 27-2). The problem created by a cleft lip and palate is usually a triple one: (1) Retardation of the consonant sounds (*p*, *b*, *t*, *d*, *k*, and *g*) is the most common finding. Because the consonant sounds are necessary for the development of early vocabulary, much prelanguage activity is omitted. As a re-

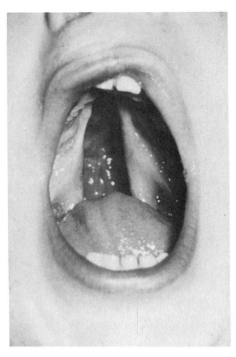

FIG. 27-2. Complete cleft of the hard and soft palates. Surgical repair and speech therapy are necessary. (Courtesy Dr. Verner V. Lindgren, Portland, Ore.)

sult, good sound discrimination is lacking by the time the palate is closed. (2) Hypernasality is usual in the patient with a cleft of the soft palate and may remian after surgery, because of insufficient closure between the soft palate and nasopharyngeal wall. (3) Dental malformation or faulty tongue placement, or both, may develop before the palate is closed and produce an articulatory problem.

The parents of children with a cleft palate should be given early instruction regarding speech development and proper treatment. Early closure of the palate may prevent hypernasality, but insufficient closure sometimes remains even after surgery. Even a small leak of air through the nasopharynx may produce as much hypernasality as a large opening. The pharyngeal flap and push-back operations are effective in preventing hypernasality in many instances. Dental correction will often prevent articulation problems. Speech therapy, when required, is again most desirable at or near 4 years of age.

PARALYSIS OF THE SPEECH ORGANS. Disease or accident that produces injury to the central nervous system may cause complete or partial paralysis of the muscles of the lips, tongue, soft palate, pharynx, or larynx. Faulty articulation, inadequate voice quality, improper or inadequate pitch, rate, or volume, or combinations of these usually result. Cooperation between the family physician, the physical or occupational therapist, and the speech therapist is very important in the proper management of these speech problems. Following paralysis caused by poliomyelitis, retraining should begin as soon as possible after the acute phase of the disease has subsided. It is important to begin work on speech problems within the first 6 months if adequate progress is to be expected. Speech therapy may be necessary for a much longer time.

Between 50% and 60% of children who have cerebral palsy will have serious speech problems. Such problems occur most often in those with the athetoid type of cerebral palsy. Accompanying hearing loss is common. The prognosis in these patients is good if the athetosis is not severe.

BRAIN DAMAGE. Lesions of the central nervous system in the areas directly affecting language function and behavior are often associated with a syndrome known as the brain damage behavior syndrome. Hyperactivity, disinhibition, catastrophic reactions, and deficiency in language and number concepts are characteristic of this syndrome. The resulting speech defect is usually manifested by a disturbance of the language-symbol association. Expressive aphasia (motor aphasia) is the most common result. The child can understand language but cannot reproduce it. Receptive aphasia (auditory aphasia) is the most common result. The child can understand language but cannot reproduce it. Receptive aphasia (auditory aphasia) is more severe. The child cannot interpret language symbols. A combination of expressive and receptive aphasia is called mixed aphasia. Most severe is global aphasia, in which both the receptive and expressive areas are totally defective. In mixed and global aphasia, all language functions are damaged, and, if language develops at all, articulation, structure, vocabulary, and reading and writing ability may all be affected. The site of damage in expressive aphasia

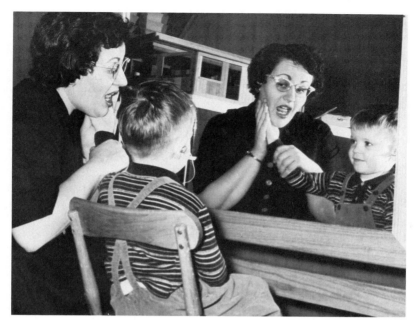

FIG. 27-3. Preschool training of the deaf or profoundly hard-of-hearing child. Note the hearing aid. The child is feeling the laryngeal sound vibrations in the teacher's neck. (Courtesy Portland Center for Hearing and Speech, Portland, Ore.)

seems to be in Broca's area in the cortex of the left frontal lobe of the brain. The exact site of damage in patients with the other types of aphasia has not been established.

MENTAL RETARDATION. Retarded language development, usually in all areas of language, may accompany mental retardation. Children whose intelligence is within the 80 or 90 IQ range usually develop adequate language if other physical or psychologic abnormalities are not present. When the IQ range is from 70 to 80, retardation in several language areas is common. When the IQ is below 70, most children show noticeable language deficiencies in all areas. Speech therapy may be beneficial, but language improvement in the mentally retarded usually closely follows the physical development and maturing process.

HEARING LOSS. The type of speech disorder that results from hearing loss depends on the amount of loss and on the time of recognition of the loss. Early recognition and proper corrective measures will prevent some speech defects (Fig. 27-3). Profound hearing loss or deafness (more than 80 decibels below normal in the speech frequencies) causes delay in language development, faulty articulation and inflection, and pitch deviations. Less severe hearing loss more often causes articulation problems and difficulty with high-frequency sounds (consonants), voiceless sounds, and word endings.

Profound hearing losses are usually detected early, but the less severe or borderline losses are frequently unappreciated. The less severe losses may cause distortion or elimination of many sounds but may not be severe enough to be recognized by the parent, teacher, or physician unless the hearing is tested with an audiometer. Speech or behavior problems, owing entirely to the hearing loss, may be misinterpreted unless the hearing loss is suspected. Children with moderate hearing losses may hear sharp sounds and respond to spoken sounds but may be unable to distinguish between many voice components and therefore may be unable to reproduce them properly.

Treatment of the speech problem caused by hearing loss should combine medical treatment to improve the hearing, when possible, with speech therapy. Often amplification, auditory training, and lipreading instruction are necessary.

ABNORMAL TONSILS AND ADENOIDS. Enlarged tonsils and adenoids rarely cause speech problems. Obstructing adenoids may occasionally produce a temporary denasal quality of the voice, but removal of tonsils and adenoids rarely eliminates a speech problem. The importance of enlarged adenoids as a possible cause of damage to hearing is a special problem.

TONGUE-TIE. A *very* short lingual frenulum can adversely affect the formation of certain consonants and may diminish the clarity of connected speech, but tongue-tie is rarely the cause of a serious speech problem. If there is an articulatory speech disorder *and* a short frenulum, speech development may improve more rapidly when the frenulum is cut.

PSYCHOLOGIC PROBLEMS. Serious speech problems may be caused by psychologic trauma such as emotional upset, unusually severe discipline, fear, rejection, or lack of a mother or father figure during a child's early years. Stuttering may result. Retardation of speech or serious delay in development of speech may occur after sustained emotional trauma. Voice and articulation defects may follow the appearance of delayed speech. Proper psychiatric evaluation and treatment may be needed before speech therapy.

ENVIRONMENTAL CONDITIONS. Certain environmental conditions may lead to speech delay or speech deviation. Among these conditions are the following: (1) abandonment and early years in a foster home, (2) major speech defect in a parent or sibling that is copied by the child, (3) lack of encouragement or motivation for speech in the home, and (4) reversion to baby talk due as a result of displacement of the child by a new, younger sibling or displacement for any reason.

Guide for checking speech. The physician should be concerned about a child's speech development when any one or more of the following conditions exist:

1. The child is not talking at all by age 2 years.
2. Speech is largely unintelligible after age 3 years.
3. Sounds are more than a year late in appearing, according to developmental sequence.
4. There are many omissions of initial consonants after age 3 years.
5. There are many substitutions of easy sounds for difficult ones after age 5 years.
6. The child uses mostly vowel sounds in his speech.
7. There are no sentences by age 3 years.
8. Word endings are consistently dropped after age 5 years.
9. Sentence structure is noticeably faulty at 5 years.
10. The child is embarrassed and disturbed by his speech at any age.
11. The child is noticeably nonfluent after age 5 years.
12. The child is distorting, omitting, or substituting any sounds after age 7 years.
13. The voice is a monotone, extremely loud, largely inaudible, or of poor quality.
14. The pitch is not appropriate to the child's age and sex.
15. There is noticeable hypernasality or lack of nasal resonance.
16. There are unusual confusions, reversals, or telescoping in connected speech.
17. There are abnormal rhythm, rate, and inflection after age 5 years.

When the child will not talk for the physician, it is risky for the physician to base an evaluation of the speech entirely on what the parents say about it. They rarely are able to report accurately concerning this aspect of their child's behavior. Generally they will give a picture of speech behavior considerably in advance of what it actually is because they read their own interpretations into what they hear. Occasionally a parent will underestimate the child's speech. Careful, detailed questioning of the parents by the physician is needed in any case in which the physician does not hear the child.

Relationship of the physician and the speech pathologist. To make a proper diagnosis of a speech disorder, the speech pathologist must know as much as possible about the probable causes underlying the defect. Only then can the speech pathologist decide how much of a problem the speech disorder will be to a child and what the child's and parents' potential is for overcoming the defect. Since the functions of language are often affected by physical, emotional, and mental factors, the speech pathologist needs information that can be supplied only by the physician who has examined the patient with the speech defect.

The important information needed from the physician includes the following: (1) prenatal, birth, or neonatal disturbances that may have produced neurologic changes; (2) congenital malformations of speech organs or allied structures; (3) injuries or serious illnesses; (4) infections that might damage hearing; (5) major defects of sight or hearing; (6) results of audiometric tests; (7) the child's general developmental pattern; (8) any malfunction of the speech organs, respiratory abnormalities, or incoordination of muscles; and (9) an opinion of the child's mental development.

After the speech pathologist evaluates all findings, speech therapy may be recommended or it may be delayed. In any event, the physician should be informed of the recommendation and his cooperation should be sought in advising the parents regarding the importance of following through with the entire program. In most instances the speech pathologist will find it necessary to reexamine the child and advise the parents further at intervals of 6 to 12 months. Such recheck consultations should continue until the child is ready for therapy or until he exhibits adequate speech.

The speech pathologist is prepared either to give speech therapy or to recommend where and by whom it should be given. Ordinarily, speech therapy is of long duration, often extending several years. The physician must recognize that speech disorders, particularly serious ones, cannot be corrected or "cured" in a few short lessons. If best results are to be obtained, the physician must counsel the parents as to the importance of following through until the speech pathologist decides that no further improvement can be accomplished or until the speech defect no longer exists.

Speech and audiology as professions. As professions, speech pathology and audiology have developed primarily in the last 40 years. Originally the major emphasis was on speech problems. The common association of hearing losses with speech disorders has given rise to the training of an increasing number of persons whose special field includes hearing testing, hearing evaluation in cooperation with the otolaryngologist, auditory training, and lipreading instruction. Thus two professional areas have developed.

The American Speech-Language Hearing Association (ASLHA) is the official certifying body in speech and hearing, at the national level. A bachelor's degree with a major in speech and hearing from an accredited institution is required for membership in the Association. Basic and advanced certificates are given in the field of either speech or hearing, or both, depending on the qualifications and experience of the individual. A number of state departments of education also grant certificates to qualified speech and hearing therapists. The requirements in general are approximately equivalent to the requirements necessary for a basic certificate in the American Speech-Language Hearing Association.

In general, five different terms are applied to persons engaged in the profession of speech and audiology. A *speech pathologist* usually holds an advanced certificate from the American Speech-Language Hearing Association and is primarily concerned with the diagnosis of pathologic speech. The *speech therapist* and *speech correctionist* perform the actual therapy after the diagnosis has been established. The *audiologist* usually designates a person with advanced certification in the field of hearing. The *audiometrist* is trained to test hearing on the audiometer but not to interpret the audiogram or to advise therapy.

These general terms are not fixed and are often used interchangeably, since many persons are trained in both speech and hearing and are competent to advise as well as to give therapy. All of them are closely allied with the medical profession by mutual interest and reciprocal needs.

SELECTED READINGS

Bernstein, L.: Treatment of velopharyngeal incompetence, Arch. Otolaryngol. **85:**67, 1967.

Bloomer, H.H., and Wolski, W.: Office examination of palatopharyngeal function, Clin. Pediatr. **7:**611, 1968.

Crikelair, G.F., Striker, P., and Cosman, B.: The surgical treatment of submucous cleft palate, Plast. Reconstr. Surg. **45:**58, 1970.

Sturim, H.S., and Jacob, C.T., Jr.: Teflon pharyngoplasty, Plast. Reconstr. Surg. **49:**180, 1972.

Yules, R.B.: Secondary correction of velopharyngeal incompetence; a review, Plast. Reconstr. Surg. **45:**234, 1970.

28 REHABILITATION OF PERSONS WITH HEARING LOSS

Although many patients with hearing loss receive benefit from medical and surgical treatment, it is evident that there are many others whose hearing cannot be improved. It is estimated that in the U.S. population of 200 million people, over 15 million will need help for a hearing problem sometime during their lives. Of these, a minimum of 5 million have a permanent hearing loss great enough to handicap them. For this segment of the population help must come from amplification of sound (hearing aids) and from speech reading. Since education, interchange of ideas, carrying out of orders, and the pure pleasure of listening and responding are important functions of living, this sort of help is essential. *The physician is the logical counselor to the patient with a hearing loss problem.*

Concept of rehabilitation. The physician's work is not completed even though hearing cannot be improved by medical or surgical methods. He must advise suitable rehabilitation. In no other field of medicine is rehabilitation as important as it is in otology. Under the guidance of otologists and with the help of medical schools, communities, and educators of the deaf, training has been given to a large number of audiologists, speech therapists, and speech teachers. There is need for still more of these specialists. In most communities the specialists in hearing and speech act as a team.

Rehabilitation resources. Many resources are available for the rehabilitation of the person with a hearing loss.

HEARING AIDS. From the time man held his cupped hand to his ear to aid hearing, there has been a constant search for better methods to amplify sound. An early (and still excellent) device was the ear trumpet. After the development of storage batteries, crude electric amplifying systems were made. They were bulky and practically chained the patient to his instrument. Following the invention of the telephone it was possible to manufacture better electric aids. They were smaller than earlier models, amplified better and distorted sound less (Fig. 28-1).

Early hearing aids contained magnets, carbon particles, and diaphragms. They were like telephones. The subsequent manufacture of hearing aids progressed from the use of vacuum tubes (similar to radio tubes) to the employment today or transistors. An electric hearing aid must have the following parts to amplify sound properly: (1) a microphone to convert sound waves into electric energy, (2) an amplifier, (3) a receiver that converts electric energy back to sound waves, and (4) a power source (batteries or transistors) that provides the electric power to run the system.

The use of transistors as a source of power has made it possible to reduce the size of hearing aids until they can be concealed in the hair, worn behind the ear, or incorporated into the temple piece of eyeglasses. (Fig. 28-2). Translucent plastics have replaced other materials in the manufacture of earpieces and connecting tubes for transmission of sound. Claims that are made in advertisements as to the efficiency of hearing aids without batteries, cords, and ear molds are usually "bait" and should be recognized as such. Manufacturers of hearing aids are proud of the advances they have made in eliminating bulk, static, and clothing noises that

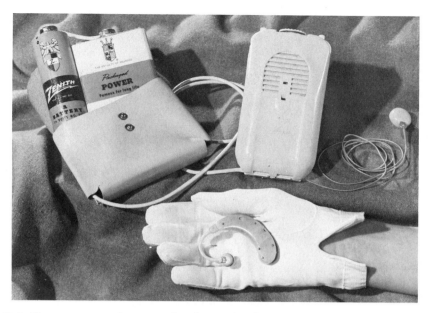

FIG. 28-1. Change in size in hearing aids. *Above,* An aid (1943) with two batteries and a microphone worn under the dress or in a vest pocket. *Below,* All components in a small aid worn behind the ear (1959). (Courtesy Zenith Radio Corp., Hearing Aid Division, Chicago, Ill.)

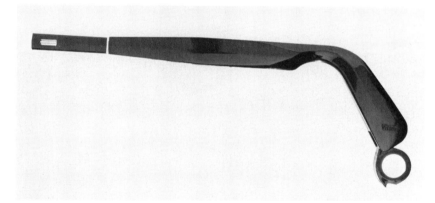

FIG. 28-2. Temple of eyeglass-type hearing aid. The swing-out ring at the right holds a transistor battery, which can easily be replaced as needed.

formerly deterred many persons from wearing a hearing aid. Improvements are constantly being made in the modern electric hearing aid.

Perhaps the greatest deterrent to more widespread use of hearing aids is the retail cost. Prices range between $125 and $400. If both ears are fitted, the cost may be more than $800.

The patient who benefits most from the use of a hearing aid is the one who has a pure conduc-

tive hearing loss. There are several reasons for this: (1) In conductive hearing loss, all tones are more likely to be affected to nearly the same degree. This is often called a flat type of hearing loss. (2) There are no problems of sound discrimination. If the sound is loud enough, the patient can understand what he hears. (3) Recruitment is not present. Therefore the person with conductive hearing impairment can receive sound over a wide range of intensities without discomfort.

The patient with a mixed or sensorineural hearing loss has more difficulty using a hearing aid. Sensorineural hearing loss in most instances involves the high tones, or the high and middle tones, and leaves the low tones nearly normal. Some compensation for low or high tones can be built into the electric circuit of a hearing aid, but it is not sufficient for patients who have wide differences between the high and low tones. In spite of these difficulties, *many persons with sensorineural hearing loss can wear a hearing aid effectively* and can understand speech. Only patients who are profoundly deaf (with a loss of 85 to 90 decibels) in both ears obtain no help in hearing understandable speech. Even some of these patients, however, benefit from a perception of tonal differences, which helps understanding when it is combined with speech reading (lipreading).

Speech and pure tone audiograms are useful in determining not only whether a patient would benefit from amplification, but also the type of amplification most suitable. Pure tone thresholds indicate whether the loss affects high frequencies, low frequencies, or all frequencies. Comfort levels and tolerance levels are important in aid selection, since the patient needs comfortable listening without noise intolerance. This level is often difficult to achieve when the range between comfort level and tolerance level may be only 10 decibels.

The patient who has damaged cochlear hair cells and exhibits recruitment is the most difficult to fit with a hearing aid. He hears weak sounds poorly or not at all, and loud sounds cause distortion of sound and pain. The intolerance of such a patient to minute increases in volume and the narrow range between comfortable loudness and uncomfortable loudness create problems that sometimes cannot be solved. One of the goals of hearing aid improvement is to develop aids to the point at which they can be fitted to individual losses as accurately as glass lenses can be made to correct individual errors of refraction.

CROS HEARING AID. The CROS (contralateral routing of offside signals) is a modified ear-level aid in either the eyeglass or the behind-the-ear

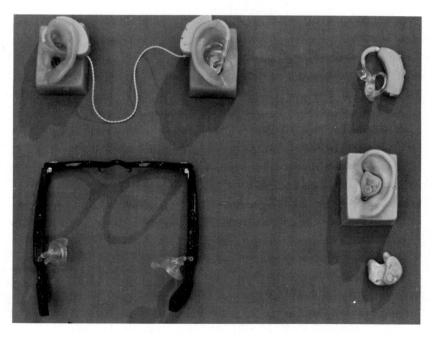

FIG. 28-3. The two aids on the left are CROS aids, one fitted into the temple of the glasses and the other connected across the head with a cord. *Upper right*, A behind-the-ear aid. *Lower right*, An all-in-ear aid.

type (Fig. 28-3). It was specially designed to reduce the listening problems encountered by patients with loss in one ear. In the CROS aid the auditory signals are picked up by a microphone placed near the poor ear and electrically routed across to an earphone mounted beside the good ear. The amplified signals are directed into the good ear either by placing a plastic tube in the ear canal or by using a special nonoccluding earpiece that holds the tube firmly in the canal. Such an arrangement should not block off the normal reception of sound in the good ear.

Although originally designed for persons with profound unilateral loss, the CROS or modifications of it (BICROS and IROS) are also useful because they separate the microphone from the earphone, thus avoiding the "feedback" that may result when both elements are close together on one side of the head.

Formerly, all earpieces were constructed to fit the canal tightly, completely occluding it, now better results are achieved in some patients by using an open insert in which only the hollow end of a small plastic tube fits into the ear canal. Still other earpieces have a tight mold for the ear canal, but with a hole in the mold, so that only a partial occlusion results. These "vented aids" affect the amplification of various frequencies, making it possible for example, to selectively amplify higher frequencies without equally amplifying lower frequencies.

LIPREADING (SPEECH READING). The ability to understand speech through the observance of lip and tongue movement and facial expression is known as speech reading or lipreading. Some persons have a natural ability to read lips and practice it as a matter of habit. Others, even after long training, never learn to read lips well.

Speech reading is an additional aid to anyone with hearing impairment. Although some patients can learn it by themselves, help from a teacher gives more satisfactory results (Fig. 28-4). The combination of a well-fitted hearing aid and good lipreading ability is the ultimate in hearing rehabilitation.

SPECIAL EDUCATION. The educational problem presented by the deaf or profoundly hard-of-hearing child is a serious one. Early recognition of hearing loss is essential for good results. The normal infant may cease his activity when he hears a sound. The deaf infant will not. Between the ages of 2 and 3 months the normal infant will turn his head toward a sound. A history of response only to loud sound suggests a hearing loss. At 1 year of age the normal child uses two or three words, and at 2 years of age he speaks in short sentences. Noticing a deviation from this normal pattern, the observant parent

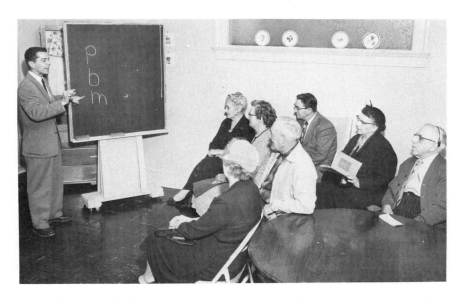

FIG. 28-4. Class of hard-of-hearing persons learning the differences in consonants. (Courtesy Portland Center for Hearing and Speech, Portland, Ore.)

or physician should be aware of serious hearing loss at least by the time the child is 2 years old.

Special training of the deaf child should begin by the age of 2 years, or sooner if possible (Fig. 28-5). Early training in sense perception, attention to the face and lips of the mother, and visual association are important foundations for later education. When serious hearing loss is recognized, most schools will begin special education when the child is 3 to 4 years old, which is 2 years before the child with normal hearing begins his schooling. Preschool training should, if possible, be started as early as 18 months of age.

Facilities for education of the profoundly hard of hearing are available in every state. There are state schools for the deaf, special municipal schools in the larger cities, and private schools. In general, early educational efforts are directed toward teaching awareness of sound and speech and attempts to elicit early speech sounds from the child.

No child born deaf is born mute. The larynx and vocal cords function normally. A deaf child is mute only because he cannot hear sounds and words. He produces sound, lots of it, but it is unintelligible unless he is given years of special training. During the early education of deaf children continuing attempts are made to determine the exact degree of hearing loss. Hearing aids are recommended for use as early as possible when there is any suggestion of residual hearing. Hearing aids have been successfully used on patients under 1 year of age. If there is enough residual hearing, children are placed in classes with normal children as soon as they can compete.

OTHER FACILITIES. The National Association of Hearing and Speech Agencies is an organization with over 100 chapters in various cities in the United States; its headquarters are in Washington, D.C. The Association conducts educational programs with an emphasis on the social and economic rehabilitation of the hard of hearing. It publishes a monthly magazine in which new information regarding all aspects of hearing loss and rehabilitation is made available.

Hearing and speech clinics are located in many cities throughout the country. Of 152 such

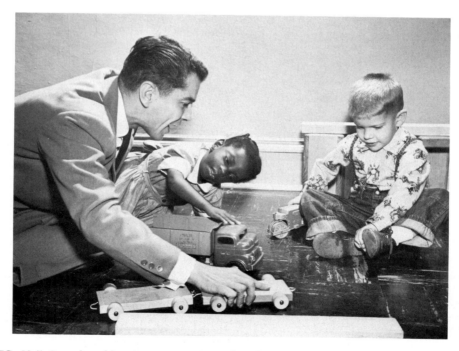

FIG. 28-5. Speech and hearing training. Note that play activity with a trained teacher involves both attention and patience in order to achieve understanding of sounds and finally repetition of words. (Courtesy Portland Center for Hearing and Speech, Portland, Ore.)

centers in the United States, more than 90 are associated with universities, medical schools, or hospitals; 26 are chapters of the National Association of Hearing and Speech Agencies; 22 are federal or state agencies (such as veterans' agencies); 8 are public agencies; and several are privately endowed. Hearing and speech clinics offer the following services: (1) audiometric and psychogalvanometric tests of all types, (2) advice regarding selection and fitting of hearing aids, (3) lipreading classes for adults and children, (4) preschool classes for deaf children, (5) classes for the parents of hard-of-hearing and deaf children, (6) recreational activities for the hard of hearing, (7) speech diagnosis and therapy, and (8) teaching of esophageal speech (see Chapter 8).

The *John Tracy Clinic* is a unique effort in education of the parents of hard-of-hearing and deaf children. This organization sends, free of charge, a step-by-step course to guide the parents of the deaf child. This course is used throughout the world. Parents, with their deaf child, are accepted during certain periods for concentrated work in adjustment problems.

The *Deafness Research Foundation* is supported by all the national otolaryngologic societies as the official fund-raising group for research in this field. The operating expenses of this organization are furnished by the ear, nose, and throat specialists, so that 100 cents of every dollar given will go to research.

Under the auspices of this foundation more than 20 Temporal Bone Banks have been established. Through this unique program many persons who have had ear disease or deafness who have had ear disease or deafness can will their temporal bones to be studied after death. Methods have been set up to immediately fix the bones, remove them, and process them for microscopic study. A record of the patient's history and hearing tests is kept at the Temporal Bone Bank Center from the time that the request is made until the bones are processed. Correlation of the known history and physical findings with the microscopic appearance of the

bone after death should add significantly to our knowledge of ear disease in the next three decades.

National medical associations contribute time and money toward the rehabilitation effort. The American Academy of Otolaryngology has a standing committee on conservation of hearing. Communications directed to this committee or to the Academy, as well as to other sources, will enable the physician to obtain information regarding rehabilitation facilities.

The names and addresses of some of the societies and agencies are as follows:

National Association of Hearing and Speech Agencies
919 18th St., N.W.
Washington, D.C. 20006

American Academy of Otolaryngology
15 Second St., S.W.
Rochester, Minn. 55901

The Deafness Research Foundation
366 Madison Ave., Suite 1010
New York, N.Y. 10017

The John Tracy Clinic
807 W. Adams Blvd.
Los Angeles, Calif. 90007

The American Speech-Language Hearing
    Association
9030 Old Georgetown Rd.
Washington, D.C. 20014

Temporal Bone Bank Center
Box 146, Faculty Exchange
University of Chicago
Chicago, Ill. 60637

SELECTED READINGS

Byrne, D.: Hearing aid selection: an analysis and point of view, Arch. Otolaryngol. **105**:519, 1979.

Glorig, A.: Hearing aids and the otolaryngologist, J.C.E. O.R.L. Allergy **41**:15, 1979.

Schiff, M., and Cohen, I.J.: What every otolaryngologist should know about hearing aids, Laryngoscope **88**:932, 1978.

Schuneman, J.R., and Viscomi, G.J.: Open canal amplification, Trans. Am. Acad. Ophthalmol. Otolaryngol. **78**: 256, 1974.

Surr, R.V., and others: Factors influencing use of hearing aids, Arch. Otolaryngol. **104**:732, 1978.

29 DIZZINESS AND VERTIGO

Dizziness indicates a disturbed sense of relationship to space. It is a subjective sensation that rises to the level of consciousness, alarming and disturbing the patient, who is often unable to describe exactly what he is feeling. The sensation may be one of turning or whirling, or it may be a less well-defined symptom of giddiness, weakness, confusion, blankness, or unsteadiness.

Dizziness may be produced by alteration in the normal physiology of the *eyes, proprioceptive system, statokinetic system* (labyrinth, eighth nerve, and vestibular nuclei), *cerebellum*, or *cerebrum*.

The interrelationship between the labyrinth, eyes, and proprioceptive system is the important mechanism (Fig. 29-1). Loss or disturbances of function of any one of these structures will upset normal equilibrium. When loss of function of one occurs, the other two may gradually compensate, so that equilibrium and locomotion are almost normal. However, loss of function of *any two* results in incapacitation. For example, the patient with tabes dorsalis whose vestibulospinal tracts are damaged may be able to walk when he can see but is unable to maintain his balance when in the dark. Similarly, a blind person who has never learned to swim may be totally unable to coordinate his muscles in the water.

A sensation of true whirling or turning means disturbed function in the end-organ, eighth nerve, or vestibular nuclei. Various other sensations that patients may describe as dizziness indicate the presence of lesions at higher levels or regions farther away. The former group of symptoms can be called *systematized vertigo*, and the latter group *nonsystematized dizziness*. The following classification is based on this premise.

Nonsystematized dizziness

I. Eyes
  A. Muscle imbalance
  B. Refractive errors
  C. Simple glaucoma
II. Proprioceptive system
  A. Pellagra
  B. Chronic alcoholism
  C. Pernicious anemia
  D. Tabes dorsalis
III. Central nervous system
  A. Mild cerebral anoxemia
    1. Arteriosclerosis
    2. Hypertensive cardiovascular disease
    3. Chronic hypertension
    4. Anemia
    5. Paroxysmal auricular fibrillation
    6. Aortic stenosis with insufficiency
    7. Heart block
    8. Carotid sinus syndrome
    9. Simple syncope
    10. Postural hypotension
  B. Infection
    1. Meningitis
    2. Encephalitis
    3. Brain abscess
    4. Syphilis
  C. Trauma
  D. Tumors
  E. Migraine
  F. Petit mal epilepsy
  G. Endocrine conditions
    1. Menstrual-pregnancy-menopause pattern
    2. Hypoparathyroidism with tetany
    3. Hypothyroidism
    4. Paroxysmal hypertension associated with adrenal medullary tumor
    5. Hypoglycemia
  H. Psychoneurosis

Systematized vertigo

I. Ear
  A. External ear
    1. Wax or foreign bodies

B. Middle ear
   1. Retracted tympanic membrane
   2. Acute disease
      a. Acute suppurative otitis media
      b. Otitis media with effusion
   3. Chronic disease
      a. Labyrinthitis
      b. Cholesteatoma (fistula reaction)
   4. Injury with hemorrhage
C. Internal ear
   1. Acute toxic labyrinthitis
   2. Vascular episodes
   3. Trauma
   4. Allergy
   5. Hydrops of the labyrinth (Meniere's disease)
   6. Motion sickness
   7. Postural vertigo

II. Eighth nerve
   A. Infection
      1. Acute meningitis
      2. Tuberculous meningitis
      3. Basilar syphilitic meningitis
   B. Trauma
   C. Tumors
III. Brain stem (nuclei)
   A. Infections
      1. Encephalitis
      2. Meningitis
      3. Brain abscess
   B. Trauma
   C. Hemorrhage
   D. Thrombosis of posteroinferior cerebellar artery
   E. Tumors
   F. Multiple sclerosis

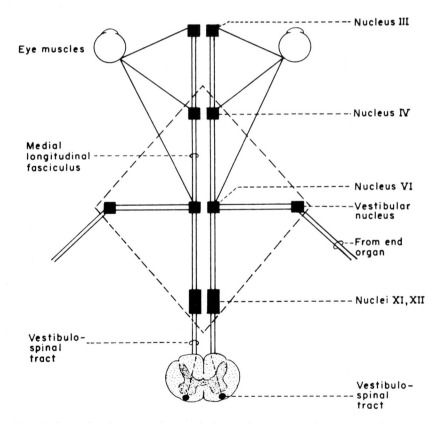

FIG. 29-1. Relationship between the vestibular nuclei, eye muscle nuclei, and proprioceptive tracts. For ease of recall, note the resemblance to a baseball diamond. (From DeWeese, D. D.: Dizziness; an evaluation and classification, Springfield, Ill., 1953, Charles C Thomas, Publisher.)

HISTORY

The evaluation of dizziness must begin with the history. It is the *most important* part of the examination. Certain diseases or syndromes present a characteristic history. In many other diseases, the physical examination, roentgenograms, and laboratory tests are normal and the probable diagnosis *must* be suspected from the *history alone*. In taking the history, the examiner should elicit the following information:

1. Whether the patient has experienced *true whirling*. The direction and character of the motion are not important. The fact that there either is or is not a real sense of motion is important. With his eyes open the patient feels that objects are moving around him, but with his eyes closed he feels that he is in motion. *Both indicate true vertigo* and narrow the field of investigation to the statokinetic system. If it is not possible to elicit a history of a sense of motion, the entire body becomes a field for investigation.

2. The *pattern of the dizziness*. A history of paroxysmal attacks with intervals of complete relief between attacks may indicate certain diseases. Similarly, a history of continued dizziness indicates other diseases. The time of occurrence may be important. The time of day and any relationship to menstrual periods, occupation, trauma, and medications may be important.

3. The *degree of dizziness*. Severe vertigo accompanied by nausea or vomiting is, in the absence of central nervous system disease, usually due to labyrinthine disease. Less severe dizziness, without a demonstrable pattern, may arise from disease in any part of the body.

4. Any *associated hearing loss* or *tinnitus*. When hearing loss accompanies the dizziness, localization of the cause is easier.

EXAMINATION

The functional examination of the ear is an essential part of the examination. An audiogram should always be made. If it is normal, further hearing tests are unnecessary. If it is abnormal, it is imperative to determine definitely whether the hearing loss is conductive or sensorineural in nature. Care must be taken in determining bone conduction. Masking of the opposite ear should be done to ensure accuracy, and the audiometric findings should be checked with tuning forks (see discussion of hearing tests in Chapter 20).

An abnormal audiogram does not always indicate that the statokinetic system is responsible for the dizziness. It may be an incidental finding unrelated to the symptom being investigated.

The function of the labyrinth can be tested in several ways (see discussion of tests for labyrinthine reactions in Chapter 21). Regardless of the technique used, and assuming that it is constant from patient to patient, the *interpretation of the reaction produced by stimulation is of primary importance*. The patient should be questioned regarding the intensity of the subjective sensation and asked (before the test is begun) to compare the sensation produced to the dizziness he usually experiences. If the response produced by labyrinthine testing is described by the patient as much more severe than the symptom being investigated, one can be sure that the patient is not suffering from an end-organ lesion of any significance. If the response is similar to, or less severe than, the patient's spontaneous dizziness, disease of the statokinetic system should be suspected. If there is definite hyperactivity of the *subjective* response without a coincident hyperactivity of the *observed* labyrinthine reactions, a neurosis should be suspected. True hyperactive responses can be anticipated from the history. A history of swing sickness, car sickness, or seasickness suggests that the labyrinths are hyperactive. If no reaction can be produced, one can safely consider that labyrinthine function is absent (that is, that the labyrinth is dead). Perverted nystagmus, such as vertical, oblique, variable, third-degree, or gretaly exaggerated nystagmus, is suggestive of central nervous system disease.

One must guard against placing too much emphasis on caloric reactions or attempting to emphasize minute deviations. Often one can be sure only of *normalcy, hyperactivity, hypoactivity*, or *complete loss of function*.

Attempts to elicit positional nystagmus should be repeated several times if postural vertigo is a possibility. Positional nystagmus cannot be reproduced every time a given change of position is assumed. When positional nystagmus can be demonstrated, the direction of the nystagmus must be noted. If nystagmus that changes direction with different head positions is elicited, it is attributed to a central lesion. If the direction of the nystagmus produced by position change is constant, either central or peripheral disease may be indicated.

Correlation of the history, physical examination, and all other examinations is necessary to arrive at the correct diagnosis as often as possible.

One must not make the error of dumping into a general "wastebasket" many cases bearing such labels as pseudo-Meniere's disease, Meniere-like syndrome, or functional dizziness. Such diagnoses, without careful examination, increase the probability of error in exact diagnosis and lead to trial-and-error management, which is often unsuccessful. If the dizziness is disturbing enough to the patient to make him seek medical advice, it may require as complete an investigation as fever of unknown origin or other obscure symptoms with few confirmatory signs.

When the symptom of dizziness is obscure, whether or not the sensation is one of motion, discovery of the cause may be difficult. Often the combined talents of the otolaryngologist, the neurologist, the ophthalmologist, and the internist are required to determine the underlying cause. Unless the cause is apparent or the symptom self-limited, close cooperation among several physicians offers the best chance for successful diagnosis. In spite of all efforts, there will still be patients in whom the cause of dizziness cannot be discovered and in whom treatment must be on an empiric, symptomatic basis.

DIFFERENTIAL DIAGNOSIS—
NONSYSTEMATIZED DIZZINESS
EYES

Normal or nearly normal vision is necessary to maintain a normal relationship of the body to the environment. The blind person has lost one of the three senses that maintain equilibrium. He must rely on the labyrinth and the proprioceptive system. Therefore a disturbance of vision may produce dizziness when all other systems of the body are normal.

Muscle imbalance. Muscle imbalance is a cause of dizziness. The dizziness is not severe, nor is it whirling in nature. Muscle imbalance should be suspected as a possible etiologic factor when a patient has mild dizziness that he has difficulty describing and that is annoying but not incapacitating. Transient diplopia may also be a symptom.

Errors of refraction. Errors of refraction may produce the same subjective complaint. They are more easily suspected, since there is more

likely to be an actual complaint of visual difficulty. Errors of refraction should be suspected if the patient complains of dizziness and his history reveals that he had a new prescription for glasses at the time of, or shortly before, the onset of dizziness. Errors of refraction should also be suspected when there is a history of frequent change of glasses.

Simple glaucoma. Simple glaucoma may also produce a sensation of dizziness.

PROPRIOCEPTIVE SYSTEM

Diseases of the proprioceptive system or of the spinal tracts carrying proprioceptive sensations to the central nervous system may be accompanied by dizziness. Advanced stages of these diseases are also associated with a disturbed sense of position. Therefore they may produce ataxia. An ataxic or staggering gait also occurs as part of the disturbance of the statokinetic system or of the cerebellum.

Pellagra. Pellagra still exists in many areas. It may produce dizziness or ataxia, or both.

Chronic alcoholism. Chronic alcoholism may produce peripheral changes in nerve pathways. It may also reduce the absorption of vitamins from the gastrointestinal tract sufficiently to produce symptoms similar to those of pellagra but less severe.

Pernicious anemia. Pernicious anemia frequently causes dizziness. When it is advanced, the dizziness may also be accompanied by ataxia, loss of motion and position sense, and loss of vibratory sense in the lower extremities.

Tabes dorsalis. Tabes dorsalis may produce symptoms identical to those produced in pernicious anemia or pellagra, since the disease process commonly involves the posterior and lateral columns of the spinal cord.

CENTRAL NERVOUS SYSTEM

Any disease of the central nervous system may irritate or partially block some part of the pathways that influence equilibrium. Certain conditions are more likely to produce dizziness as a single presenting complaint.

Mild cerebral anoxemia. Mild cerebral anoxemia is produced by a wide variety of conditions and may be of short or long duration. Frequently the underlying condition will give rise to a sensation of dizziness that lasts a few moments or rises to the conscious level at any time of the day or night.

In none of these conditions do we find tinnitus or hearing loss as part of the picture. Both tinnitus and hearing loss may be present in patients with cerebral anoxemia, but they are not part of the symptomatology.

ARTERIOSCLEROSIS, HYPERTENSIVE CARDIO-VASCULAR DISEASE, AND CHRONIC HYPOTEN-SION. Arteriosclerosis, hypertensive cardiovascular disease, and chronic hypotension may all produce the picture described. The complaint is usually one of a feeling of imbalance or insecurity that the patient finds difficult to describe. It is not present constantly but usually occurs several times a day for varying periods of time and with varying intensity. It may be influenced by fatigue, emotional upset, or overwork.

ANEMIA. Anemia may produce cerebral anoxemia. Any condition that produces a low hemoglobin, from simple iron deficiency to leukemia, may be the underlying cause of dizziness.

CARDIAC DISEASE. Paroxysmal auricular fibrillation, aortic stenosis with insufficiency and regurgitation, heart block, and carotid sinus syndrome are important causes of dizziness. The dizziness is sudden, paroxysmal, and separated by variable intervals during which there are no symptoms. Because of the paroxysmal nature of these symptoms, the underlying condition may easily be misinterpreted as Meniere's syndrome unless care is taken with the history and examination. In heart block and carotid sinus syndrome the onset of symptoms may be so sudden that the patient falls to the ground without a chance to seek support. The onset of symptoms in heart block and carotid sinus syndrome is usually more abrupt than in Meniere's syndrome. Simple syncope also causes sudden light-headedness (or dizziness) and, of course, loss of consciousness.

POSTURAL HYPOTENSION. Many persons, particularly in the later decades of life, complain of dizziness when they rise from bed or a sitting position. The dizziness lasts only a few moments and is rarely severe enough to cause falling. It is followed by complete recovery until the next sudden change of posture. Such dizziness is caused by failure of the blood pressure to rise when the person stands and is commonly referred to as postural hypotension. Recordings of the blood pressure while the patient is in the recumbent position and immediately after he rises will usually demonstrate that the blood pressure falls sharply. Treatment consists of educating the patient to make a habit of rising slowly.

Inflammation. Inflammation may be the underlying cause of dizziness.

MENINGITIS, ENCEPHALITIS, AND BRAIN AB-SCESS. Meningitis, encephalitis, and brain abscess are frequently accompanied by dizziness. The dizziness is not violent or paroxysmal but is usually slowly progressive. Spontaneous nystagmus may be present. Postural vertigo should be expected, and perversion of caloric response from the labyrinths may occur. Encephalitis may involve the cochlear or vestibular nuclei and may be associated with hearing loss. The diagnosis is established from signs such as fever, disturbance in function of other cranial nerves, increased intracranial pressure, papilledema, and so forth.

SYPHILIS. For centuries syphilis has been known as the great imitator. In many areas of the central nervous system it can cause changes that will produce dizziness or nystagmus, or both. There is nothing characteristic about the dizziness produced by syphilis.

Trauma. Trauma to the central nervous system is a frequent cause of dizziness. Dizziness without whirling occurs frequently. Fortunately, this form of dizziness is mild, recedes slowly (up to 6 or 8 months), and usually does not have a tendency to recur. The sensation is one of unsteadiness, giddiness, or weakness. It is often made worse by a change of position or by exertion and frequently is accompanied by blackouts. Other symptoms, such as headache, fatigue, and difficulty in concentration, are common. The exact location of the disease producing this dizziness is unknown. It may be due to multiple small hemorrhages of the central nervous system or to concussion alone, as well as to disturbance of the normal neuron pathways. The ultimate prognosis is good, and reassurance should be given to the patient to prevent the development of a neurosis on the basis of fear from continued insecurity.

Tumors. Brain tumors may cause dizziness. When they arise in or near the statokinetic system, they may produce whirling (systematized) vertigo. When they originate in other areas of the central nervous system, they produce nonsystematized dizziness. Dizziness of this type is neither characteristic nor diagnostic. Other evidence of a brain tumor is necessary before the diagnosis can be established.

Migraine. Migraine may be preceded by an aura of dizziness, or it may be accompanied by dizziness. The typical pattern is a unilateral headache associated with scotoma, nausea, and vomiting for 1 to 4 days. In some persons dizziness is the outstanding symptom and the headache is secondary. When dizziness predominates, it is often referred to as a migraine equivalent.

Petit mal epilepsy. Petit mal epilepsy may cause dizziness. A careful history will help to establish that such dizziness is actually a sudden, momentary loss of consciousness without aura or after symptoms. No nystagmus, tinnitus, or hearing loss accompanies this condition.

Endocrine conditions. Endocrine dysfunction can give rise to dizziness. The mechanism by which this is produced is unknown.

MENSTRUATION, PREGNANCY, MENOPAUSE. Clinical observation reveals many instances in which dizziness is part of the menopausal pattern or is associated with pregnancy, menstruation, or the administration of hormone substances, particularly estrogens. In obscure cases of dizziness the patient's case history should be carefully taken and evaluated in an effort to determine whether there is a relationship between the dizziness and the menstruation-pregnancy-menopause pattern.

HYPOGLYCEMIA. Hypoglycemia may be the cause of nonsystematized dizziness. It should be suspected when there is a definite time relationship between dizziness and hunger or ingestion of food. The dizziness resulting from a low level of blood glucose comes on gradually over a period of 15 to 30 minutes and lasts from 1 to 2 hours (until food is ingested or the level of blood glucose rises again). It is usually accompanied by a feeling of fatigue. The symptoms may progress to apprehension, overexcitability, and convulsive movements such as those seen in a diabetic patient who has had an overdose of insulin. Hypoglycemia can be proved only by a glucose tolerance test. Management of dizziness caused by hypoglycemia consists of a high-protein, high-fat diet and thorough follow-up study. A possible diagnosis of islet cell tumor of the pancreas should be considered.

OTHER ENDOCRINE CONDITIONS. Hypoparathyroidism with tetany, hypothyroidism, or paroxysmal hypertension associated with adrenal medullary tumor may also give rise to dizziness.

Psychoneurosis. Psychoneurosis undoubtedly accounts for many instances of nonsystematized dizziness. There is nothing characteristic about this type of dizziness. In the absence of disease of the ear, it is not accompanied by hearing loss and tinnitus. Tinnitus may have a functional basis, but its association with dizziness on this basis is probably coincidental. In these cases the physician can make no definite rules except to be aware of the possibility. The practice of labeling any set of symptoms the physician cannot explain as "functional" not only dulls the investigative powers of the physician but also may lead to errors in diagnosis or to neglect of organic disease. *The physician should form the habit of searching for organic causes first.* Furthermore, even when organic disease cannot be demonstrated, the diagnosis of functional dizziness should be made only when it is supported by other symptoms and signs of psychoneurosis.

DIFFERENTIAL DIAGNOSIS— SYSTEMATIZED VERTIGO

The characteristic of dizziness caused by disturbance of the statokinetic system is a *sense of motion.* The direction or character of the sense of motion is not as important as the fact that there is a feeling of whirling or propulsion. The patient's feeling that he is turning, which occurs with the eyes closed, is of no more significance than his feeling that the environment is turning around him, which occurs with the eyes open.

Systematized vertigo is frequently accompanied by nausea or vomiting. It is often accompanied by either loss of hearing or tinnitus, or both. Spontaneous nystagmus is frequently present with whirling vertigo. It may be present only at times of severe vertigo, or it may not be seen, because the patient consults the physician between attacks of vertigo. However, *when it is seen, it is indicative of disease, and in most cases the disease is in the statokinetic system.*

EAR

External ear and middle ear. Vertigo may be caused by disease of the external ear and middle ear.

WAX AND FOREIGN BODIES. Disease of the external ear may produce vertigo. It is usually mild and most commonly is caused by wax firmly impacted against the tympanic membrane. Foreign bodies against the drum membrane may also produce vertigo.

NEGATIVE PRESSURE IN THE MIDDLE EAR. Negative pressure in the middle ear from eustachian tube blockage may cause vertigo. The vertigo may be constant or paroxysmal, mild or severe.

ACUTE SUPPURATIVE OTITIS MEDIA. Acute suppurative otitis media and its complications can be the cause of vertigo. The vertigo is mild when it accompanies uncomplicated otitis media. It is whirling when it is associated with mastoiditis complicated by labyrinthitis. Purulent invasion of the labyrinth usually causes severe loss of perceptive hearing in the involved ear and almost always results in a dead labyrinth. Vertigo associated with suppurative middle ear disease is always a danger signal.

Destruction of the inner table of the mastoid, which produces an epidural abscess on the anterior face of the cerebellum, can give all the signs of labyrinthitis.

These complications are rare today because of the advances in chemotherapy, but they still occur in patients who have been undertreated or untreated.

OTITIS MEDIA WITH EFFUSION. Otitis media with effusion is often accompanied by dizziness. The dizziness is a feeling of imbalance rather than a whirling sensation and is usually more noticeable when the patient changes position. It is not as severe as postural vertigo, the dizziness that occurs suddenly during changes of position.

CHRONIC SUPPURATIVE OTITIS MEDIA. Chronic suppurative otitis media and its complications may be the cause of systematized vertigo. Acute exacerbations of chronic disease may produce labyrinthitis identical to that seen with acute mastoiditis.

CHOLESTEATOMA. A cholesteatoma causes erosion and enlargement of the attic of the middle ear, as well as erosion of the mastoid antrum and of the horizontal semicircular canal. If erosion of the labyrinth occurs, the patient may experience sudden severe vertigo that throws him to the floor. Typically, the onset is so rapid that the patient cannot protect himself. However, the vertigo is over in a few moments, and there are no after-symptoms. There may be a history of such episodes immediately following sneezing or blowing of the nose. An attack may occur if the patient puts his finger into the ear canal to scratch the canal or if he cleans the ear with an applicator or with an irrigating solution. This history is pathognomonic of a fistula in the labyrinth and can be confirmed by the fistula test (see the discussion of tests for labyrinthine reactions in Chapter 21).

INJURY. Injury to the middle ear can produce vertigo. Blows over the ear with the open hand may rupture the eardrum and dislocate the ossicles, which would cause temporary vertigo. Fractures through the middle ear produce vertigo and may be accompanied by bleeding or leaking of cerebrospinal fluid from the middle ear.

Internal ear. Many conditions of the middle ear give rise to vertigo.

ACUTE TOXIC LABYRINTHITIS. Acute toxic labrinthitis is probably the most frequent syndrome of whirling vertigo the physician sees. Typically, there is a gradual onset of whirling vertigo that reaches a maximum in 24 to 48 hours. At its height the vertigo is accompanied by nausea and vomiting. Then it gradually regresses to normal over a 3- to 6-week period. *Tinnitus and hearing loss do not occur.*

The patient suffering from acute toxic labyrinthitis is frequently incapacitated for 3 to 5 days, during which time any motion of the head brings on the symptoms. He seeks the supine position. During the period of recovery, a less severe sensation of whirling occurs when the head is turned suddenly in any direction. This syndrome may accompany acute febrile diseases such as pneumonia, cholecystitis, or influenza. In many patients it follows the ingestion of drugs, overindulgence in alcohol, allergy, or extreme fatigue. Reassurance of recovery is important in management.

The inclusion of this syndrome with the discussion of internal ear dysfunction may be open to argument. The exact area of irritation of the statokinetic system that gives rise to acute toxic labyrinthitis is unknown. The severity of the vertigo and the added irritation from any movement suggest the end-organ as the probable site of the disturbance. The use of the word "toxic" is in itself an admission of ignorance and should be recognized as such. In most cases it means that we are assuming the presence of a toxic irritation from some source without having any proof that such is true. Nevertheless, the syndrome is common and characteristic. The name given to it is descriptive and must serve until the exact mechanism of this condition is discovered. This sequence of symptoms is also commonly called "vestibular neuronitis."

VASCULAR EPISODES. Vascular episodes of several types can disturb the physiology of the internal ear and produce vertigo. Arterial spasm may reduce the blood supply to the labyrinth and produce transient whirling vertigo with nystagmus. It is most frequently seen with hypertensive cardiovascular disease. Rupture of a vein or artery with hemorrhage into the labyrinth produces a sudden, dramatic, incapacitating vertigo. This is accompanied by loud tinnitus and sudden loss of hearing. Complete loss of hearing and loss of caloric response are evident early and are permanent. In 3 to 4 weeks equilibrium is well established and nearly normal physical activity can be resumed, although some instability remains.

TRAUMA. Trauma to the internal ear may result from fracture through the internal ear, concussion, or sudden loud noise. Fracture through the cochlea and vestibule may give a picture exactly like hemorrhage into the internal ear. The seventh cranial nerve will frequently be injured, and facial paralysis will follow. Head injuries producing sudden linear motion of the head may tear the membranes of the internal ear and cause vertigo. In both situations hearing loss and usually tinnitus accompany the vertigo.

When head injury results in systematized vertigo that is associated with hearing loss but no visible damage to the middle ear or eardrum, the vertigo occurs early and may persist for years. The dizziness disappears and recurs in varying degrees of severity. Caloric stimulation frequently shows a delay in response and a decrease in the amplitude of nystagmus.

The physician is often asked to estimate the duration of probable incapacity or to evaluate the extent of disability as a basis for determining unemployment compensation. The prognosis as to the duration of the disability should always be guarded, and the patient should be followed at intervals to determine at what stage his return to work will be safe. Such a patient should be warned regarding the dangers of working in high places and driving a car.

Malingering, or compensation neurosis, must constantly be borne in mind when one is evaluating the condition of patients with evidence of trauma to the internal ear. In the absence of other evidence of a neurosis, when malingering is suspected, the patient should be given the benefit of doubt until further observations are carried out.

ALLERGY. Allergy may produce whirling dizziness. There is nothing characteristic about this dizziness.

HYDROPS OF THE LABYRINTH (MENIERE'S SYNDROME). Hydrops of the labyrinth, which is usually called Meniere's disease or Meniere's syndrome, is a common cause of *paroxysmal, whirling vertigo*. In this condition a triad of symptoms is seen: (1) *attacks of whirling vertigo*, (2) *tinnitus*, and (3) *sensorineural hearing loss*. Early in the disease one or two of the symptoms may occur without the third. A final diagnosis of labyrinthine hydrops *should not be made*, however, until all three symptoms are present. In most patients the vertigo, the tinnitus, and the hearing loss exhibit certain patterns that are characteristic of labyrinthine hydrops.

Isolated attacks of severe whirling vertigo, with no dizziness or instability between attacks, is the most characteristic symptom of Meniere's syndrome. Each attack begins abruptly, but not so suddenly that a patient falls. In the typical attack the vertigo increases for 10 minutes to an hour, persists for several hours, and subsides. It is *important to remember* that the vertigo lasts *hours, not days or weeks*. Continuous vertigo for several days is *not* typical of labyrinthine hydrops.

The attacks may be several weeks or months apart. If the patient is not treated, the attacks become more frequent and more severe until they may occur once every 2 or 3 days. Rarely, in the most severe cases, they may occur daily, *but* they remain paroxysmal, and there are periods of complete relief between attacks. Most episodes of this type of vertigo are associated with both nausea and vomiting for several hours. Nausea without vomiting may be seen in mild attacks.

The hearing loss associated with Meniere's syndrome is typically a sensorineural loss of *low tones* (Fig. 25-6). It is present in only one ear in most instances. Rarely, there is bilateral endolymphatic hydrops. The loss of hearing tends to fluctuate abruptly, but when the patient is not treated, the hearing loss progresses slowly to severe cochlear damage. A sense of fullness or pressure in the involved ear is a frequent complaint when the hearing is impaired. Distortion of certain words and diplacusis (see p. 289) are common.

The typical audiogram of patients with labyrinthine hydrops reveals the low-tone character of the loss. In patients with other types of sensorineural hearing loss the *high* frequencies are most often impaired. Recruitment of loudness in some degree is almost always present. This condition may be suspected when a patient complains that loud, sharp sounds are annoying or painful in the ear that has poor hearing (see pp. 287-288 and Fig. 20-8).

The tinnitus that accompanies endolymphatic hydrops is typically a low buzz, and it fluctuates. It is frequently louder preceding or during the attack of vertigo. Both hearing loss and tinnitus remain between attacks of vertigo.

Caloric stimulation of the involved ear may produce normal responses, but more often the reaction is hypoactive. Sometimes the response is hypoactive in the impaired ear alone, but not infrequently it is hypoactive in both ears. A hyperactive response to caloric stimulation should make one doubt the presence of labyrinthine hydrops.

One may see patients with attacks of vertigo that are without hearing loss or tinnitus but that otherwise are typical of labyrinthine hydrops. In these patients the diagnosis should not be made until hearing loss or tinnitus appears.

In 1938 Hallpike and Cairns first reported the pathologic changes in hydrops. These changes have since been confirmed by several others from postmortem examination of temporal bones of patients known to have labyrinthine hydrops. They consist of gross distention of the endolymphatic system and consequent degeneration of the neural end-organ of both the labyrinth and the cochlea. The underlying cause is not yet known. It has been attributed to many things, including sodium retention, allergy, vascular spasm, abnormal production of endolymph, and toxicity. It is likely that each of these conditions may play a part in producing the syndrome. Some recent experimental evidence indicates that the attacks of vertigo may be caused by the sudden rupture of small vesicles that form in the walls of the endolymphatic system. This theory, however, still does not explain the underlying cause of the vesicle formation.

Too often Meniere's syndrome has been another "wastebasket" into which unclassified cases of vertigo are carelessly thrown. Regardless of its cause, the syndrome presents a clear-cut history and functional changes in the ears. Both elements of the syndrome should be rigidly demanded before paroxysmal vertigo is labeled Meniere's disease.

MEDICAL TREATMENT. Although most patients with Meniere's syndrome are seen between attacks and the attacks are self-limited without treatment, there are times when the acute vertiginous attacks should, and can, be stopped. This is accomplished effectively by the following methods:

1. Atropine, given subcutaneously, will often stop an attack in 20 to 30 minutes. The dose should be 1/75 grain.
2. Epinephrine (Adrenaline), given intravenously at a very slow rate, may stop the attack. Usually 3 to 5 minims of a 1:1000 solution will suffice. The least amount necessary should be used.
3. Histamine diphosphate (beta-imidazolylethylamine diacide phosphate), which is prepared in ampules of 2.75 mg., can be given in 250 to 500 ml. of 5% glucose solution. The drip should be slow, giving the total dose in approximately 1 hour; it should be given at a slower rate if there is excessive flushing, headache, or precordial pressure.
4. Diphenhydramine hydrochloride (Benadryl) is also effective when given intravenously. The dosage is up to 100 mg., given slowly in full strength as supplied for intravenous use (10 ml.), or added to an intravenous solution of glucose.

Strong reassurance should be given to all patients to help them realize that the attacks will ultimately stop of their own accord or that they can be stopped. Control of the anxiety caused by the violence of the vertigo and of the retching will make any other treatment more effective.

The most successful method of managing continuing vertigo of Meniere's syndrome is still that of restricting salt intake. A neutral ash, salt-free diet, when properly controlled, and ammonium chloride will give relief of vertigo to more than 75% of patients. The disappointment of some physicians with the results of salt restriction and the use of ammonium chloride is due, we believe, to the fact that they either have been lax in controlling the diet or have not given large enough doses of the ammonium chloride. To obtain good results, salt must be completely eliminated from the diet. This means preparation of food without salt, the use of salt-free bread and salt-free butter, and abstinence from food high in sodium content. In our experience, the following diet (the Furstenberg diet) has been effective.

Diet for Meniere's disease (Furstenberg diet)

1. Fluids not restricted; however, excessive quantities of water discouraged
2. Proteins unrestricted or forced; calories permitted as indicated; sodium allowance low
3. All foods to be prepared and served without salt
4. The following foods to be eaten daily:
   a. Eggs, meat, fish, and fowl as desired
   b. Bread as desired
   c. Cereal, one of the following: farina, oatmeal, rice, puffed rice, or puffed wheat
   d. Potato and at least one of the following: macaroni, spaghetti, rice, corn, plums, prunes, or cranberries
   e. Any fruit and any vegetable not listed below
   f. Milk as desired
   g. Butter, cream, honey, jellies, jam, sugar, and candy (except chocolate) as desired
5. The following foods to be avoided at all times:

Salted meats and fish	Carrots	Cheese
	Spinach	Condensed
Bread, crackers,	Endive	milk
and butter pre-	Cow peas	Olives
pared with salt	Clams	Raisins
	Oysters	Caviar

6. The following foods may be eaten no more than twice weekly:

Chard	Radishes	Muskmelon
Kohlrabi	Celery	Dried currants
Pumpkin	Cantaloupe	Dried coconut
Watercress	Strawberries	Buttermilk
Beets	Limes	Peanuts
Cauliflower	Peaches	Horseradish
Turnips	Figs	Mustard
Rutabagas	Dates	

For best results, the ammonium chloride must be given in large doses and in capsule form. Enteric-coated capsules often pass through the gastrointestinal tract unchanged. The initial dosage should be six capsules of 0.5 gm. each with each meal for 3 days; then no ammonium chloride is taken for 2 days. This provides 9 gm. of ammonium chloride for 3 out of every 5 days. Most patients can tolerate this dosage without gastric discomfort if the capsules are taken at intervals throughout the meal rather than in a single dose. If too much gastric irritation occurs, the dosage can be reduced to 1 or 2 gm. per meal, instead of 3 gm.

Insistence on this rigid regimen frequently gives immediate good results. Many patients have no further vertiginous attacks after starting the diet. If an immediate result is obtained, the program should be continued for 2 or 3 months, after which time the ammonium chloride can be stopped. If the vertigo does not recur after the patient has had no ammonium chloride for 3 or 4 weeks, small amounts of salt can be allowed in the diet. However, the patient can never resume intake of the amount of salt commonly used.

Potassium chloride in large doses has been advised as a substitute for salt restriction. It has been shown, however, that salt restriction is necessary if the potassium is to have a beneficial effect.

Vasodilating drugs of many kinds have been effective in controlling the symptoms of Meniere's syndrome. They are perhaps more effective than salt restriction in improving tinnitus and hearing loss. For many patients a vasodilator is a worthwhile addition to the salt-free program. For the many patients who are unable to follow a strict salt-free program, vasodilators must be used as the main method of controlling the vertigo.

The most effective vasodilator is nicotinic acid. It is relatively inexpensive, has no injurious side effects, and accomplishes good vasodilation. Administration of the drug is usually started with 50 mg. three times a day *20 minutes before meals*. The dosage may be raised successively to 100 or even 200 mg. three times a day. The desired effect is obtained when there is flushing of the peripheral skin. Although this flushing need not occur after every dose of nicotinic acid, it should follow the majority of the doses. In other words, if flushing occurs half the time with 50-mg. doses, it is unnecessary to increase the dosage.

Nicotinic acid amide does not produce dilation or increased blood flow either intracranially or peripherally. Therefore it cannot be used in place of nicotinic acid.

Roniacol tartrate (beta-pyridyl-carbinol) can be used successfully in a dosage of 25 to 50 mg. four times a day and can be increased, if necessary, to produce flushing. It has no particular advantage over nicotinic acid.

Tolazoline hydrochloride (Priscoline) produces a similar effect when given orally or intramuscularly.

Other vasodilators, such as neostigmine or magnesium sulfate, have been used experimentally and have had good results. Again, however, they offer no advantages over nicotinic acid.

Methantheline bromide (Banthine) has been effective when used either alone or in conjunction with salt restriction and vasodilators, or both. In some instances it appears to have a dramatic beneficial effect on tinnitus and hearing loss. The initial dose may be either 50 or 100 mg. every 6 hours. If 100 mg. is used, the dosage should be dropped to 50 mg. every 6 hours after a therapeutic effect has been achieved. Propantheline bromide (Pro-Banthine) in doses of 15 mg. every 6 hours will occasionally give the same results.

There are a few patients with Meniere's syndrome whose attacks appear to be initiated by fluid retention during the premenstrual period. They frequently will notice weight gain and puffiness of the hands and feet during the 10 days preceding menstruation. It may be necessary to give them vitamin B or diethylstilbestrol (1 mg. daily) and thyroid extract in small doses. Any such program must be adapted to the needs of the individual patient.

The use of histamine has been advised as a means of controlling the continuing symptoms of Meniere's syndrome. Horton's method of successive daily intravenous injections of histamine in the dosage already described for treatment of the acute vertiginous attack has been advised. There is considerable valid controversy regarding the supposition that a patient can be desensitized to histamine. The effectiveness of histamine as a general treatment seems exaggerated. Whatever beneficial results are obtained must be explained on a basis other than desensitization to histamine. The probable effect of histamine is that of vasodilation.

Benadryl and dimenhydrinate (Dramamine) in the ordinary doses of 50 to 100 mg. every 4 to 6 hours have been used in the management of Meniere's syndrome and have had varying degrees of success. In any patient who gives a history of other episodes of allergic reactions, the antihistamine drugs may be of benefit and occasionally may be all that is necessary for control. Williams said that in only 5% of patients with Meniere's syndrome is there an allergic cause. Dramamine raises the threshold of labyrinthine irritability and therefore may be successfully used without other treatment in patients with mild vertigo. In patients with severe vertigo it does not appear to be equally effective.

In addition to these specific methods of controlling the continuing symptoms of Meniere's syndrome, attention must be given to the tension factors produced by the severity of the vertiginous attacks. Therefore phenobarbital in small doses may be given to these patients. The *sodium barbiturates*, such as pentobarbital (Nembutal) and secobarbital (Seconal), *should never be used*. Because nicotine is known to have a vasospastic action, some patients should be advised to stop the use of tobacco.

SURGICAL TREATMENT. Surgical destruction of the labyrinth may be both necessary and justifiable when (1) medical management fails, as it will in 10% to 20% of patients; (2) the attacks continue and are severe; or (3) a patient's occupation makes it either imperative that he take no chance on having an attack or impossible for him to carry out medical management. Most patients chosen for the operation have failed to respond to any type of medical management. The syndrome these patients present is progressive, and the hearing in the affected ear is seriously and permanently damaged.

Surgical destruction of the labyrinth has in recent years slowly supplanted partial or complete eighth nerve section. The procedure is not formidable for anyone trained in temporal bone surgery. The morbidity from the operation is low, and there should be no mortality.

One procedure consists of a simple mastoidectomy. Enough mastoid cells are removed to uncover the horizontal semicircular canal. Then a window is made in the anterior end of the canal, as a fenestration surgery. Through this window the canal and the vestibule of the labyrinth are destroyed either by careful electrocoagulation, after the method of Day, or by mechanical destruction, as described by Cawthorne. The latter procedure, performed with small forceps, fine-wire probes, or dental nerve broaches, is less dangerous because it avoids the possibility of damage to the facial nerve by the electrocoagulating current.

A second procedure is to reflect the tympanic membrane (as is done in operations on the stapes), remove the stapes, and destroy the labyrinth through the oval window. This procedure has been more common since the advances in middle ear surgery during the past 20 years.

Further destruction of the cochlea has been advocated in the hope of stopping tinnitus, but this approach has not always been successful. Cervical sympathetic ganglionectomy and a stellate ganglion block have been tried. However, results are not yet certain, and there seem to be no advantages to these procedures over labyrinthine destruction. Ultrasonic vibrations have been used successfully as a method of labyrinthine destruction.

Endolymphatic pressure has been relieved by a "shunt" procedure. In selected patients it has been possible to insert a plastic tube or button between the endolymphatic sac and the subarachnoid space. Careful case selection is important. It is not always possible to create a "shunt" between the endolymph and the subarachnoid space. Surgical decompression of the endolymphatic sac without shunting has often been successful in controlling vertigo and preserving hearing.

In other carefully selected patients a "tack" has been successful in controlling vertigo in endolymphatic hydrops. In this procedure the middle ear is exposed, with the patient under local anesthesia, in a manner similar to that of a stapes operation. Under magnification of platinum "tack" (specifically made as to shape and length) is inserted through the footplate of the stapes and remains in place permanently. The success of this procedure is dependent on temporary relief of endolymphatic pressure each time the point of the "tack" ruptures the utricular membrane as it expands under increased endolymphatic pressure.

Streptomycin, administered systemically and carefully controlled by serial audiometry and caloric testing, has been used to decrease labyrinthine activity and prevent attacks of vertigo caused by labyrinthine hydrops. Such treatment is difficult to control and obviously has the disadvantage of causing a depressing and toxic effect on *both ears*, even though treatment is intended for only one ear.

COGAN'S SYNDROME. In 1945 Cogan described a condition of nonsyphilitic interstitial keratitis with symptoms of a vestibuloauditory disorder, including tinnitus, vertigo, and hearing loss. They were essentially the triad of Meniere's disease plus interstitial keratitis. Other bodily findings were negative. Many investigators believe that Cogan's syndrome is only a part of a larger complex, possibly a variant of periarteritis nodosa or other collagen disease. If the patient is seen early, large doses of steroids might be expected to help halt the rapidly progressive hearing loss, tinnitus, and vertigo.

MOTION SICKNESS. Motion sickness is the term applied to the disturbance of equilibrium caused by repeated motion, such as occurs aboard a ship on the ocean. It has been recognized for many years.

During stimulation the patient has almost continuous dizziness and nausea and frequent vomiting. The symptoms last until some hours after stimulation ceases. A large number of persons who are otherwise normal experience motion sickness when they are on a merry-go-round or a swing or are riding for any distance in the rear seat of an automobile. Many of these people find riding for even a few blocks impossible.

A question regarding motion sickness should be included in the history of every patient complaining of dizziness. Dramamine and other such drugs have provided a method of controlling motion sickness.

BENIGN POSITIONAL VERTIGO. Benign positional vertigo produces a sudden sensation of severe whirling that occurs when the person changes position and that lasts from 5 to 30 seconds. It is accompanied by nystagmus, occasionally by nausea, and rarely by vomiting. It may occur when a person changes position in any direction, but it occurs most frequently when the person lies down or turns over while lying down. It does not occur every time the person assumes the inciting position. It should be noted that this sensation is *true vertigo* (that is, whirling) and should not be confused with postural hypotension, which produces a feeling of lightheadedness or mild syncope.

Benign positional vertigo occurs rarely in persons with central nervous system disease, and for the most part the lesion is peripheral; it is common, although often overlooked. Usually it is self-limited, and no specific cause can be demonstrated.

One theory says that the disorder is caused by a deposit, probably mineral, on the cupula of the posterior semicircular canal, which sensitizes this organ to gravitational force and thus to stimulation with changes in head position. This theory is supported by histologic evidence in the temporal bones of at least two patients. When positional vertigo is observed, it is necessary to investigate both ears and the central nervous system. It is often seen after head injuries. Tests for positional nystagmus, when positive, help establish the diagnosis (see discussion of tests for labyrinthine reactions in Chapter 21).

EIGHTH NERVE

Irritation or destruction of the eighth nerve pathways to the brain stem may cause dizziness, which is often accompanied by some disturbance of hearing. Frequently the damage to hearing is total.

Inflammation. Inflammation, such as meningitis, may cause irritation to the nerve during the active stage and produce dizziness, tinnitus, and hearing loss. Permanent damage to the nerve with residual permanent reduction in hearing acuity may result, but dizziness occurs only during the irritative phase. The dizziness so produced is frequently accompanied by spontaneous nystagmus.

Trauma. Trauma to the eighth cranial nerve occurs as a result of basilar skull fracture, usually through the petrous apex. Such trauma usually produces severe and often total hearing loss that is not recovered. The dizziness produced is whirling in nature, but it lasts only during the period immediately following the damage. If total section of the nerve is the result, immediate symptoms last 2 to 3 weeks, during which time the opposite labyrinth assumes control, as in hemorrhage of the internal ear. Frequently the sixth and seventh cranial nerves are damaged at the same time because of their close anatomic relationship to the eighth nerve. Therefore facial paralysis and lateral rectus palsy are frequently seen with trauma to the eighth nerve.

Tumors. Tumors of the posterior fossa or cerebellopontile angle produce systematized vertigo that is often accompanied by spontaneous nystagmus. In patients with cerebellar tumors the symptoms are most likely to be slowly progressive dizziness, ataxia, incoordination, and headache. In those with tumors of the cerebellopontile angle, dizziness is similar and is accompanied by progressive hearing loss. Acoustic neuroma usually produces cochlear symptoms first, and these symptoms precede the onset of dizziness.

The hearing loss that accompanies tumors of the cerebellopontile angle is sensorineural in nature and progressive in degree, and it fre-

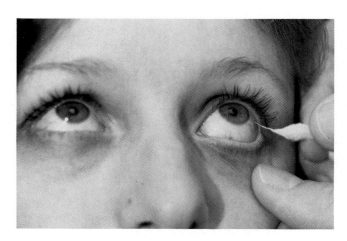

FIG. 29-2. Testing corneal reflex.

quently shows an early complete loss of bone conduction, while the air conduction threshold may still be in the region of 50 to 60 decibels. Response to caloric stimulation becomes progressively more hypoactive and is finally lost.

As such tumors enlarge, other cranial nerves are involved. The fifth nerve is most commonly involved. The earliest and most common sign is partial or complete corneal anesthesia on the involved side. It takes but a moment to test the corneal reflex, and it should never be overlooked in the routine examination (Fig. 29-2).

BRAIN STEM (NUCLEI)

Involvement of the brain stem in the region of the vestibular nuclei, regardless of origin, may produce whirling vertigo. When the lesion is small, vertigo occurs without hearing loss or tinnitus. Larger lesions cannot affect the vestibular nuclei alone because of the close proximity of the nuclei of other cranial nerves. Therefore lesions of the brain stem producing vertigo and hearing loss together are accompanied by signs of dysfunction of adjacent cranial nerves.

TABLE 11. Comparative characteristics of central and peripheral vestibular disease

Central vestibular disease	Peripheral vestibular disease
Insidious onset	Sudden onset
Continuous episode	Intermittent episodes
Duration: months	Duration: seconds, minutes, or at most a few days
Mild disequilibrium	True vertigo and intense disequilibrium during episodes
Little aggravation with head motion	Marked aggravation with head motion
Absence of associated unilateral auditory phenomena	Auditory phenomena (fullness, unilateral hearing loss, and tinnitus)
Presence of other neurologic or vascular signs and symptoms	Absence of other neurologic signs and symptoms
Positional nystagmus: immediate onset, no fatigue, does not adapt, direction changing with different head positions	Positional nystagmus: latent period, fatigue, adapts, direction fixed or changing
Spontaneous nystagmus: horizontal, rotary, or vertical	Spontaneous nystagmus: horizontal, rotary, *not* vertical
Caloric reaction: normal, perverted, or dissociated, rarely hypoactive	Caloric reaction: normal or hypoactive, not perverted or dissociated

TABLE 12. Comparative characteristics of central and peripheral spontaneous nystagmus

	Peripheral	Central
Form	Horizontal/rotatory	Horizontal, vertical, diagonal rotatory, multiple, pendular, alternating
Frequency	.05 to 6 times per second	Any frequency, usually low or variable, of long intervals (weeks to months)
Intensity	Decreasing intensity	Constant
Direction of fast component	Toward "stimulated" labyrinth or away from "destroyed" labyrinth	Toward side of CNS *lesion*
Duration	Minutes to weeks	Weeks to months
Dissociation between eyes	None	Possible
Unidirectional	Present	Seldom present
Multidirectional	Seldom present	Present
Past pointing and falling	Direction of slow phase	Direction of fast phase

Inflammations and trauma. Inflammations such as encephalitis, meningitis, and brain abscess or trauma may cause damage to the brain stem directly or through pressure.

Hemorrhage. Bleeding into the brain stem cannot cause dizziness alone because of the close proximity of other nuclei. Small petechial hemorrhage might conceivably do so, but this theory is unproved.

Thrombosis of the posteroinferior cerebellar artery. Thrombosis of the posteroinferior cerebellar artery produces sudden vertigo associated with other signs. The onset typically is sudden. In addition to vertigo and nystagmus, examination shows dysphagia, weakness of the palate, impairment of sensations of pain and temperature on the face, Horner's syndrome, and cerebellar signs in the arm and leg on the same side as the lesion. Impairment of sensations of pain and temperature on the opposite side of the body accompanies these signs.

Tumors. Tumors of the brain stem produce symptoms and signs similar to those of other brain stem damage, but progression is less rapid. Diagnosis depends on careful neurologic examination.

Multiple sclerosis. Multiple sclerosis may cause vertigo, which will be the only complaint. Here the picture is similar to that described as acute toxic labyrinthitis. A maximum is reached in hours or a day. The dizziness may then last several days or even several weeks, following which it gradually subsides. Tinnitus and hearing loss are not associated. The only assistance one may gain from the history is that most patients who have had acute toxic labyrinthitis relate that they were well on the way to recovery in 10 days. The symptoms from multiple sclerosis are more prolonged.

When there is a suspicion of multiple sclerosis, a detailed history should be taken with regard to any past neurologic episodes, such as a sudden blurring of vision followed by recovery. Temporal pallor of the optic discs is characteristic but may not appear until last.

CENTRAL AND PERIPHERAL VERTIGO

In Tables 11 and 12 some guidelines are suggested to assist in the differentiation of central and peripheral vertigo. These general guidelines will not replace the specific, careful history and other studies, which are essential to an accurate diagnosis.

SELECTED READINGS

Anson, B.J.: Endolymphatic hydrops; anatomic aspects, Arch. Otolaryngol. **89**:70, 1969.

Arslan, M.: Treatment of Meniere's disease by apposition of sodium chloride crystals on the round window, Laryngoscope **82**:1736, 1972.

Arslan, M.: New hypothesis on plurifactorial etiology of Meniere's disease, Acta Otolaryngol. (suppl. 357):1, 1978.

Barber, H.O.: Positional vertigo and nystagmus, Otolaryngol. Clin. North Am. **6**(1):169, 1973.

Basek, M.: Ultrasound for Meniere's disease, Arch. Otolaryngol. **97**:133, 1973.

Berman, J.M., and Fredrickson, J.M.: Vertigo after head injury: five-year follow-up, J. Otolaryngol. **7**:237, 1978.

Bhatia, P.L., and others: Audiologic and vestibular function tests in hypothyroidism, Laryngoscope **87**:2082, 1977.

Caparosa, R.J.: Diagnosis of posterior fossa tumor, Laryngoscope **88**:1209, 1978.

Clemis, J.D., and Becktr, G.W.: Vestibular neuritis, Otolaryngol. Clin. North Am. **6**(1): 139, 1973.

Cushing, H.: Tumors of the nervus acusticus, Philadelphia, 1947, W.B. Saunders Co.

Erickson, L.S., Sorenson, G.D., and McGavran, M.H.: Review of 140 acoustic neurinomas (neurilemmoma), Laryngoscope **75**:601, 1965.

Furnstenberg, A.C., Lashmet, F.H., and Lathrop, F.: Meniere's symptom complex; medical treatment, Ann. Otol. Rhinol. Laryngol. **43**:1035, 1934.

Glasscock, M.E.: Middle fossa approach to the temporal bone, Arch. Otolaryngol. **90**:15, 1969.

Glasscock, M.E.: Vestibular nerve section, Arch. Otolaryngol. **97**:112, 1973.

Glasscock, M.E., and others: One-state combined approach for management of large cerebellopontine angle tumors, Laryngoscope **88**:1563, 1978.

Hallpike, C.S., and Cairns, H.: Observations on the pathology of Meniere's syndrome, Proc. R. Soc. Med. **31**: 1317, 1938.

House, W.F.: Acoustic neuroma perspective, 1977, Laryngoscope **88**:816, 1978.

Hybels, R.L.: Drug toxicity of the inner ear, Med. Clin. North Am. **63**:309, 1979.

Jongkees, L.B.W.: Vestibular tests for the clinician, Arch. Otolaryngol. **97**:77, 1973.

Kimura, R., and Schuknecht, H.: Effect of fistulae on endolymphatic hydrops, Ann. Otol. Rhinol. Laryngol. **84**:271, 1975.

Lindsay, J.R.: Paroxysmal postural vertigo and vestibular neuronitis, Arch. Otolaryngol. **85**:544, 1967.

Meyerhoff, W.L., Paparella, M.M., and Shea, D.: Meniere's disease in children, Laryngoscope **88**:1504, 1978.

Pulec, J.L.: Meniere's disease; results of a two and one-half year study of etiology, natural history and results of treatment, Laryngoscope **82**:1703, 1972.

Rubin, W.: Whiplash with vestibular involvement, Arch. Otolaryngol. **97**:85, 1973.

Schuknecht, H.: Cupulolithiasis, Arch. Otolaryngol. **90**:765, 1969; Acta Otolaryngol. **69**:17, 1970.

Schuknecht, H.: Destructive labyrinthine surgery, Arch. Otolaryngol. **97**:150, 1973.

Schuknecht, H.F.: Delayed endolymphatic hydrops, Ann. Otol. Rhinol. Laryngol. **87**:743, 1978.

Shambaugh, G.: Effect of endolymphatic sac decompression on fluctuant hearing loss, Otolaryngol. Clin. North Am. **8:**537, 1975.

Singleton, G.T., and others: Perilymph fistulas: diagnostic criteria and therapy, Ann. Otol. Rhinol. Laryngol. **87:** 797, 1978.

Smith, J.L.: Cogan's syndrome, Laryngoscope **80:**121, 1970.

Turner, J.S., Jr., Saunders, A.Z., and Per-Lee, J.H.: A 10-year profile on Meniere's disease and endolymphatic shunt surgery, Laryngoscope **83:**1816, 1973.

Williams, H.L., Horton, B.T., and Day, L.A.: Endolymphatic hydrops without vertigo; its differential diagnosis and treatment, Trans. Am. Otol. Soc. **35:**116, 1949.

Wolfson, R., and Cutt, R.: Long-term results with cryosurgery for Meniere's disease, Arch. Otolaryngol. **93:** 483, 1971.

Wood, C.D., and Graybiel, A.: The antimotion sickness drugs; symposium on vertigo, Otolaryngol. Clin. North Am. **6**(1):301, 1973.

30 THE FACIAL NERVE

ANATOMY AND PHYSIOLOGY

Facial nerve. The facial, or seventh cranial, nerve leaves the pons, travels a short distance, and enters the internal auditory meatus together with the eighth cranial nerve. This close relationship of the seventh (*petrous* portion) and eighth nerves is maintained throughout the petrous portion of the temporal bone. Leaving the eighth nerve, where it is distributed to the cochlea and labyrinth, the seventh nerve, with the chorda tympani, continues laterally and emerges on the anterior and superior aspect of the medial wall of the middle ear. Here the nerve turns sharply, posteriorly and inferiorly, to make a bend known as the genu of the facial nerve and to traverse the medial wall of the middle ear, superior to the oval window and the stapes (*intratympanic* portion). The geniculate ganglion is located 2 to 3 mm. proximal to the genu of the facial nerve.

At the stapes the seventh nerve makes an arch posteriorly and passes inferiorly to the prominence of the horizontal semicircular canal (*pyramidal* portion), bringing the nerve deep into the bone of the external auditory canal. It continues vertically downward (*vertical* portion) and emerges from the skull through the stylomastoid foramen (Fig. 30-1).

On leaving the stylomastoid foramen, the facial nerve turns forward, passes immediately lateral to the base of the styloid process, crosses the posterior belly of the digastric muscle (*cervical* portion), and enters the parotid gland. In the parotid gland it travels between the superficial and deep lobes and divides into three trunks that fan out between the lobes (Fig. 30-2). The point of division is called the *pes anserinus*, or goose's foot. After traversing the gland, the branches of the facial nerve emerge from the anterior and superior borders of the gland to sup-

ply the muscles of facial expression. The cervical branch of the facial nerve is in close relationship with the posterior facial vein (Fig. 30-3).

SURGICAL LANDMARKS. The facial nerve can be located in the temporal bone because of its constant relationship to the oval window, horizontal semicircular canal, and stylomastoid foramen (Figs. 30-1 and 30-3). In its cervical portion it can be located by its relationship to the styloid process and digastric muscle. The facial nerve can also be located by its relationship, lateral but adjacent, to the posterior facial vein (Fig. 30-3).

FUNCTION. The facial nerve supplies motor fibers (Figs. 30-2 and 30-4) to the muscles of facial expression, that is, those of the lips, nose, cheeks, eyelids, and forehead. Motor fibers from branches of the facial nerve go to the stapedius, extrinsic auricular, stylohyoid, and platysma muscles as well as to the posterior belly of the digastric muscle.

The facial nerve also has sensory fibers. Exact sensory pathways have not been proved. A portion of the outer one third of the external auditory canal and a portion of the concha of the external ear receive cutaneous branches from the facial nerve. These sensory branches have connections with the trigeminal, glossopharyngeal, and vagus nerves. Sense of taste to the anterior two thirds of the tongue and secretory fibers to the sublingual and submaxillary salivary glands are carried by the chorda tympani (Fig. 30-5).

Chorda tympani nerve. The chorda tympani (special visceral efferent) nerve accompanies the facial nerve to a point just below the horizontal semicircular canal. Here the two nerves separate. The chorda tympani leaves the facial (fallopian) canal through a small foramen (iter chordae posterius) and then crosses the tympanic membrane between the fibrous and mucous lay-

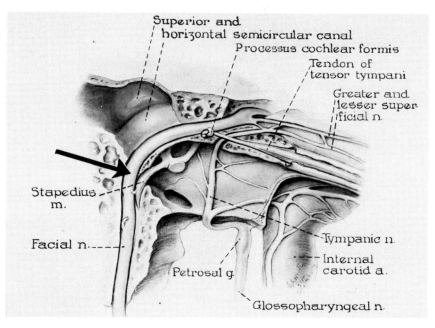

FIG. 30-1. Medial wall of the middle ear showing the facial nerve and other structures. Arrow points to the most common site of injury during an operation on the temporal bone.

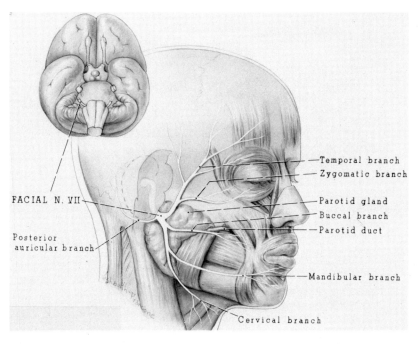

FIG. 30-2. Distribution of the facial nerve after its exit from the stylomastoid foramen. (From Jacob, S.W., and Francone, C.A.: Structure and function in man, Philadelphia, 1970, W.B. Saunders Co.)

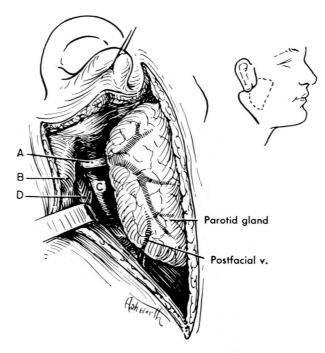

FIG. 30-3. Relationships of the facial nerve at the stylomastoid foramen. *A*, Main trunk of the facial nerve. *B*, mastoid tip. *C*, styloid process. *D*, posterior belly of the digastric muscle. Note the relationship of the posterior facial vein. *Inset*, Incision to expose parotid gland and facial nerve.

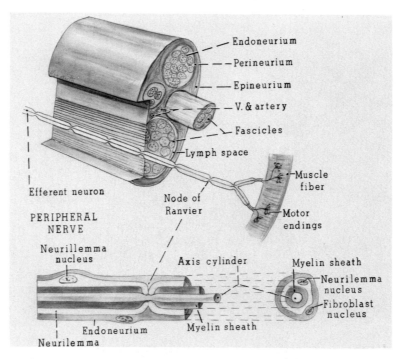

FIG. 30-4. Peripheral motor nerve, such as the seventh nerve. (From Jacob, S.W., and Francone, C.A.: Structure and function in man, Philadelphia, 1970, W.B. Saunders Co.)

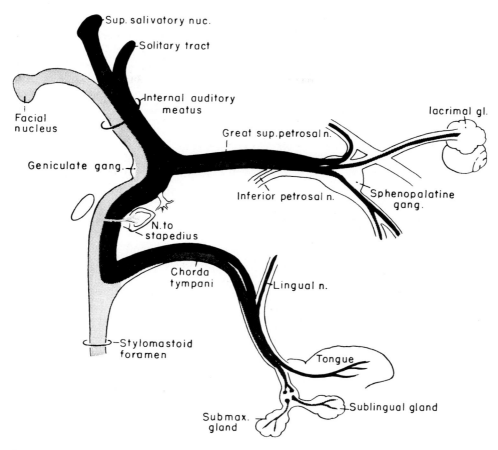

FIG. 30-5. Components of the facial nerve. (Adapted from Mielhke, A.: Die Chirurgie des Nervus facialis, Berlin, 1960, Urban & Schwarzenberg.)

ers of the eardrum at the level of the malleolar folds and between the incus and the neck of the malleus. Leaving the ear through a small foramen (iter chordae anterius), the chorda tympani joins the lingual nerve medial to the mandible and is distributed to the tongue and to the sublingual and submaxillary salivary glands.

SENSORY DISTURBANCES

Disturbance of the sensory function of the facial nerve produces pain in and around the ear. It may also impair the sense of taste in the anterior two thirds of the tongue. Other conditions incident to disturbed sensory function of the facial nerve are herpes zoster oticus and geniculate neuralgia.

Herpes zoster oticus (Ramsay Hunt syndrome) (Fig. 30-6). Some otolaryngologists believe that herpes zoster oticus is due to inflammation of

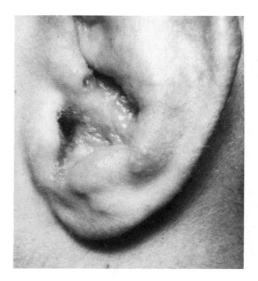

FIG. 30-6. Herpes zoster oticus. Note vesicles.

the geniculate ganglion. It produces severe pain in the ear, vesicles in the external auditory canal, and facial paralysis. The pain and vesiculation may, however, be present without paralysis. The cutaneous area involved is supplied by fibers from the fifth, ninth, and tenth cranial nerves as well as fibers from the facial nerve. It also receives fibers from the cervical plexus. Consequently, it is impossible to establish which nerve is responsible for the inflammation.

Treatment of herpes zoster oticus consists of narcotics for pain, topical anesthetic ointments such as dibucaine (Nupercaine), and, occasionally, local or systemic antibiotics if the vesicles become infected. Systemic corticosteroids may shorten the duration of the inflammatory episode. The majority of patients recover completely in 7 to 21 days and have no residual symptoms. Some patients, however, have persistent postherpetic pain. It can sometimes be controlled by the use of vitamin B_{12} or by Protamide given intramuscularly, or by both. Either or both must be taken daily for at least 10 to 14 days. In an occasional patient the facial paralysis may persist and will not recover, even after decompression of the facial nerve.

Geniculate neuralgia. In geniculate neuralgia syndrome, the primary site of pain is deep in the ear. The pain occurs in paroxysms, and its severity is comparable with that of tic douloureux. It may radiate to the jaw, face, and neck. The drug of choice is carbamazepine (Tegretol), 200 mg., three or more times daily. Prolonged and intractable pain can be completely relieved by intracranial section of the *nervus intermedius*.

MOTOR DISTURBANCES

Irritation to or injury of the motor portion of the facial nerve produces twitching, spasm, weakness, or paralysis of the facial muscles. Paralysis is the most important. If uncorrected, the resultant deformity of the face not only is disfiguring but also may be accompanied by serious psychologic trauma, particularly in women.

Hemifacial spasm. Hemifacial spasm is manifested by repeated twitching of one or more muscles supplied by the facial nerve. Although not painful, it is annoying and difficult to manage. It does not progress to paralysis of the nerve. Blocking of individual branches of the nerve with alcohol may give some relief. Decompression of the facial nerve has been successful for only short periods. A few patients have been relieved by careful partial sectioning of the seventh nerve (Fig. 30-7), but a more effective technique seems to be avulsion of the branches of the facial nerve going to the spastic musculature along with the anastomotic branches from the other rami.

Peripheral facial paralysis. On the involved side of the face the buccinator and other muscles are completely paralyzed, so that there is a total lack of motion. Consequently, on this side of the face mastication of food is difficult. Saliva nay drool from the corner of the mouth. Irritation of the lids and cornea occurs. Foreign bodies may easily enter the eye, since the lids will not close to protect the cornea (Fig. 30-8, *B*). Smiling, laughing, and frowning on the uninvolved side of the face produce a one-sided

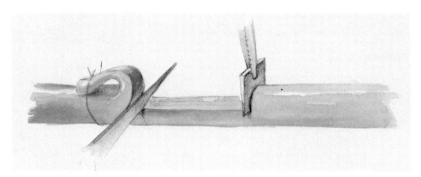

FIG. 30-7. Partial section of the seventh nerve for hemifacial spasm. This procedure is sometimes effective. It must be done under high magnification. (Adapted from Mielhke, A.: Die Chirurgie des Nervus facialis, Berlin, 1960, Urban & Schwarzenberg.)

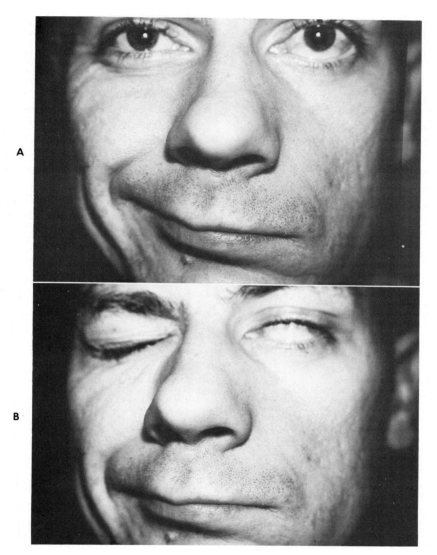

FIG. 30-8. A, Facial paralysis on the left side. **B,** Facial paralysis on the left side during an attempt at motion. Note that the eye does not close.

grimace. A lesion at or proximal to the geniculate ganglion decreases lacrimation.

Congenital facial paralysis. Facial paralysis may be present at birth. When it is caused by a disorder of embryologic development or by intracranial hemorrhage before birth, the prognosis for recovery is poor. Associated with this type of facial paralysis may be paralysis of the abducens, oculomotor, trigeminal, glossopharyngeal, and hypoglossal nerves. Paralysis may also be caused by pressure from obstetric forceps and other trauma during delivery. In these instances the prognosis is usually good.

Central facial paralysis. The frontalis muscles receive a bilateral supranuclear innervation (Fig. 30-9). When there is a lesion superior to the nucleus of the seventh nerve, usually a brain tumor or abscess, the lower half of the face on the contralateral side is paralyzed. Forehead motions (frowning and raising of the eyebrows) are retained. Awareness of this aids in localization of the cortical lesion.

Thalamic lesions influence involuntary motions, such as laughing and crying. When a lesion of this type is present, the face is paralyzed or weak during these involuntary acts, but the face moves normally when voluntary motion is attempted. Remember, in peripheral paralysis the face does not move at all on the involved side. The involuntary emotional motions are retained in central lesions not involving the thalamus.

Bell's palsy. Spontaneous facial paralysis without evidence of other disease or injury is known as Bell's palsy. It affects all ages with a peak incidence between the ages of 20 and 40 years. Bell's palsy is not rare; the overall annual incidence is between 10 and 20 per 100,000 population. The incidence in pregnant women is a little more than three times the general incidence. The reason for this is unknown.

Paralysis occurs suddenly or gradually over a period of 24 to 48 hours. Symptoms of disturbance of the chorda tympani are impaired taste

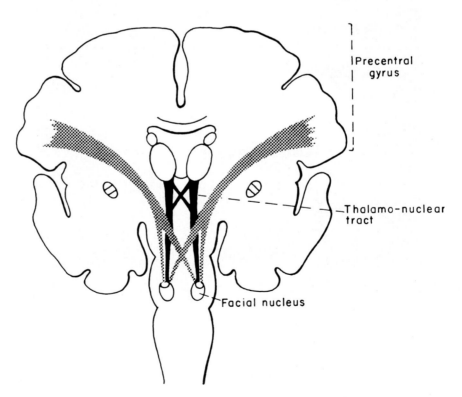

FIG. 30-9. Supranuclear facial tracts. Note bilateral supranuclear innervation. (Adapted from Mielhke, A.: Die Chirurgie des Nervus facialis, Berlin, 1960, Urban & Schwarzenberg.)

and dryness of the mouth, which may or may not occur simultaneously and which precede the paralysis by 2 to 7 days. Pain behind the ipsilateral ear occurs in 20% of Bell's palsy sufferers, and numbness of the face occurs in 20%, both often preceding the paralysis.

Although the specific cause of Bell's palsy is unknown, it is recognized that swelling of the facial nerve (whether traumatic or idiopathic) causes ischemia, which in turn leads to more swelling and more ischemia. The edema produced may seriously compress the nerve, which has a long course through the temporal bone in a rigid canal. There is some evidence that the original insult in Bell's palsy is viral in origin. Between 30% and 50% of patients with Bell's palsy have a prodrome of viral nature. One extensive study has indicated that two thirds of Bell's palsy victims have other cranial nerve symptoms, including evidence of dysfunction of the fifth, ninth, or tenth nerves. The viral origin is as yet unproved.

Neurophysiologists have described three degrees of damage that can occur when a nerve is injured:

1. *An injury that causes no degeneration of the nerve distal to the injured site.* There may, however, be some interruption of the continuity of the myelin sheath at the site of injury. This slightest of the three degrees of damage is known as *neuropraxia.* Recovery from this type of injury is usually rapid and complete.

2. *An injury that causes division of the axon with degeneration of both the axon and the myelin sheath peripheral to the injury but no degeneration proximally or toward the parent nerve cell.* Some changes do take place in the nerve cell, but the cell does not degenerate. The other components of the nerve (neurilemma and endoneurium) remain normal. A person who has this amount of injury may also recover without serious sequelae; however, the recovery is slow, since the myelin sheath and axon must re-form and grow out to the nerve end. This degree of injury is called *axonotmesis.*

3. *An injury that completely disrupts all the essential elements of the nerve with subsequent degeneration of the axon and myelin sheath and sometimes of the parent cell itself.* When this degree of damage has occurred, a new sheath and axon must grow from the cell (provided that it has not degenerated) and traverse the entire length of the nerve. This type of injury results in the most severe degree of damage, which is known as *neurotmesis.* The term does not necessarily imply physical severance of the nerve, but regeneration in this situation carries some hazards. The axons and sheath cells may not regrow into the same channels from which they originated. They may grow part of the way to the extremity of the nerve, or they may grow out of the sheath if an aperture is present through which they can travel.

All three degrees of injury can, and do, occur in Bell's palsy. Some of the nerve fibrils may show a minor degree of injury, and others a severe degree. There is no specific method of determining the type of degeneration that has occurred in a patient with Bell's palsy. It is ascertained only by evaluating the amount and rapidity of recovery. Note that the term "injury" as related to Bell's palsy is used here in its broadest sense. Traumatic injury is not implied.

There is general agreement on the immediate treatment of Bell's palsy, which should be medical. Many different medical treatments have been recommended, but currently the use of cortisone is regarded as most effective. The recommended course of treatment is with prednisone, 5 mg. four times daily for 4 days followed by a decreasing dosage to three times, then twice, and finally once daily for a total treatment time of 8 days. Although this will not cause cessation of the palsy, there is some evidence that it may reduce the percentage of patients whose condition progresses to complete nerve degeneration.

Under such conservative treatment, and also, of course, with no treatment at all, 80% to 85% of patients suffering from Bell's palsy will recover completely or with so little residual weakness that no further management is required. The majority of the remaining patients recover only partially. A few do not recover at all.

The problem is to determine what, if anything, can be done for the 15% to 20% of patients who are to recover only partially or not at all.

Certain rules or guides to management can be presented with the full recognition that some are subject to controversy. If the facial muscles are degenerated by the physiologic block produced in Bell's palsy, changes take place that can be partially evaluated by electric testing. In complete paralysis, response to faradic stimulation may be absent after the first few days but usually remains 10 to 14 days. The reaction of degeneration, which is evidenced by lack of faradic response plus a slow, wormlike galvanic response on both contraction and relaxation of the muscle itself, does not appear for 10 to 14 days.

When expertly performed and interpreted, electromyography may add information, but it is of little value until 21 days after the injury. Basically, electromyography is valuable because there is a readily discernible difference in the electrical silence of a normal muscle and the spontaneous potentials that can be recorded from a denervated muscle. Electromyography is valuable later, since it may be helpful in predicting recovery. When an injured or repaired nerve is recovering, electromyography can demonstrate early electric potential in the muscles several weeks before any motion of the facial muscles can be seen. Controversy begins, and the ability of the person interpreting the testing becomes important when different electric manifestations occur that may or may not indicate beginning regeneration.

If the patient suffering from Bell's palsy has no pain and begins to show slight motion in the face by the end of 3 to 4 weeks, his chances of recovery are good. Surgical decompression (see pp. 420-421) should be *considered*, however, if there is no sign of returning function at the end of 3 weeks, if response to faradic current is absent, if a reaction of degeneration is demonstrated, and if electromyography indicates the activity characteristic of denervated muscle. Kettel has shown that when complete denervation is present, it may be dangerous to wait for further electromyograms a week or two later, because during that time a persistent pressure on the nerve in the canal may change a reversible block of conduction (neuropraxia) into an irreversible condition (axonotmesis or neurotmesis).

If recovery is to be *complete*, there should be some signs of response in 3 to 4 weeks. Cawthorne, Kettel, and Sullivan, who have the largest series and the most experience with Bell's palsy, seem agreed that *complete* recovery is *never* seen when there is no sign of beginning recovery at the end of 2 months. Partial recovery may, of course, occur.

Surgical decompression of the facial nerve in its vertical portion (and sometimes in its horizontal portion) may be indicated at any time after paralysis is *complete*. The proper time for the operation varies according to careful observation of the patient and the results of electric testing of the nerve.

One practical method by which facial nerve function can be followed is to test both sides of the face daily or at intervals of 2 or 3 days. The nonparalyzed side is tested to determine the number of microvolts necessary to produce a response. The paralyzed side is similarly tested, and if it responds, the strength of current necessary to produce a contraction is recorded. The normal side is used as the control. If the paralyzed side requires only slightly more current, the prognosis is good; if it requires a much larger amount of current, the prognosis may be poor. However, day-to-day changes in reaction can be followed. In general, if the face requires less and less current to produce a contraction, the prognosis is good. If, however, there is a sudden change that requires more current to produce a reaction, immediate decompression of the nerve may be indicated.

Best overall results will be obtained if decompression is the rule when there is no physical or electric evidence of recovery after 8 weeks. Following this rule will mean that some patients will be subjected to the operation who may have recovered 60% to 70% of normal function at a later date without the operation. The decompression must be done skillfully and with minimal trauma to the nerve. Poor technique can only add further insult to an injury already present.

Measurement of the rate of flow of saliva from the submaxillary gland may be of prognostic value. When there is ischemia of the facial nerve, there is also impairment of function of the chorda tympani. This impairment results in a decrease of salivary flow on the involved side. Measurement of the rate of flow seems to indicate that when there is marked reduction in the rate, the prognosis for spontaneous recovery is poor.

In this test both submaxillary gland ducts are cannulated intraorally with a small plastic tube, and the rate of flow from each is measured. A reduction in flow to 70% on the involved side is considered abnormal, and a reduction to 25% or less indicates a poor prognosis for spon-

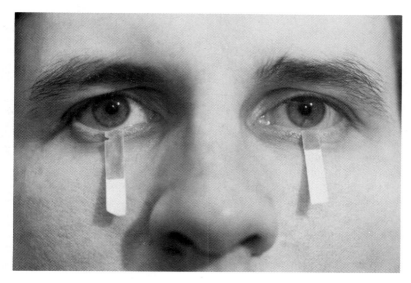

FIG. 30-10. Schirmer test. Note the diminution of wetting from the left eye (the involved side).

taneous regeneration. Some studies also suggest that if the pH of the saliva collected is 6.4 or higher, the prognosis is good, and if it is 6.2 or lower, the prognosis is poor.

The Schirmer test is also used to aid in localization of the level of nerve compression and, possibly, to aid in prognosis. In this test a piece of dry litmus paper is lightly placed on each lower eyelid. The amount of moistening of the litmus paper is observed (Fig. 30-10). Wetting of the litmus paper for a distance of at least 1.5 cm. is considered to be normal. Less than 1.5 cm. indicates the probability that edema, compression, or injury is present at or proximal to the geniculate ganglion. A *marked* diminution of wetting, or a dry eye, indicates a poor prognosis.

A further test of facial nerve function is the stapedius reflex. Since the stapedius muscle is innervated by the seventh nerve and will contract when stimulated by a short sharp sound (motivated by the sound being produced in the opposite ear, since there are bilateral crossing neural connections), the reflex will not be initiated if the facial nerve is not functioning properly at the level of the branch to the stapedius muscle (pyramidal portion of the nerve).

It may be necessary to carry out any or all of these tests to localize the exact injury to the nerve or to assist in judging the prognosis. None of the tests by itself is prognostic. Only when all tests agree (and they do not always agree)

can the physician be reasonably sure of the prognosis.

Although electric stimulation of the nerve has been advocated as a method of early treatment of Bell's palsy, there is no rationale that this procedure will help the nerve recover. During a prolonged period of paralysis after known injury or repair, electric stimulation of the facial muscles will prevent some disuse atrophy of the muscle fibers. They will then be in better condition to receive and react to nerve impulses when regeneration occurs. This treatment may give a better final result, but it does not benefit the nerve directly.

Melkersson's syndrome. Melkersson's syndrome is rare. It produces unilateral facial edema—supposedly lymphedema. Often it is accompanied by facial paralysis. The cause is unknown. Usually the paralysis clears, but the edema may persist.

Tumors of the facial nerve. Tumors of the facial nerve are rare. The majority that have been reported are benign neurinomas (schwannomas) or neurofibromas. Most of them arise within the fallopian (facial) canal. Very rarely, a meningioma may occur. This tumor originates from the displacement of meningeal tissue laterally during early embryonic development, grows attached to the sheath of the facial nerve, and may compress the nerve or invade it. *In these locations (either the vertical or horizontal portion of the nerve) the only symptom of* *the presence of a tumor is a slowly progressive facial paralysis.*

If the tumor arises distal to the stylomastoid foramen, it can be palpated. A tumor in this location does not produce facial paralysis until late. Benign tumors grow slowly. It may take several months or a year or two before there is clinical evidence of a tumor in the middle ear and before erosion occurs in the bony external auditory canal. Diagnosis of tumors of the facial nerve is more exact when polytomography is used. Sometimes this may be the only way one can distinguish between Bell's palsy and tumors of the nerve.

Treatment demands adequate surgical excision of the tumor, with end-to-end anastomosis when possible. When anastomosis is not possible, grafting must be done to replace the resected segment of nerve.

Injury to the facial nerve. The facial nerve may be compressed or severed either intracranially or in the petrous portion of the temporal bone by (1) brain stem tumors, (2) acoustic neuromas, or (3) fractures of the base of the skull.

Repair of the nerve in the petrous portion of the temporal bone after skull fracture is possible. The repair is accomplished by way of a combined mastoid and middle fossa approach to the superior portion of the temporal bone, location of the injury, and decompression or suture of the nerve as indicated by the extent of the injury. Most often the facial nerve is damaged in the middle ear or in its descending vertical portion. Injuries in these areas usually occur during operations on the mastoid. Damage to the facial nerve outside the skull is caused by trauma, such as in war or automobile injuries (Fig. 30-11). Invasion of the nerve by a malignant tumor of the parotid gland also causes paralysis. *A benign tumor of the parotid gland rarely causes facial paralysis.* Another source of injury is resection of the nerve during partial or total parotidectomy (see Chapter 31).

When facial paralysis is caused by a parotid tumor, the tumor must be considered to be malignant until proved to be nonmalignant. Frozen sections of such tumors at the time of operation, when indicated, will determine whether the tumor can be removed safely without sacrificing the nerve. Safe removal can be accomplished when the tumor is benign. If a frozen section reveals malignancy, however, *the*

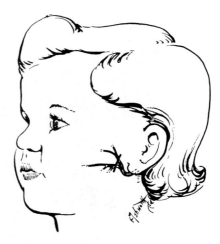

FIG. 30-11. The dark line across the facial nerve shows the usual site of external trauma to the nerve.

nerve must be sacrificed and removed with the tumor. One or several grafts (usually from the anterior femoral cutaneous nerve) can be sutured in place during the same operation to give the best chance for the return of facial tone and motion.

REPAIR OF THE FACIAL NERVE

The facial nerve has remarkable powers of regeneration. Even after complete section, which causes, as in other nerves, wallerian degeneration to the nucleus, recovery can and does take place if the tunnel back to the muscle end-plates is intact and not compressed.

Electric tests of the nerve and facial muscles aid in determining whether repair can be performed successfully or should not be attempted. If the facial muscles still react to a faradic current applied to the skin over the nerve trunk, there is no actual interruption of continuity. In this event, surgical measures are delayed. When the nerve will not react to faradic stimulation but the muscles will still respond to galvanic current, continuity of the nerve has been interrupted. Attempt at surgical repair is then the procedure of choice. If the muscles fail to respond to a galvanic stimulus at all, nerve repair is useless.

Decompression. When there is pressure on the nerve from edema, a tumor, or depressed bone, causing paralysis, decompression of the facial nerve is indicated. Decompression can be performed from the petrous portion to and in-

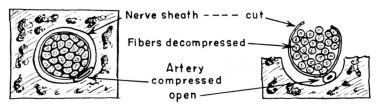

FIG. 30-12. Facial nerve before and after decompression (schematic).

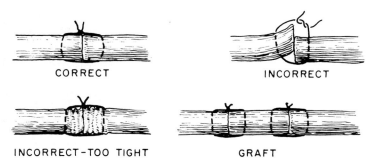

FIG. 30-13. Suturing technique used in injuries or grafts of the facial nerve. No. 6-0 silk is used on an atraumatic needle.

cluding the stylomastoid foramen. It is accomplished by careful uncapping of the nerve in its bony canal in the temporal bone. At the end of the dissection the nerve is no longer encased in a solid bony tunnel but lies in a trough of bone, with three sides uncovered (Fig. 30-12). The sheath of the nerve is then slit to remove all pressure. Decompression allows the return of normal blood supply, reduces edema, and provides an unobstructed pathway through which the regenerating nerve fibers can grow.

End-to-end anastomosis. When the nerve has been severed, the best results are obtained by end-to-end anastomosis. The procedure must be performed with care so that the approximation of the severed nerve ends is firm but not too tight. Careful suturing with a single No. 6-0 suture gives optimal results (Fig. 30-13).

Nerve grafts. When it is not possible to accomplish end-to-end anastomosis, nerve grafts are used. Fresh grafts, taken at the time of the surgical exposure for the repair, allow results as good as, or better than, prepared grafts. The greater auricular nerve or the femoral cutaneous nerve is used most often. Either can be dissected to give a single- or a multiple-branched graft. Both are about the size of the

facial nerve. Successful grafting has been performed between the main trunk and all branches after extensive removal of the nerve during an operation on the parotid gland.

Substitution anastomosis. When the facial nerve is damaged so that it cannot be repaired, substitution anastomosis may be performed. Either the spinal accessory or the hypoglossal nerve is used (Figs. 30-14 and 30-15). When the spinal accessory nerve is sacrificed for anastomosis to the facial nerve, the resulting shoulder drop and atrophy of muscles create an undesirable deformity. Although this nerve is sometimes used for such a repair, most surgeons prefer to use the hypoglossal nerve. Use of the latter causes loss of motion and some atrophy of the tongue on the side of anastomosis, but the resulting disability is less than when the spinal accessory nerve is used as the donor.

Substitution anastomosis gives less satisfactory results than decompression, end-to-end anastomosis, or grafting, but it improves muscle tone and allows some motion, which is far more desirable than permanent paralysis.

Plastic procedures. When the facial muscles have so atrophied that they will no longer re-

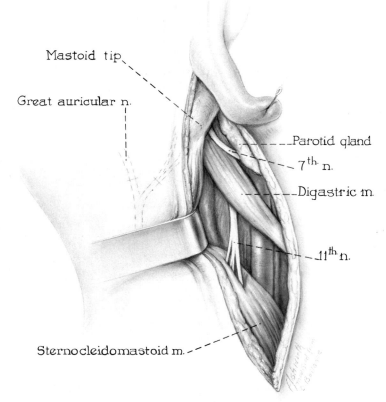

FIG. 30-14. Relationship of the facial nerve to the spinal accessory nerve in the neck.

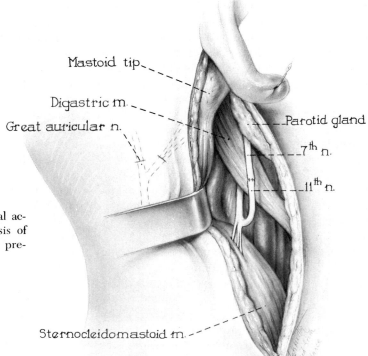

FIG. 30-15. Anastomosis of the spinal accessory and facial nerves. Anastomosis of the hypoglossal and facial nerves is preferred.

spond to stimulation of any kind, none of the procedures mentioned is of value. Some cosmetic improvement can be gained by slings, or face-lifting, which is accomplished by the use of wire or fascia lata to support the facial tissues from the zygoma. Portions of the masseter muscle can be used. The temporalis muscle can also be dissected from the skull and turned down into the cheek to increase bulk and supply an appearance of tone. Slight motion can be learned by clenching the teeth when either the masseter or the temporalis muscles are used. These muscles have their motor nerve supply from the fifth cranial nerve.

With the advent of microsurgery, other muscles from other parts of the body can also be used. These types of muscle-nerve-vessel transplants require meticulous anastomosis of arteries, veins, and nerves under high magnification.

When the facial distortion is significant, it may be advisable to combine the above procedures with blepharoplasty, tarsorrhaphy, face-lift, brow lift, or lip transplantation to obtain the best cosmetic result. Although these procedures may improve the appearance of the face at rest and correct sagging of the soft tissues, no motion of the face occurs, except as noted above.

SELECTED READINGS

Adour, K.K., and others: Surgical and nonsurgical management of facial paralysis following closed head injury, Laryngoscope **87:**380, 1977.

Adour, K.K.: The true nature of Bell's palsy: analysis of 1,000 consecutive patients, Laryngoscope **88:**781, 1978.

Alford, B.R., Sessions, R.B., and Weber, S.C.: Indications for surgical decompression of the facial nerve, Laryngoscope **81:**620, 1971.

Baker, D., and Conley, J.: Regional muscle transposition for rehabilitation of the paralyzed face, Clin. Plast. Surg. **6:**317, 1979.

Baker, D., and Conley, J.: Facial nerve grafting: a thirty year retrospective review, Clin. Plast. Surg. **6:**343, 1979.

Blatt, I.M.: Bell's palsy. I. Diagnosis and prognosis of idiopathic peripheral facial paralysis by submaxillary salivary flow—chorda tympani nerve testing; a study of 102 patients, Laryngoscope **75:**1070, 1965.

Boyle, W.: Evaluation of facial nerve decompression in experimental facial nerve paralysis in monkeys, Laryngoscope **77:**1168, 1978.

Conley, J.: Hypoglossal crossover—122 cases, Trans. Am. Acad. Ophthalmol. Otolaryngol. **84:**763, 1977.

Conley, J., and others: Hypoglossal-facial nerve anastomosis for reinnervation of the paralyzed face, Plast. Reconstr. Surg. **63:**63, 1979.

Crabtree, J.A.: Herpes zoster oticus (Ramsay Hunt syndrome), Laryngoscope **78:**1853, 1968.

DeWeese, D.: Facial nerve problems, Laryngoscope **62:**693, 1962.

Ekstrand, T., and Glitterstam, K.: Bell's palsy—prognostic value of the stapedius reflex with contralateral stimulation, J. Laryngol. Otol. **93:**271, 1979.

Ekstrand, T.: Bell's palsy: prognostic accuracy of case history, sialometry, and taste impairment, Clin. Otolaryngol. **4:**183, 1979.

Ewing, J., and Endicott, J.: Rehabilitation of the face after facial-nerve paralysis, Ear Nose Throat J. **57:**288, 1978.

Fisch, U.: Guidelines for management of traumatic injury to facial nerve, O.R.L. Allerg. Dig. **38:**42, 1976.

Fisch, U.: Total facial nerve decompression and electroneuronography. In Silverstein and Marrell, editors: Neurological surgery of the ear, Birmingham, Ala., 1977, Aesculapius Publishing Co.

Fisch, U.: Current surgical treatment of intratemporal facial palsy, Clin. Plast. Surg. **6:**377, 1979.

Freeman, B.S.: Review of long-term results in supportive treatment of facial paralysis, Plast. Reconstr. Surg. **63:**214, 1979.

Hardin, W.B.: Facial palsy: interpretation of neurologic findings, Trans. Am. Acad. Ophthalmol. Otolaryngol. **84:**710, 1977.

Jonkees, L.B.W.: Peripheral facial nerve paralysis and its surgical treatment, Eye Ear Nose Throat Mon. **49:**16, 1970.

Katz, A.D., Passy, V., and Kaplan, L.: Neurogenous neoplasms of major nerves of face and neck, Arch. Surg. **103:**51, 1971.

Kumagami, H.: Neuropathological findings of hemifacial spasm and trigeminal neuralgia, Arch. Otolaryngol. **99:**160, 1974.

Lathrop, F.D.: Facial nerve grafting, Trans. Am. Acad. Ophthalmol. **68:**1060, 1964.

Maxwell, J.H.: Repair of the facial nerve after facial lacerations, Trans. Am. Acad. Ophthalmol. **58:**733, 1954.

May, M.: Anatomy of the facial nerve (spatial orientation of fibers in the temporal bone), Laryngoscope **82:**1311, 1973.

May, M.: Bell's palsy: progressive ascending paralysis, therapeutic implications, Laryngoscope **88:**61, 1978.

May, M.: Submandibular salivary flow test in facial paralysis, Ann. Otolaryngol. **87:**279, 1978.

May, M.: Total facial nerve exploration: transmastoid, extralabyrinthine, and subtemporal indications and results, Laryngoscope **89:**906, 1979.

May, M., and Schlaepfer, W.M.: Bell's palsy and the chorda tympani nerve: a clinical and electron microscopic study, Laryngoscope **85:**1957, 1975.

May, M., and others: Natural history of Bell's palsy: the salivary flow test and other prognostic indicators, Laryngoscope **86:**704, 1972.

McCabe, B.F.: Management of hyperfunction of the facial nerve, Ann. Otol. Rhinol. Laryngol. **79:**252, 1970.

McCabe, B.F., Some evidence for the efficacy of decompression for Bell's palsy: immediate motion postoperatively, Laryngoscope 246, 1976.

McGovern, F.H.: Facial nerve injuries in skull fractures; recent advances in management, Arch. Otolaryngol. **88:**536, 1968.

Mechelse, K., and others: Bell's palsy; prognostic criteria and evaluation of surgical decompression, Lancet **3**:57, 1971.

Olson, N.R., and others: Adverse effects of facial nerve decompression for Bell's palsy, Trans. Am. Acad. Ophthalmol. Otolaryngol. **77**:67, 1973.

Pulec, J.: Bell's palsy: diagnosis, management and results of treatment, Laryngoscope **84**:2119, 1974.

Saito, H., and others: Submandibular salivary pH as a diagnostic aid for prognosis of facial palsy, Laryngoscope **88**:663, 1978.

Taverner, D.: Electrodiagnosis in facial palsy, Arch. Otolaryngol. **81**:470, 1965.

Tschiassny, K.: Topognosis of lesions of the facial nerve, J. Int. Coll. Surg. **23**:381, 1955.

Wakasugi, B.: Facial nerve block in the treatment of facial spasm, Arch. Otolaryngol. **95**:356, 1972.

Yanagihara, N., and others: Transmastoid decompression of the facial nerve in Bell's palsy, Arch. Otolaryngol. **105**:530, 1979.

31 THE SALIVARY GLANDS

The major salivary glands, through their respective ducts, supply saliva to the oral cavity. Produced in the parotid, submaxillary, and sublingual glands, saliva is necessary for the initial digestion of starch. It also assists in keeping the mouth moist. Minor salivary glands are scattered abundantly throughout the palate.

Parotid gland. The parotid gland, located over the mandible and in front of and below the external ear, has two components. One is the superficial lobe, and the other is the deep lobe. The superficial lobe lies on the masseter muscle and extends to the zygoma superiorly. The deep lobe has an inner prolongation that lies posterior and medial to the angle of the mandible and extends medial to the styloid process. The duct of the parotid gland (Stensen's duct) passes through the buccinator muscle and opens opposite the upper second molar (Figs. 31-1, 31-2, and 31-4).

Submaxillary gland. The submaxillary gland is located in the submaxillary triangle, medial and inferior to the ramus of the mandible and at the junction of the anterior and posterior bellies of the digastric muscle. The gland and its duct (Wharton's) are in close relationship to the lingual nerve. The gland lies on the hyoglossus muscle. Wharton's duct opens into the floor of the mouth through a small papilla a few millimeters lateral to the frenum of the tongue (Fig. 31-5).

Sublingual glands. The sublingual glands, of which there are several, are located beneath the tongue. The ducts of the sublingual glands enter the mouth under the tongue through several minute openings. Occasionally one or more sublingual ducts will open into Wharton's duct.

• • •

The salivary glands are of particular concern to the physician when they are injured by infection, trauma, or neoplasm. The diagnosis of disease of the salivary glands requires special methods. Management requires special operative techniques.

Diagnostic procedures. In addition to inspection and palpation of the salivary glands, other procedures are available to aid in correct diagnosis of salivary gland abnormalities.

PHYSICAL EXAMINATION. Often disease of the salivary glands may be diagnosed by physical examination alone. However, the examination must include inspection of the nose, nasopharynx, oropharynx, larynx, neck, ears, cheeks, and oral cavity. The presence of dissimilar metallic fillings in teeth may account for sialorrhea (excessive salivation) and drooling. Bimanual palpation may demonstrate a stone lodged in a duct. Palpation will also express any pus or mucus that may be present in a duct. Usually any tumor can be felt.

PROBING. If the diagnosis cannot be established on the basis of the history and physical examination, the duct must be probed. This procedure is an important addition to the diagnostic armamentarium because it may reveal stones, strictures, or other obstruction. When there is acute pain and swelling without pus, epidemic parotitis (mumps) should be suspected. Probing of the duct in this instance is contraindicated.

A punctum dilator is used to stretch the orifice of a duct. Then a small lacrimal probe is inserted. In Wharton's duct the probe is directed laterally and inferiorly toward the submaxillary gland. In Stensen's duct, because of its course around the masseter muscle, the probe is inserted at right angles to the buccal

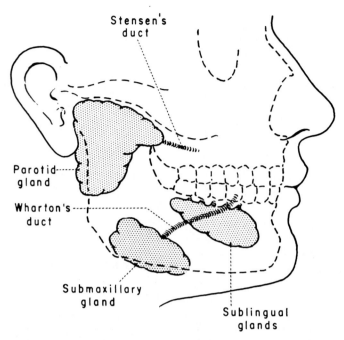

FIG. 31-1. Location of the salivary glands and their ducts.

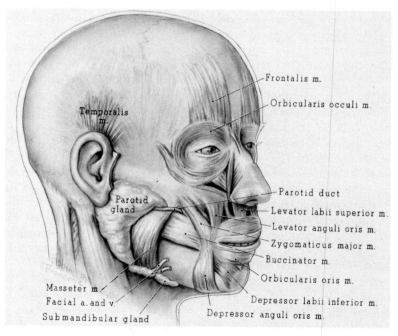

FIG. 31-2. Relationship of the parotid and submandibular glands to the face and jaw. (From Jacob, S.W., and Francone, C.A.: Structure and function in man, Philadelphia, 1970, W.B. Saunders Co.)

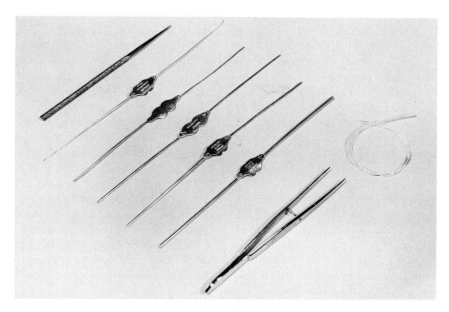

FIG. 31-3. Instruments for examination of the salivary glands. *Left to right*, Punctum dilator, lacrimal probes, thumb forceps, and polyethylene tube.

FIG. 31-4. Lacrimal probe in Stensen's duct *(right)*. Note that the orifice is opposite the upper second molar.

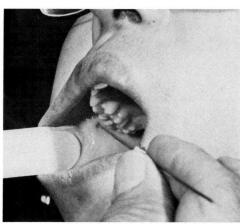

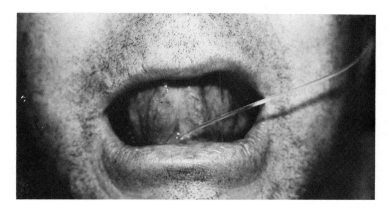

FIG. 31-5. Polyethylene tube (No. 60) in Wharton's duct.

mucosa. After it has been advanced a distance of 5 to 8 mm., it is turned toward the ear, which permits advancement of the probe to the hilus of the gland (Fig. 31-4).

INSPECTION OF THE SALIVA. Removal of the probe is usually followed by a copious flow of saliva, which at times contains flakes and strings of mucus or other material. The saliva should therefore be carefully inspected as it flows out. If flakes or strings are noted, they should be smeared and stained, and examined for the presence of leukocytes.

If there is a question of a recurrent allergic plug in the duct, saliva should be collected and stained to see if eosinophils are present. Specimens of saliva should also be taken for culture and for antibiotic sensitivity test if there is a history of recurrent or chronic infection.

SIALOGRAPHY. If a diagnosis is not obtained despite the measures discussed, sialography is indicated. It demonstrates strictures and calculi, the most common abnormalities. In adults, as well as in children, sialography demonstrates pathologic conditions of the peripheral ducts and acini, such as Mikulicz's disease, Sjögren's syndrome, and recurrent pyogenic parotitis. It reveals fistulas, and it defines the stages of sialectasis.

By means of the sialogram it is possible to determine whether a mass in the region of the parotid gland is within or outside the gland and also whether it is inflammatory, neoplastic, encapsulated, or invasive. An extrinsic tumor does not interfere with normal emptying of the duct system. An intrinsic benign tumore produces some retention of the radiopaque material. An invasive malignant tumor causes varying degrees of damage to the duct system.

Before the sialogram is made, a simple roentgenogram is made of the gland region. Preparations for the sialogram are preferably carried out in the physician's office and consist of the following procedures.

Stensen's or Wharton's duct is dilated with lacrimal probes (Fig. 31-3). A No. 60 polyethylene tube is then placed in the duct (Fig. 31-5). Prior to its placement a wire stylet is inserted into the tube for a distance of about 10 cm. The wire gives the tube sufficient rigidity to facilitate its introduction into the duct.

As soon as the tube is in the duct, the wire is removed. A flow of saliva follows, and it can be collected for examination if necessary. The flow of saliva is stopped by plugging the exposed end of the polyethylene tube with a toothpick, and the patient is taken to the x-ray department. There the toothpick is removed, and Pantopaque is injected into the tube until minimal pain is produced. At this point, the exposed end of the polyethylene tube is again plugged with a toothpick and roentgenograms are made. Finally, the polyethylene tube is withdrawn and the patient is given a piece of lemon to suck. Normally, the salivary stimulation evacuates the gland. Five minutes after the tube is removed, another set of roentgenograms is made. If the second set shows any residual dye, still another set is made. If the third set shows any residual dye, still another roentgenogram is made, in 1 hour.

ADDITIONAL STUDIES. In mumps, there is lymphocytosis; in leukemia, there is leuckcytosis. A roentgenogram of the chest may show the hilar nodes of Boeck's sarcoidosis. Examination of the eyes sometimes reveals enlargement of the lacrimal glands, which suggests Mikulicz's disease. It may also show minimal uveitis, which would be indicative of uveoparotitis. Neurologic examination is also of value because cranial nerve palsies are often associated with uveoparotitis. If all other procedures fail to establish the diagnosis, a biopsy may be of value.

Inflammation of the salivary glands. Inflammation of the salivary glands may be suppurative or nonsuppurative. The most common example of nonsuppurative disease is epidemic mumps.

Mumps (epidemic parotitis) is one of the common diseases of childhood. It occurs less often in adults. The childhood variety usually runs a benign course. The typical patient has swelling of one or both parotid glands. The swelling is accompanied by local pain and tenderness over the gland and pain when the patient attempts to chew or open the mouth. The temperature varies from 100° to 103° F. The white blood cell count is usually low, and the differential count of the white blood cells reveals a preponderance of lymphocytes. There is pouting and sometimes inflammation of the buccal opening of Stensen's duct. The entire gland is involved in the inflammatory process.

Mumps also occurs in the submaxillary glands. Symptoms are similar to those of mumps in the parotid glands.

Since mumps is a generalized viral disease, malaise is common. The virus may cause encephalitis or damage the cochlea, the seventh nerve, the ovaries, the testes, or the pancreas.

Treatment is conservative. Heat, fluids, control of pain, and bed rest are the only measures necessary, except when complications occur. In a few patients there is suppuration of the gland, and antibiotics must be given. Bed rest for 2 or 3 weeks is recommended when mumps occurs in an adult (after puberty). If viral inflammation develops in the testes or in the ovaries, sterility may ensue.

Recurrent, nonsuppurative enlargement. Recurrent obstruction of Wharton's or Stensen's duct gives rise to recurrent, nonsuppurative enlargement of the submaxillary or parotid gland. The obstruction may be caused by thick *mucus* plugs, the cause of which is unknown. Allergy is thought to be a cause, but this theory has not been proved.

Calculi of the salivary glands. Stones in the ducts of the salivary glands are common. Although they are found in the ducts of the parotid and sublingual glands, they are observed more often in the ducts of the submaxillary gland. Most statistical surveys agree that approximately 85% occur in Wharton's duct, about 10% to 12% in Stensen's duct, and the remainder in the sublingual ducts.

Stones have been observed in all age groups and as early as 3 weeks after birth. They may be small or large. A stone weighing 67 gm. has been reported. Usually there is only one stone, but sometimes several are found in a duct and more in the gland. Such patients have recurrent stones unless the gland (usually submaxillary) and duct are excised.

Although the pathogenesis is not known, several factors appear to account for the fact that stones usually occur in the submaxillary duct. Among them are the following:

1. The greater exposure of the submaxillary duct to trauma during mastication.
2. The irritation of the papilla that results from tartar formation on the lower teeth.
3. The slower flow of saliva from the submaxillary gland than from the parotid gland because (a) the submaxillary duct is larger in diameter and longer than the parotid duct; (b) the flow of saliva from the submaxillary gland is upward, against gravity; (c) there are frequently diverticula of the submaxillary duct near the papilla, which lead to stasis of saliva; and (d) the submaxillary gland secretion is high in mucin, whereas the secretion of the parotid gland is entirely serous. It has been shown that mucin enhances the chemical deposition of calcium on bacterial or epithelial debris. The lingual nerve and the external maxillary artery also cause slight constrictions along the course of the submaxillary duct.

The patient who has a stone in the submaxillary duct usually gives a characteristic history. He complains of swelling under the ramus of the mandible that comes on suddenly while he is eating. It may be painful but is not accompanied by local inflammation. The swelling usually subsides over a period of 30 minutes to 2 hours. It does not occur with every meal and may not recur for intervals of several days, weeks, or months. It may continue over a period of years before the patient seeks medical attention. All episodes are exactly alike, however. Such a history is pathognomonic of a submaxillary duct stone. Nevertheless, the diagnosis is frequently not suspected. Often a diagnosis of tumor or of enlarged cervical lymph gland is erroneously made.

Deviations from the typical picture are seen. Occasionally a stone may become lodged in a narrow portion of the gland and allow little or no saliva to pass. In these cases, some degree of swelling of the submaxillary gland may persist and additional swelling may occur at irregular intervals.

Sometimes the duct and gland become infected. In such an event the acute inflammatory process is evidenced by increased swelling, subjective pain, fever, and exquisite tenderness over the gland. Throughout its course along the floor of the mouth the duct is also edematous, tender, and enlarged. At times it is possible to obtain purulent material from the orifice of the duct by pressure over the gland. Untreated infection may lead to serious cellulitis of the neck.

Parotid duct stones give rise to widely varied clinical pictures. At one extreme are patients with complaints of pain and swelling in the involved cheek. As a rule, these symptoms occur suddenly during meals. The pain usually disappears promptly, whereas the swelling may persist for a few hours to several days. If the duct is completely blocked, the swelling may not subside until the blockage is relieved. At the other extreme are patients with no symptoms. Either such a patient finds a mass in his cheek or the physician encounters it on routine examination. Between these extremes are patients with various combinations of symptoms. Their parotid calculi may be misdiagnosed and called mumps.

When the patient presents an atypical picture, consideration must be given to a diagnosis of tumor, tuberculosis, or actinomycosis of the gland, as well as cervical lymph node disease.

The presence of a stone in the submaxillary gland is determined by bimanual palpation of the floor of the mouth, probing of the duct, and x-ray examination. This last procedure is the most reliable. Many stones in Wharton's duct can be felt by placing the index finger of one hand under the tongue and compressing the soft tissue of the floor of the mouth against the other hand, which is pushing upward from the outside. However, small or deep stones sometimes are missed in bimanual examination.

The x-ray technique used to demonstrate submaxillary duct stones is extremely important. Too often the roentgenologist makes a diagnosis from lateral and oblique views of the soft tissue of the jaw and upper neck. Large stones can be demonstrated, but small stones are missed half the time. Frequently the stones are not demonstrated, because they are obscured by the overlying mandible and also because some are not sufficiently radiopaque.

A much more staisfactory technique for demonstrating submaxillary duct stones, regardless of their size, is to *have the patient hold an occlusal dental x-ray film (2 ¼ × 3 inches) between the upper and lower teeth and to project the x-rays through the floor of the mouth from below* (Fig. 31-6). To demonstrate stones deep in the duct or in the gland, the tube may have to be angulated. This technique shows most stones. Unless the physician insists that the roentgenologist use this technique, the physician is likely to receive a report of no stones when stones are present.

Parotid duct stones are seen more often in men than in women. Although they occur anywhere from the parenchyma of the parotid gland to the buccal papilla, their most common location is between the hilus of the gland and the point where the duct turns medially around the masseter muscle.

Palpation may reveal swelling that involves the entire gland in front of and below the ear. There may be minimal saliva or no saliva at all. Pus may come from the papilla of Stensen's duct.

Often sialography will show whether the obstruction is due to stenosis, a stone, or a tumor. Each condition gives a different pattern. Eighty percent of parotid duct stones are radiopaque. They are usually composed of calcium carbonate and calcium phosphate.

A stone in Stensen's duct can be demonstrated by the use of the same type of dental x-ray film used to visualize a stone in the submaxillary duct. The film is placed inside the cheek but outside the teeth, and the x-rays are projected through the cheek.

An operation is often required in treatment of calculi of the salivary glands. Dilation of Stensen's or Wharton's duct followed by milking of the gland or duct with the fingers may deliver small stones into the mouth. Some stones will pass spontaneously without treatment. When neither of these procedures is possible, the duct must be opened from within the mouth and the stone removed.

Although an external approach for removal of submaxillary duct stones is advised in many surgical textbooks, it is seldom necessary. A better and more practical approach is from inside the mouth. The technique is not difficult, provided that one works in good light and opens the submaxillary duct along its entire course to the stone. General anesthesia is unnecessary. As a rule, procaine hydrochloride (Novocain), 3 to 5 ml., injected along the duct in the floor of the mouth provides excellent anesthesia. The steps of the surgical procedure are as follows:

1. The submaxillary duct papilla is raised with thumb forceps, and the papilla is cut across with small scissors and then discarded (Fig. 31-7, A).
2. A grooved or round probe is placed in the submaxillary duct. With small, sharp scissors, the duct is cut wide open along its lumen. This approach also implies incision of all the soft tissue of the floor of the mouth superficial to the duct. The line of incision is parallel to the duct (Fig. 31-7, B).

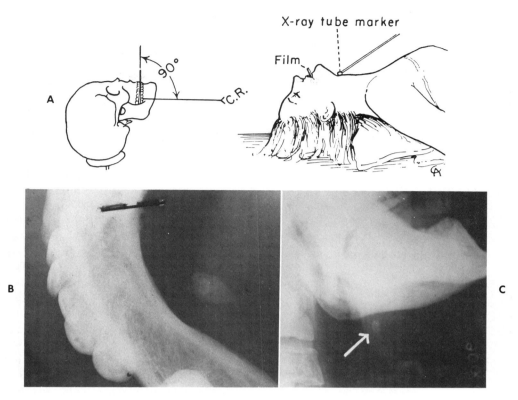

FIG. 31-6. **A,** Technique for making roentgenograms of a submaxillary duct stone with dental film. **B,** Stone in the submaxillary duct as demonstrated by the dental film technique. **C,** Stone in the submaxillary duct as demonstrated by the usual technique. Arrow points to stone. Small stones often are not seen because of the shadow of the mandible. (**A,** From DeWeese, D.D.: Portland Clin. Bull, **7:**1, 1953.)

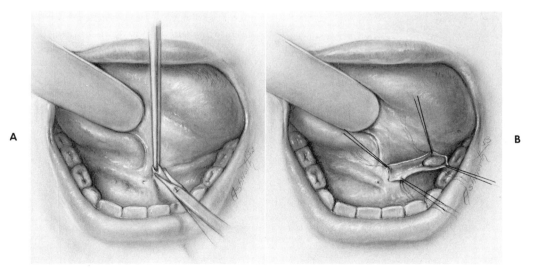

FIG. 31-7. **A,** Cutting off the submaxillary duct papilla. **B,** Submaxillary duct stone exposed before removal. (From DeWeese, D.D.: Portland Clin. Bull. **7:**1, 1953.)

3. When the stone is visualized, it should be grasped with cupped forceps and removed with this instrument. The stone has a chalky white color.

4. The wound should not be closed. However, one loose suture may be placed if a deep stone necessitates a long incision. Leaving the wound open is important because tight closure will result in either secondary infection or stenosis of the duct, or both.

Antibiotics are unnecessary after this procedure unless infection is already present. Usually there are minimal local reactive symptoms, and the duct will recannulize without stenosis even though the new orifice may be several millimeters from the papilla that has been sacrificed. Some authorities still advise cutting down directly over the stone to remove it without opening the duct along its full length. In our experience, this has led to postoperative stenosis of the duct in a high percentage of cases.

To remove a parotid duct stone, a U-shaped incision with a posterior base is made in the mucous membrane around the papilla (Fig. 31-8). The buccinator muscle is identified, and the incision is carried through it. By dissection, the mucous membrane flap is elevated posteriorly until the parotid duct is encountered. The duct is followed to the point of obstruction, where it is incised (Fig. 31-9). If only stricture is present, a polyethylene tube is passed into the duct through the papilla. The tube is approximately the size of the duct and extends slightly beyond the incision in the duct. If a stone is found, it is removed, after which a polyethylene tube is placed in the duct.

No sutures are taken in the duct. The mucous membrane flap is replaced and sutured with nonabsorbable material. A suture with nonabsorbable material anchors the polyethylene tube to the buccal mucosa.

The length of time the tube is allowed to remain in the duct depends on whether there was a stone or stenosis alone, or whether both were present. Accordingly, the time may vary from 5 days to 2 weeks.

When a calculus is embedded in the substance of either the parotid or submaxillary gland, excision of the gland may be necessary. Ordinarily this is not done unless the calculus is associated with recurrent or chronic suppuration of the gland.

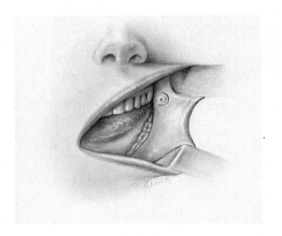

FIG. 31-8. Incision for exposure of a parotid duct stone. (From DeWeese, D.D.: Portland Clin. Bull. **11:**9, 1957.)

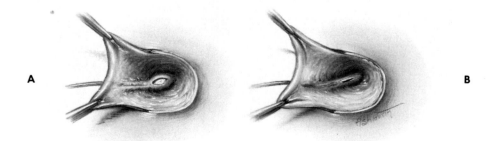

FIG. 31-9. Removal of a parotid duct stone. **A,** Stone exposed. **B,** Polyethylene tube in Stensen's duct after removal. (From DeWeese, D.D.: Portland Clin. Bull. **11:**9, 1957.)

Chronic bilateral enlargement of the parotid glands. It is possible to have chronic bilateral enlargement of the parotid glands without pain or other symptoms. Such enlargement may be caused by lead or mercury poisoning, by the use of iodides or thiouracil, by vitamin deficiencies, or by lymphoma and lymphoblastoma. The treatment depends on the cause of the enlargement. In some instances the cause is unknown.

Acute suppurative parotitis. Acute suppurative parotitis is characterized by painful swelling and tenderness of the entire parotid gland, high fever, and leukocytosis. Pus is visible at, or can be expressed from, the orifice of Stensen's duct. When tissue breakdown is present, as often happens, multiple abscesses are formed (Fig. 31-10). General toxicity and delirium are also frequently observed.

Acute suppurative parotitis is often a complication after a prolonged operation on a debilitated patient. In this event, dehydration, oral sepsis, or trauma to the gland from pressure exerted during administration of the anesthetic may be the cause.

In the early stage of the infection (24 to 48 hours) treatment consists of hydration, full dosage of an antibiotic, and radiation. Later, when the abscesses have formed, incision and drainage are necessary. A small incision will not allow access to the multiple separate abscesses. It is best to make a vertical incision that starts immediately anterior to the ear and extends downward, under the angle of the mandible. A skin flap is then turned forward, and each abscess is drained. If the incision is made close to the cartilage of the external auditory canal, the facial nerve will not be injured.

Chronic suppuration of the salivary glands. Repeated obstruction of the duct of either the parotid or submaxillary gland may cause chronic suppuration (Fig. 31-11). Relief of the obstruction and conservative treatment are recommended. Culture of the purulent secretion is important. If the purulent process fails to respond to conservative measures, the gland should be excised. *Because of the danger of injury to the facial nerve, total removal of the parotid gland should not be attempted until all conservative methods have been used.* In removal of the submaxillary gland, injury to the facial nerve is not a hazard.

Chronic granulomas of the salivary glands. In differential diagnosis, tuberculosis sarcoidosis (Boeck's sarcoid), and actinomycosis must be considered. All are rare. Often the diagnosis is not established until a palpable nodule is removed and the tissue studied microscopically.

Sarcoidosis is a chronic granulomatous disease affecting several organ systems of interest to the otolaryngologist—especially the salivary glands, the larynx, and the sinuses. It is characterized by discrete epithelioid granulomas with giant cells of the Langhans and foreign body types. Fibrinoid necrosis, often indistinguishable from caseating granulomas of tuberculosis, may occur. The etiology of the disease remains unknown. Theories for its origin include a relationship to tuberculosis, an altered immune

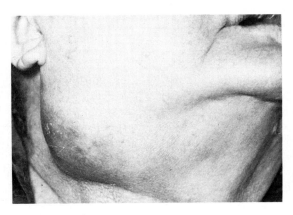

FIG. 31-10. Acute parotid abscess. Note diffuse swelling of the entire gland and brawny thickening over most of the swollen portion.

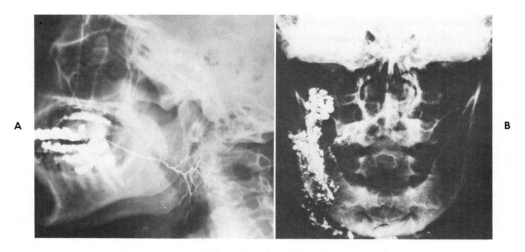

FIG. 31-11. A, Sialogram of a normal parotid gland, lateral view. **B,** Sialectasis of the parotid gland, anterior view.

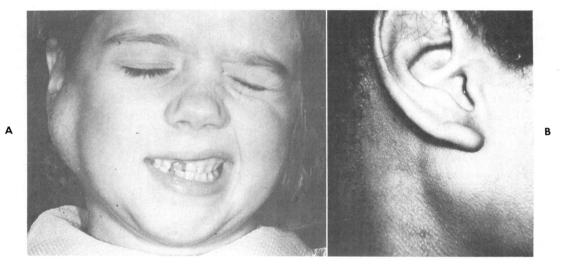

FIG. 31-12. A, Malignant parotid tumor with partial facial paralysis. **B,** Typical position of a mixed salivary gland tumor of the parotid gland.

response to an unknown external agent, environmental causes, parasites, an autoimmune relationship, and a viral etiology.

Symptoms include weight loss, fatigue, cough, dyspnea, and chest pain. The lungs, skin, lymph nodes, bones, liver, spleen, parotid glands, and uveal tract are usually involved. Sarcoidosis may also affect the nasal mucosa, pharynx, larynx, eyelids, cardiovascular system, or gastrointestinal tract. The disease may present to the otolaryngologist as lymphadenopathy, parotid swelling, voice change or hoarse-

ness, chronic cough, or nonhealing nasal ulcer. The diagosis is based on clinical appearance, x-ray film, biopsy, and laboratory data. Sarcoidosis is treated with corticosteroids, but relapse upon cessation of the drug therapy can be expected.

Neoplasms of the salivary glands. Neoplasms of the parotid and submaxillary glands may be benign or malignant. The presenting complaint is a palpable lump or mass either in the face in front of the ear or in the neck under the mandible. Benign neoplasms enlarge slowly and are

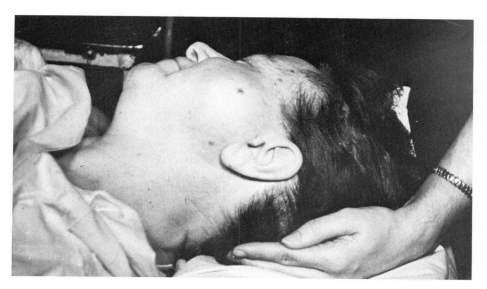

FIG. 31-13. Mixed salivary gland tumor of the parotid gland. No facial paralysis.

painless. Some may be present for years without being discovered. Malignant growths enlarge more rapidly than do benign growths. A neoplasm in the inner prolongation of the parotid gland may be visible in the lateral wall of the pharynx before it is noticeable in the soft tissue under the ear.

A neoplasm should be suspected when any mass persists in the area of the parotid or submaxillary gland. Palpation will determine whether the tumor is fixed or movable. A tumor that can be moved easily and seems to have movable soft tissue beneath it is usually benign. A rapidly growing tumor is usually malignant. Associated weakness or paralysis of the facial nerve is almost certain evidence of malignancy (Fig. 31-12, *A*). Roentgenograms are of little value unless contrast media is introduced into the duct and a sialogram is made. Sialography may outline the tumor and give some indication of its size and the extent of the damage to the duct system. Removal of tissue for biopsy generally is considered contraindicated, but some authorities do advocate the use of needle biopsy in all cases. The malignant tumor of the parotid or submaxillary gland is poorly encapsulated, and incision into it may adversely affect the final result.

Differential diagnosis of a tumor of the salivary glands is difficult until microscopic slides are examined. Many classifications of these tumors have been made; the one offered by

Maxwell in 1954 is widely accepted. It is given here as a basis for differential diagnosis.

Benign epithelial tumors

  I. Mixed tumors (Fig. 31-13)
    A. Cylindromatous type (stromal elements predominate)
    B. Canalicular type (epithelial elements predominate)
  II. Mucoepidermoid tumors
  III. Adenomas
    A. Serous cell
    B. Acidophilic cell
      1. Papillary lymphoid cyst adenoma

Malignant epithelial neoplasms

  I. Carcinomas
    A. Squamous cell
      1. Cornifying
      2. Noncornifying
      3. Lymphoepithelioma
    B. Gland-celled carcinomas
      1. Pseudoadenomatous basal cell carcinoma—cylindromatous canalicular, medullary, and cystic forms
      2. Acidophilic gland-celled carcinoma
      3. Serous cell adenocarcinoma
    C. Mucoepidermoid carcinomas
    D. Unclassified carcinomas

A neoplasm of the salivary glands demands total excision not only of the lesion itself but of its capsule and a wide area of surrounding normal tissue. The initial operation is the most important. Attempts to shell out a tumor from in-

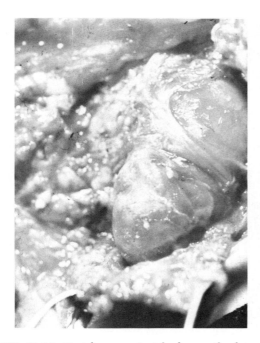

FIG. 31-14. Facial nerve stretched over the lateral surface of a mixed salivary gland tumor. Resection was accomplished without injury to the nerve in this instance. (Courtesy Dr. James Maxwell, University of Michigan, Ann Arbor, Mich.)

side its capsule will result in recurrence in almost every instance, unless the lesion is a simple fibroma or a lipoma. When there is doubt regarding the extent of a large tumor, the entire gland should be removed.

Complete removal of the submaxillary gland presents few problems either from the standpoint of operative technique or from the standpoint of postoperative care. The lingual nerve may have to be sacrificed. If so, only a sensory disturbance follows.

Complete removal of the parotid gland may require removal of the facial nerve if malignancy is present. When the tumor is benign, every effort should be made to preserve the facial nerve (Fig. 31-14). The tympanomastoid fissure has proved to be a constant landmark, pointing directly to the main trunk of the facial nerve as it leaves the stylomastoid foramen and therefore providing a safe and reliable method of locating the nerve. Dissection of the main trunk and its branches can be performed (see discussion of nerve grafts in Chapter 30, p. 421). If portions of the nerve are injured or removed, grafts can be placed to restore function.

A second or third operation may be necessary for recurrence after inadequate removal. With each successive procedure, the prognosis for cure becomes poorer. Radical dissection of glands in the neck may be required if there is evidence of metastasis. This should be done at the same time as the resection of the gland and with tissue continuity between the tumor and soft tissue of the neck, when possible.

Trauma to the salivary glands. Trauma to the salivary glands and their ducts is most often the result of lacerating and penetrating injury to the face or neck. Automobile accidents and military injuries account for most of these instances of trauma.

The primary concern of treatment is reestablishment of continuity of the main duct, if it has been severed, and resuture of the facial nerve, if it has been cut. Repair of the facial nerve is discussed in Chapter 30.

Polyethylene, Teflon, or silicone tubes threaded into Stensen's or Wharton's duct through the mouth and left in place 7 to 14 days are ideal splints around which ducts will reform. Other repair requires only restoration of soft tissue and bone continuity that is as nearly normal as possible in each situation.

Gustatory sweating. Gustatory sweating, also called Frey's syndrome, occurs after trauma to the parotid gland (such as partial parotidectomy). The patient sweats, often profusely, in the area of the cheek innervated by the auriculotemporal nerve. The patient has symptoms when he eats or thinks about eating, and sweating is induced over a localized area on the side of the face. Several theories have been proposed to account for this phenomenon, and the most widely accepted is that of misdirected axons. The mechanism is similar to what happens in a patient with Bell's palsy who later exhibits mass motion—all muscles on one side of the face contract when he intends to activate only one muscle.

Usually no special treatment is necessary for Frey's syndrome, unless symptoms are severe. Then it may help to resect the tympanic plexus in the middle ear, since it is through this pathway that parasympathetic motor fibers from the petrosal ganglion reach the otic ganglion and finally the auriculotemporal branch of the mandibular nerve. The auriculotemporal nerve lies just medial to the parotid gland and is prone to injury at the time of parotidectomy or other facial trauma.

Parotid duct transplant. A unique use of the salivary secretion—to moisten a totally dry eye—can be successfully initiated by transplanting the duct of the parotid gland in the conjunctiva. The procedure has been used in the treatment of total xerophthalmia to prevent recurrent corneal ulceration and serious loss of vision.

A rectangular flap of mucous membrane is incised around Stensen's duct. The duct is dissected, usually without difficulty, to the hilus of the parotid gland. An incision is made in the lateral aspect of the conjunctiva of the lower lid on the same side. A subcutaneous tunnel is made by blunt dissection between the conjunctival incision and the area of the hilus of the gland. Stensen's duct is then pulled through the tunnel, and mucosa is sutured to the conjunctival opening. The defect in the buccal mucous membrane is closed. This procedure has, at present, not stood the test of time and is seldom recommended. It is mentioned here to indicate that the procedure can be successfully done; if, in the future, new indications for its use are found, the technique will not be forgotten.

SELECTED READINGS

Blatt, I.M., and others: Studies in sialolithiasis. I. The structure and mineralogical composition of salivary gland calculi, Ann. Otol. Rhinol. Laryngol. **67**:595, 1958.

Castro, E.B., and others: Tumors of the major salivary glands in children, Cancer **29**:312, 1972.

Cummings, C.W.: Adenoid cystic carcinoma (cylindroma) of parotid gland, Ann. Otol. Rhinol. Laryngol. **86**(pt. 1):280-292, 1977.

Devine, K.: Sarcoidosis and sarcoidosis of the larynx, Laryngoscope **75**(4):533-569, 1965.

Eneroth, C.M., and others: Preoperative facial paralysis in malignant parotid tumors, Otolaryngology **39**:272-277, 1977.

Fee, W.E., Goffinet, D.R., and Calcaterra, T.C.: Recurrent mixed tumors of the parotid gland: results of surgical therapy, Laryngoscope **88**:265-273, February, 1978.

Frable, W.J., and Elzay, R.P.: Tumors of minor salivary glands; a report of 73 cases, Cancer **25**:932, 1970.

Furstenberg, A.C., and Blatt, I.M.: Intermittent parotid swelling due to ill-fitting dentures, Laryngoscope **68**:1165, 1958.

Hays, L.L.: Frey syndrome: review and double-blind evaluation of topical use of new anticholinergic agent, Laryngoscope **88**:1796-1824, November, 1978.

Kaban, L.B., Mulliken, J.B., and Murray, J.E.: Sialadenitis in childhood, Am. J. Surg. **135**:570-576, April, 1978.

Kassan, S.S., and others: Increased risk of lymphoma in sicca syndrome, Ann. Intern. Med. **89**:888-892, December, 1978.

Krippaehne, W.W., and others: Acute suppurative parotitis; a study of 161 cases, Ann. Surg. **156**(2):251, 1962.

Leegaard, T., and Lindeman, H.: Salivary gland tumors; clinical picture and treatment, Acta Otolaryngol. **263**:155, 1970.

Maxwell, J.H.: Chronic lymphoepithelial sialadenopathy with sialodochiectasis, Trans. Am. Acad. Ophthalmol. Otolaryngol. **64**:225, 1960.

Saberman, M., and Tenta, L.: The Melkersson-Rosenthal syndrome, Arch. Otolaryngol. **84**:74, 1966.

Schuller, D.E., and McCabe, B.F.: Firm salivary mass in children, Laryngoscope **87**:1891-1898, November, 1977.

Skolnik, E.M., and others: Malignancies of the parotid gland, Arch. Otolaryngol. **93**:256, 1971.

Spiro, R.H., Huvos, A.G., and Strong, E.W.: Acinic cell carcinoma of salivary origin: clinicopathologic study of 67 cases, Cancer **41**:924-935, March, 1978.

Spiro, R.H., and others: Mucoepidermoid carcinoma of salivary gland origin: clinicopathologic study of 367 cases, Am. J. Surg. **136**:461-468, October, 1978.

Tabb, H.G., Scalco, A.N., and Fraser, S.F.: Exposure of the facial nerve in parotid surgery, Laryngoscope **80**:559, 1970.

32 CYSTS AND TUMORS OF THE HEAD AND NECK AND RELATED CONDITIONS

Various tumors and cysts of the head and neck not discussed in previous chapters are discussed in this chapter. Also, several related conditions to be considered in the differential diagnosis of these tumors and cysts are included.

MAXILLARY CYSTS

Several types of cysts form in the maxilla (some also in the mandible) that can be confused with one another. All these cysts are the result of developmental anomalies.

Median palatine cyst. In the embryo there are two palatine processes that eventually fuse in the midline. They also fuse with the nasal septum above. Thus, at one stage in the embryo, the oral and nasal cavities communicate. When the palatine processes fuse, mesenchyme invading the fusion line normally obliterates all epithelium (Fig. 32-1, A). Sometimes, however, epithelial cells remain, and eventually a cyst may form (Fig. 32-1, B). As might be expected, such median palatine cysts can have either a squamous or a respiratory type of epithelium. Some have both.

Nasopalatine duct cyst. Clinically similar to the median palatine cysts but embryologically different, the nasopalatine duct (incisive canal) cyst arises from epithelium left behind when the two palatine processes join the premaxilla. Normally, there are two nasopalatine ducts that remain for a time and then obliterate. If their lining persists, a cyst may form. Again, the lining may be of either squamous or respiratory type.

Nasoalveolar cyst. The nasoalveolar cyst causes a swelling at the junction of the nasal ala and the upper lip. Thus it may appear in the floor of the nose or, anteriorly, above the lip. This cyst is also of the fissural type. Epithelium is entrapped where the nasal and maxillary processes join.

Dentigerous cyst. Dentigerous cysts are associated with enamel-forming epithelium and are found about the crowns of unerupted teeth. Sometimes the cysts grow very large.

Periodontal cyst. Periodontal cysts form about the roots of teeth in response to inflammation. Sometimes an abscess cavity at the apex of a tooth becomes epithelized and forms such a cyst, or epithelial cells remaining in the periodontal membrane may proliferate in response to infection of the dental pulp.

MANDIBULAR TUMORS

A number of benign tumors and cysts affect the mandible. Treatment is dependent on correct diagnosis, and this is aided greatly by adequate radiographs and biopsy techniques. Adamantinoma is discussed on p. 449. Most benign tumors are correctable by excision of only a partial thickness of the mandible, so that continuity of the jaw is not lost.

Malignant tumors, on the other hand, require wide resection of the mandible and adjacent tissues, such as the gingiva, floor of the mouth, often a part of the tongue, and radical neck dissection. The deformity produced is not great if only the angle of the mandible and part of the horizontal ramus are excised. When the symphysis must be taken, the patient is apt to have an "Andy Gump" appearance postoperatively unless particularly skillful reconstructive surgery is done. Some surgeons reconstruct part of the mandible using an iliac bone graft, a rib

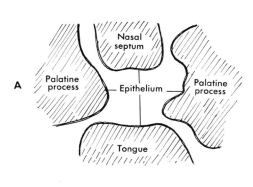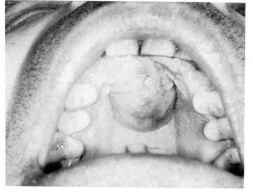

FIG. 32-1. **A,** Fusion of the palate, showing how epithelium is entrapped. **B,** Large median palatine cyst.

graft, or a steel rod. Others may elect not to use grafts, at least not at the time of the original surgery.

CERVICAL CYSTS

Thyroglossal duct cyst. Remnants of the embryonic thyroglossal duct may be found anywhere from the base of the tongue to the thyroid gland. Most thyroglossal cysts, however, are found at the level of the thyrohyoid interval under the deep cervical fascia (Fig. 32-2). They are midline, or just off the midline, and move up and down when the patient swallows.

The cyst may be connected with the foramen cecum, or a tract of cells may lead upward from the cyst and then end in tongue muscle. Often no tract can be demonstrated.

Because in the embryo the hyoid bone forms around the thyroglossal duct, the surgeon should remove the body of the hyoid and then core out a tract of tongue muscle toward the foramen cecum. Otherwise there may be a recurrence. Removal of the central portion of the hyoid (Fig. 32-3), even though this bone affords attachment to many muscles, is not disabling.

The thyroglossal cyst is lined by columnar epithelium. Malignancies in thyroglossal remnants, most of which were papillary adenocarcinomas, have been reported in at least 43 cases.

Ranula. A ranula (Fig. 32-4, *A*) is caused by obstruction of one of the ducts of the sublingual salivary gland; in some instances it may represent a congenital cyst. The term means "little frog"; the name has been given because of the appearance of the tense, bulging cyst under the

tongue, resembling a frog's belly. The tongue is displaced upward when the cyst becomes large. Treatment is surgical *excision* (Fig. 32-4, *B*)—mere incision and drainage is not sufficient.

Dermoid cysts. Dermoid and epidermoid cysts also cause midline swellings. They occur most often under the chin, just above the hyoid (Fig. 32-5). If large enough, a cyst may fill the floor of the mouth and push the tongue upward. Except for their size, dermoid cysts are asymptomatic. Treatment is surgical.

The only difference between dermoid and epidermoid cysts is their lining. In the dermoid cyst there are skin structures such as hair follicles and sweat glands, whereas only squamous epithelium lines the cavity of the epidermoid cyst (Fig. 32-6). The dermoid cyst in the neck is not to be confused with the ovarian teratologic anomaly.

Branchial cysts and remnants. Persistence of branchial remnants is fairly common. Many times the anomaly is asymptomatic; but occasionally, especially when a cyst or fistulous tract becomes infected, symptoms develop.

FIRST BRANCHIAL APPARATUS. A small dimple just above and anterior to the tragus may mark the site where the first branchial cleft failed to close completely (Fig. 32-7). Occasionally a sinus tract leads a short distance subcutaneously. Rarely, the sinus tract may extend deeply. Ordinarily, unless infection causes drainage, excision is unnecessary.

Another anomaly of development related to the first branchial region is found in the tongue. The anterior part of the tongue derives from the first branchial arches bilaterally and also from a

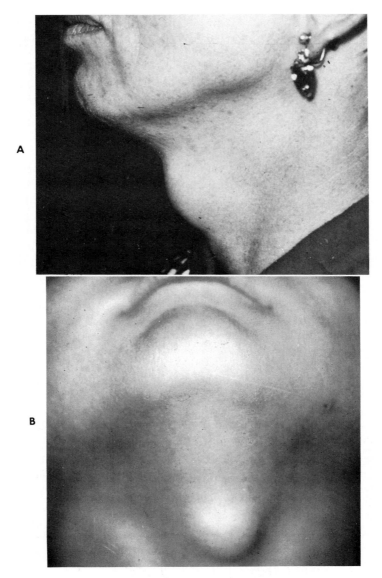

FIG. 32-2. A, Lateral view of a thyroglossal duct cyst. **B,** Most typical position of a thyroglossal duct cyst—the thyrohyoid space.

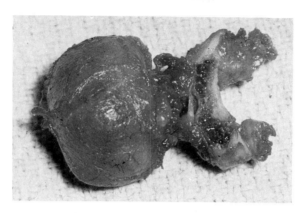

FIG. 32-3. Gross specimen (including the body of the hyoid) of the cyst shown in Fig. 32-2, *A*.

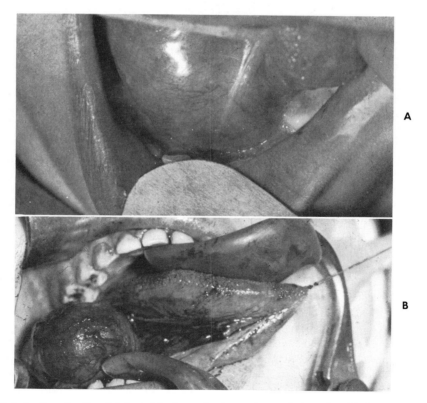

FIG. 32-4. A, Ranula. One blade holds down the lower lip, and the other blade holds up the tongue. **B,** Patient shown in **A** at time of surgery.

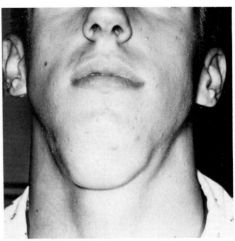

FIG. 32-5. Epidermoid cyst in the typical location. The tumor cannot be differentiated from a dermoid cyst.

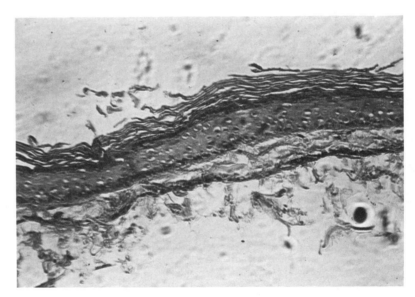

FIG. 32-6. Epidermoid cyst. Note absence of any dermal elements—hair follicles, sebaceous glands, or sweat glands.

median part where the arches join. This median part is called the *tuberculum impar*. As development progresses, the two lateral halves of the first arch fuse and cover the tuberculum impar. In anomalous development, however, the tuberculum impar occasionally persists as a surface structure. Since it never grows papillae, it looks different from the rest of the tongue. In the adult it is seen as a diamond-shaped red area just anterior to the foramen cecum. The

condition is known clinically as median rhomboid glossitis (Fig. 2-1).

SECOND BRANCHIAL APPARATUS (Fig. 32-8). The essentials of the second branchial apparatus are simple. Look at your left fist. Let each knuckle (ignore the thumb) represent a *branchial arch*—there are four. The depression between the knuckles represents the *branchial grooves*. The bars and grooves, being external, are covered with ectoderm. Now open your

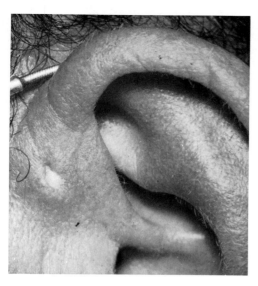

FIG. 32-7. Squamous debris in a preauricular fistula, a remnant of the first branchial apparatus.

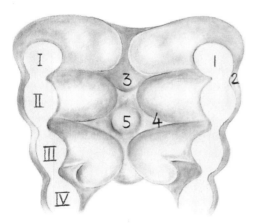

FIG. 32-8. Branchial apparatus from which numerous adult anomalies may develop. *1*, Arch. *2*, Groove. *3*, Tuberculum impar. *4*, Pouch. *5*, Copula.

fist so that the fingers are together and outstretched. The palmar surfaces of your fingers represent the inner surfaces of the branchial arches, and the spaces between the fingers represent the *branchial pouches*. The pouches are lined by entoderm. Between ectoderm and entoderm is mesoderm.

In the fish, ectoderm and entoderm meet and the epithelial membranes rupture. The breakthrough from the outside to the inside forms a

gill cleft. However, in humans, except in anomalous developments, mesoderm continues to separate ectoderm and entoderm. Eventually the ectodermal grooves on the outside and the entodermal pouches on the inside smooth out.

Sometimes, when development goes awry, a branchial groove connects with a branchial pouch. In later life the patient with this anomaly has a branchial fistula; an opening on the skin connects with the pharynx.

Most branchial cysts and fistulas are related to the second branchial apparatus because the second branchial arch grows farther downward than the others and overlaps them. A persistent branchial fistula may be lined by either squamous or columnar epithelium, depending on whether the entrapped lining derives from the branchial groove (ectoderm) or the branchial pouch (entoderm). Usually there is a squamous lining with dense collections of lymphoid tissue underneath. The association of lymphoid tissue and squamous epithelium is logical when one considers that the pharyngeal orifice opens near the faucial tonsil.

When a branchial fistula becomes infected, pus oozes from its orifice and there may be tenderness along the tract. The pharyngeal opening is not visible, but occasionally one can press on the neck and see pus ooze from behind the faucial tonsil. The cutaneous openings of the branchial fistulas are usually found lower in the neck than are branchial cysts (Figs. 32-9 to 32-11). This arrangement is reasonable when one considers that the cyst is caused by epithelial secretions from the middle portion of the tract; the distal end of the tract (and sometimes the proximal end) is obliterated. When removing a fistulous tract, the surgeon finds that the upper end passes between the internal and external carotid arteries.

THIRD BRANCHIAL APPARATUS. The third branchial apparatus seldom leaves a remnant that is clinically demonstrable. When it does, the tract leads to the pyriform sinus.

Aberrant thyroid. *Lingual thyroid* (Fig. 32-12) is a rare condition in which thyroid tissue, persisting near the foramen cecum, forms a tumor at the base of the tongue. There is usually additional thyroid tissue in the neck, but it should be remembered that sometimes all of the thyroid tissue may be at the base of the tongue. In such a case, excision of the tumor would leave a

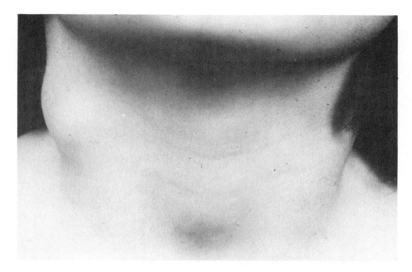

FIG. 32-9. Branchial cyst in the usual location. This cyst had no upper or lower tract.

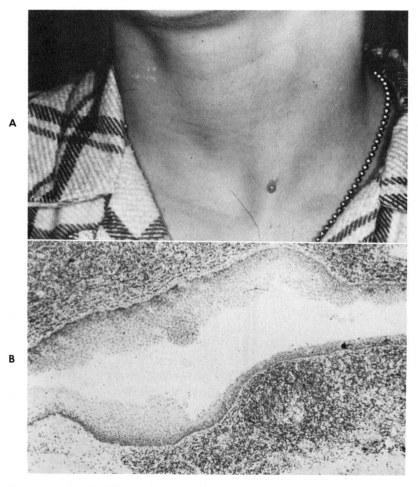

FIG. 32-10. A, Branchial fistula. The tract was easily traced all the way to the supratonsillar fossa. **B,** Lining of the fistula. Note the lymphoid nodules in close relationship to squamous epithelium.

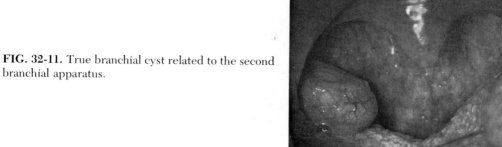

FIG. 32-11. True branchial cyst related to the second branchial apparatus.

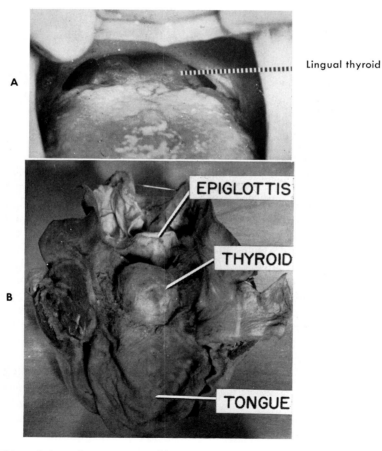

Lingual thyroid

A

EPIGLOTTIS

THYROID

B

TONGUE

FIG. 32-12. A, Lingual thyroid in a 60-year-old woman. This tumor had been asymptomatic except for some muffling of the voice. **B,** Cadaver specimen from patient shown in **A.** She died of pulmonary tuberculosis and laryngeal carcinoma. (From Adornato, S.G., and Saunders, W.H.: Ann. Otol. Rhinol. Laryngol. **71:**959, 1962.)

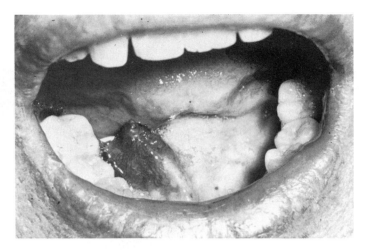

FIG. 32-13. Unusual instance of thyroid tissue in the floor of the mouth. A normal thyroid gland is present in the neck.

serious deficiency. Preliminary examination using radioactive uptake methods will help settle the matter.

Aberrant thyroid tissue may also occur in the floor of the mouth (Fig. 32-13) and in various parts of the neck, unattached to the main gland. Such aberrant tissue sometimes represents a metastatic growth of thyroid carcinoma.

THYROID CANCER

Both the otolaryngologist and the general surgeon perform thyroid surgery. Familiarity with the surgical anatomy of the thyroid gland, its blood supply, and especially laryngeal innervations are essential.

The thyroid gland arises from the pharyngeal floor between the first and second branchial pouches and descends to its adult location from the foramen cecum. It is served by 2 pairs of arteries (superior and inferior), 2 pairs of veins (superior and inferior), an inconstant artery (thyroid ima), and an inconstant vein (middle thyroid). As the inferior thyroid artery passes medially behind the gland, it crosses the recurrent laryngeal nerve (in front, behind, or on either side). The superior thyroid artery is in relation to the external branch (motor) of the superior laryngeal nerve medially. One of the artery's branches (the laryngeal branch) enters the larynx with the internal (sensory) branch of the superior laryngeal nerve. All of these nerves (especially the recurrent laryngeal) are important to identify during thyroidectomy.

Thyroid storm, a potentially life-threatening syndrome characterized by fever and by central nervous system, gastrointestinal, and cardiovascular symptoms, can occur in hyperthyroid patients not properly treated before surgery. Prophalaxis with antithyroid drugs prior to thyroidectomy has almost eliminated this syndrome. Treatment is supportive; glucose, fluids, electrolytes, steroids, antithyroid drugs, propranolol, and digitalis are given as needed.

Thyroid malignancy is relatively rare. It occurs twice as often in females as in males, and its incidence increases with age. It is more frequent in persons with a history of radiation therapy to the head and neck area. Thyroid malignancy is diagnosed by thyroid scan, where it shows up as a cold area, and by physical examination, usually as a nodule in the gland. Studies have shown that as many as 27% of cold spots in scans of patients who do not have palpable nodules represent malignancy. Treatment is by means of surgery or ^{131}I ablation. There are four main types of thyroid carcinoma.

Papillary thyroid carcinoma. Papillary thyroid carcinoma is the most common type of thyroid carcinoma, comprising 60%-70% of cases. It is unencapsulated and most often multifocal; its spread is local, usually via lymphatics. Distant metastasis occurs in less than 5% of cases. Conversion to anaplastic thyroid carcinoma can occur in approximately 5% of cases. Psammoma bodies on histologic section are diagnostic.

Treatment is by lobectomy on the involved side and subtotal thyroidectomy contralaterally or total thyroidectomy. Postoperative radioiodine is indicated for distant spread. "Node plucking" or radical neck dissection also may be indicated, according to some authorities.

Follicular thyroid carcinoma. Next most common is follicular carcinoma, which accounts for 15%-20% of thyroid malignancies. It is usually solitary and encapsulated and only occasionally multicentric. It is divided into high and low grades, with the low-grade form usually being noninvasive and most likely to be characterized by functioning follicles. The prognosis depends on whether the condition is angioinvasive and on whether capsular invasion occurs. Metastasis is usually to lung or bone, by way of the bloodstream. Life expectancy is close to normal in the noninvasive type; in the invasive type, the 5-year survival rate is 60% and the 10-year survival rate is 10%.

Total lobectomy on the involved side with subtotal lobectomy contralaterally is the usual treatment. Because of the low incidence of nodal spread, radical neck dissection is rarely indicated. For disease with distant spread, total thyroidectomy and postoperative radioiodine are indicated.

Medullary thyroid carcinoma. Medullary thyroid carcinoma is derived from C cells (calcitonin secretory parafollicular cells). It is rare, accounting for only 5%-10% of thyroid malignancies. Its presentation is sporadic or as an autosomal dominant part of MEA II (MTC, pheochromocytoma, parathyroid hyperplasia) or MEA III (or MEA IIb) with marfanoid habitus. Amyloid seen in the stroma is characteristic. Medullary thyroid carcinoma is usually bilateral, and it is sharply circumscribed but unencapsulated. Cervical metastases occur in 50% of clinically palpable lesions. The prognosis is related to stage, with occult involving a near normal life expectancy and the 5- and 10-year survival rates in nodal involvement being 60% and 40% respectively. Total thyroidectomy is the best surgical treatment.

Anaplastic thyroid carcinoma. Anaplastic thyroid carcinoma comprises 5% to 15% per cent of thyroid cancer. The most aggressive of all types, it results in death within a few months in nearly all instances. The 5-year survival rate is less than 3%. Anaplastic thyroid carcinoma is a poorly marginated lesion that occurs in the older individuals. There is no effective treatment.

TUMORS OF THE NECK

Branchiogenic carcinoma. A squamous cell carcinoma of the neck (for which no primary lesion can be found) is sometimes erroneously ascribed to malignant degeneration of the epithelium in previously unrecognized branchial cleft tissue.

Rather than assuming neck cancer to be branchiogenic carcinoma, *one should regard the neck mass as metastatic and continue to search for the primary lesion, even after years.* Almost always, patients with carcinoma of the neck in whom no primary lesion can be found eventually die of a cancer that was overlooked because of its small size or submucosal location.

Metastatic carcinoma in the neck (or cervical metastases). One of the more common neck lesions is metastatic carcinoma. The usual primary sites from which malignant cells break loose and seed in lymph nodes of the neck are the larynx, lip, tongue, tonsil, nasopharynx, and parotid and thyroid glands. Less commonly, lesions from below the clavicle metastasize to the neck. Often there is only one palpable node, but sometimes several are palpable, and then the prognosis is worse. The patient with cancer originating in one of the areas just mentioned may be unaware of the primary lesion and consult his physician because of a lump in the neck. The primary lesion may cause no symptom, because of its small size or submucosal position. On the other hand, in another patient the metastatic lesion in the neck may appear months or even years after the primary lesion has been discovered and treated.

In examining the neck for metastasis, the physician should palpate carefully beneath the sternocleidomastoid muscle along the course of the internal jugular vein. The submaxillary area is another common place for metastasis to occur. The supraclavicular region, although a less common site of metastasis, should not be overlooked. *Nasopharyngeal carcinomas have a habit of producing a large node in the posterior triangle, even when there is only a tiny primary lesion.* Too much emphasis cannot be placed on careful periodic examinations of the neck in patients known to have malignant disease of the head and neck.

Silverman needle biopsy. Silverman needle biopsy with the patient under local anesthesia is particularly applicable to tumors of the head and neck. A small skin incision is made over the lesion. The needle, with its obturator in place, is then inserted into the mass and a core of tissue carefully removed and placed in formalin, 10%. False biopsies are not likely to occur, and failure to provide a positive diagnosis is due to absence of the lesion in the tissue submitted. Some surgeons prefer open biopsy to the use of the Silverman needle because they think that a representative section may not be obtained.

Radical neck dissection. In radical neck dissection the entire contents of one side of the neck are removed. Only the carotid artery; the vagus, sympathetic, and phrenic nerves; and the scalene and prevertebral muscle groups are spared. Removed are the sternocleidomastoid muscle, the jugular vein with its associated lymph nodes, and the contents of the submaxillary triangle. The eleventh cranial nerve is sectioned, but the hypoglossal and lingual nerves are preserved.

The purpose of the operation is to remove from the neck malignant disease that has metastasized from adjacent areas. Chief among the primary sites and the larynx, tonsil, lip, tongue, and thyroid and parotid glands. Sometimes a metastatic node is not palpable, but the surgeon elects to do a radical neck dissection in continuity with, for example, a laryngectomy. This is done because certain lesions are prone to have metastasized even though the metastasis may still be microscopic. Usually, however, the operation is done for readily palpable metastases. All too often the patient is found inoperable because a large node is fixed to the internal carotid artery or to the base of the skull.

As an operation for removal of lymph nodes, neck dissection is more effective than either axillary or inguinal dissection.

With radical neck dissection the patient usually experiences shoulder pain for at least several months after surgery. There is a downward and forward drooping of the shoulder, and he may have difficulty in raising his arm above his head. These alterations in function are caused by loss of the nerve supply to the trapezius muscle. It is possible at the time of surgery to place a graft between the cut ends of the eleventh cranial nerve so that this disability is not permanent.

Supraclavicular masses. An isolated mass in the supraclavicular fossa is most likely to be a metastasis from a primary lesion below the clavicle. Although cancer of the lung is the most common source, malignant neoplasms of the stomach, kidney, bladder, and gallbladder may produce an isolated supraclavicular metastasis. These latter sources should be thoroughly investigated, especially if the supraclavicular metastasis is adenocarcinoma rather than epidermoid carcinoma.

Blood volume determination. The patient with recent weight loss caused by carcinoma is expected to have a reduced blood volume. Recognition of this point is extremely important to the preoperative preparation of the patient. If his blood volume is not restored by transfusion of whole blood or packed red cells, the patient is likely to become severely hypotensive when given a general anesthetic. The student is reminded that there is *no constant relationship between either the hemoglobin level or the hematocrit and the patient's blood volume.* The patient may, for example, have a hemoglobin level of 14 gm./100 ml. but still be in need of transfusion. A handy rule of thumb is as follows: for each 10 lb. of weight loss, transfuse 1 unit of whole blood or its equivalent in packed red cells. Determination of the blood volume by laboratory methods is, of course, recommended, but when there is a discrepancy between an obvious weight loss and the laboratory report, transfuse according to weight loss.

UNCOMMON TUMORS

The following tumors, although uncommon, are important because their correct diagnosis often permits effective treatment.

Adenoid cystic carcinoma. Adenoid cystic carcinoma (or cylindroma) is a particularly distressing tumor when it arises in the head and neck area. The primary lesion is apt to appear in salivary gland tissue, especially in the minor salivary glands of the tongue, palate, or floor of the mouth. Early cure rates are good, but long-term rates (over 10 years) are uniformly poor. Metastases occur to distant organs, especially the lungs. In the lung great "snowball" lesions may be present for several years without producing any marked symptoms, but eventually death does occur as a result of the disease.

The best results have come from extreme surgical removal of the local lesion, including a very wide "cuff" of apparently normal tissue, to try to encompass perineural invasion, which is so common with this tumor. Thus a lesion of the submandibular gland, even though small, would necessitate a mandibular resection, resection of the floor of the mouth and anterior tongue, and radical neck dissection at the very least. Irradiation therapy does cause the original lesion to regress or disappear, but the intermediate and long-term survival rates are not as good as with radical surgery.

Carotid body tumor. Carotid body tumors are rare. Also known as a nonchromaffin paraganglioma (or chemodectoma) and resembling the glomus jugulare tumor of the middle ear and mastoid, the carotid body tumor grows at the bifurcation of the common carotid and enlarges very slowly over many years. These tumors are movable laterally, but because they are attached to the carotid, they cannot be displaced up or down. The chief symptom is a lump in the neck. The diagnosis is made by detecting a bruit (when present) and by making a *carotid arteriogram* that will demonstrate the tumor clearly and establish its relationship to the three adjacent carotid vessels. Treatment is surgical removal.

Neurofibroma. Neurofibroma is an uncommon tumor that can form along the sheath of any nerve. In the neck the sympathetic trunk and vagus nerves have been involved. Fig. 32-14 shows a large tumor formed in association with the vagus nerve. Preoperatively the diagnosis was suspected, since the patient had laryngeal paralysis and a long history of a slowly enlarging, painless neck mass.

Adamantinoma. Adamantinoma (or ameloblastoma) is a tumor of the jaws, usually the mandible. It is benign. Most adamantinomas remain small, but an occasional tumor may deform the jaw and interfere with nutrition and speech (Fig. 32-15). Cystic areas develop as the tumor outgrows its blood supply. Treatment is surgical excision.

Aneurysm. Aneurysm of the carotid or subclavian artery is uncommon but must be kept in mind. Because of the pulsating and expanding nature of the tumor, the diagnosis is not likely to be overlooked. A carotid angiogram, if necessary, will help in diagnosis. Treatment is surgical removal; it is fraught with danger because of the likelihood of permanent interruption of one internal carotid artery. Both external carotids may be ligated without hazard, but ligation

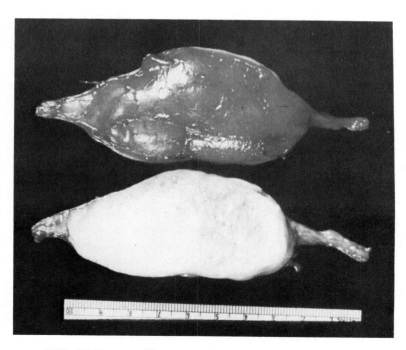

FIG. 32-14. Neurofibroma appearing as a lateral neck mass.

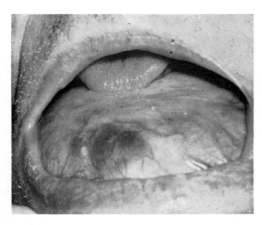

FIG. 32-15. Adamantinoma. Patient drooled and had to swallow like a chicken. The tongue is pushed into the back of the mouth.

of either the common or the internal carotid artery produces a discouraging incidence of hemiplegia and sometimes death. Apparently, some patients have good cerebral anastomosis between branches of the two internal carotids and others do not.

Cystic hygroma. Cystic hygroma (or cavernous lymphangioma) is a congenital defect of the lymphatic system. It involves the neck or the lower part of the face (tongue, lip, cheek, and parotid area). The infant with cystic hygroma has a greatly swollen neck, jaw, and cheek (Fig. 32-16); the region feels soft, with occasional firm areas. It is not tender. It is not easily reduced by pressure, as is a hemangioma. Treatment is surgical excision. Sometimes various forms of irradiation are tried—usually unsuccessfully. The growth tends to become larger if left alone and may encroach on structures that leave a functional defect if excised, such as the eyelids or the lips.

Lymph nodes seen in Hodgkin's disease. Hodgkin's disease (Fig. 32-17) frequently causes cervical lymphadenopathy. Often such adenopathy is so massive as to cause great swelling in both sides of the neck. With such extensive involvement there is usually disease in other parts of the lymphatic system, and the diagnosis is readily confirmed by biopsy. Sometimes, however, a patient's only sign may be a single node in the neck. In such instances radical neck dissection has been used as treatment. Generally, however, treatment is by irradiation therapy

or sometimes by medical means. The prognosis is always grave.

Hodgkin's disease is potentially curable if treated promptly and if the patient has the more curable, localized form of the disease. *Every patient who appears for treatment with a seemingly innocent enlarged gland in the neck that persists for more than a few weeks deserves to have the gland examined by biopsy or removed.* He may have a curable disease.

Lymph nodes seen in leukemia. Leukemia may occur in several forms, and by the time the patient is seen by the otolaryngologist the diagnosis is usually known. Lymph nodes enlarge in the neck and about the face. They may ulcerate. Under treatment the lymphadenopathy regresses and then may reappear within weeks. Sometimes there are longer remissions. The prognosis is extremely poor. The otolaryngologist's chief services are to do what he can to heal ulcerated mucous membranes, occasionally incise suppurating lymph nodes, and once in a while perform tracheotomy.

Midline lethal granuloma. Midline lethal granuloma (Fig. 32-18) is a disease of unknown etiology that is slowly progressive over a period of months or years and that usually causes the death of the patient. The ulcerative granulation tissue that appears in the nose, sinuses, palate, and other midline structures of the head gives the disease its name. The patient may also have pulmonary and renal manifestations, although often they are less apparent and may not be discovered until autopsy.

The disease once was considered the same as Wegener's granulomatosis, but the latter disorder is now classified as one type of midline lethal gramuloma.

Pathologists may be confronted with the problem of differential diagnosis between midline lethal granuloma and undifferentiated reticulum cell sarcoma.

Treatment with corticosteroids is of great benefit to many patients, although the help is usually only temporary. The dosage of the medication has to be increased until finally it is of no value and the patient dies, wasted and with part of the facial structures eroded. There are no diagnostic tests, either laboratory or clinical, that absolutely establish the diagnosis, which is made clinically by excluding other diseases.

Wegener's granulomatosis is considered an

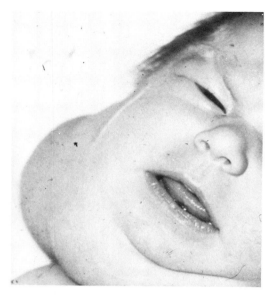

FIG. 32-16. Cystic hygroma.

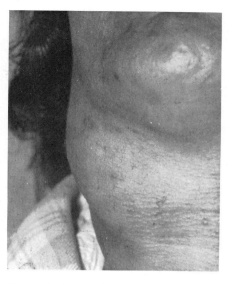

FIG. 32-17. Hodgkin's disease. Usually the diagnosis is not difficult to make, but the condition must be included in the differential diagnosis of cervical swellings. This tumor, for example, could represent a number of different diseases.

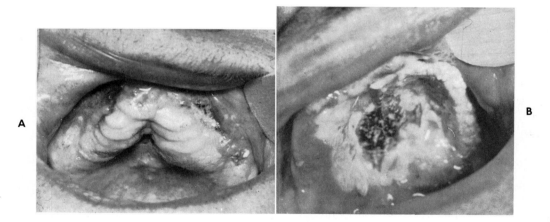

FIG. 32-18. **A,** Midline lethal granuloma. Similar lesions were present in the nose and maxillary sinuses. **B,** Hard palate showing extensive ulceration in another patient with midline lethal granuloma.

autoimmune disorder—a hypersensitivity reaction to an antigen as yet unknown. It is one of the three lethal midline granulomas, the other two being *midline malignant reticulosis* and *malignant lymphoma*. Differentiation is important, as treatment, for the latter two consists of radiation therapy and not cytotoxic drugs. Wegener's granulomatosis is characterized by necrotizing granulomatous vasculitis of the upper and lower respiratory tract, and glomerulonephritis. All organ systems may be involved, but the nasopharynx, the paranasal sinuses, the lungs, and the kidneys are most commonly affected. Mucosal ulcerations and saddle-nose deformities are the usual nasal manifestations. Sinusitis, caused by necrotizing granulomas, and secondary bac-

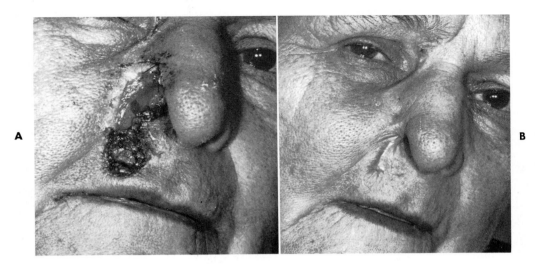

FIG. 32-19. **A,** Factitial dermatitis. Patient picked and scratched at the cheek and nose for years. Such lesions are usually confused with malignancy. Prompt healing occurred after a dressing was applied that sealed the wound from her fingernail for 2 weeks. These lesions may be inflicted by the patient as the result of a nervous habit of scratching, or they may be caused maliciously as a form of malingering. **B,** Same patient after healing.

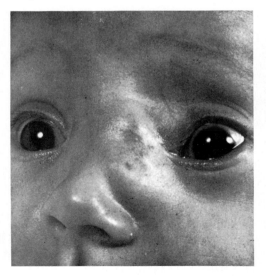

FIG. 32-20. Encephalocele. Any newborn infant with such a swelling or with a nasal polyp must be investigated for herniation of the brain and meninges through a defect in the region of the cribriform plate.

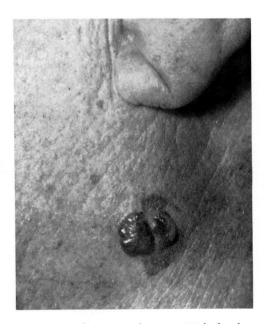

FIG. 32-21. Malignant melanoma. Wide local excision and skin grafting are indicated. Although the prognosis must always be guarded, it is probably better than is sometimes supposed. Neck dissection may also be indicated, but it was not done for this patient.

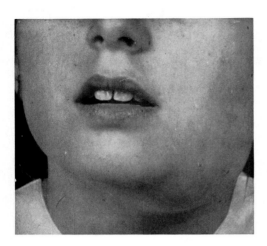

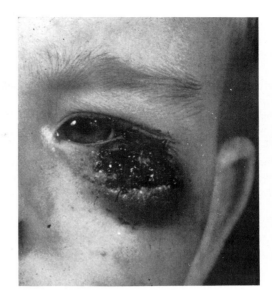

FIG. 32-22. Tuberculous adenitis. Now relatively infrequent since pasteurization of milk has become common, this disease must be kept in mind in any patient with cervical adenopathy. A more common cause of adenopathy like this is *cat-scratch fever.*

FIG. 32-23. Eosinophilic granuloma of bone. The lesion cleared promptly with local curettement and irradiation therapy. (Courtesy Dr. A.C. Furstenberg and Dr. J.H. Maxwell, Ann Arbor, Mich.)

terial infections occur in 95% of cases. Pulmonary manifestations are varied, but bilateral nodular and cavitary infiltrates with necrotizing granulomatous vasculitis are classic. The male-female ratio is 2 to 1, with persons of all ages being involved. Presenting complaints to the otolaryngologist include rhinorrhea, paranasal sinus pain and drainage, nonhealing nasal ulcers, serous or purulent otitis media, and cough. Abnormal laboratory values indicate anemia, leukocytosis, hyperglobulinemia (especially IgA), elevated erythrocyte sedimentation rate, and proteinuria.

Treatment is with cytotoxic agents, especially cyclophosphamide, 1 to 2 mg./kg., and prednisone. The natural course of the disease without therapy usually leads to death within 5 months of clinical onset, as a result of renal failure. With current therapy, long remissions are expected.

Midline malignant reticulosis is characterized by an infiltrate of neoplastic cells with normal inflammatory cells. It is a local, indolent ulceration that usually ends in death as a result of pneumonitis, meningitis, or hemorrhage. Dissemination is possible unless the patient is treated with radiation at levels of 4000 to 6000 rads. *Malignant lymphoma,* in contrast to mid-line malignant reticulosis, is characterized by tumor cells that are relatively uniform. Treatment with radiation therapy and surgery results in a 40% 5-year survival. Distant metastasis is the rule.

• • •

Figs. 32-19 to 32-23 show other pathologic conditions of the head and neck that should be considered in the differential diagnosis of cysts and tumors of this region.

ARTERIAL EMBOLIZATION IN THE HEAD AND NECK

There are three main indications for arterial embolization in head and neck lesions. It may be used preoperatively to reduce the vascularity of a lesion. This is especially useful in vascular lesions like nasopharyngeal angiofibromas, chemodectomas, capillary angiomas, and arteriovenous malformations. Arterial embolization may also be used in palliation of symptoms such as pain or hemorrhaging in unresectable malignant tumors. Finally, internal maxillary embolization has been used for uncontrollable epistaxis or arteriovenous malformations.

Various materials are used: some are permanent (such as silicone rubber, silicone spheres, tantalum powder, and detachable balloons), and others are resorbable (such as Gelfoam). The material is introduced into the feeder vessel through a catheter. The purpose is not to obstruct the vessel, as in arterial ligation, but to provoke retrograde thrombosis in the distal vessels by a reaction within the vessel's wall. Surgery is usually performed 2 to 15 days after embolization, before recanalization has occured.

Embolization is not performed prior to radiation therapy for malignant or benign tumors, since success in radiation therapy depends on tissue oxygenation. Embolization can, however, be performed after radiation therapy.

Complications may be severe. They include stroke or death as a result of retrograde flow of material, cranial nerve palsies, and skin sloughs and necrosis. Complications occur more frequently with liquid materials, which occlude vessels down to the capillary level.

SELECTED READINGS

Batsakis, J.G., and McBurney, T.A.: Metastatic neoplasm to the head and neck, Surg. Gynecol. Obstet. **133**:673, 1971.

Black, M.B.: Surgery for Graves' disease, Mayo Clin. Proc. **47**:966, 1972.

Blady, J.V.: The present status of treatment of cervical metastases from carcinoma arising in the head and neck region, Am. J. Surg. **111**:56, 1971.

Brooks, J.E.: Cystic hygroma of the neck, Laryngoscope **83**:117, 1973.

Conley, J., and Dingman, D.L.: Adenoid cystic carcinoma in the head and neck (cylindroma), Arch. Otolaryngol. **100**:81, 1974.

Conley, J., and Hamaker, R.C.: Melanoma of head and neck, Laryngoscope **87**(pt. 1):760-764, May, 1977.

Crawley, W.A., and Levin, L.S.: Treatment of ameloblastoma: a controversy, Cancer **42**:357-363, July, 1978.

Crile, G., Jr.: Diagnosis and management of thyroid cancer, Hosp. Medicine, July, 1977, pp. 48-63.

Deane, S.A., and Telander, R.L.: Surgery for thyroglossal duct and branchial cleft anomalies, Am. J. Surg. **136**:348-353, September, 1978.

Dedo, D.D., Alonso, W.A., and Ogura, J.H.: Povidone-iodine: adjunct in treatment of wound infections, dehiscences and fistulas in head and neck surgery, Trans. Am. Acad. Ophthalmol. Otolaryngol. **84**:68-74, January-February, 1977.

Donaldson, R.C.: Chemoimmunotherapy for cancer of the head and neck, Am. J. Surg. **126**:507, 1973.

Dozios, R.R., and others: Surgical anatomy and technique of thyroid and parathyroid surgery, Surg. Clin. North Am. **57**:4, August, 1977.

Edir, A.J.: Surgical treatment for thyroid cancer, Surg. Clin. North Am. **57**:3, June, 1977.

Feldman, D.E., and Applebaum, E.L.: The submandibular triangle in radical neck dissection, Arch. Otolaryngol. **103**:705-706, 1977.

Furci, A.S., and others: NIH conference: the spectrum of vasculitis: clinical, pathologic, immunologic, and therapeutic considerations, Ann. Intern. Med. **89**(pt. 1):660-676, 1978.

Goodwin, W.J., and Chandler, J.R.: Indications for radical neck dissection following radiation therapy, Arch. Otolaryngol. **104**:367-370, 1978.

Harwood, J., Clark, O.H., and Dunphy, J.E.: Significance of lymph node metastasis in differentiated thyroid cancer, Am. J. Surg. **136**:107-112, July, 1978.

Jaffe, B.F., and Jaffe, N.: Head and neck tumors in children, Pediatrics **51**:731, 1973.

Jesse, R.H., Ballantyne, A.M., and Larson, D.: Radical or modified neck dissection: therapeutic dilemma, Am. J. Surg. **136**:516-519, October, 1978.

Jesse, R.H., and Lindberg, R.D.: Evaluation of clinically negative neck; squamous cell carcinoma of oral cavity and faucial arch, J.A.M.A. **217**:453, 1971.

Kolson, H., and others: Epidermoid carcinoma of the floor of the mouth, Arch. Otolaryngol. **93**:280, 1971.

Krugman, M.E., Canalis, R., and Konrad, H.R.: Sternomastoid "Tumor" of infancy, J. Otolaryngol. **5**:523-529, December, 1976.

Lingeman, R.E., and others: Neck dissection: radical or conservative, Ann. Otol. Rhinol. Laryngol. **86**:737-744, 1977.

MacComb, W.S.: Diagnosis and treatment of metastatic cervical cancerous nodes from an unknown primary site, Am. J. Surg. **124**:441, 1972.

Macklin, J.F., and others: Current concepts: thyroid storm and its management, N. Engl. J. Med. **291**(26):1396-1398, 1974.

Martin, D.S.: The necessity for combined modalities in cancer therapy, Hosp. Pract. **8**:129, January 1973.

McGuirt, W.F., and McCabe, B.F.: Significance of node biopsy before definitive treatment of cervical metastatic carcinoma, Laryngoscope **88**:594-597, April, 1978.

Michaels, L., and Gregory, M.M.: Pathology of nonhealing (midline) granuloma, J. Clin. Pathol. **30**:317-327, April, 1977.

Montgomery, W.W.: Surgery of the upper respiratory system, vol. 2, Philadelphia, 1973, Lea and Febiger, pp. 315-371.

Morton, D.L.: Immunotherapy of cancer, Cancer **30**:1647, 1972.

Nahum, A.M., Bone, R.C., and Davidson, T.M.: The case for elective prophylactic neck dissection, Laryngoscope **87**:588-599, 1977.

Newton, H.T.: First panel discussion: embolization material, Neuroradiology **16**:402-412 (1978).

Northrop, M., and others: Evolution of neck disease in patients with primary squamous cell carcinoma of the oral tongue, floor of mouth, and palatine arch, and clinically positive neck nodes either fixed or bilateral, Cancer **29**: 23, 1972.

Quick, C.A., and Lowell, S.H.: Ranula and sublingual salivary glands, Arch. Otolaryngol. **103**:397-400, July, 1977.

Rothman, K.J.: Epidemiology of head and neck cancer, Laryngoscope **88**:435-438, March, 1978.

Sako, K., Razack, M.S., and Kalnins, I.: Chemotherapy for advanced and recurrent squamous cell carcinoma of the head and neck with high and low dose cis-diaminodichloroplatinum, Am. J. Surg. **136:**529-533, October, 1978.

Saunders, W.H., and Johnson, E.W.: Rehabilitation of the shoulder after radical neck dissection, Ann. Otol. Rhinol. Laryngol. **84:**812-816, 1975.

Schottenfeld, D., and others: Epidemiology of thyroid cancer, CA **28**(2):66-86, 1978.

Sessions, D.G., and others: Total glossectomy for advanced carcinoma of the base of the tongue, Laryngoscope **83:**39, 1973.

Shamblin, W.R., and others: Carotid body tumor (chemodectoma), Am. J. Surg. **122:**732, 1971.

Simmonds, W.P.: Chemotherapy in recurrent head and neck cancer, Otolaryngol. Clin. North. Am. **7**(1):205, 1974.

Simpson, W.J., and Carruthers, J.S.: Role of external radiation in management of papillary and follicular thyroid cancer, Am. J. Surg. **136:**457-460, October, 1978.

Skinner, M.D., and Schwartz, R.S.: Immunosuppressive therapy, N. Engl. J. Med. **287:**221, 281, 1972.

Southwick, H.W.: Elective neck dissection for intraoral cancer, J.A.M.A. **217:**454, 1971.

Spiro, R.H., and Strong, E.W.: Epidermoid carcinoma of the mobile tongue; treatment by partial glossectomy alone, Am. J. Surg. **122:**707, 1971.

Spiro, R.H., and Strong, E.W.: Surgical treatment of cancer of the tongue, Surg. Clin. North Am. **54**(4):759, 1974.

Stell, P.M.: The management of cervical lymph nodes in head and neck cancer, Proc. R. Soc. Med. **68:**83-85, 1975.

Thibant, A., and Collignon, J.: Embolization and surgical removal of nasopharyngeal angiofibromas, Neuroradiology **16**, 418-419, (1978).

Ward, P.H., Jenkins, H.A., and Hanafee, W.N.: Diagnosis and treatment of carotid body tumors, Ann. Otol. Rhinol. Laryngol. **87:**614-621, 1978.

Ward P.H., and others: The many faces of cysts of the thyroglossal duct, Surgery **67:**281, 1970.

Wetmore, S.J., and others: Idiopathic midface lesions, Ann. Otolaryngol. **87:**60-69, 1978.

Wizenberg, M.J., and others: Treatment of lymph node metastases in head and neck cancer; a radiotherapeutic approach, Cancer **29:**1455, 1972.

33 PLASTIC AND RECONSTRUCTIVE SURGERY OF THE HEAD AND NECK

Facial plastic and reconstructive surgery is a branch of surgery that involves procedures performed for cosmetic and functional reasons. These procedures include rhinoplasty, rhytidectomy (facelift), blepharoplasty, mentoplasty, otoplasty, dermabrasion, scar revision, and mandibular or maxillary osteotomy. Reconstructive procedures of the head and neck are often necessary after surgical ablative procedures or traumatic tissue losses. They often require extensive relocation of skin and/or tissue from other sites.

Patient selection. Before cosmetic or reconstructive procedures of the head and neck are performed, it is essential that the surgeon carefully evaluate the patient psychologically as well as physically. Many patients who seek facial plastic surgery have ulterior motives such as attracting a mate, becoming more popular, preventing the breakup of a marriage, or pleasing a family member. If there is a question about the psychological stability of the patient, it is important that there be psychiatric consultations. The surgeon must also evaluate his abilities and listen to the patient's desires to decide *if the result will match the patient's expectations.* If the patient is not realistic in his expectations or the surgeon is not realistic regarding the surgical outcome, the result may be an unhappy or even hostile patient.

Rhinoplasty. Rhinoplasty is done for cosmetic as well as physiologic reasons. Many persons have grossly deformed noses as a result of either injury or growth processes. Some persons are unconcerned about such a deformity. Others, however, suffer psychologically and seek surgical correction of the deformity. Also, there are some patients, with or without an external de-

formity, who find breathing difficult because of internal obstruction caused by a septal deformity. It should be noted that the presence of a deformed nasal septum does not *necessarily* mean that the patient has symptoms; if the patient does not complain of nasal obstruction, he should not be encouraged to have an operation merely to straighten the septum. The aims of rhinoplasty are, first, to correct an external nasal deformity and, second, to relieve obstruction of the nasal airway when necessary.

A typical rhinoplasty is done with the patient under local anesthesia. The nasal vibrissae are clipped short. Incisions are made on each side of the nose between the upper and lower lateral nasal cartilages and are extended downward just in front of the septal cartilage to separate the cartilaginous portion of the columella from the membranous portion. These incisions afford access to the dorsum of the nose all the way up to the frontal bone and also afford access to the nasal septum and the front of the nose. The upper lateral cartilage is cut free from the septum to give better access to the nasal dorsum. Also, this cartilage is freed so that it can be shortened.

The skin is elevated over the dorsum and a little over the upper sides of the nose by working through the intercartilaginous incisions with a knife or scissors. The periosteum of the nasal bones is elevated. A saw is introduced through the intercartilaginous incisions to remove a hump (if present) or to lower the dorsum, which may be too high. A chisel is admitted through the same incision and driven upward in order to separate the nasal bones from the septum.

At this stage of the operation the nose is without its hump, but because the hump has been removed, the dorsum is flat and broad. Therefore, the lateral walls must be sawed through in order to press the nasal bones (and nasal processes of the maxillary bones) inward to close the "open" top of the nose. The same procedure narrows the bridge. Another incision is made on each side in the lateral part of the nasal vestibule, and the periosteum of the maxillary bone is raised to the inner canthus. A saw is inserted through this incision, and each maxillary bone is sawed through where it meets the nose. Then the surgeon places his thumbs along the sides of the nose; as he presses hard, the bones snap inward.

When the nasal tip is too large, when it droops, or when it is otherwise unattractive, additional incisions are made just inside the rim of the vestibule. The lower lateral cartilages (both medial and lateral crura) are exposed, delivered, and trimmed as required.

As a final step (or at first if the operator wishes), the nasal septum is corrected. This step is not always necessary. Some surgeons perform two operations, several months apart, rather than doing septal reconstruction and rhinoplasty at the same time.

When every member of the nose is in position, a few catgut sutures are used to approximate the cartilaginous and membranous parts of the columella, and a small amount of nasal packing is placed in the vestibule. Then an external dressing and a splint are applied. The packing and external dressing are removed in 4 days.

There are a great many variations in rhinoplastic techniques, and the procedures are constantly being revised.

Unfortunately, not every rhinoplasty gives the results hoped for by the surgeon and the patient. Sometimes the results after a week and those after a year are noticeably different. Pre-

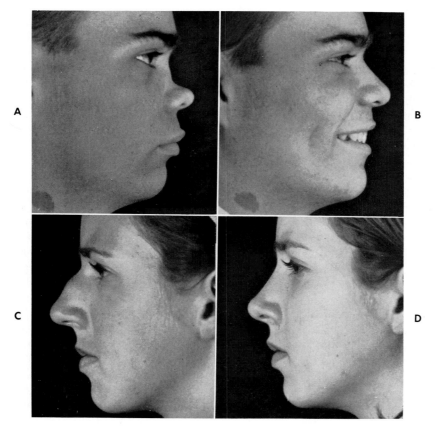

FIG. 33-1. A and **B,** Saddle nose following infection at 8 years of age—repaired with a silicone rubber nasal implant. **C** and **D,** Nasal convexity and chin retrusion repaired by combined rhinoplasty and chin augmentation. (Courtesy Dr. Trent Smith, Columbus, Ohio.)

operative photographs are essential for careful planning of the operation and also for medicolegal reasons. (Fig. 33-1).

Complications from rhinoplasty include bleeding and infection in the early postoperative period. Later complications include recurrence of the preoperative deformity and "polly-beak" deformity.

• • •

For many years surgeons have sought substances for implantation in various bodily parts that would provide satisfactory shape—for example, to the chin or nose—and which would not absorb, calcify, or be rejected. Paraffin has been tried and found unsatisfactory, as have ivory implants. Autogenous cartilage and bone have been satisfactory in some instances; but their shape tends to change, and they become infected and extrude in some patients.

Silicone rubber (Silastic*) is a product currently very much in demand for augmentation of the nose and chin. There is very little postoperative reaction, and a preformed prosthesis can be inserted through a small incision under the chin or through the mouth of a patient with micrognathia, or through an intranasal incision in a patient with a saddle nose, for example. The correction of micrognathia by means of a preformed curved block of Silastic to augment the chin is of great help in restoring confidence to a patient whose retruded chin has been a lifelong embarrassment (Fig. 33-1). A similar product, made of Teflon, is also available. It comes in the form of a thick liquid that can be injected into an atrophic vocal cord to relieve hoarseness.

Rhytidectomy (Facelift). Facelifts have in recent years become an acceptable surgical procedure. Today, with many celebrities and nationally known people openly having facelifts, it is an acceptable procedure for both women and men, especially in our youth-oriented culture.

The ideal candidate is the middle-aged woman who is of average weight, with high cheek bones, and sagging in the jowl area and the neck-chin line. Deep nasolabial folds and a double chin or a poorly defined neck-chin line are only slightly improved by a classical facelift procedure. Overweight individuals should be

---

*Dow Chemical Co.

encouraged to lose weight prior to surgery to maximize the result. Men must be warned of the change in position of beard and sideburns postoperatively. With a good result, the patient should look very much as he did several years earlier. The results will last 5 to 10 years, and the procedure may be repeated. The results of a second or third operation may last longer, since it is performed over a scar tissue base.

The procedure may be performed under local anesthesia and sedation or under general anesthesia. The incision starts 4 to 5 cm. above the root of the helix and extends inferiorly and anteriorly in a skin crease to the auricle, under the earlobe, superiorly behind the ear in the postauricular crease to the posterior auricular muscle, and then posteriorly into the hair or parallel to the hair line. Elevation of a skin flap is then carried subcutaneously superficial to the level of the platysma muscle and parotid fascia to avoid the branches of the seventh nerve. The elevation is carried forward to the malar eminence, nasolabial fold, and midportion of the mandible and cervical skin. The flap is then rotated posteriorly and superiorly to remove the wrinkles. A subcutaneous stay suture (to hold the tension) is placed posterior to the auricle, and a second one is placed just superior to the root of the helix. The excess skin is then removed, and the skin is closed with nylon sutures. A drain is placed subcutaneously. A light pressure dressing of cotton and gauze bandage is applied.

The most common complication is a hematoma, which occurs in approximately 10% of cases. Other, more serious complications are paralysis of some portion of the seventh nerve, wound separation, infection, and skin slough.

To enhance the results, some patients may require auxiliary procedures such as dermabrasion, chemical peels, or submental lipectomy. These procedures supplement the facelift in areas where it does not do well, especially in the area of fine perioral rhytides and double chins.

Browlift. In contrast to the facelift, which involves an extensive amount of surgery for a small amount of cosmetic gain, the browlift provides the most benefit for the least surgery. The intent of this procedure is to correct brow ptosis and to eliminate the squinting look that the sagging brow produces. The direct browlift offers excellent control to the surgeon and little risk of nerve damage, hematoma, hair loss, or skin slough.

Blepharoplasty. Blepharoplasties are performed for persons with excessive skin of the upper and/or lower eyelids. As a person ages, there may be excessive wrinkling of the skin, laxity of the orbicularis oculi muscle, and/or excessive periorbital fat. Frequently a blepharoplasty may be performed at the same time as a facelift.

As in other cosmetic procedures, various techniques are used, depending on the patient's specific problem and the surgeon's preference. Basically, in upper lid blepharoplasty, a lower incision is made at the upper edges of the tarsal plate, 4 to 6 mm. above the lash line; it is carried out in a crow's foot. The *amount of excess skin is estimated*, and an upper incision is made roughly parallel to the lower edges of the eyebrow, in a scimitar shape; this incision is carried out in the crow's foot to meet the lower incision. The skin between the two incisions is then removed. If there is excess periorbital fat, a small stab incision is made through the orbital septum, parallel to the orbicularis oculi muscle fibers, and the excess fat is teased out. The skin is closed with a running subcuticular suture using 6-0 nylon.

In lower lid blepharoplasty, an incision is made 2 to 3 mm. below the lash margin and parallel to it and carried out laterally into a crow's foot line. After elevating the skin from the orbicularis oculi muscle, the surgeon rotates the skin laterally and upward with a minimum of traction. The excess skin is then removed, and the skin is closed laterally with interrupted sutures and along the eyelid with a running subcuticular suture. If necessary, fat may be removed as described for the upper eyelid. If there is excess laxity of the orbicularis oculi, the surgeon may choose to make a skin-muscle flap, removing orbicularis oculi muscle with the skin. The resultant scars fall nicely into the natural skin lines and are essentially unnoticeable after 3 or 4 weeks.

The most common complication of blepharoplasties is formation of an ectropion as a result of too much lower lid skin be removed and/or excessive scarring. This complication is avoided by being conservative in lower lid skin removal. The most devastating complication is blindness, which fortunately is rare. Usually the development of blindness related to removal of fat; the complication is believed to result from a periorbital hematoma. Other possible complications include keloid formation and hematoma formation.

Otoplasty. Children who have protruding or "lop" ears are frequently teased in school by being referred to as "Dumbo" and "big ears." (Fig. 22-1). This usually occurs early in the school years but may be carried into the teen years. Such teasing can, and often does, cause considerable psychological damage to the child. Frequently parents are unaware that a surgical procedure may correct the condition.

The most common defect is the lack of an anthelical fold, a situation that allows the ear to stand out from the head. Other defects may be various deformities of the auricular cartilage or a deep, wide concha. The helical rim should be less than 2 cm. from the side of the head. If it is farther from the head, the patient has the appearance of lop ears.

There are many different techniques for correction of lop ears. The most widely used is the Mustarde mattress suture technique. An eliptical skin incision is made in the postauricular area, and about 1 cm. of skin in the widest area is removed. The new anthelical fold is marked with tattoos or needles to make a guide for the sutures. Clean nylon or white braided cotton suture material is most often used. Three or four horizontal mattress sutures are placed through the cartilage and the anterior perichondrium, with the knots posterior. The sutures are placed from inferior to superior and tightened to give the desired sharpness to the anthelical fold. The skin is then closed posteriorly with a running subcuticular suture. The ears are well cushioned with cotton balls soaked in mineral oil, and a mastoid dressing of fluffs and bandage is applied. The mastoid dressing is kept in place for 10 to 12 days. The patient should then wear a protective elastic dressing such as a ski ear protector day and night for 2 more weeks and at night for another 2 weeks.

Other procedures may be used to reduce the size of the concha: sacrificing the cartilage to break its spring; excising the concha, the helix, or extra skin; or incising the cartilage.

Complications include postoperative hematoma or infection. These should be treated promptly to prevent a cauliflower ear or chondritis (see Fig. 22-4). Occasionally sutures may pull out, causing recurrence of the deformity. Revision is possible if this should occur.

Mentoplasty. Mentoplasties are most commonly requested by patients who have micrognathia or retrognathia, giving the appearance of a weak chin. Such a chin is most noticeable in profile. Infrequently, someone with a protruding chin may ask to have it reduced.

The most common procedure for the receding chin is to apply an onlay to the mentum to build out the point of the chin. This is the type of procedure in which alloplastic materials such as Silastic, acrylic, Supramid mesh, and Proplast have been the most satisfactory. The surgeon may also use autograft material of cartilage or bone. The degree of deformity is calculated by taking lateral soft tissue x-ray films or facial cephalometric x-ray films. The material chosen to build the area up is either preformed or carved at the time of surgery. It is inserted through a small incision in the submental crease, or it is inserted transorally.

Complications include infection, assymetry, shifting of the implant, bony erosion (with hard implants) and extrusion.

Dermabrasion. Dermabrasion is used to remove depressed scars or pitted areas caused by car accidents or acne. It does not remove the scar but planes the epithelial surface to a uniform level, reducing the shadows from the deep scar and breaking up the light pattern on the skin. Dermabrasion will improve but not clear deep pitted scars. It may also be used as an adjunct to scar revisions or in facelifts in patients who have many fine circumoral wrinkles. Dermabrasion is a useful technique in removing ground-in dirt or debris at the time of initial treatment of soft tissue injuries.

The technique involves the use of a rotating burr with various sizes of sandpaper disks, diamond burrs, or wire wheels to scarify the superficial epithelium. The surgeon must leave the deep dermis, hair follicles, and sweat glands to regenerate a new epithelial surface. Initially there will be a scabbed surface, but in 7 to 14 days this will peel off, leaving a fresh, pink, regenerating epithelium.

Complications include excess scarring if dermabrasion is carried too deep, keloid formation, superficial infection, and variable degrees of hypopigmentation and hyperpigmentation. Hyperpigmentation may occur if the patient goes out in the sun too soon after the procedure.

Scar revision. Scar revisions are done for depressed scars, wide scars, unsightly scars, and scars not lying in the relaxed skin tension lines. Many patients are under the impression that by means of "plastic surgery" one can remove the scars. It must be pointed out that one cannot cut the skin without leaving a scar behind. A scar revision is an attempt to change the direction of a scar, place it in a more favorable position, or make it less conspicuous by closing it meticulously to prevent a depressed or wide scar. One technique is breaking a long straight scar up by using a W-plasty or geometric broken line closure. Dermabrasion performed after healing will break up highlights and further help to camouflage a scar.

In general, one would like to rotate scars so that the longest axis lies in relaxed skin tension lines. Long straight scars should be broken up into shorter lines to make a random pattern that the eye is less likely to follow. The skin edges should be closed carefully with good buried subcutaneous sutures to remove the tension from the skin edge. Fine approximation of the skin edges with mutiple sutures will give the best result. These last, superficial sutures are removed in 2 to 4 days to prevent crossnotching of the skin.

Reconstructive surgery for cancer. Plastic and reconstructive surgery as done for patients with malignancy differs from the more definitive surgery done for patients with congenital malformations or deformities following trauma. In the cancer patient the cardinal aim is elimination of malignant disease; relatively less consideration is given to an excellent cosmetic or even excellent functional result. Nevertheless, careful preoperative planning many times leads to a far better result than would occur if the procedure for cancer were considered separately from the reconstruction. There is some difference of opinion as to whether the reconstructive procedure should be postponed until there is reasonable assurance of permanent eradication of malignant disease. Every surgeon has been frustrated, at one time or another, by the recurrence of malignant disease in the midst of a reconstructive procedure. On the other hand, early reconstruction reduces the length of time the patient must endure his deformity, often provides protection for vital structures that otherwise are left exposed, and reduces the number of operations needed to repair the defect and thus the total economic burden to the patient.

Virtually all major defects of the head and neck can be closed by one of three or four commonly used *pedicle flaps* (Figs. 33-2 to 33-4). Many other flaps, each dependent on its own particular blood supply, also are available (Figs. 33-5 to 33-8). Pedicle flaps for reconstruction are used ideally in a one-stage repair to prevent contraction and malposition of structures in the operative site, but the same techniques are also useful in late repairs. Close proximity of the donor and recipient sites and good blood supply are advantages working in favor of pedicle flaps formed in the head and neck areas, as contrasted to some other parts of the body.

Pedicle flaps are sometimes raised and then replaced ("delayed") for 10 to 20 days to ensure their blood supply more adequately, or they can be raised and transferred in a one-stage procedure. The forehead flap is particularly safe in one-stage transfers (Fig. 33-4). The donor site may be grafted with split-thickness skin taken from the abdomen or thigh, or it may be dressed with an antibiotic nonadherent covering such as nitrofurazone (Furacin) and allowed to granulate until such time, usually 3 weeks, as the excess pedicle can be returned. In general, the ratio of the length of a graft to its width should not be greater than 3:1, although there are exceptions.

Myocutaneous flaps are a recent innovation based on the fact that in certain areas of the body the skin is supplied with blood by perforators from the underlying muscle, in contrast to an axial blood supply from subcutaneous vessels. The advantage of the myocutaneous flap is that a surgeon can turn relatively large areas of skin and muscle on a relatively small muscle-vessel pedicle. It is possible to take an island of skin, and it therefore is not necessary to leave a skin bridge. This means that intraoral defects may be closed in one stage. Large skin defects may be resurfaced without the necessity of cutting the pedicle of the flap.

The survival of any tissue flap depends on the adequacy of the blood supply. There are two basic classifications of vascular-based skin flaps,

axial and random. The *axial* flap is based on a named artery in its longitudinal axis. The length of the flap is determined by the length of the vessel. The *random* flap, on the other hand, gets its blood supply from the dermal-subdermal plexus. Therefore, viability is dependent on width (the longer the flap, the wider it must be) and its position in the body. Like pedicled skin flaps, random flaps useful in grafting in a poorly nourished recipient bed, such as an irradiated area, since they carry their own vascular supply. Myocutaneous flaps, like skin flaps, may be of either type: pectoralis major, trapezius, and latissimus dorsi, being flat muscles, are all axial, while round muscles like the sternocleidomastoid are random.

The myocutaneous flap most often used in head and neck reconstructive procedures is the pectoralis myocutaneous flap. The main blood supply is the pectoralis branch of the thoracicoacromial artery, which lies on the deep surface of the pectoralis major muscle. Myocutaneous flaps like the pectoralis major offer several advantages over traditional skin flaps. They provide more bulk for filling defects; the donor site often may be closed primarily; they usually do not require staging. Creation of a so-called island flap, with skin only at the end of the flap, is also possible with the myocutaneous flap. A disadvantage of the myocutaneous flap is that the added bulk sometimes makes later palpation for recurrent tumor difficult. Myocutaneous flaps are particularly useful in reconstruction of the floor of the mouth, the tonsillar fossa, the tongue, the pyriform sinus, and orbital and temporal bone. The trapezius myocutaneous flap has as its main blood supply the transverse cervical artery. A useful modification of this flap is to include the scapular spine with the muscle to reconstruct the mandible.

The use of pedicle flaps is making the application of free grafts and anastomosis rarely necessary in head and neck reconstructive procedures. Axial flaps such as the deltopectoral flap will be used less frequently, and may be combined with myocutaneous flaps.

Free grafts, of either split or full thickness, are also widely used in the repair of defects about the head and neck (Figs. 33-10 and 33-11). They do not, of course, carry their own blood supply and cannot provide the thickness

Text continued on p. 468

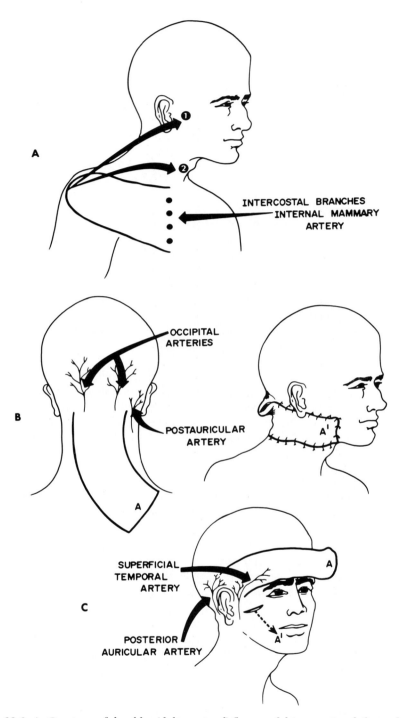

FIG. 33-2. A, One type of shoulder (deltopectoral) flap, useful in covering defects of the face or neck and, when tubed, in reconstructing the cervical esophagus. **B,** Nape-of-neck flap, useful in covering defects of the upper neck, jaw, or face. The "dog ear" is not removed at this stage for fear of interrupting some of the blood supply to the flap. The donor site requires spit-thickness grafting. **C,** Forehead flap. A will be inserted through the cheek incision to line the floor of the mouth at A' (or adjacent area).

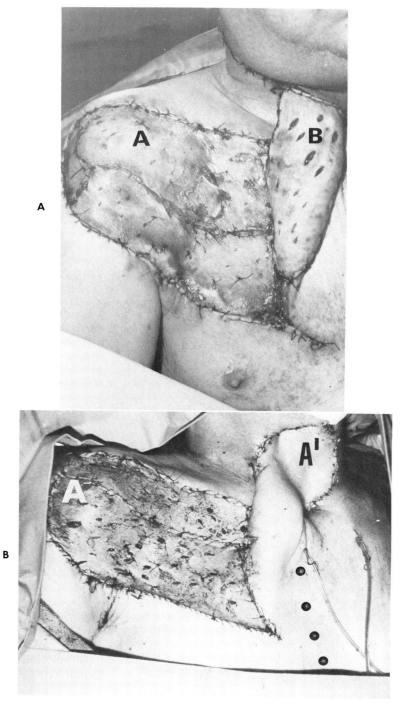

FIG. 33-3. A, Deltopectoral pedicle flap for reconstruction of the esophagus. **A,** Split-thickness skin graft to donor site. **B,** Tubed pedicle graft with skin surface inside. Grafting has been done externally with split-thickness skin, leading to pharyngostome above and esophagus (end-to-side anastomosis) posteriorly. Later the excess tube will be reopened and placed back on the donor site. **B,** Another use for deltopectoral pedicle flap—resurfacing the anterior neck after total laryngectomy. Tumor had extended through the thyroid cartilage to skin. The skin at A′ originally was at A. The small circles indicate a source of blood—perforating branches of the internal mammary artery.

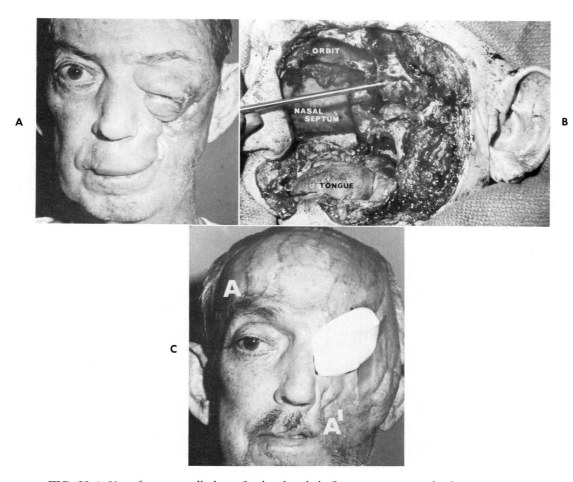

FIG. 33-4. Use of an unusually large forehead pedicle flap to reconstruct the face. **A,** Extensive carcinoma of the maxilla, orbit, and facial area—after irradiation therapy. **B,** Radical excision of the maxilla, ethmoid, orbit, part of the mandible, and entire side of the face for advanced carcinoma after cobalt therapy. **C,** Reconstruction of the face using a previously lined forehead pedicle flap. Another minor adjustment or two will reduce the bulk of the flap. The skin at *A* was shifted to *A'*, and a split-thickness skin graft was applied to the forehead.

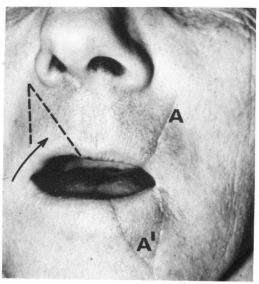

FIG. 33-5. Lip-switch operation for carcinoma of the lower lip. Tissue at A' came from A. Diagram shows the direction of the blood supply and an incision in the upper lip designed to leave a pedicle attached to the blood supply—later divided. (Courtesy Dr. A.W. Miglets, Jr., Columbus, Ohio.)

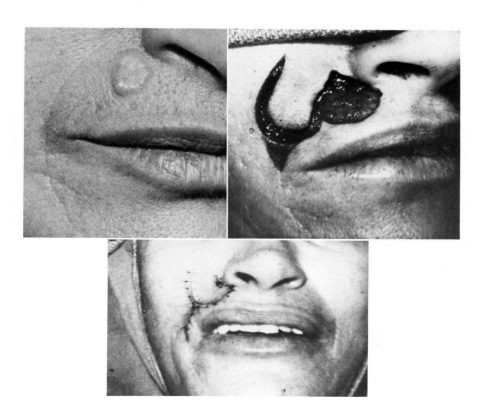

FIG. 33-6. Carcinoma of the upper lip and repair after excision by rotation of a local cheek flap.

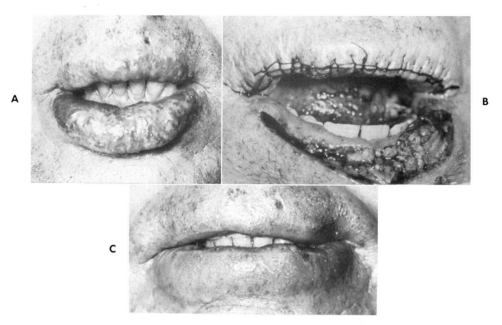

FIG. 33-7. Lip-shave procedure in patient with hereditary hemorrhagic telangiectasia—an unusual application. **A,** Masses of abnormal vessels weighted the lips. **B,** Upper lip completed. Upper lip cut to muscular layer and stripped of mucosa and underlying masses of vessels. Mucosa will be joined to skin. **C,** Postoperative appearance. The same procedure is used more commonly for superficial carcinoma, hyperkeratosis, and leukoplakia. Patient shown in Fig. 2-21, *C,* was treated in this fashion.

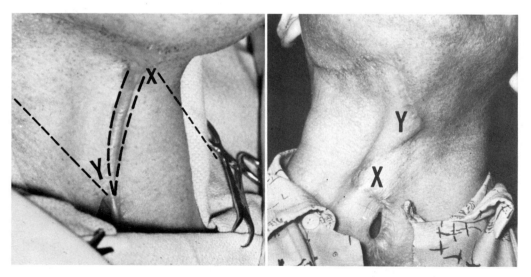

FIG. 33-8. Z-plasty. One of the most versatile techniques to release a linear scar contracture. Two triangular flaps are transposed so that a vertical scar becomes oblique. The usual angle is 60 degrees.

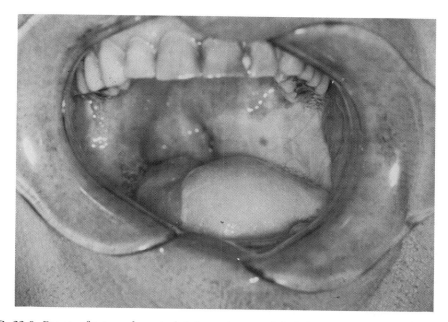

FIG. 33-9. Repair of intraoral surgical defect using a pedicled skin graft. Note that the lateral wall of the pharynx, more than half of the floor of the mouth, and more than half of the tongue have been reconstructed.

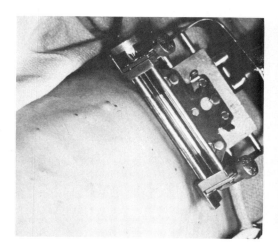

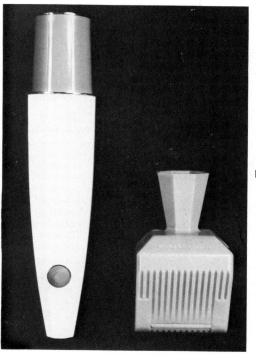

FIG. 33-10. A, Brown electric dermatome in use. Screw settings adjust thickness and width of the cut. **B,** Battery-powered fixed-thickness (0.015 inch) dermatome with a disposable head. Useful for minor office procedures.

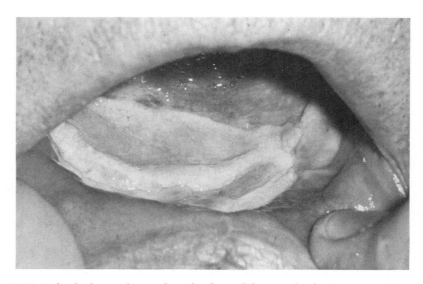

FIG. 33-11. Split-thickness skin graft in the floor of the mouth after resection of carcinoma.

or bulk of a pedicle graft. Where applicable, however, they are simple and generally successful. Typically, a split-thickness graft is between 0.008 and 0.015 inch. They can be cut freehand or, more commonly, with the aid of a calibrated dermatome, driven electrically or by air pressure.

A *dermal graft* is occasionally employed in otolaryngology to provide thickness for a subcutaneous structure, as in building up a saddle deformity of the nose, or to serve as protection for the carotid artery after laryngectomy and neck dissection. After a dermatome has been used to remove the epidermis with its glands and hair follicles, the dermal layer is removed with a second cut of the dermatome. Then the epidermis is replaced.

SELECTED READINGS

Alonso, M.R., and Bailey, B.J.: Reconstruction of the mandible, Otolaryngol. Clin. North Am. **5**:501, 1972.

Conley, J., and Schuller, D.: Reconstruction following temporal bone resection, Arch. Otolaryngol. **103**:34-37, January 1977.

Farr, H.W., Jean-Gilles, B., and Die, A.: Cervical island skin flap repair of oral and pharyngeal defects in the composite operation for cancer, Br. J. Plast. Surg. **23**:173, 1970.

Gullane, P.J., and Arena, S.: Palatal island flap for reconstruction of oral defects, Arch. of Otolaryngol. **103**:598-599, October, 1977.

Johnson, C.M., Jr., and others: The brow lift 1978, Arch. Otolaryngol. **105**:124-126, March, 1979.

McGregor, Ian A.: Problems of reconstructive surgery of oral cavity, J. Laryngol. Otol. **91**:445-465, June, 1977.

McGregor, I.A.: The temporal flap in intraoral reconstruction. In Gaisford, J.C., editor, Symposium on cancer of the head and neck, vol. 2, St. Louis, 1969, The C.V. Mosby Co.

Montgomery, W.W.: Surgery of the upper respiratory system, vol. 2, Philadelphia, 1973, Lea and Febiger, pp. 315-371.

Mustarde, J.C.: The use of flaps in the orbital region, Plast. Reconstr. Surg. **45**:146, 1970.

Myers, E.N.: Reconstruction of the oral cavity, Otolaryngol. Clin. North Am. **5**:413, 1972.

Sessions, D.G., and others: Total glossectomy for advanced carcinoma of the base of the tongue, Laryngoscope **83**:39, 1973.

Skolnik, E.M., Tardy, M.E., Jr., and Stagman, R.G.: Rehabilitation following anterior jaw resection, Laryngoscope **80**:1580, 1970.

Spiro, R.H., and Strong, E.W.: Surgical treatment of cancer of the tongue, Surg. Clin. North Am. **54**(4):759, 1974.

Terz, J.J., and Lawrence, W., Jr.: Primary reconstruction of oropharyngeal surgical defects with forehead flap, Surg. Gynecol. Obstet. **129**:533, 1969.

34 ALLERGY IN OTOLARYNGOLOGY

Allergic reactions and symptoms, either as the primary cause or as an underlying additive, are common in many ear, nose, and throat problems. The physician who diagnoses and treats diseases of the ear, nose, throat, and head and neck must be constantly aware of the possibility that sensitivity (or hypersensitivity) to some external or internal agent may cause or alter the problem being investigated and treated.

Allergy has been defined as "an acquired altered reactivity of the tissues of the body to a specific antigen or allergen" (Hansel). It is probable that most allergic reactions are not hereditary but are due to past exposure to allergens. Such reactions occur in persons who have an inborn tendency toward dysfunction of usual protein metabolism. In other words, an allergic individual may *overreact* when challenged or insulted by a given substance to which he has become "allergic" by a previous exposure. This process or overreaction is called sensitization or sensitivity.

An antigen is usually considered to be a bacterial product or some other protein that is intentionally administered to a person in order to produce antibodies. By this method it is possible to initiate future protection against such diseases as measles, diphtheria, and tetanus.

Immunology can be defined as "the study of those processes with which the host maintains *constancy of his internal environment* when confronted with substances which are recognized as foreign, whether from the external environment or from within the host" (Hansel). Immunology recognizes the effects of external sources as well as internal conditions. Each may have some relationship to allergy, infection, nutrition, or malignancy, as well as to autoimmune and connective tissue disease.

While it is true that "previous exposure" may occur as a result of injection of a medication or a vaccine, most sensitizations occur from inhaled, ingested, or directly contacted substances. It is not, therefore, a coincidence that allergic problems are common in ear, nose, and throat and head and neck pathology. The mouth, throat, esophagus, and stomach are the route of all ingested materials. The nose, nasopharynx, pharynx, larynx, trachea, and bronchi are the route of all inhalants. The skin of the face, eyelids, lips, ears, and scalp are usually exposed to most external irritants, and these parts of the body are the areas most frequently exposed to soaps and cosmetics, as well as to dust, smoke, and other environmental irritants. If allergic disease is as common as it seems to be and if previous exposure is a necessary foundation for the development of allergic symptoms, it would be unusual for this area of the body not to be frequently involved. Therefore the physician should be constantly aware that allergy may play an important role in ear, nose, and throat disease. This is particularly true in disorders of the nose and paranasal sinuses but may also be important in vertigo, headache, otitis media, hearing loss, head and neck pain, hoarseness, and bronchitis. Some otolaryngologists confine their entire practice to otolaryngic allergy, and many general allergists, whose training is in internal medicine or pediatrics, find a high percentage of their problems in the head and neck and the digestive and respiratory systems.

In general, it is reasonable to say that whenever ear, nose, and throat symptoms seem to be exaggerated and possible complications have been investigated and ruled out, an allergic overlay may be the cause of the overreaction. The same is true of symptoms that tend to "hang on" beyond the time when resolution is expected. Allergy should also be suspected when symptoms are recurrent without obvious cause. A constant high index of suspicion regarding allergy as a factor in ear, nose, and throat symptoms is necessary for accurate diagnosis and proper treatment.

ALLERGIC SYMPTOMS

The primary tissue reactions to an allergic stimulus are edema and urticaria. There may also be an inflammatory reaction, caused by capillary dilation, that mimics low-grade infection. Therefore swelling, itching, and sometimes redness are the common symptoms. Since the lymphatic system is commonly involved in an allergic reaction and the pharynx, hypopharynx, nasopharynx, and neck are rich in lymphoid tissue, enlargement of the lymphoid tissue of the throat, lateral pharyngeal bands, and nasopharynx is frequent. The same is true of the cervical lymph glands. These basic reactions are responsible for the symptoms that comprise the patient's chief or secondary complaint.

Mouth and throat. Swelling of the lips, and sometimes cracking, occurs. Itching of the lips or of the throat or palate should lead a physician to suspect an allergy. The tongue may show intermittent swelling, glossitis, or, occasionally, ulceration. Recurrent vesicles or "canker sores" are often caused by a specific food or medication. Low-grade sore throat, usually of short (hours) duration and without systemic reaction, can be entirely an allergic manifestation. Mild inflammation of the pharynx with swelling of the tonsils, the lateral pharyngeal bands, and the pharyngeal lymphoid islands is common. There may be coincident, painless swelling of the cervical lymph glands. These lymphoid changes can easily be misinterpreted as chronic infection and, on this basis, suggest the need for tonsillectomy. Careful observation over time is necessary to avoid surgical removal of the tonsils if the problem is allergic rather than inflammatory.

Nose and sinuses. The classical symptoms of nasal allergy (inhalant) are well known—sneezing, copious nasal discharge, and a stuffy nose. These symptoms are characteristic of the typical, seasonal "hay fever" as well as of some other nasal allergic episodes. However, nasal allergy that is perennial and present most of the time—not in acute or seasonal episodes—also causes

nasal itching, occasional sneezing, increased nasal discharge or "postnasal drip," and a stuffy or blocked nasal passage. The severity of symptoms depends on how much of the allergen is contacted and the general status of the patient. Fatigue, intercurrent illness, chilling, or other stress may allow symptoms to surface that otherwise would be absent or minimal. For example, a patient who is allergic to two different foods might have few symptoms, or no symptoms, from a small serving of one of the foods but might have definite symptoms when both are eaten together. He might have minimal symptoms, or none, from his own house dust most of the time but always have symptoms during "spring house cleaning" or when he works in a particularly dusty area or in a damp, moldy basement. Intermittent or constant stuffiness of the nose, increased nasal discharge, whether thick or thin, and nasal irritation are still the primary symptoms of nasal allergy. A constantly blocked nose may—and often does—cause a low-grade frontal or temporal headache.

Examination of the nose in nasal allergy usually reveals a mucosa that shows edema and that is paler than normal. Small pale polyps may be present (see Chapter 15). The nasal discharge is mucoid in the absence of upper respiratory infection or of sinusitis. If either of these conditions is present, the discharge may be purulent.

Since the mucosa of the sinuses is continuous with the nasal mucosa, and similar histologically, one expects that the mucosa of the paranasal sinuses may be equally as involved as the nasal mucosa, and such is the case. Roentgenograms of the sinuses will show thickening of the mucosa lining the sinuses. Sometimes the sinuses will also contain fluid which, however, when collected by antral washing, will be mucoid and not purulent. The management of chronic sinusitis, when nasal and sinus allergy are also present, becomes much more difficult than when infection alone is the cause. When infection and allergy are present concomitantly, successful management will usually not result unless or until *both* are treated. Complications of sinus infections are more common when infection and allergy are present at the same time.

Ears. Allergic manifestations in the ear most commonly occur in dermatitis of the skin of the pinna and/or the external auditory canal. Such dermatitis is similar to all contact dermatitis, with characteristic itching, scaling, and cracking of the skin and edema of the soft tissue. Often the dermatitis is accompanied by infection of the skin and subcutaneous tissues as a result of the trauma of constant scratching. The process may be limited to the external canal, or it may spread and involve the entire pinna and parts of the surrounding skin. Again, successful management *must* be directed at *both* the infection and the allergen.

Serous otitis media may occur because of nasopharyngeal blocking of the eustachian tubes as a result of nasal and sinus allergy. Serous otitis media that fails to respond to early treatment by routine measures (see Chapter 24) may be controlled only after the underlying allergic problem has been suspected, proved, and treated. There are no specific differences between the symptoms of serous otitis media when it is caused by allergy and the symptoms of the disease when it is caused by antecedent infection or viral inflammation.

Although allergy is not the usual cause of sudden or fluctuating hearing loss, severe vertigo, or tinnitus, each may be caused by an allergic hypersensitivity. (The usual and most common causes of hearing loss and vertigo are discussed in Chapters 25, 26, and 29.) A certain percentage of cases of each disorder can be caused by allergy to certain foods and drugs. If a complete investigation of the possible causes of hearing loss, vertigo, or tinnitus has not resulted in a specific diagnosis, allergy should be investigated as a possible cause—particularly in Meniere's syndrome, fluctuating hearing loss, and sudden unexplained hearing loss.

DIAGNOSIS

History. The allergic history, rather than skin tests or laboratory tests, may often be the most important part of an allergic investigation. The number of known (or suspected) allergens is so large that all methods possible must be used in an attempt to find the substance to which a hypersensitivity may have developed. The preliminary step is an adequate history. It must be detailed and specific. For this reason it is often initiated with an allergy history questionnaire. Such a questionnaire is designed either to discover or to eliminate certain possibilities by means of a series of questions that can be an-

swered by the patient with a simple "yes" or "no." The questions cover the main complaint, onset, acute episodes, seasonal occurrence of symptoms, specific symptoms relating to the ears, nose, throat, chest, gastrointestinal tract, skin, and so on. Family and childhood allergic episodes are covered, as well as dietary habits, employment history, vacation habits, hobbies, and general medical, social and psychiatric history. Any of these questions may lead the way to a probable cause or to several possibilities. Within the questionnaire are clues to the physician that help to indicate whether inhalants, ingestives, or contacts should have further investigation. After the allergy history questionnaire has been completed, the physician can proceed to specific, conventional one-on-one questions.

Cytologic examination. The immense value of the microscopic study of cells in all areas of diagnosis is well known. Smears, scraping of skin lesions, washing of bronchial secretions, or tissue biopsy may often provide the final definitive findings in establishing the diagnosis in tuberculosis, malignancy, and many other disease processes. In cases of allergic patients, microscopic study is done primarily from nasal smears. Such smears, when properly prepared and examined with high-power, oil immersion microscopy, will clearly show the presence and the proportion of neutrophils, eosinophils, basophils (or mast cells), epithelial cells, and bacteria. While each of these data has some diagnostic significance, the presence or absence of eosinophils is of utmost importance in an allergic investigation, particularly in the very common nasal allergies. A few eosinophils are present in normal nasal secretions. During an infection such as the common cold or sinusitis the cell content of a smear is often 100% neutrophils. During a purely allergic episode, and usually even between acute allergic episodes, the nasal secretion will show a high percentage of eosinophils, often in clumps. Such a finding is almost diagnostic of nasal allergy. Those who work often with a variety of nasal smears in a variety of conditions are able to make further assumptions from the various types of cells studied, but for practical diagnosis the presence of numerous or clumped eosinophils confirms a suspicion of allergy. One must remember that in the presence of acute, subacute, or chronic infection eosinophils may be absent and another smear should be done at a later time after the infection has been controlled. In allergic situations the eosinophils will again be present in greater than expected numbers.

A cytologic examination is easily done in the physician's office. It is not necessary to send the slide to a laboratory. The procedure is as follows: (1) the patient is asked to blow his nose in a piece of waxed paper (glassine) or a piece of cellophane. (2) The mucus is easily transferred to a clean glass slide and spread to produce a thick smear. (3) The smear is allowed to air dry without heating. (4) The slide is covered with Hansel's stain for 30 seconds. (5) The slide is covered with distilled water for an additional 30 seconds. (6) The slide is tilted and washed free of excess stain with distilled water. (7) The slide is briefly decolorized by being washed quickly with ethyl alcohol or 75% methyl alcohol. (8) The slide is air dried and examined under high power.

Skin tests. Skin testing has been used in allergic investigations for many years. The original "scratch tests" have been supplemented by intracutaneous tests, patch tests, passive transfer tests, provocative tests, and immunoassay tests. Each has a place in allergic investigations, and all are subject to false positives, false negatives, delayed reactions and untoward systemic reactions. They should be used only by persons who have been thoroughly trained in proper interpretation and who have the ability to handle the possible systemic reactions. When properly used and interpreted, the skin tests are most valuable in pollen sensitivities (diagnostic in approximately 95% of cases). They are less valuable in other inhalant allergies (approximately 75%) and least valuable in food allergies (approximately 30%). They are, however, in spite of some limitations, an important tool in allergic investigation.

Physical examination. In addition to the history, the cytologic examination, and skin tests, a complete physical examination is necessary to indicate any other abnormalities and to evaluate the lymphatic system generally. Roentgenograms, particularly of the sinuses, the chest, and sometimes the temporal bones, may be needed to complete a total evaluation of the allergic patient. A complete blood count and an immunoglobulin assay should also be done.

Food allergies. When food allergies are suspected a different approach is necessary. There are no specific symptoms that indicate that food may be the cause. However, certain clues do occur that should alert the physician to the likelihood of food as the allergen. Suspicious are foods that always cause the same symptoms when eaten, foods that can be eaten raw but not cooked (or vice versa), foods that can be eaten in small amounts without trouble but not in large amounts, foods that are particularly liked and eaten very often, and foods that are strongly disliked. The further investigation of food allergy demands very close cooperation between the physician and the patient and may require that a careful diet diary be kept for weeks or longer (with notation of symptoms), as well as certain elimination diets and food challenges. Again, thorough training and constant experience are necessary in order to discover the offending food or foods.

Allergy to medications. All physicians are aware that when drugs are given to alleviate symptoms or to control a disease, the patient may develop a sensitivity to a drug. This is particularly true of patients who already have a history of allergic symptoms. In otolaryngology it is not uncommon to see symptoms produced by medications. Symptoms can occur in cases in which drugs are used locally and in cases in which they are taken systemically. While some of these symptoms may not be true allergic reactions, they do simulate the symptoms and signs that result from allergic insult. It is not necessary to document here all of the possible drugs or drug reactions that can and do occur, but the physician should be aware of those symptoms of the ears, nose, and throat that can be caused either by an allergy to a medication or by the side effects of that medication. Stomatitis or dry mouth can be caused by chemotherapeutic drugs, adrenergic drugs, or anticholinergics. Nasal stuffiness and congestion are often caused by antithyroid drugs, decongestants, estrogens, progestins, and reserpine drugs. Anosmia can be caused by locally used tyrothricin. Dizziness, tinnitus, and hearing loss can be caused by chloroquine, streptomycin and dihydrostreptomycin, quinine, quinidine, salicylates, an all of the aminoglycoside drugs such as neomycin, kanamycin, and gentamicin, as well as some antihypertensives, central nervous system depressants, and estrogens. Hoarseness can be caused by antithyroid drugs, gingival hyperplasia by phenytoin (Dilantin), and tooth discoloration by tetracyclines. This is, of course, a partial list and must be constantly updated as new drugs are continually discovered and used for treatment of a variety of medical problems.

It is important to add to the allergic history a *very specific history of drugs* taken in the past and being taken currently, since many drugs can cause symptoms that either simulate allergy or that actually are allergic. Occasionally a physician who is suspicious of such reactions can solve a questionably allergic problem by stopping the administration of a medication or switching to a medication with different side effects.

MANAGEMENT

The control of allergic symptoms or the complete control of the allergic problem in otolaryngology can be rapid and very satisfactory when a single allergen is recognized and then avoided. Control can be difficult, time-consuming, and frustrating when the cause cannot be definitely found or when symptoms are caused by several different substances. When the physician is certain that the presenting problem has an allergic basis, it becomes necessary to promptly attempt to find the allergen. As mentioned earlier in this chapter, a very detailed history, by questionnaire sometimes, is required. Often the patient will begin to "look back" when questioned carefully and will supply the clue to the offending allergen. This is most likely to be true of contact allergies, such as external otitis caused by nail polish, hair spray, permanent wave solutions, hair dyes, and so on or lesions of the lips and oral cavity caused by mouthwashes, gargles, toothpaste or tooth powders, lozenges, and so on. A drug used locally— salve, lotion, ear drops—or systemically is frequently the *only* causative agent. The early recognition of this type of allergy will, by elimination of the specific cause, allow the most rapid and most satisfactory control.

Allergic symptoms that occur only sporadically and that last only a short time or allergic symptoms that are seasonal *and* of short duration are most often controlled with the antihistamine drugs, often in combination with ephed-

rine or pseudoephedrine. Many combinations of antihistamine ephedrine, theophylline, and/or phenobarbital are available to control symptoms for the short term, but continued use over a long period of time may be detrimental. Long-term use may thicken secretions or mask other allergic symptoms, or a combination of drugs may include something to which the patient is also allergic. Antihistamines often have annoying side effects—most often drowsiness—and thus substitute another set of symptoms for the original ones. The physician may have to change medications, on a trial-and-error basis, until the proper control without side effects is found. When such a procedure is necessary, the physician should be certain that a new regimen involves a *different class* of drug, since many of the available capsules have similar ingredients under different trade names. The *PDR* (*Physician's Desk Reference*, published by Medical Economics Company) can be used to advantage in these situations; it can provide an accurate description of the ingredients of a given combination, proper dosage, and a description of side effects.

Cortisone has been used effectively for several years in most allergic problems. It is particularly valuable in severe, acute allergic problems; combined with the proper use of epinephrine where indicated, cortisone can be lifesaving. Cortisone is a valuable adjunct in the management of many otolaryngologic problems of an allergic nature. It is used both systemically and locally, depending on the problem. In general, when infection and allergy exist simultaneously, as they may in sinusitis or external otitis, cortisone and an antibiotic administered at the same time can produce rapid and dramatic control of the problem. A proper antibiotic should be given in full dosage for as long as indicated. Cortisone is given in *descending* doses over 3 to 5 days, beginning with the first day of treatment. The long-term use of cortisone in the treatment of otolaryngic allergies should be considered only as a last resort, when other methods of management have failed and the symptoms are disabling. The long-term adverse effects of cortisone must always be considered. Cortisone and hydrocortisone are frequently used in lotions and salves for allergic dermatitis of the lips, face, eyelids, and external ear and external auditory canal. They are very effective.

No attempt has been made in this book to discuss the details and problems of various skin tests or details of desensitization techniques. The student is advised to become aware of these methods by referring to standard texts on allergy and immunology and to be alert to situations that should be managed by the trained allergist or by the otolaryngologist who specializes in allergy. The general principles outlined in this chapter are guidelines only; they should alert the student to otolaryngologic problems most likely to have an allergic component, so that proper consultation will be sought.

SUGGESTED READINGS

Bellanti, J.A., and Frenkel, L.S.: Adverse reactions to immunizing agents. In Middleton, E., Jr., Reed, C.M., and Ellis, E.F., editors: Allergy: principles and practice, St. Louis, 1978, The C.V. Mosby Co.

Bendixen, G.: Food allergy, editorial, Allergy 33:163, 1978.

Byrom, N.A., and Tinlin, D.M.: Immune status in atopic eczema: a survey, Br. J. Dermatol. 100:491, 1979.

Clemis, J.S., and Derlacki, E.L.: Allergy of the upper respiratory tract, Otolaryngol. Clin. North Am. 3:265-276, June, 1970.

Davison, F.W.: The antibody deficiency syndrome, Arch. Otolaryngol. 86:685-690, 1967.

DeWeese, D.D.: Stop the medicine? Trans. Am. Acad. Ophthalmol. Otolaryngol. 78:ORL 5-14, January-February, 1974.

Hansel, F.K.: Allergy and immunology in otolaryngology, Rochester, Minn., 1975, American Academy of Ophthalmology and Otolaryngology.

Henson, P.M.: Mechanisms of tissue injury produced by immunologic reactions. In Bellanti, J.A.: Immunology II, Philadelphia, 1978, W.B. Saunders Co., Ch. 13.

Houri, M., and others: Correlation of skin, nasal and inhalation tests with IgE in the serum, nasal fluid and sputum, Clin. Allergy 2:285, 1972.

Kaufman, H.S., and Frick, O.L.: Immunological development in infants of allergic parents, Clin. Allergy 6:321, 1976.

May, C.D., and Block, S.A.: A modern clinical approach to food hypersensitivity, Allergy 33:166, 1978.

Miglets, A.: The experimental production of allergic middle ear effusion, Laryngoscope 88:1355, 1973.

Randolph, T.G.: Comprehensive environmental control with special reference to advanced otologic conditions, 12:11-26, 1972.

Reports of the committee on provocative food testing, Ann. Allergy 31:375-381, 1973.

Rinkel, H.J.: The management of clinical allergy. II. Etiologic factors and skin titration, Arch. Otolaryngol. 77:42, 1963.

Rinkel, H.J.: The management of clinical allergy. IV. Food and mold allergy, Arch. Otolaryngol. 77:302-326, 1963.

Rowe, A.H., and Rowe, A.H., Jr.: Food allergy: its manifestations and control by the elimination diets, Springfield, Ill., 1972, Charles C Thomas, Publisher.

Shambaugh, G. E., Jr.: Allergy in otology, Trans. Am. Acad. Ophthalmol. Otolaryngol. 12:7-10, 1972.

Sipilä, P., Ryhänen, P., and Karma, P.: T cells as marked with acid α-naphthyl acetate esterase staining in secretory otitis media, Acta Otolaryngol. [Suppl.] [Stockh.] 360:216, 1979.

Symposium on food allergy, Trans. Am. Acad. Ophthalmol. Otolaryngol. 13:31-42, 1973.

Wilson, W.H.: Acute suppurative otitis media: a method of terminating recurrent episodes, Laryngoscope 86(9):1401, 1971.

INDEX